W. J. Huk
G. Gademann
G. Friedmann

Magnetic Resonance Imaging of Central Nervous System Diseases

Functional Anatomy – Imaging
Neurological Symptoms – Pathology

With Contributions by
I. Baer D. Baleriaux G. M. Bydder W. L. Curati
M. Deimling H. Goetz R. Haerten W. Heindel
R. H. Hewlett E. Kraus J. W. Lotz G. Michelozzi
U. Mödder T. Pasch J. M. Pennock W. Schajor
W. Steinbrich H.-J. Weinmann F. E. Zanella

With 614 Figures in 822 Separate Illustrations

Springer-Verlag Berlin Heidelberg New York
London Paris Tokyo Hong Kong

Translated by Terry Telger

ISBN-13:978-3-642-72570-8 e-ISBN-13:978-3-642-72568-5
DOI: 10.1007/978-3-642-72568-5

Library of Congress Cataloging-in-Publication Data
Huk, W.J. (Walter Josef), 1939- Magnetic resonance imaging of central nervous system diseases : functional anatomy, imaging, neurological systems, pathology / W.J. Huk, G. Gademann, G. Friedmann ; with contributions by I. Baer ... [et al.] ; translated by T. Telger. Includes bibliographies and index.ISBN-13:978-3-642-72570-8 (U.S.:alk.paper)1.Central nervous system-Magnetic resonance imaging. 2. Central nervous system - Diseases - Diagnosis. I. Gademann, Günther, 1952- . II. Friedmann, Gerd. III. Title. [DNLM: 1. Central Nervous System - anatomy & histology. 2. Central Nervous System - pathology. 3. Central Nervous System Diseases - diagnosis. 4. Magnetic Resonance Imaging. WL 141 H911m]
RC386.6.M34H85 1989 616.8'04754-dc 19 89-5927 CIP

Softcover reprint of the hardcover 1st edition 1990

Reproduction of the figures: Gustav Dreher GmbH, Stuttgart

2121/3130-543210 - Printed on acid-free paper

Preface

Magnetic resonance imaging (MRI) is a new and still rapidly developing imaging technique which requires a new approach to image interpretation. Radiologists are compelled to translate their experience accumulated from X-ray techniques into the language of MRI, and likewise students of radiology and interested clinicians need special training in both languages. Out of this necessity emerged the concept of this book as a manual on the application and evaluation of proton MRI for the radiologist and as a guide for the referring physician who wants to learn about the diagnostic value of MRI in specific conditions.

After a short section on the basic principles of MRI, the contrast mechanisms of present-day imaging techniques, knowledge of which is essential for the analysis of relaxation times, are described in greater detail. This is followed by a demonstration of functional neuroanatomy using three-dimensional view of MR images and a synopsis of frequent neurological symptoms and their topographic correlations, which will facilitate examination strategy with respect to both accurate diagnosis and economy.

The clinical sections include all categories of diseases of the central nervous system. We are fully aware that these chapters are incomplete and that the value of a clinical assessment of MRI at this early stage is rather transient. Nevertheless, we have tried to depict the present state of knowledge, drawing on the literature, on our own clinical experience since the early days of MRI and on experience in other institutions. In order to improve the diagnostic evaluation of MR images as to the underlying disease, abnormal signal intensities and histopathological findings are presented for comparison. Since the clinical background is often also important for decisions as to diagnosis on the basis of MRI, it is described in the text and in the figure legends.

It is our goal to familiarize the reader with the diagnostic tool MRI and to provide the knowledge needed for the understanding of future technical advances and the resulting improvement in the morphologic information gained.

W. J. Huk
G. Gademann
G. Friedmann

Acknowledgements. The authors are grateful to all those people who helped them to write and publish this book. The following deserve special thanks:

Dr. Buchholz, Dr. Holik, and their colleagues (Private Radiological Institute, Erlangen, FRG), the Siemens AG Medical Engineering Group (Erlangen, FRG), and Philips Medical Systems (Eindhoven, The Netherlands) for their willingness to examine a large number of our patients in their MR units or laboratories. Dr. H. König, Siemens AG Medical Engineering Group (Erlangen, FRG), for the arrangement and surrender of the 3 D images.

Drs. Kuhn, Steen, and Terwey (Private Radiological Institute, Oldenburg, FRG), T. Beydoun, M. D. (Director, Department of Diagnostic Imaging, Dr. Erfan-Bagedo Hospitals, Yedaah, Saudi Arabia), and Dr. P. Sneider (Parklane Clinic, Johannesburg, South Africa) for contributing a variety of important cases.

P. Haesendonck, M. Lemort, C. Segebarth, C. Christophe, S. Louryan, and G. Rodesch (Cliniques Universitaires des Bruxelles, Hospital Erasme Service de Radiologie et Neuroradiologie, Bruxelles, Belgium) for their cooperation in the chapter on lesions of the posterior fossa.

The Medical Research Council of South Africa for the use of the scanner and the generous assistance of their personnel and Prof. J. C. de Villiers, Head of the Department of Neurosurgery of Cape Town University Medical School, South Africa, for the case referrals which provided important clinical information in the chapter on inflammatory disease.

The *Bundesministerium für Forschung und Technologie* for their support (contract no. 01 VF 1427) of the research on MR contrast media (Sect. 1.3.3) and the *Deutsche Forschungsgemeinschaft* for its financial support of the MR unit of the University of Cologne, FRG.

Dr. D. Kömpf, Professor and Head of the Dept. of Neurology of the University of Lübeck Medical School, for his critical review of Chapter 4 (Symptoms and Pathologic Anatomy, a Tabular Listing).

Mrs. U. Seidl and Mr. Baden (Siemens, UB Med, Erlangen, FRG), Mrs. M. Schmied (Philips, Hamburg, FRG), Mrs. G. Schreier and Mr. M. Bischofsberger (Department of Radiology, University of Cologne Medical School, FRG), and Mr. Seebach (Neurosurgical Hospital of the University of Erlangen, FRG) for their excellent photographic work. Mr. B. Zimmerman for the excellent cooperation in sketching the drawings of Chaps. 1 and 2.

The staff of the MR units involved for their unselfish help in performing numerous examinations.

Dr. Ute Heilmann of Springer-Verlag for her generous assistance during the preparation of the manuscript and the production of this book.

Contents

List of Authors

Prof. Dr. med. W. J. Huk
Neurosurgeon, Head of the Neuroradiological Department of the Neurosurgical Hospital of the University of Erlangen-Nürnberg, Schwabachanlage 6, 8520 Erlangen, FRG

Dr. med., Dipl. Phys. G. Gademann
Radiological Clinic of the University of Heidelberg Medical School, Im Neuenheimer Feld 400, 6900 Heidelberg, FRG

Prof. Dr. med. G. Friedmann
Head, Department of Radiology of the University of Cologne Medical School, Joseph-Stelzmann-Str. 9, 5000 Cologne 41, FRG

Dr. med. I. Baer
Department of Diagnostic Radiology, University Hospital Nürnberg, Flurstraße, 8500 Nürnberg, FRG

Prof. Dr. D. Baleriaux
Chef de Service Neuro-Radiologie, Hôpital Erasme, Université Libre de Bruxelles, Rue Lennex, Bruxelles, Belgium

G. M. Bydder, M. D.
Department of Diagnostic Radiology, Royal Postgraduate Medical School, Hammersmith Hospital, Du Cane Road, London W12 OHS, Great Britain

W. L. Curati, M. D.
Department of Diagnostic Radiology, Royal Postgraduate Medical School, Hammersmith-Hospital, Du Cane Road, London W12 OHS, Great Britain

Dr. rer. nat. M. Deimling
Siemens AG, Medical Engineering Group, Henkestr. 127, 8520 Erlangen, FRG

Dr. med. H. Goetz
Institute of Anaesthesiology of the University of Erlangen-Nürnberg, Universitätsstr. 12, 8520 Erlangen, FRG

Dr. rer. nat. R. HAERTEN
Siemens AG, Medical Engineering Group, Henkestr. 127,
8520 Erlangen, FRG

Dr. med. W. HEINDEL
Department of Radiology of the University of Cologne Medical School,
Joseph-Stelzmann-Str. 9, 5000 Cologne 41, FRG

R. H. HEWLETT, PhD, MRCPath
Department of Pathology, University of Stellenbosch Medical School &
Tygerberg Hospital, Cape Town, South Africa

Dr. med. E. KRAUS
Institute of Anaesthesiology of the University of Erlangen-Nürnberg,
Universitätsstraße 12, 8520 Erlangen, FRG

J. W. LOTZ, FRCR
Department of Radiology, University of Stellenbosch Medical School &
Tygerberg Hospital, Cape Twon, South Africa

Dr. G. MICHELOZZI
Service Neuro-Radiologie, Hôpital Erasme, Université Libre de
Bruxelles, Rue Lennex, Bruxelles, Belgium

Prof. Dr. U. MÖDDER
Department of Radiology, Hospital of the University of Düsseldorf,
Moorenstr. 5, 4000 Düsseldorf, FRG

Prof. Dr. med. T. PASCH
Head, Institute of Anaesthesiology of the University of Zürich Medical
School, Rämistr. 100, 8091 Zürich, Swisse

J. M. PENNOCK, M. D.
Department of Diagnostic Radiology, Royal Postgraduate Medical
School, Hammersmith Hospital, Du Cane Road, London W12 OHS,
Great Britain

Dr. rer. nat. W. SCHAJOR
Siemens AG, Medical Engineering Group, Henkestr. 127,
8520 Erlangen, FRG

Priv.-Doz. Dr. med. W. STEINBRICH
Department of Radiology of the University of Cologne Medical School,
Joseph-Stelzmann-Str. 9, 5000 Cologne 41, FRG

Dr. rer. nat. H.-J. WEINMANN
Schering AG, Müllerstr. 170–178, 1000 Berlin 65, FRG

Dr. med. F. E. ZANELLA
Department of Radiology of the University of Cologne Medical School,
Joseph-Stelzmann-Str. 9, 5000 Cologne 41, FRG

1 Physical Principles and Techniques of MR Imaging

1.1 Physical Principles

G. Gademann

1.1.1 Historical Background

Magnetic resonance (MR) imaging is based on the principle of nuclear magnetic resonance (NMR), which has long been known to physicists. As early as 1939, Rabi and his colleagues demonstrated the phenomenon of NMR in the deflection of a molecular beam [113]. Seven years later, Purcell and coworkers of Harvard University [111] and Bloch and coworkers of Stanford University [15] independently demonstrated the phenomenon in larger bodies. The implications of the discovery for physics and chemistry were quickly recognized and earned Purcell and Bloch a Nobel Prize in 1952. The earliest well-known application of MR to clinical medicine came in 1971, when Damadian noted significant differences in the MR properties of tumors and normal tissues [37]. In 1973 Lauterbur published initial experiments on the use of MR to generate an image [78]. Since that time, progress has been very rapid [25] and has enabled the adoption of MR imaging as a standard procedure in medical diagnosis (Table 1.1).

Table 1.1. Highlights in medical NMR history

1939	Molecular beam resonance	Rabi et al. [113]
1946	First successful nuclear induction experiments	Purcell et al. [111], Bloch et al. [14, 15]
1952	Nobel Prize for physics to Felix Bloch and Edward Purcell	
1971	First NMR experiments with tumors	Damadian [37]
1973	First NMR image of two water-filled tubes	Lauterbur [78]
1974	NMR image of a living mouse	Lauterbur, Hutchison
1976	NMR image of the human thorax	Damadian
1980	First application of surface coils	Ackerman et al. [2]
1982	Clinical NMR imaging of the brain: 140 cases	Bydder et al. [26]
1984	First clinical use of gadolinium-DTPA as contrast agent	Schörner et al. [124], Carr et al. [29]
1986	Rapid NMR images	Haase et al. [61]

1.1.2 Properties of Atomic Nuclei

The physics of MR can be accurately described only in terms of quantum mechanics [1, 129]. For our purposes, however, it will be sufficient to consider models drawn from classical physics [14]. First, it must be understood that the electron cloud is not the only structure responsible for the magnetic properties of atoms, molecules, and bodies. Approximately two-thirds of positively charged atomic nuclei possess a very small magnetic moment by virtue of their intrinsic mechanical rotation, called *spin*. This magnetic moment can exist only if the nucleus contains an odd number of protons or neutrons (nucleons), because even numbers of nucleons

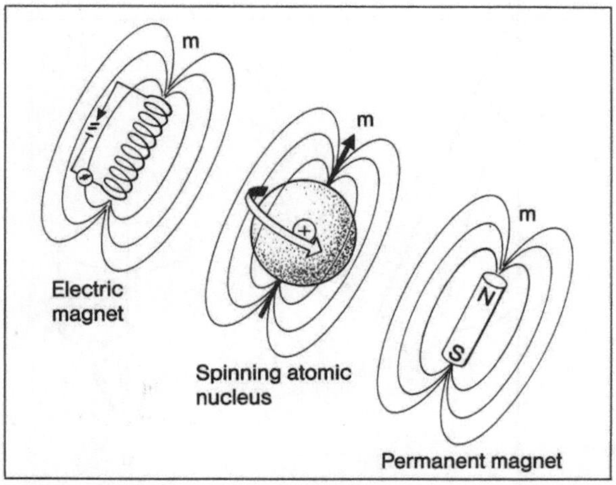

Fig. 1.1. Examples of magnetic dipoles

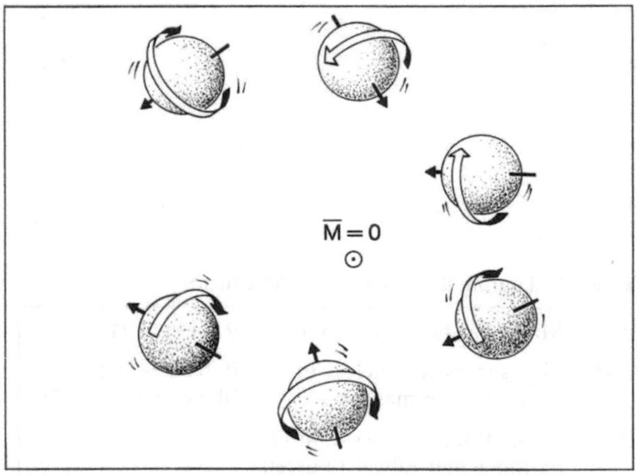

Fig. 1.2. Nuclei in the absence of an applied magnetic field: randomized orientation and no net magnetic moment $\vec{M}$

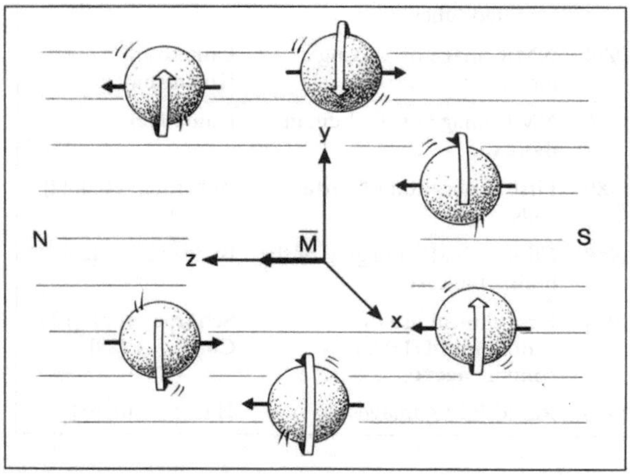

Fig. 1.3. Nuclei in the presence of an applied magnetic field $\vec{B}_0$ *(horizontal lines)*: alignment parallel to the field causing a net magnetic moment $\vec{M}$

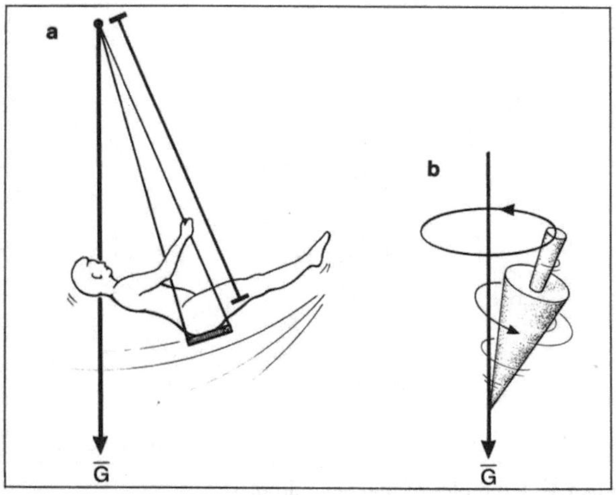

Fig. 1.4 a, b. Classic examples of swinging systems. **a** The swing; **b** the spinning top

tend to align such that their spins and magnetizations cancel. The micromagnetic field of nuclei with a spin of 1/2 is very similar to the field produced by a bar magnet or by a coil that is carrying electric current (an electromagnet), with the lines of magnetic flux emerging and entering at the poles of the spinning nucleus (Fig. 1.1). The strength of the magnetic moment depends on the type of nucleus and is described in terms of the gyromagnetic ratio γ. The hydrogen nucleus, consisting of one proton, possesses the largest gyromagnetic constant (after deuterium); that fact, plus its ubiquitous occurrence in tissues, makes the proton especially well suited for imaging applications. Unless stated otherwise, the discussions below will pertain exclusively to hydrogen nuclei.

1.1.3 Situation in the Absence of an Applied Magnetic Field

In the absence of an external magnetic field, the weak magnetic properties of nuclei are not accessible to measurement because the spin axes of the many tiny "magnets" are oriented randomly so that the sample as a whole does not possess a net measurable magnetic moment $\overline{M}$ (Fig. 1.2).

1.1.4 Situation in the Presence of an Applied Magnetic Field

When the sample is placed into an external magnetic field $\overline{B}_0$, the nuclei become oriented either parallel or antiparallel to the direction of the applied field (Fig. 1.3). The energy difference between the two orientations is extremely small. Out of several million aligned nuclei, only a few will form an excess in the direction of the applied field, depending on the field strength (SI unit: tesla) and temperature. The extremely weak net magnetic moment $\overline{M}$ resulting from these few nuclei must suffice for measurement purposes. The direction parallel to the applied field $\overline{B}_0$ is defined as the z axis of the three-dimensional coordinate system.

1.1.5 Resonance

Resonance is a property common to all systems that can vibrate. It is utilized for the measurement of nuclear magnetism. Such a system can be made to oscillate by external excitation. Resonance exists when the excitation frequency coincides with the *natural* frequency of the system. Energy transfer is greatest at this time, and so is the amplitude of the oscillations. A classic example is the pendulum or swing (Fig. 1.4a). When a push is imparted to the swinging body in phase with its *natural* motion, very large oscillations can be induced with a minimum of energy input. The properties of such a system are most readily observed when the resonance condition is satisfied.

Nuclei aligned in a magnetic field can oscillate in a manner analogous to the way a spinning top wobbles about its spin axis under the force of gravity (Fig. 1.4b), moving in a path that describes the wall of a cone. In physics, this type of motion is called precession. An electromagnetic pulse applied perpendicular to the aligned nuclei can act on the magnetic dipoles of the nuclei and induce a precessional motion by tipping them out of alignment with the main field (Fig. 1.5).

The frequency of the oscillation depends entirely on the oscillating system itself. While in a pendulum this frequency is inversely proportional to the root of the length of the pendulum, in MR it increases linearly with the strength of the applied field. The proportionality factor is the aforementioned gyromagnetic ratio γ. The resonance condition of the MR experiment is defined by the equation

$$f = \gamma B_0 / 2\pi \tag{1.1}$$

which states that for every NMR nucleus, excitation can occur only at a certain frequency which depends on the magnetic field strength. The quantity f is also termed the Larmor frequency. The gyromagnetic constant γ of protons is equal to 42.5659 MHz/T. Actually the classical model is not valid for individual nuclei, because the spin directions are quantized; it is valid, however, for describing the motion of the net magnetization vector $\overline{M}$. The "flip angle" of $\overline{M}$ (α) relative to the main field direction increases with the strength and duration of the excitation pulse. The direction of $\overline{M}$ can even be inverted so that $\alpha = 180°$.

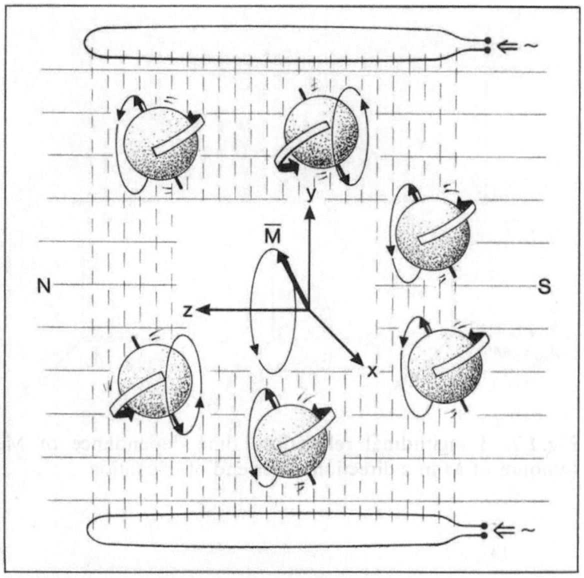

Fig. 1.5. Nuclear magnetic resonance. The nuclei behave - classically - like tiny tops when excited by a RF pulse of their resonance frequency *(vertical dotted lines)*, a precessional motion of $\bar{M}$ results

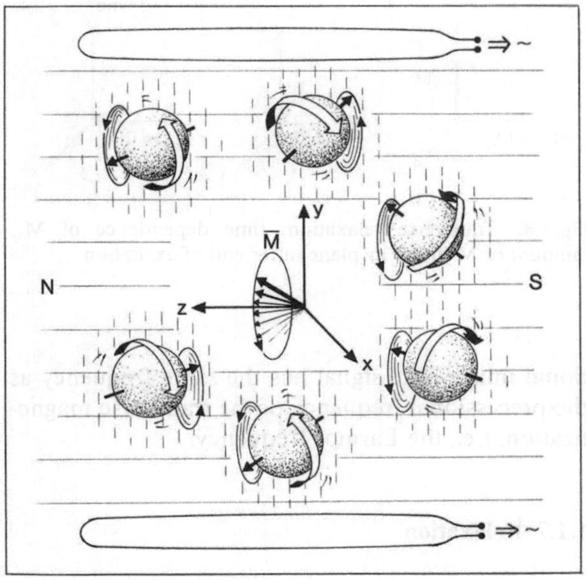

Fig. 1.6. Induction and relaxation. The precessional motion of $\bar{M}$ induces an alternating voltage in the receiver coil. Relaxation tends to realign the spin axis

1.1.6 Induction

The net magnetization vector $\overline{M}$, which precesses at the Larmor frequency after excitation, has a component that is perpendicular to the main field $\overline{B}_0$. This component is called the transverse magnetization, M_{xy}. It persists even after the excitation pulse has been turned off, and it induces an alternating voltage in a receiver coil mounted perpendicular to the main field, similar to the principle of an electric generator (Fig. 1.6). The signal induced in the coil is processed by a computer to ultimately yield a sec-

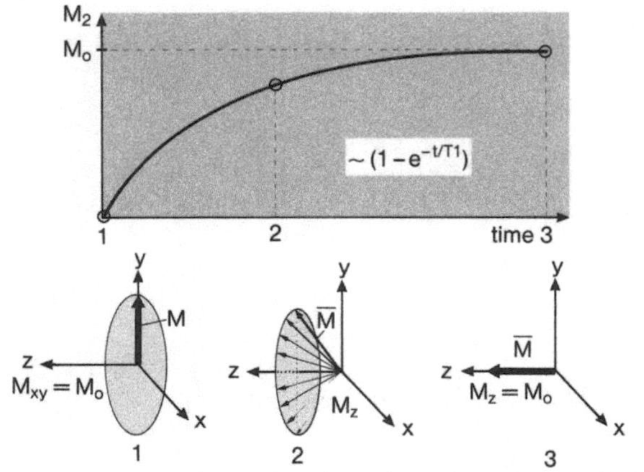

Fig. 1.7. Longitudinal relaxation: time dependance of M_z (amount of $\bar{M}$ in *z* direction) after end of excitation

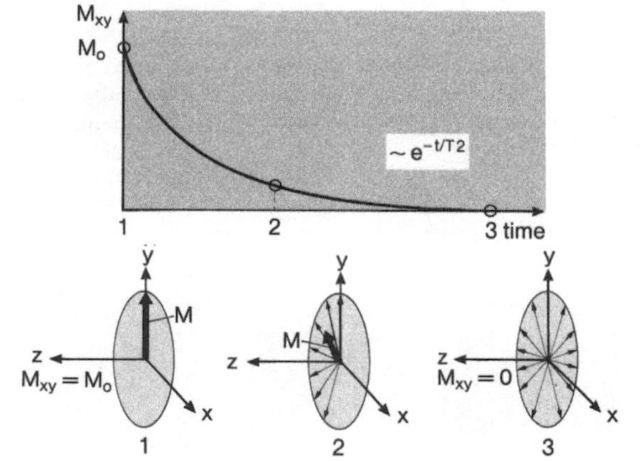

Fig. 1.8. Transverse relaxation: time dependence of M_{xy} (amount of $\bar{M}$ in the *xy* plane) after end of excitation

tional image. The signal has the same frequency as the precessional frequency of the transverse magnetization, i.e., the Larmor frequency.

1.1.7 Relaxation

The energy absorbed by oscillating systems is gradually released. The pendular motion of a swing, for example, becomes progressively smaller in amplitude through frictional losses and heat generation. In a similar way, the precessing nuclei release their kinetic energy to the surrounding molecules and lattice structures as their magnetic axes return to alignment with the field $\overline{B}_0$. This is accompanied by an exponential rise in the longitudinal magnetization M_z, the component of $\overline{M}$ in the field direction *z*, which recovers 63% of its initial value (1/e) after a time T1. This form of realignment is called spin-lattice or longitudinal relaxation (Fig. 1.7).

The large numbers of nuclei that are precessing give rise to a second effect known as spin-spin or transverse relaxation. Interactions among nuclear spins and local inhomogeneities in the applied field cause the individual nuclei to precess at slightly different rates and to deviate from the uniform motion they had on initial excitation. A similar phenomenon occurs when several swings given the same initial impetus are allowed to swing freely as their motions decay. The result of this spin-spin relaxation is a rapid exponential fall of the transverse magnetization M_{xy}, leading to a decay in the included signal intensity even though the nuclei remain in an excited state (Fig. 1.8). This is called the free induction decay (FID). Figure 1.6 shows that, despite the applied field $\overline{B}_0$, the situation is similar to that in the absence of an external field, i.e., a state of disorder in which a resonance signal cannot be received and reexcitation cannot occur. This form of relaxation takes place without energy loss. Its time constant is designated T2.

1.1.8 Significance of Relaxation Times

The two relaxation mechanisms, normally described in terms of the time constants T1 and T2, are chiefly responsible for the high level of contrast seen in MR images. Their importance in the study of molecular motions has been recognized for many years [16]. However, it is difficult to account for the large variations in relaxation times (several hundred percent) that are observed in MR investigations of living tissues.

Spin-lattice relaxation is essentially a thermal phenomenon. The kinetic energy of the precessing particles, which may be called the "spin temperature," is released to the surrounding molecular structures (the lattice), which likewise undergo rotational or translational motions (the "lattice temperature"). The energy transfer from the nucleus to the lattice also exhibits resonant behavior. Small molecules, like those in free water, move much more rapidly at the same temperature than do large molecules such as proteins and lipids. Their *natural* frequencies are much higher than the usual Larmor frequencies, and so relaxation occurs more slowly than in the more inert macromolecules. The latter vibrate at rates closer to the Larmor frequencies, resulting in a more rapid energy release and shorter relaxation times. Water molecules that are bound to such large structures by hydrogen bonding or that are undergoing exchange with them (e.g., diffusion) likewise shorten the spin-lattice relaxation time T1 in comparison with free water. As a result, water occurring in different compartments of the body (interstitial, intracellular, free fluid) exhibit different relaxation properties.

A parallel usually exists between the spin-spin and spin-lattice relaxations. Again, the rate of dephasing (loss of uniform motion) depends on resonance with the environment - in this case with the spins of neighboring nuclei. Localized inhomogeneities in the applied field lead to local differences in the Larmor frequencies, causing a decrease in T2, which is then designated T2*.

The spin-lattice relaxation time exhibits two extreme values in living tissues: very long T1 times on the order of several seconds in free water, and very short T1 times of approximately 200 ms in lipids and proteins. The T2 values are substantially shorter and range from about 30 to 500 ms. Both relaxation times carry information on viscosity, bonding conditions, diffusional processes, and paramagnetic ion concentrations, and both vary with temperature and with the external magnetic field. The predominant role of the T1 and T2 relaxation times for contrast production in MR images is described in greater detail in Sects. 1.3 and 1.4.

1.1.9 Chemical Shift

The signals emitted by the precessing nuclei also carry information on the structure of the molecules containing the nuclei. The resonance condition defined in Eq. 1.1 actually is valid only for free nuclei. The magnetic shielding effect of the electron clouds

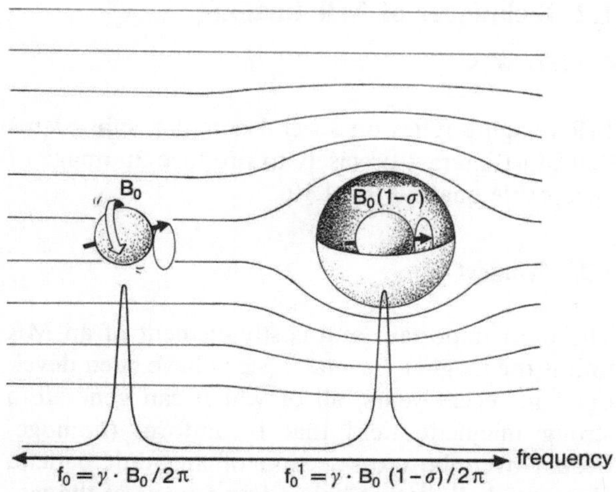

Fig. 1.9. Chemical shift: small change in resonance frequency by magnetic shielding effect of the electron cloud

in the molecule gives rise to a "chemical shift," which can change the resonant frequency by several parts per million (ppm), depending on the site at which the nucleus is bound in the molecule (Fig. 1.9). We can describe this change by introducing the shielding constant σ:

$$f = \gamma B_0 (1-\sigma)/2\pi \tag{1.2}$$

The spectral shifts of the signals can be measured and provide important information on the chemical structure of the compound. The technique of MR spectroscopy has been used in chemistry for three decades to analyze complex molecular structures. Its medical applications are just beginning to be appreciated and will be discussed briefly in Sect. 1.4.4. Already, means are available for producing a pictorial record of the chemical shift.

1.2 Techniques of MR Imaging

G. GADEMANN

MR imaging relies on several complex subsystems that must interact precisely to produce an image of acceptable quality (Fig. 1.10).

1.2.1 Magnet

The most important and costly element of an MR unit is the magnet. Several designs have been developed in recent years, all of which can generate a strong magnetic field that is uniform (homogeneous) over the cross-section of an adult patient. Here we shall discuss only a few aspects of the major types. The reader may consult Morris [97] for a more detailed account.

Usually the primary magnet consists of large, current-carrying coils which generate a field pattern similar to that of a bar magnet, i.e., a magnetic dipole with a north and south pole (see also Fig. 1.1). At the center of these coils - the bore of the "tunnel magnet" - the lines of magnetic flux are very densely arranged and parallel to one another, creating a strong, homogeneous field in that region. The patient is positioned so that the field lines traverse his body in the craniocaudal direction. The generated field is many thousands of times stronger than the earth's magnetic field, which averages 0.06 mT. Field strengths up to 0.3 T can be produced by resistive magnets, which must be water-cooled to remove the heat generated by the circulating current (low-field magnets) [100, 127].

Superconducting magnets can produce even higher field strengths in the range from 0.35 to 2 T or even more (high-field magnets). The conductive material in the coils consists of a special alloy that behaves as a superconductor at very low temperatures. Under these conditions an electric current will flow without any resistance losses. Superconducting magnets have a relatively complex design. The coils must be cooled to only 4.2° above absolute zero by immersion in liquid helium, and additional liquid-nitrogen and vacuum shielding must be provided to achieve adequate insulation.

Permanent magnets also are employed. They are assembled from individual blocks of magnetic material, and most have a "horseshoe" configuration. The patient lies between the pole pieces so that the field lines run at right angles to the body axis [45]. Roughly the same conditions are created by setting a coil magnet on end and positioning the patient between the turns of the coil, as practiced by the Aberdeen group [85].

Electromagnets that use iron guides to return the flux lines or extra superconducting coils to screen off fringe fields are in use [108, 128]. "Hy-

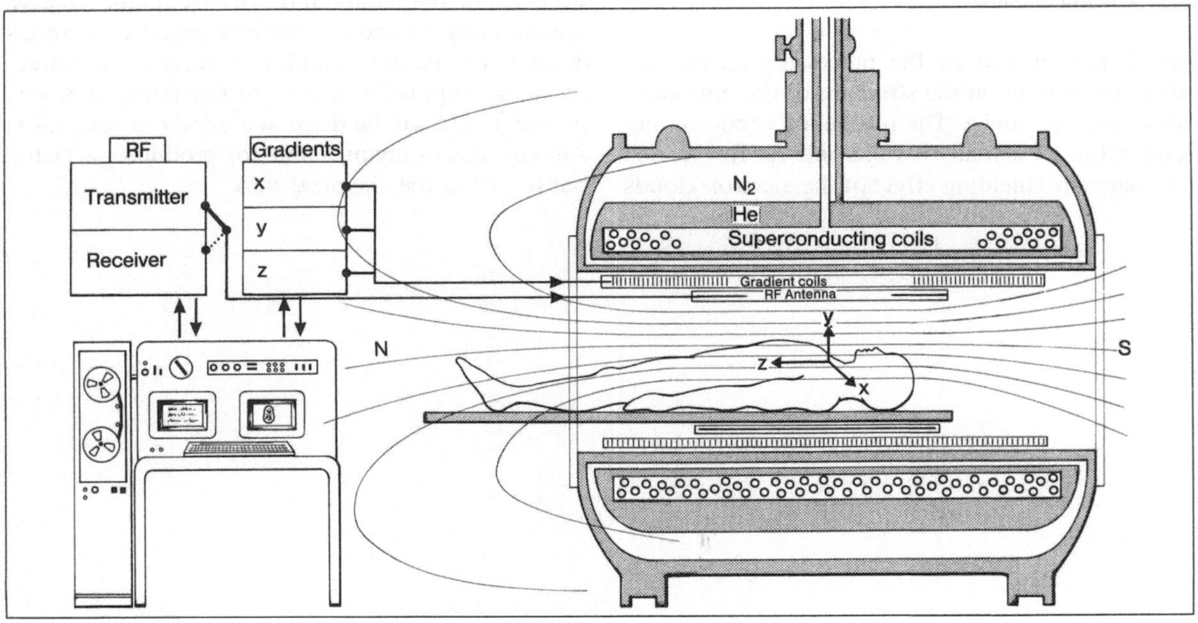

Fig. 1.10. Diagram of generic MR system using a superconducting magnet

brid" magnets employ an iron core to amplify the field strength.

Each of these techniques has its advantages and disadvantages. Most manufacturers of MR imagers currently offer superconducting magnets. The main advantage of a high field strength is a stronger MR signal and thus a sharper image [13]. Units operating at about 1.5 T or more additionally permit the MR spectroscopy of other nuclei. Disadvantages are the dependence on expensive superconducting technology and the relatively high operating costs because of the helium consumption. Resistive magnets have a lower initial cost and are less costly to operate. Their greatest disadvantage is that their field strength is limited to about 0.3 T, leading to sacrifice of image quality. Permanent magnets consume no energy, do not require cooling, and operate at field strengths up to 0.3 T, but the weight of the system (up to 90 tons) can be a problem. The main advantage of permanent magnets is that they produce almost no fringe fields, and the vertical direction of the flux lines permits the use of solenoid receiver coils, resulting in a better MR signal.

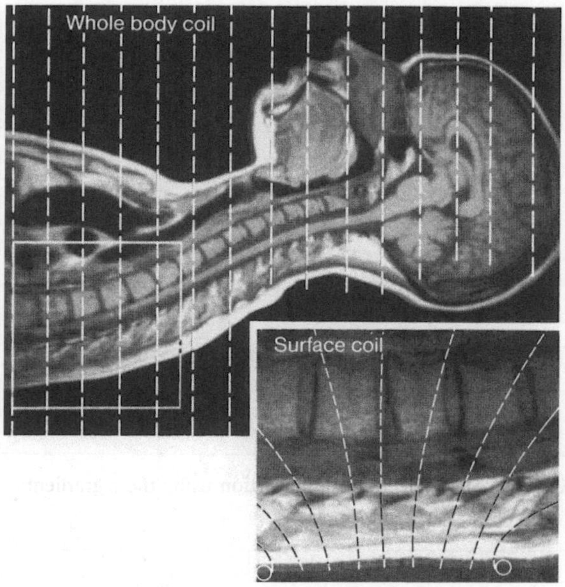

Fig. 1.11. RF field (B_1) of the whole body saddle coil and of a circular plane surface coil

1.2.2 Radiofrequency Equipment

Resonance frequency depends on the magnetic field strength (see Eq. 1.1). It lies in the medium frequency range of about 4–15 MHz for low-field magnets, and in the short-wave or low VHF range (up to about 85 MHz) for higher-field imaging. A powerful radio transmitter is required for excitation of the nuclei, and a sensitive radio receiver for detection of the MR signals. The transmitter and receiver operate through separate or common antenna coils that surround the region of interest. The more closely these coils enclose the body region to be examined, the greater the intensity of the received signal, and the more favorable the ratio of the MR signal to the thermal and electronic background noise (signal-to-noise ratio). That is why larger coil diameters of about 60 cm are used for imaging of the trunk (body coils), and smaller diameters of about 30 cm for imaging of the head (head coils). Saddle-shaped coils are used in tunnel magnets to produce a highly uniform radiofrequency (RF) field.

1.2.3 Surface Coils

The imaging of superficial structures is improved by the use of flat or contoured coils that are applied directly to the body region of interest [2, 73]. These are called surface coils. The better filling factor gives an excellent signal-to-noise ratio in proximity to the coil, but the signal intensity falls off sharply with distance from the coil (Fig. 1.11). The image looks as if a cross-section of the body were being illuminated with a flashlight, owing to the highly nonuniform sensitivity of these coils. Therefore surface coils are mostly used for detection only, while the body coil is used for excitation. This arrangement can cause coupling problems to occur between the two coils, leading to attenuation of the signal or even to a dangerous amplification of the RF field in the region of the surface coil [18]. Coupling can be minimized by positioning the coil parallel to the RF excitation field or by use of active electronic switching. The manufacturer's instructions should be followed with utmost care (see also Sects. 3.1 and 3.4). The range of surface coils is approximately equal to the diameter of the coil. Thus, for imaging of the central nervous system, surface coils provide especially good detail of the spinal cord (Sects. 2.9, Chap. 17), the orbit (Sect. 2.6), and the inner ear (Sect. 2.7).

1.2.4 Gradient System

As we saw in Sect. 1.1, a uniform magnetic field and RF equipment are all that are needed to perform an

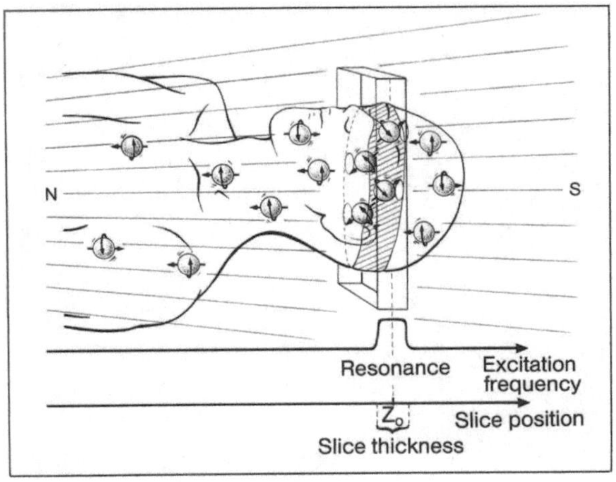

Fig. 1.12. Slice selection in *z* direction using the *z* gradient

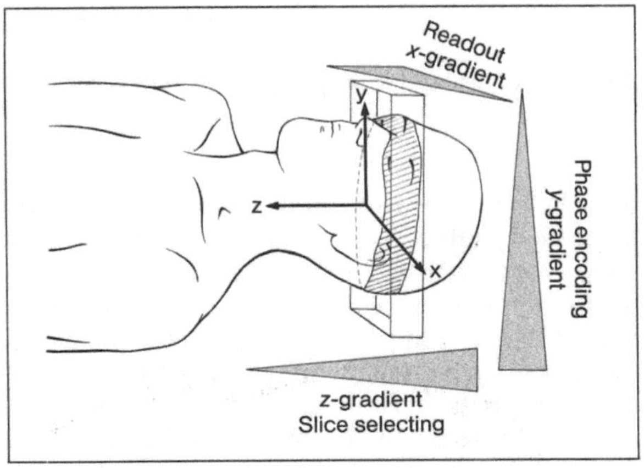

Fig. 1.13. Forming an image line by line: the two-dimensional Fourier transform technique (2DFT) with phase encoding and readout gradient

MR experiment. However, the long radio waves (wavelengths in the meter range) are unable to produce an image directly, as light or X-rays can. We are forced to apply entirely new principles to the problem of spatial encoding of the MR signals. To produce an image, each signal must carry explicit information on its site of origin. This is achieved by manipulating its frequency and phase angle Φ by adding linear magnetic field gradients $\overline{G}$ generated by resistive coils within the imaging volume of the magnet. For simplicity, these linear field gradients are also known as the *x, y,* and *z* gradients. These coils can uniformly (linearly) alter the main field $\overline{B}_0$ in its three dimensions *x, y,* and *z* in a way that causes neighboring points to have different resonance frequencies, in accordance with Eq. 1.1.

From $\overline{B}(z) = \overline{B}_0 + \overline{G}_z \cdot z$ with $\overline{G}_z = \frac{\partial B_z}{\partial z}$ follows

$$f(z) = \gamma(\overline{B}_0 + \overline{G}_z \cdot z)/2\pi \quad (1.3)$$

Figure 1.12 shows schematically the effect of the *z* gradient coil on the field lines, which take a diverging path when the coil is switched on.

1.2.5 Forming an Image

Several techniques are available for reading the spatial information in the signals and making an image. An image can be reconstructed using the back-projection method known from computed tomography [68], but today it is more common to use the two-dimensional Fourier transform (2DFT) technique first suggested by Kumar et al. in 1975 [74]. Below we shall illustrate this technique for a tunnel magnet with a horizontal flux pattern:

For transverse images, the *z* gradient functions as the slice selection gradient during the excitation (preparation) phase. The transmitter pulse is given a frequency spectrum which enables it to excite nuclei only in the plane in which the resonance condition is satisfied (Fig. 1.12). The MR signal, which can occur only on that plane, becomes spatially encoded in the *x* direction by switching on the *x* gradient during the detection phase, so that a mixture of frequencies is received (Fig. 1.13). The range of the different resonance frequencies depends on the strength of the *x* gradient and represents one line in the *x* direction. The *x* gradient is also called the readout gradient or line gradient in this context. The third dimension, representing the columns of the image, is encoded by the phase relationship of the received signal. For this purpose the *y* gradient, known as the phase encoding gradient or column gradient, is switched on between excitation and detection (see also spin-echo techniques, Sect. 1.3.2). Varying the gradient field strength between the individual acquisitions of each line alters the precession of the net magnetization vector $\overline{M}$. In this way the vector determines the phase relationship of the signal, which in turn defines the columns of the image (Fig. 1.13). As many individual acquisitions must be made as there are columns in the image matrix; a single acquisition is sufficient to provide the information needed for a complete image line. Thus, the total imaging (acquisition) time for an MR examination is determined by the interval between the excitation pulses, called the repetition time TR, and by the number of columns in the image matrix (MA). When the signal-to-noise ratio is poor, it is possible to measure the same line repeatedly (AC times), so that the total image acquisition time t_m is given by the equation

$$t_m = TR \times MA \times AC \quad (1.4)$$

Because the same slice is many times during a complete image acquisition excited, the repetition time TR is an important and freely selectable parameter for image contrast (see Sect. 1.3). The cyclic process of image formation (pulse sequence) is represented schematically in Fig. 1.14. After the interval TR, the entire slice is again excited with the slice selection gradient *(z)* turned on. Shortly thereafter the phase gradient *(y)* is switched on, followed by signal reception while the readout gradient *(x)* is activated. Generally TR is much longer than the delay time TE until the signal is received, with total imaging times ranging from 1 to 15 min. This is because of the relatively long T1 relaxation times of the tissues and the resulting image contrasts (see Sect. 1.3). One way to shorten total imaging time is by using the multislice method proposed by Crooks et al. in 1982 [34]. During the long intervals between pulse applications (see Fig. 1.14) other parallel slices are selectively excited, enabling data to be acquired from a number of slices, rather than just one, during the total imaging time t_m. Figure 1.15 illustrates the overlapping sequence of excitation and acquisition of the individual sections. It is necessary only to change the frequency spectrum of the excitation pulse during slice selection and read the measured values into different sets of raw data. These resemble holograms (or better, interferogram) in that they contain both amplitude and phase information on the wave field (Fig. 1.16). An initial Fourier transform converts the frequency encoding of the lines into spatial form. A second transform along the columns completes the image formation process.

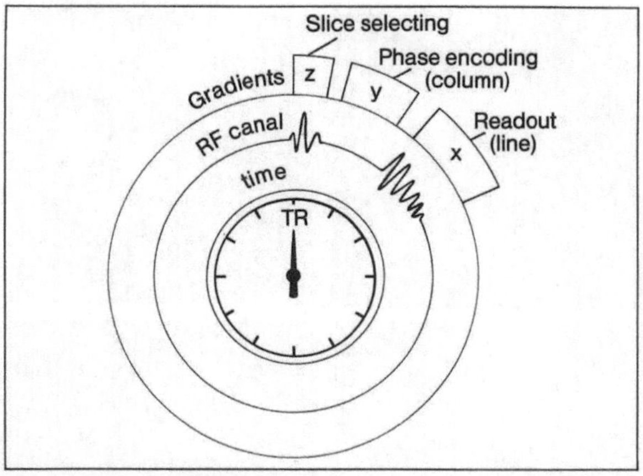

Fig. 1.14. Imaging pulse sequence: cyclic process of excitation and signal detection with rhythmic switching of gradient fields

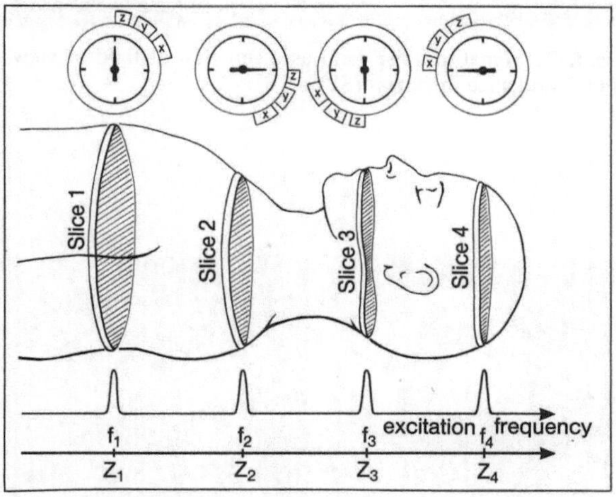

Fig. 1.15. Multislice method: overlapping of excitation and data acquisition for several individual slices within one cycle period

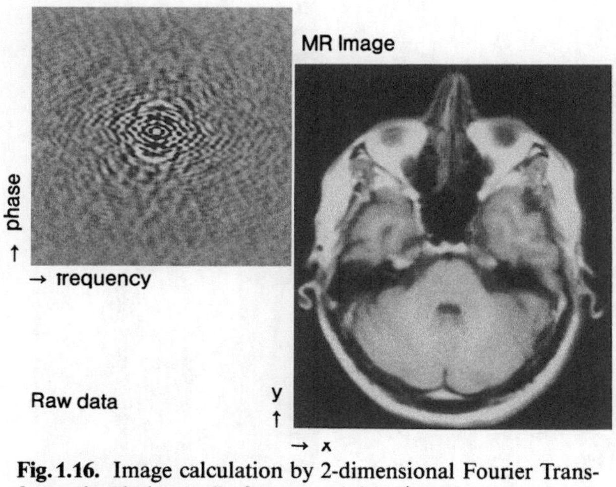

Fig. 1.16. Image calculation by 2-dimensional Fourier Transform; the "hologram" of measured data (raw data) is converted to the MR image

1.2.6 Central Control Unit

As we have seen, the production of an MR image relies on a complex sequence of RF excitation and reception, the rapid switching of strong electric currents to pulse the gradient fields on and off, and finally a complex image reconstruction process. Only a powerful computer system can handle the associated tasks of coordination, image computation, evaluation, and storage. This is illustrated in Fig. 1.10.

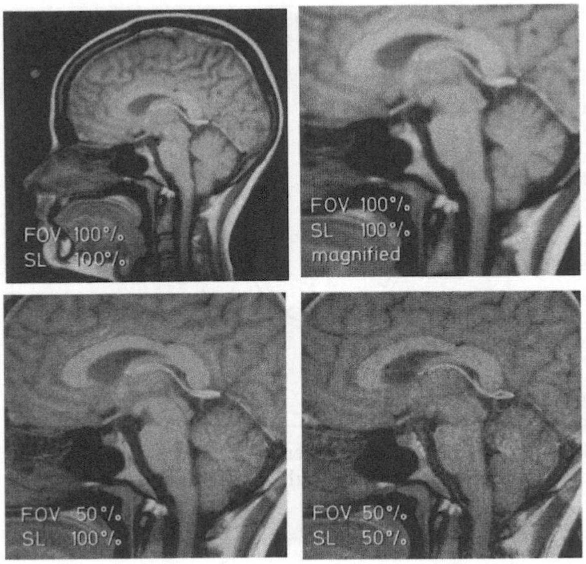

Fig. 1.17. Signal-to-noise ratio as a function of field of view (FOV) and slice thickness (SL).

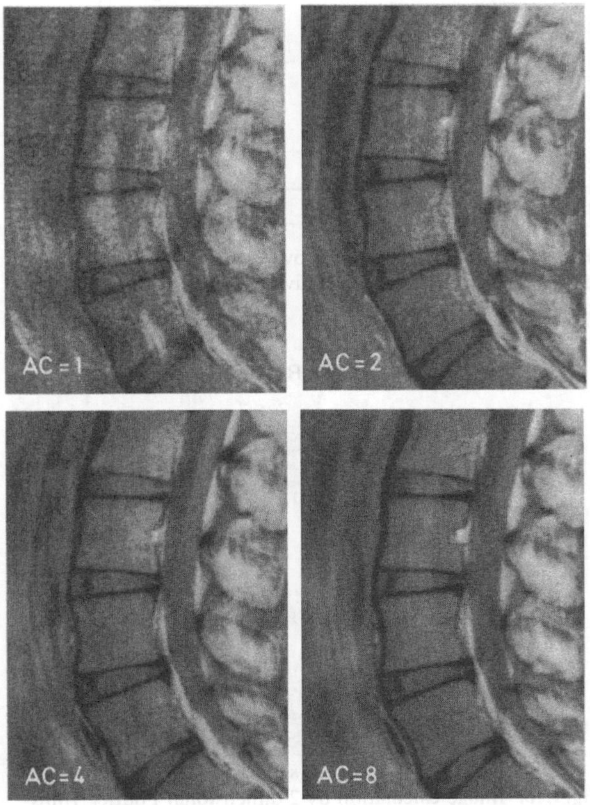

Fig. 1.18. High-resolution imaging using surface coil and multiple measurements (AC).

1.3 Pulse Sequences and Image Contrasts

The quality of MR images for medical diagnosis is determined by several factors, such as the MR signal intensity, the signal-to-noise ratio, the spatial resolution (Sect. 1.3.1), the inherent (Sects. 1.3.2 and 1.4.1) and artificially enhanced (Sect. 1.3.3) contrast between tissues, flow (Sect. 1.3.4), and the absence of artifacts (Sect. 1.3.5).

1.3.1 Aspects of MR Image Quality

R. HAERTEN

The signal intensity measured by MR carries information on the relaxation characteristics of tissues (Sect. 1.1). The signal intensity is proportional to the magnetization induced in a volume element ("voxel") by the static magnetic field.

Image quality is affected by the level of random noise in the MR measurement. The noise level is basically determined by the square root of the bandwidth of the MR signal detector circuits, i.e., the range of resonance frequencies measured at a given readout gradient field strength (Sect. 1.2). A sufficiently high signal-to-noise ratio is necessary for reliable tissue discrimination.

The signal intensity measured in MR imaging is proportional to the number of protons contributing to the magnetization of a voxel. Thus, for a given static magnetic field strength, signal intensity depends on the choice of the pixel resolution and the slice thickness. For a given matrix size, such as 256×256, pixel resolution is determined by the choice of the field of view (FOV). When the pixel resolution (in mm) is halved, the voxel size and thus the signal intensity are reduced by a factor of four. Halving the slice thickness reduces signal intensity by another factor of two. As a result, gains in spatial resolution can be achieved only at the cost of the signal-to-noise ratio (Fig. 1.17), and contrast between different kinds of tissue may be lost if the selected pixel resolution or slice thickness is too small.

Several approaches exist to maintaining a sufficiently high signal-to-noise ratio in high-resolution imaging. Averaging over two, four, or more complete measurements (Ac), for example, would allow for small-FOV images (Fig. 1.18), where a single measurement would yield a signal-to-noise ratio sufficient only for a large-FOV image.

Thus, the differentiation of small anatomic structures in the image can be improved at the cost of extended patient examination time (Eq. 1.4). Alternatively, special surface coils, which offer high sensitivity within a limited volume defined by the size and shape of the coil, can be utilized for high-resolution imaging of small organs and superficial structures (Sect. 1.2.3).

The signal-to-noise ratio is, after all, a function of the magnetic field strength of the MR imaging system. Under otherwise equal experimental conditions, the achievable signal is roughly proportional to the magnetic field strength: twice the field strength will yield twice the signal intensity.

However, in situations where waterlike and fatty compounds are present, as in the orbit, spine, abdominal organs, and joints, the gradient strength must be increased with increasing field strength to avoid chemical shift artifacts in the image (see Sect. 1.3.5). Consequently, the bandwidth of the MR signal detector has to be adjusted to the field strength, and the increase in the signal-to-noise ratio is proportional to the square root of the field strength rather than to the field strength itself [143]. Doubling the field strength will increase the signal-to-noise ratio by 40% in these situations, and not by a factor of 2.

Magnetic field strengths ranging from 0.02 T to 1.5 T are presently used in clinical MR. The upper limit is determined by the power density, which for proton imaging should not exceed 0.4 W/kg (see Sect. 3.4). At field strengths less than 1.0 T, a sufficiently high signal-to-noise ratio is obtained by averaging over multiple acquisitions, whereas at high field strengths of 1.0 T or above, good imaging results can be achieved with a single acquisition, thereby shortening the examination time (Figs. 1.19–1.21).

For a given image acquisition time, the gain in signal-to-noise ratio at a field strength of 1.0 T or above will allow for higher spatial resolution and thinner slices. While 1.0 T has been found to be a reasonable choice for high-resolution MR imaging [67], 1.5 T or more is necessary for efficient MR spectroscopy.

The aforementioned tissue parameters, the relaxation times T1 and T2, and the spin density determine the intensity of the MR signal for a given field strength, image matrix, and slice thickness. T1 increases with the strength of the static magnetic field, and this can influence image contrast [36, 49, 69]; T2 is essentially unchanged with increasing field strength. Table 1.2 shows the tissue parameters

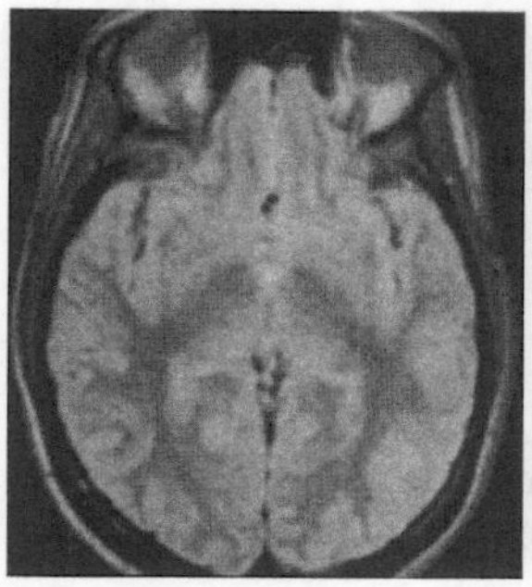

1.19

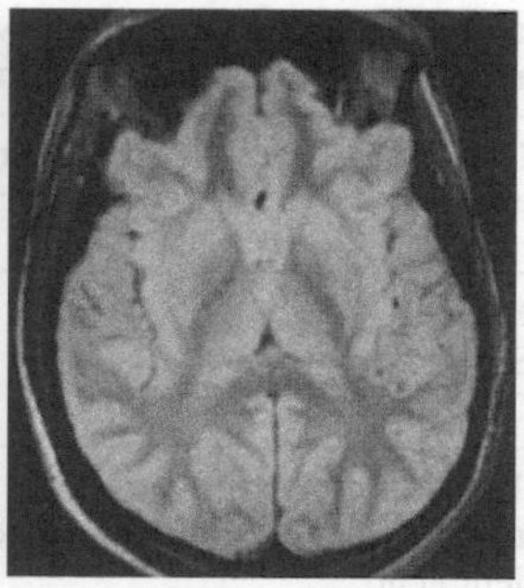

1.20

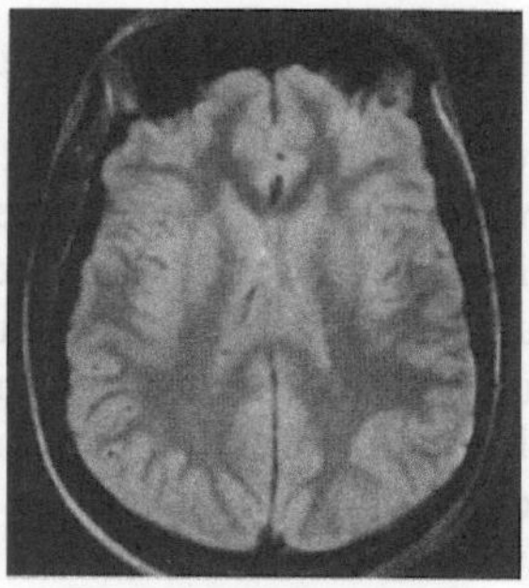

1.21

Figs. 1.19–1.21. Comparison of MR images obtained at different field strengths B_0. **1.19** Single measurement at 0.5 T; **1.20** single measurement at 1.0 T; **1.21** single measurement at 1.5 T

of the major types of central nervous system tissue for field strengths of 0.15, 0.5, 1.0, and 1.5 T.

The contrast between different tissues can be critically influenced by manipulation of the RF pulse sequences. Through proper selection of the pulse sequence, it is possible to accentuate specific tissue parameters, resulting in images that are

Table 1.2. MR parameters of central nervous system tissues

Tissue	T1 (ms)	T2 (ms)	N(H) (%)	B_0 (T)
White matter	350	90	73	0.15
	530	90	73	0.5
	675	90	73	1.0
	710	90	73	1.5
Gray matter	450	100	87	0.15
	650	100	87	0.5
	800	100	87	1.0
	910	100	87	1.5
CSF	2200	900	100	1.0
Fat	170	84	80	0.15
	210	84	80	0.5
	240	84	80	1.0
	255	84	80	1.5

From ref [33], [138], and [19] cited in Bydder 1985 [26]

Table 1.3. Image weighting with various combinations of preparation pulses and detection methods

Detection method	Preparation pulse		
	SR	IR	A
FID	N(H)	T1	(T1)
SE	N(H), T2	T1	(T1, T2)
GE		See Table 1.6	

SR, saturation recovery; IR, inversion recovery; LA, low angle; FID, free induction decay; SE, spin echo; GE, gradient echo

"weighted" toward T1, T2, spin density N(H), or a mixture of these parameters. This offers the possibility of enhanced tissue differentiation, but at the same time it requires a knowledge of complicated contrast mechanisms. Contrast may be lost completely if unfavorable sequence parameters are selected.

1.3.2 Pulse Sequences

G. GADEMANN

An increasing number of pulse sequences are becoming available for use in clinical MR and scrutting of the literature discloses a lack of uniformity in the designation and description of these sequences. Every MR sequence consists of a preparation phase and a detection phase. The classification presented in Table 1.3 is based on the definitions of the Subcommittee of the American College of Radiology [3] (see also Glossary). It shows the different weightings that result from the various combinations of preparation and detection pulses. The three pulse sequences mainly used for preparation are saturation recovery (SR), inversion recovery (IR), and, recently, low-angle excitation (LA). While these preparation sequences most strongly affect the T1 and spin-density weighting of the image, the detection phase is of significance for T2 weighting. The pure FID signal provides no T2 weighting, and that mode is seldom used in present-day imaging. On the other hand, the spin-echo detection sequence has enjoyed great popularity for some time. The related gradient echo permits substantially shorter delay times and, together with low-angle excitation is commonly used for fast imaging sequences (see Sect. 1.4). The contrast mechanisms of these sequences are variable and not yet completely understood (see Table 1.7).

The two most important clinical sequences - SR spin echo and IR spin echo - are described below in greater detail.

Saturation-Recovery Spin-Echo Technique (SE)

The SR spin-echo technique, also known simply as the spin-echo (SE) sequence, was developed in 1950 by Hahn [62]. There are several reasons for its popularity in MR imaging: (1) It provides T2 weighting of images, (2) it largely eliminates the effect of field inhomogeneities, and (3) the time window of the MR signal is easily determined.

The resonance signal induced at the end of a 90° excitation pulse (the FID) disappears very rapidly when the phase gradient is turned on, because the spins go out of phase. Several milliseconds after the initial excitation (TE/2), a second pulse is applied which is strong enough to tip the spins through 180° (Fig. 1.22). This causes the individual dephasing moments to become "reflected" on the *xy* plane, so that the dephasing process converts to a rephasing one, the transverse magnetization M_{xy} increases again, and a strong signal, the echo, can be detected at the time TE/2 after application of the 180° pulse. Compared with the initial amplitude of the FID, the echo amplitude is reduced by a factor characterized by the true T2 relaxation at echo time TE (Fig. 1.23). Additional echoes can be elicited by applying several 180° pulses in succession. An echo train of this type generated by a Carr-Purcell-Meiboom-Gill (CPMG) sequence [30, 91] permits the most accurate calculation of the T2 times of tissues, for the amplitudes of the individual echoes decline exponentially with T2 as a time constant due to the increase of the phase angle Φ. The longer the T2 time, the longer an echo can be traced. Figure 1.24b shows the exponential curves for the T2 decay of some tissues listed in Table 1.2 at a field strength of 1.0 T. These curves correspond to the time course of the transverse magnetization M_{xy} (Fig. 1.8). Increasing the echo time TE, and thus delaying echo production, increases the degree of T2 weighting in the image [44, 117].

The echo time TE is a specific sequence parameter for the SE technique. It may be arbitrarily chosen within a range limited from below by the speed with which the gradients can be switched on and off (10-35 ms) and from above by the second major sequence parameter, the repetition time TR (see Sect. 1.2). Generally the TE interval is chosen to correspond roughly to the T2 times of the tissues to be discriminated.

The repetition time TR most strongly affects the T1 contribution to image contrast, for it represents the interval in which the magnetization $\bar{M}$ is allowed to realign with the external field $\bar{B}_0$ before the next excitation is applied. If recovery of the *z* component of magnetization M_z is incomplete, the intensity of the next MR signal will be deceased. A sequence in which the TR is shorter than the T1 time of the tissue is called a partial saturation (PS) sequence and produces images that are weighted more heavily toward T1.

Figure 1.24a shows how the signal intensities (S) vary with the repetition time TR for a constant echo time TE. The curves illustrate the situation for a field strength of 1.0 T (Table 1.2). They correspond to the time course of the longitudinal magnetization M_z (Fig. 1.7). With a short TR, fatty tissue gives a relatively strong MR signal because of its very short T1 (ca. 250 ms). Materials that relax more slowly, such as cerebrospinal fluid (CSF), have undergone only partial relaxation and consequently give little or no signal. As a result, fatty tissue appears brightest an T1-weighted images of this type, while fluids appear very dark. The slopes of the curves in Fig. 1.24a become flatter as the TR intervals are prolonged, and all tend asymptotically toward a value that depends solely on the proton density (spin density) of the tissue. Thus, long TR intervals (3 × T1, i.e., 2s or longer) produce images that are weighted toward spin density provided that TE is very short. CSF gives a signal intensity comparable to that of fatty tissue, and excellent contrast is seen between the gray and white matter of the brain. T1 and T2 weighting have opposite effects on contrast. From Figs. 1.24a and b, which show real sequences with finite values of TR and TE respectively, we can appreciate the complexity of the contrast mechanisms. With certain combinations or TR and TE, the contrast between tissues may vanish despite differences in their T1 and T2 times, and the tissues may appear identical. This crossover effect tends to occur in "mixed" images with moderate TR and TE, which is why extreme TR and TE values are usually chosen for clinical imaging [22, 110].

The contrast produced by the SE technique can be represented as a two-dimensional map. Figure 1.25 shows the same coronal section as a function of TR (horizontal axis) and TE (vertical axis) measured at a field strength of 1.0 T. It is obvious that as the T1 contribution to image contrast declines, the contribution of T2 increases. CSF appears dark on T1-weighted images but bright on T2-weighted images. We observe a similar reversal

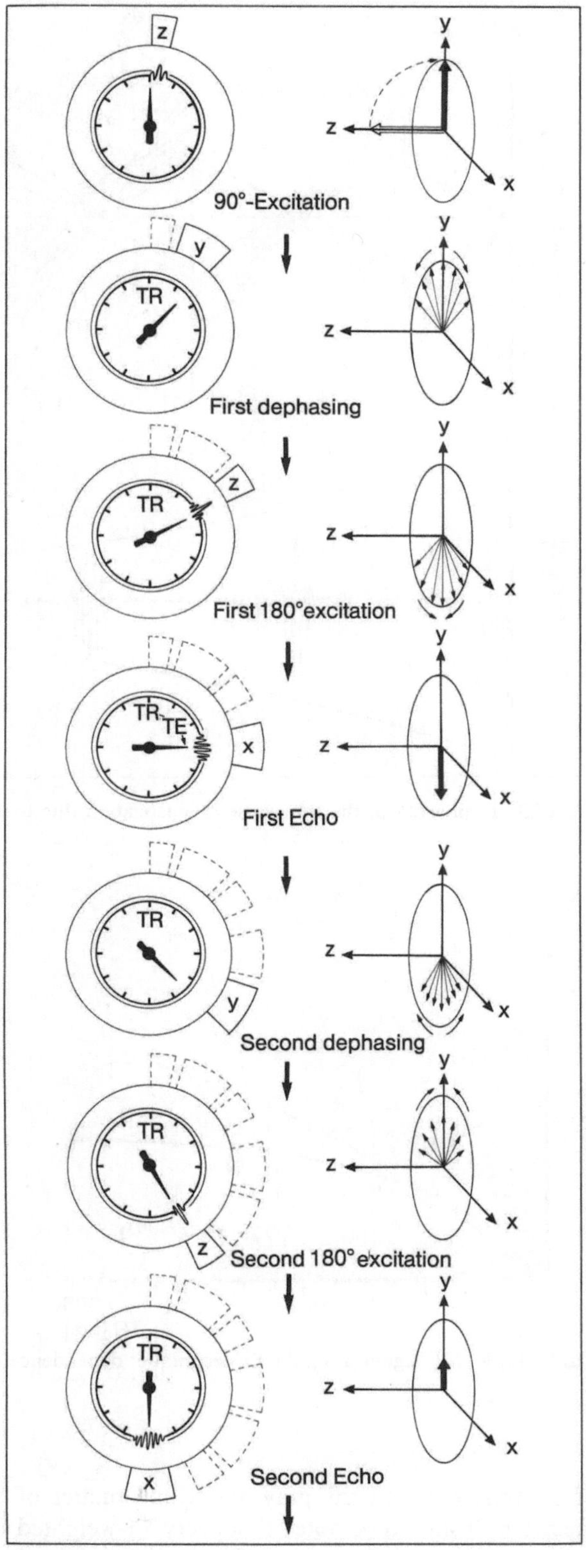

Fig. 1.22. Saturation-recovery spin-echo pulse sequence (SE). See text page 12

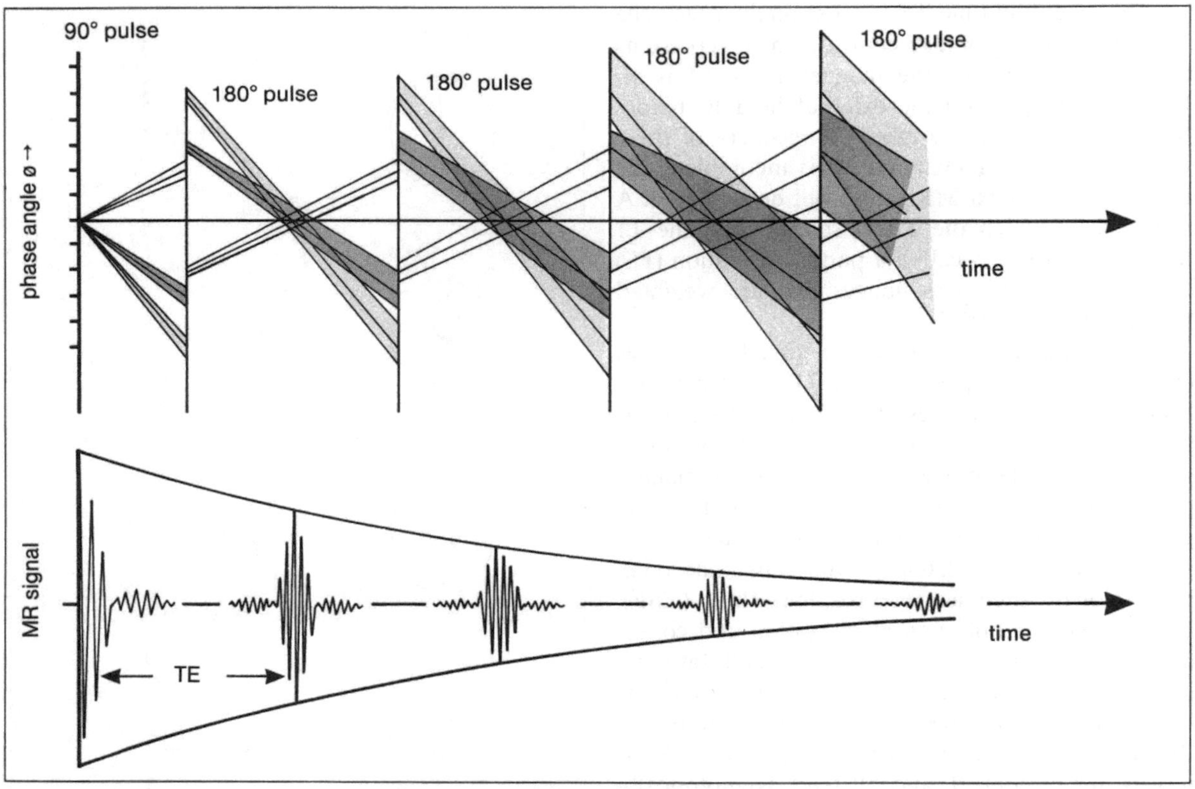

Fig. 1.23. Dephasing of the transverse magnetization due to the T2 relaxation shown with a multiecho sequence

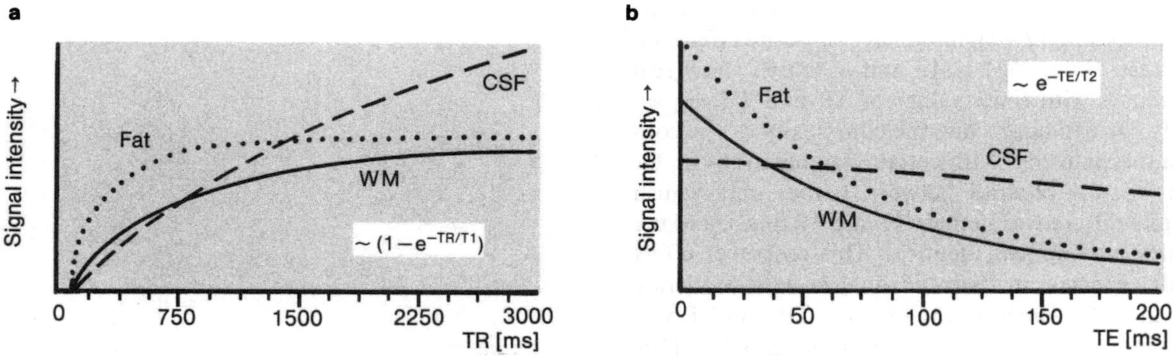

Fig. 1.24 a, b. MR signal using the SE technique: dependence on **(a)** TR and **(b)** TE. *WM* = white matter

of contrast between the gray and white matter of the brain. It should be noted that every T1-weighted image and especially every spin density-weighted image shows some T2 dependence due to the necessary presence of an echo time TE. The increase in T1 relaxation times with magnetic field strength theoretically requires longer repetition times for the same contrast in T2-weighted and spin density-weighted images. In practive, however, this does not have the significance that was originally believed.

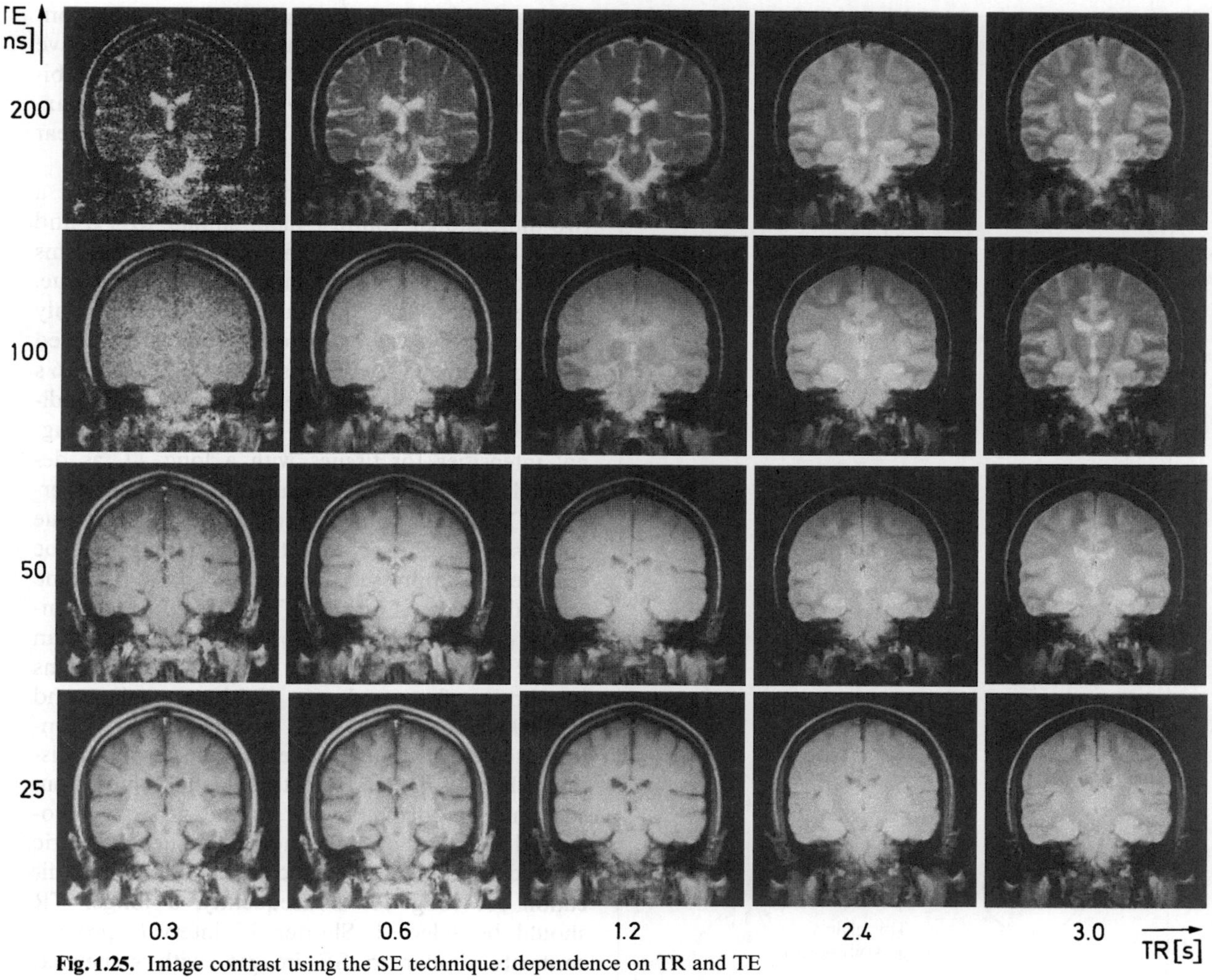

Fig. 1.25. Image contrast using the SE technique: dependence on TR and TE

Inversion Recovery Spin-Echo Technique (IR)

The IR sequence was introduced in MR as a means of accurately measuring T1 relaxation times. It provides a much greater T1 weighting of images than the SE technique.

An initial 180° pulse is applied to invert the longitudinal magnetization M_z to $-M_z$ and place the nuclear spins in an excited state where T2 relaxation cannot occur, since there is no transverse magnetization (Fig. 1.26). Accordingly, the time course of the longitudinal magnetization M_z begins at $-M_z$ (Fig. 1.27). After an interval TI (interpulse time) during which the magnetization $\vec{M}$ undergoes some degree of recovery determined by the local T1, a signal is acquired, usually by means of an SE sequence. We see in Fig. 1.27 that the inversion leads to a doubling of the T1 contrast between the CNS tissues (Table 1.2) in the IR image. Tissues that relax completely during TI yield a normal SE signal. Regions with a long T1 relax very little from inversion during the interpulse time, and so the phase of the signal is shiftet by 180°, since the 90° excitation occurs from that position. Regions whose T1 is in the range of the TI delay (TI ~ T1 × log 2) pass through the zero point and cannot be detected. Maximum contrast is achieved when the TI interval is between the T1 times of two tissues to be discriminated. With phase-dependent imaging, tissue with a shorter T1 will yield a positive signal and a bright image, while tissue with a longer T1 will yield a negative signal and a dark image. If phase is

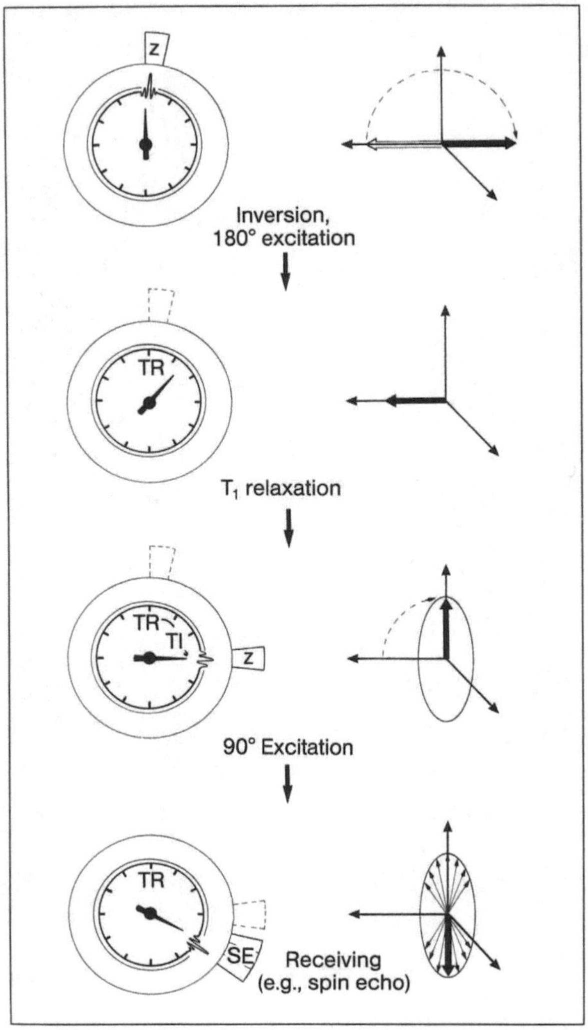

Fig. 1.26. Inversion-recovery spin-echo pulse sequence (IR). See text page 15

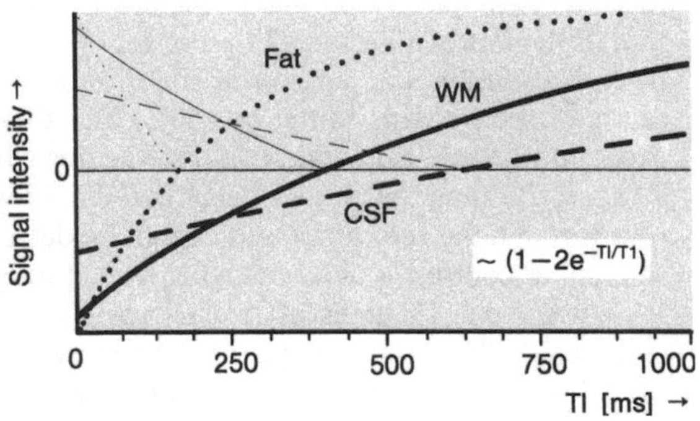

Fig. 1.27. MR signal using the IR technique: dependence on TI. *WM* = white matter

disregarded in image processing (magnitude reconstruction), the latter values also will appear positive (see narrow lines in Fig. 1.27). The result is an ambiguity of image content in which tissues with relaxation times in the range of the TI interval appear dark.

Both imaging parameters, TI and TR, define a two-dimensional contrast map, similar to TE and TR in the SE technique. The contrast mechanisms are more complicated than in the SE technique. The repetition time TR influences contrast only slightly above a value where the spins are allowed to relax completely within each cycle. A TR of 1.6 s or more is generally sufficient to satisfy this condition. Using a TR that is too short results in low signal intensities for tissues with a long T1, as described for the SE technique, and in signal reversals. Depending on the selection of TI, tissue contrasts may be accentuated or signals may be completely suppressed. Figure 1.28 shows the same coronal section as Fig. 1.25. The effect of the TI interval (vertical axis) is substantially greater than that or TR (horizontal axis). Usually a TI of 400 ms is chosen for moderate field strengths, and 500–600 ms for fields of 1.5 T or higher. Longer interpulse delays are used when it is necessary to distinguish gray matter from tumor and tumor from surrounding edema, owing to the generally prolonged T1 values of the pathologic tissues. Pediatric brain development studies constitute another indication for long TI. Consequently, a longer TR should be selected. Shorter TI intervals provide contrasts similar to SE images, with somewhat greater weighting toward T1 due to the steeper angle of the M_z alignment. Bydder and Young (1985) [26] recommended an IR sequence with a short TI (STIR) for the suppression of fatty tissue and the detection of periventricular lesions. Even on IR images, T2 makes a slight contribution to contrast owing to use of the SE technique for data acquisition; the echo time TE should therefore be as short as possible.

The necessity for a relatively long TR makes it extremely difficult to shorten the total acquisition time, and only a few sections can be imaged by the multislice method due to the long TI interval. That is why the SE technique is used more often clinically, while the IR technique is most commonly used for the differentiation or improved delineation of lesions that have already been diagnosed. However, this in no way negates the importance of the IR sequence, which continues to be a mainstay in neurologic investigations.

Fig. 1.28. Image contrast using the IR technique: dependence on TR and TI

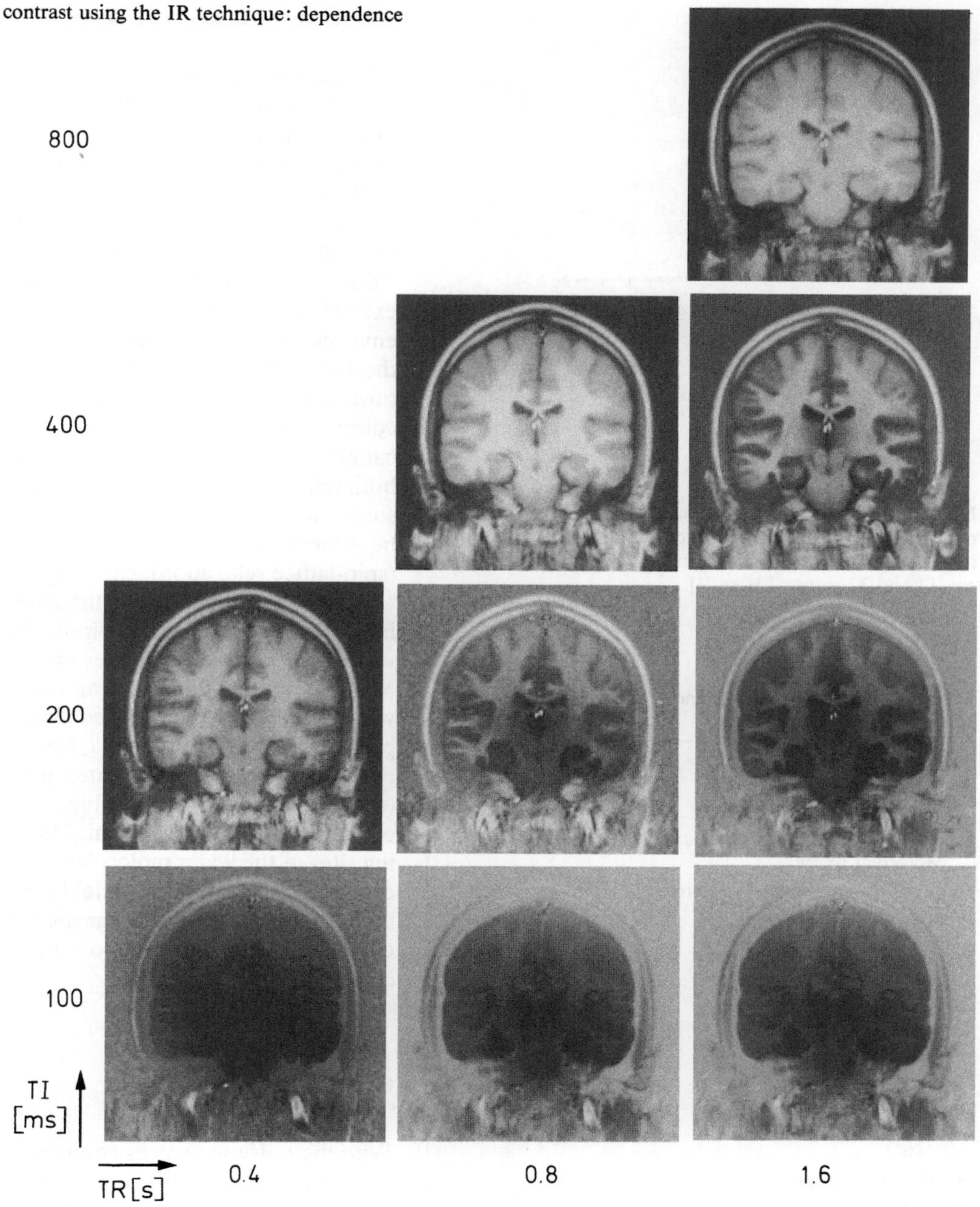

1.3.3 Contrast Agents

H. Weinmann

MR tomography has not only brought a new dimension to diagnostic imaging but has also set a milestone in contrast media research. Initially there was doubt concerning the need to administer exogenous materials, owing to the many existing ways of influencing and manipulating MR images. Conventional media that produce contrast by the increased absorption of X-rays are useless for this modality, because, unlike radiography, the source of the signal lies within the body itself. The introduction of extra protons is not a reasonable means for enhancing contrast because of the extremely high proton concentrations in the body (approximately 100 mol/l).

Lauterbur in 1978 noted the possibility of using paramagnetic ions to shorten the relaxation times of protons und thereby alter signal intensities on MR

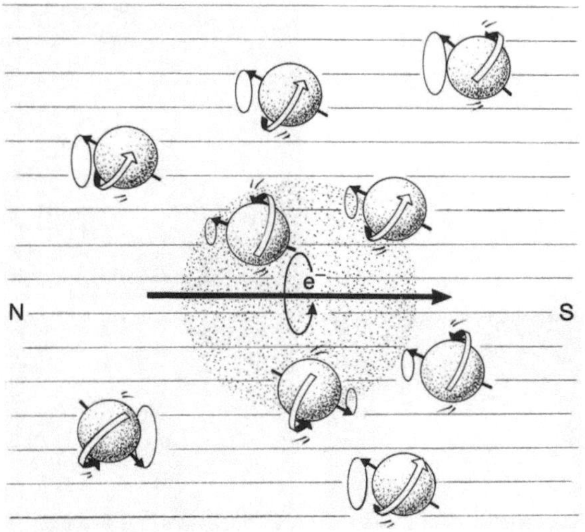

Fig. 1.29. Proton relaxation enhancement. A paramagnetic molecule (spinning unpaired electron) tends to enhance proton relaxation of nearby hydrogen nuclei and therefore shortens T1 and T2 values. [After 23]

Table 1.4. Paramagnetic substances with unbalanced electron spins

Unpaired electrons
Nitric oxide (NO)
Nitrogen dioxide (NO_2)
Paired electrons with parallel spins
Molecular oxygen
Ions containing unpaired electrons
Transition metal series
Mn^{2+}, Mn^{3+}
Fe^{2+}, Fe^{3+}
Ni^{2+}
Cr^{2+}
Cu^{2+}
Lanthanide series
Gd^{3+}
Eu^{2+}
Actinide series
Pa^{4+}
Stable free radicals
Nitroxyles
Triphenylmethyl

images [79, 92]. Intolerance to the metal ions was considered a serious drawback to this approach. Nevertheless, the method appeared feasible since even very small concentrations of the paramagnetic materials, such as ions of the transition elements and lanthanide series, as well as nitroxyl compounds, do have the effect of shortening relaxation times.

Shortening of Relaxation Times

Paramagnetic compounds have at least one unpaired electron. That electron has a magnetic moment approximately 1000 times stronger than the magnetic moment of a proton. As a result of motion (diffusion, rotation, etc.), the paramagnetic compound acts on the atomic level to produce a rapid fluctuation in the local magnetic field (Fig. 1.29). This process facilitates energy transfer among the excited protons and also from the protons to their environment (lattice), and the magnetic moments of the hydrogen nuclei deflected by the RF pulse return more rapidly to their initial state. Paramagnetic compounds can only shorten relaxation times; they cannot prolong them. Moreover, they always affect both relaxation times, usually to an equal degree. In some circumstances T2 (spin-spin relaxation) may be shortened to a much greater degree than T1 (spin-lattice relaxation); the reverse is never true.

The relaxation times of the hydrogen nuclei are influenced by a magnetic dipole-dipole interaction with the paramagnetic center of the contrast agent. Many complex factors determine the degree to which relaxation is shortened [50]. Thus, for example, the "correlation time" (τ_c) and the distance between the paramagnetic center and water molecule (a sixth-power function) influence the effectiveness of the paramagnetic material. The number of binding sites of the water molecules to the paramagnetic central atom is another crucial factor. The paramagnetic effect may show a magnetic-field and frequency dependence, depending on the size of the molecule [77].

Contrast Enhancement

With the pulse sequences commonly used in practical MR, shortening the T1 relaxation time tends to increase the intensity of the MR signal (Sect. 1.3.2). This effect is most pronounced in heavily T1-weighted images. For signal amplification to occur, the protons located in the compartment must have suitable properties. The spin-spin relaxation times must not act in a way that negates the enhancement of signal intensity. A short T2 always leads to a lower signal, regardless of how short T1 may be. This fact is significant when we consider that all paramagnetic compounds not only affect T1 but also shorten T2. When a paramagnetic agent is used in very high concentration, the shortening of

T2 becomes predominant, and the signal is weakened. This effect increases with the degree of T2 weighting of the pulse sequence. Because of the exponential relationship, the T2 effect causes the greatest signal loss when the T2 relaxation time is less than or equal to the echo time (TE). The T1 and T2 effects can shown together in Fig. 1.30. Initially the T1 effect is predominant. After reaching a maximum, the signal intensity declines because of the predominance of T2 and can even fall below the initial signal intensity if T2 is short enough. Thus, imaging sequences that have the smallest possible T2 weighting (very short TE) generally are best for enhancing contrast. Figure 1.31 a, b shows how the concentration of a paramagnetic agent alters the relaxation times and the relaxation rate (1/T).

SE sequences with a TR less than 0.8 s and a very short echo time TE (<40 ms) show contrast enhancement much more clearly than sequences that are spin-density weighted or T2 weighted, for example. IR sequences also are suitable but are disadvantageous because of their poor signal-to-noise ratio and long acquisition time.

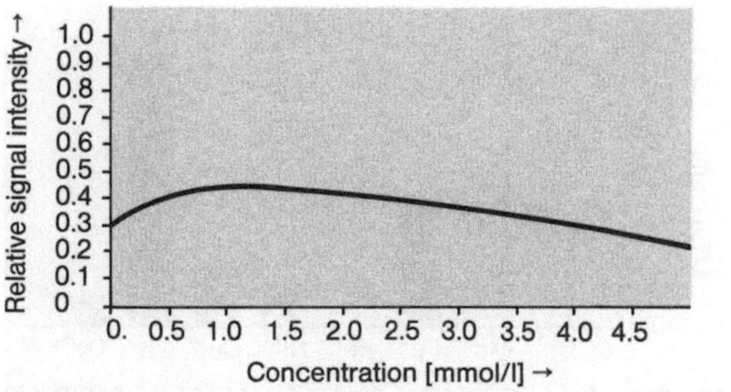

Fig. 1.30. Dependence of signal intensity on the concentration of a paramagnetic medium (gadolinium-DTPA) using a SE sequence

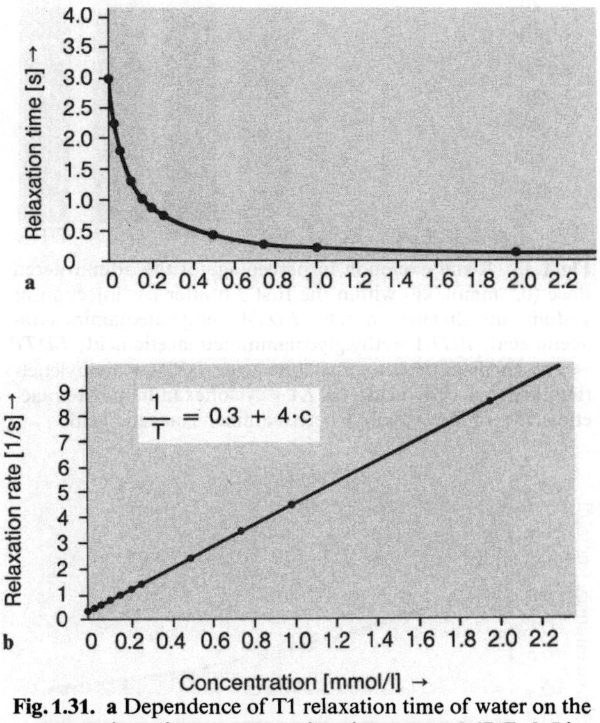

Fig. 1.31. a Dependence of T1 relaxation time of water on the concentration of a paramagnetic substance at 0.47 T. **b** Linear dependence of the T1 relaxation rate (1/T) of water on the concentration of a paramagnetic substance. The gradient of the line is a measure of the paramagnetic effect (relaxivity c)

Paramagnetic Contrast Agents

The first publications on the value of paramagnetic contrast agents appeared in the early 1980s [92, 54, 23, 119]. Some of these agents are listed in Table 1.4.

Brasch and Runge [23, 119] described the criteria for an "ideal" contast enhancer. The agent should be nontoxic and highly effective, with its effect confined to specific areas for selective tissue targeting. It should also have good water solubility, should not harm the body in any way, and should be rapidly excreted.

A major goal has been to find the most effective paramagnetic element and improve its tolerance by binding it to other molecules. A comparison of the relaxation-shortening properties of different elements shows that the manganese and gadolinium ions have the greatest potency (Fig. 1.32). Of all the elements, the gadolinium ion has the strongest effect on T1 relaxation times by virtue of its seven unparied electrons. Gadolinium is an element of the lanthanide series. (The term "rare earths," also applied to these elements, is somewhat misleading in that the concentration of lanthanides in the earth's crust is some 100 times higher than that of iodine.)

Tolerance

The body has a very low tolerance to metal ions, but these can be detoxified by administering them in suitable compounds. Compounds from the class of ethylenediaminetetraacetic acid (EDTA) derivatives show the most favorable chelating properties.

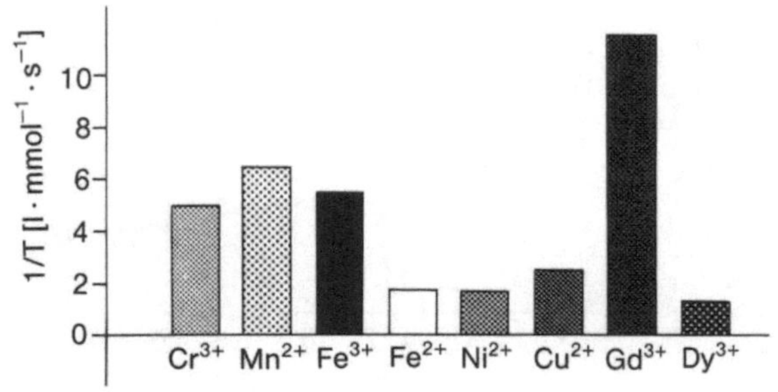

Fig. 1.32. Relaxivity of paramagnetic chlorides of different elements

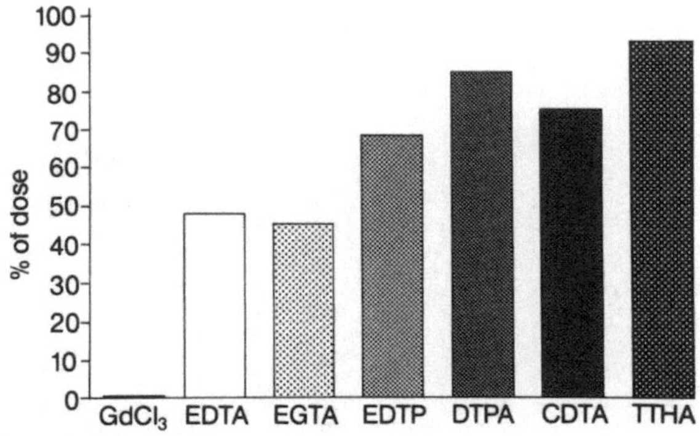

Fig. 1.33. Renal excretion in percentage of the administered dose (0.1 mmol/kg) within the first 3 h after i.v. injection of gadolinium chelates in rats. *EDTA* = ethylenediaminetetraacetic acid; *EGTA* = ethylglycolaminotetraacetic acid; *EDTP* = ethylenediaminetetraphosphone acid; *DTPA* = diethylenetriaminepentaacetic acid; *CDTA* = cyclohexandiaminetetraacetic acid; *TTHA* = triethylenetetraaminehexaacetic acid

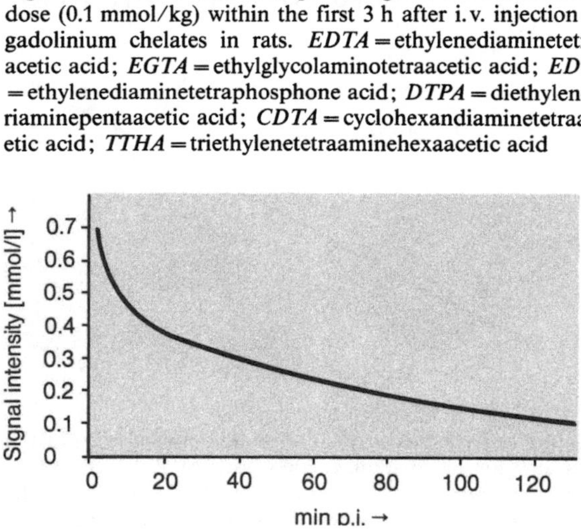

Fig. 1.34. Time course of gadolinium-DTPA plasma level after i.v. administration (0.1 mmol/kg body weight)

Chelation of the metal ions greatly improves their pharmacologic and toxicologic properties [23, 139]. In the form of their sodium or meglumine salts, the metallic chelates are water-soluble in the neutral range. Chelation provides for rapid renal excretion following i.v. injection and eliminates the undesired toxic effects of the free metal ions (Fig. 1.33).

Experiments in animals have shown that toxic effects occur only at very high doses. In subacute tests in which the substance was administered to rats and dogs by i.v. injection in daily doses up to 5 mmol/kg, the major adverse effect was an acute, diffuse tubular nephrosis. In another study this diffuse tubular nephrosis was found to be reversible. This is not surprising, since compounds with similar physicochemical properties (X-ray contrast media, inulin, mannitol, etc.) produce the same effect. So far no toxicity tests have demonstrated the intolerance phenomena typically associated with metal ions.

Remarkably good neurologic tolerance has been seen following intracisternal injection in rats. For reasons yet unknown, this tolerance is significantly greater than that to known ionic X-ray contrast media.

Pharmacology

The gadolinium ions forms an extremely stable complex with the DTPA ligand (stability constant of 10^{22}). The complex is highly stable under physiologic conditions, and this is reflected in the tolerance studies cited above. The ions occurring in plasma do not displace the gadolinium atom from its complex. Chelation has a negligible impact on the paramagnetic effect of the gadolinium ion. Measurements have shown T1 and T2 relaxivity values of 4 $lmmol^{-1}s^{-1}$ at 20 MHz. As the relaxivity does not show significant frequency dependence, it may be assumed that gadolinium-DTPA can be successfully used as a contrast agent at low as well as high field strengths.

Inert, strongly hydrophilic substances such as gadolinium-DTPA/dimeglumine cannot permeate intact plasma membranes and cannot cross the blood-brain barrier. Indeed, no appreciable increase of signal intensity is seen in T1-weighted sequences after the i.v. injection of gadolinium-DTPA/dimeglumine. If the blood-brain barrier is disrupted, the contrast agent can diffuse through it and enter the brain tissue.

In contrast to the free, nonchelated gadolinium ion, gadolinium-DTPA given intravenously is excreted from the body within a few hours in the administered form. Its pharmacokinetic behavior is essentially the same as that of known urographic and angiographic media: Following a rapid intravascular distribution and diffusion into the extracellular space, the compound is excreted via the kidneys. Extrarenal excretion is minimal. The rate of excretion is determined by the glomerular filtration rate. The half-life of gadolinium-DTPA in the human body is approximately 90 min [140]. More than 90% of the administered dose is excreted in the urine within 24 h after i.v. injection. Figure 1.34 shows the time course of the plasma concentration of gadolinium-DTPA following the i.v. injection of 0.1 mmol/kg in man. The concentration immediately after injection is slightly less than 1 mmol/l plasma and falls rapidly to lower levels through interstitial dispersion. Values of about 0.5 mmol/l are reached at 10 min. The fall of plasma levels after that point depends on the rate of renal excretion. Pharmacokinetic studies in man have shown that the half-life and the distribution pattern are independent of the administered dose. The plasma and interstitial concentrations in the first hour after injection are sufficient to exert a significant effect on MR relaxation times.

The first clinical trials of gadolinium-DTPA in humans were performed in late 1983 [124] and were paralleled by initial studies in patients with brain tumors [29, 32]. Since then the agent has been tested clinically in more than 1500 patients in Europe, Japan, and the United States. Studies using doses up to 0.2 mmol/kg have confirmed good tolerance of the paramagnetic contrast agent. To date there have been no reports of severe side effects such as nausea, circulatory changes, or even allergic reactions.

In March, 1988, the West German health authorities (BGA) were the first to approve Gd-DTPA/dimeglumine as a contrast agent for magnetic resonance imaging under the trade name Magnevist. The United States of America, Japan, and other European Countries followed.

New types of organ-specific contrast agents may yield additional diagnostic information. Superparamagnetic compounds (e.g., magnetites) are extremely effective in shortening T2. The i.v. injection of even very small amounts of these iron-containing compounds produces selective extinction of signals from the liver and spleen parenchyma [121]. Lesions show no change in signal intensity, for the compounds become concentrated only in organs that contain cells of the reticuloendothelial system. This type of compound does not appear well suited for the contrast enhancement of other organs like the heart or brain. However, it may be used as an perfusion agent.

Paramagnetic compounds add new information to the MR image. One day it may be possible not only to enhance contrast and highlight specific structures but also, by the use of new compounds, to demonstrate physiologic processes that are not presently accessible to any other modality.

1.3.4 Flow Phenomena

W. J. Huk

The time dependence of MR image sequences results in marked contrast between flowing blood and stationary tissue. This provides opportunities for demonstrating blood flow without the use of contrast media: MR angiography (see Sect. 1.4.2).

Here we shall give particular attention to the practical aspects of these phenomena for diagnostic imaging as we understand them in the light of current technology and prior clinical experience (see also Sect. 5.3).

The velocity of blood flow ranges from 5 to 20 cm/s in arteries and from 1 to 3 cm/s in veins [137]. The physical MR properties of resting blood at 0.5 T are as follows [116]:

T1 = 1150 ms ± 150 ms
T2 = 130 ms ± 10ms
Spin density N(H) = ca. 0.7 that of water

Flowing blood can give either a very low signal on MR images ("flow void") or a high signal through the phenomenon of "paradoxical enhancement" [35]. Factors that influence the signal intensity of moving protons are:

- The velocity, direction, and nature of the flow
- The repetition time TR
- The echo time TE
- The slice thickness
- The position of the slice relative to the flow direction
- The imaging technique

To aid our understanding of the MR signals obtained from moving fluids, it is helpful to distinguish between two theoretical directions of flow: flow perpendicular to the image plane, and flow parallel to the image plane. In reality, of course, the course of the blood vessel is subject to any number of variations. The considerations that follow apply to conventional SE sequences.

The *flow perpendicular to the image plane* (Fig. 1.35), an increased signal is observed in the range of low flow velocities for a short TR (curve a in Fig. 1.35). Higher flow velocities lead to an almost linear fall of signal intensity, until the vessels appear dark (empty) when the "cutoff" velocity is

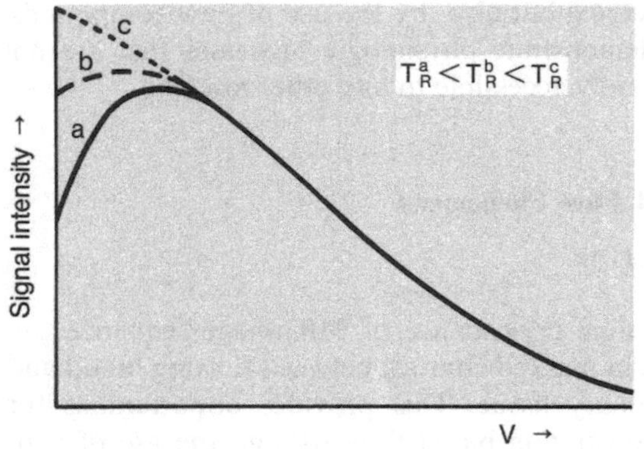

Fig. 1.35. Flow perpendicular to the image plane for the SE technique: MR signal intensity of fluid as a function of flow for three different repetition times TR (curves *a–c*). [After 116]

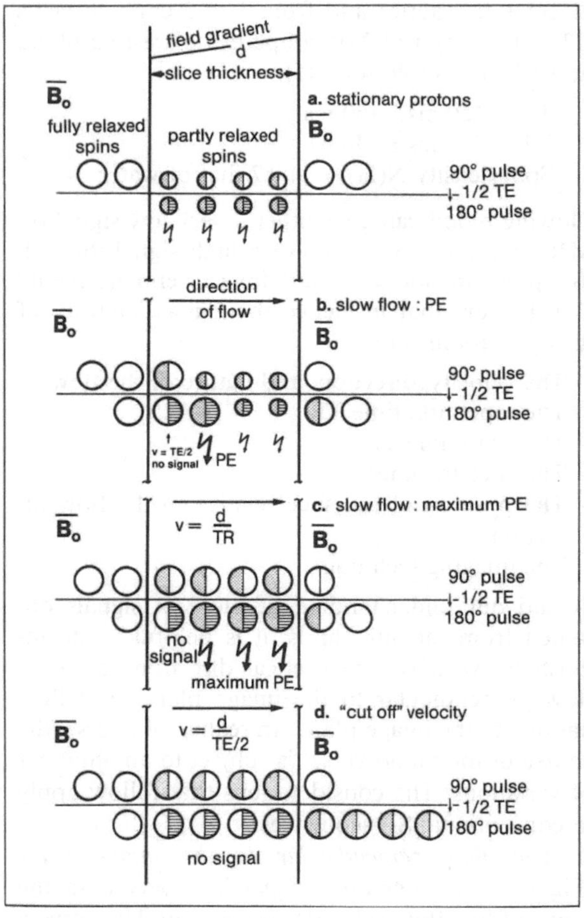

Fig. 1.36 a–d. Flow perpendicular to the image plane in SE sequences. Diagram of tagged spins in the slice. **a** For stationary protons; **b, c** for slow flow; **d** for the "cutoff" velocity. *PE* = paradoxical enhancement. [After 116]

reached. The motion-related signal increase above the value of stationary spins is called "paradoxical enhancement". It occurs when fully relaxed spins are washed into the slice during the pulse sequence, replacing the partially relaxed spins (Fig. 1.36 b, c). Thus, slow flow appears to shorten the T1 of the blood due to the presence of these fully relaxed spins. Paradoxical enhancement is most commonly seen in the bridging veins, the venous sinuses, and angiomatous masses (see also Sect. 2.8 and 5.3). As TR increases, the spins of the selected slice are able to relax completely so that no comparable signal enhancement is observed (Fig. 1.36 c, d). Flow velocity can be estimated when the repetition time TR is adjusted to maximal enhancement ($v = \frac{d}{TR}$) [72]. A "bull's-eye" pattern may be seen in venous vessels with laminar flow [21], as signals emanate from the slower peripheral flow, while flow at the center of the lumen exceeds the cutoff velocity and does not produce a signal (parabolic velocity profile). Pulsations of the blood (and the CSF) associated with cardiac and respiratory activity can disrupt the laminar flow pattern [52] and cause large artifacts to appear in adjacent tissues. These artifacts can be reduced or eliminated by ECG triggering, which ensures that the measurements are always made in the same phase of the cardiac cycle. With triggering in the diastolic phase, an increased signal is measured in the arteries, which usually have an inherently higher flow velocity.

With slow flow perpendicular to the image plane, the cutoff velocity decreases with increasing *echo time TE,* as increasing numbers of spins leave the section before the signal is received. This results in an apparent shortening of the T2 of the flowing blood and even occurs in multiecho sequences like the CPMG sequence (Fig. 1.37) (see also Sect. 1.3.2) [72].

Increasing the *slice thickness* leads to an increased signal, i.e., raises the cutoff velocity. Paradoxical enhancement also is observed at higher velocities (Fig. 1.38).

So far we have considered single-slice acquisition. With *multislice* imaging, paradoxical enhancement still occurs in the slice that the blood first enters [21, 96]. The downstream slices are increasingly populated by partially saturated spins, leading to a further decrease of signal intensity in each successive, parallel section (Fig. 1.39). This yields information on the direction and velocity of the flow and thus provides a means for the differentiation of arteries and veins. Correct image interpretation relies on knowing the relationship between the image sequence and the flow direction. The effect is used in special saturation pulse sequences which prepare the slices above and below the image slice in order to define the flow direction by differentiation of the low signal intensity of saturated spins from the high signal of nonsaturated spins [48]. This method is paricularly sensitive with gradient echo sequences (see below) [61, 106].

For *flow in the direction of the image plane,* we note a different dependence of signal intensity on flow velocity (Fig. 1.40). The signal is not influenced by the transport of the spins through the plane but by phase effects. Spins moving in the time between the excitation and the echo are effected by different gradient field strengths so that an additional phase angle is accumulated. Assuming a parabolic velocity profile inside the vessel, the signal of a voxel is decreased because of volume averaging; in the case of pulsating flow, phase artifacts in phase encoding direction occur. These artifacts can be diminished effectively by using ECG gating (see also Sect. 1.3.5). Pulsative flow creates the appearance of an "empty" vessel at velocities of only a few mm/s [7]. The visual effect is that the large cervical vessels, the carotid artery and jugular vein, appear dark on coronal and sagittal SE images (first echo) regardless of the blood flow. The spins dephase so completely during the relatively long TE of approximately 30 ms that a signal can no longer be acquired. This is true for all values of TR. As a result, stationary lesions in the vessel wall or lumen (thrombi, tumors, atheromatous plaques) contrast strongly with the blood flowing in the plane of the image slice. There is a potential for error, however, due to partial volume effects in smaller vessels and vessels with pulsatile flow.

For blood flow in the image plane, every even-numbered echo in a multiecho sequence gives a stronger signal than the odd-numbered echo that precedes it (Fig. 1.41). The explanation for this phenomenon, known as "even-echo rephasing," lies in the phase shift of the spins that are flowing along the phase gradient. As we saw in Sect. 1.1, the precessional frequence and thus the phase of the precession is linked to the field strength. Any change of position in the field gradient also produces a change of phase, and these disturbances prevent the formation of an MR signal during the first echo interrogation. It can be shown that the linearity of the field gradients leads to a refocusing exactly on the second (symmetrical echo [135].

Finally, the *type of pulse sequence* (SE, IR, fast imaging) has a significant effect on the imaging of

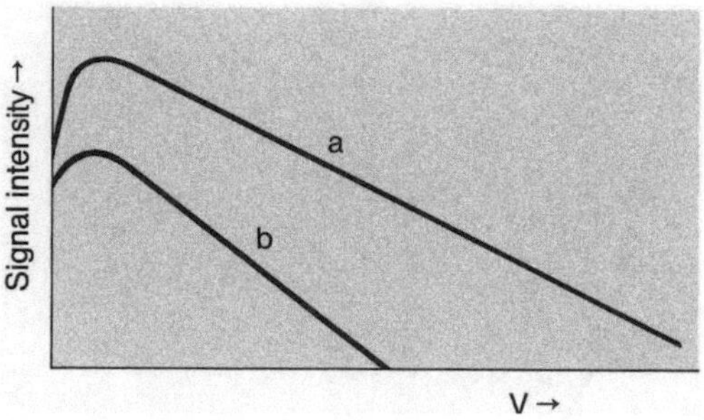

Fig. 1.37. Influence of echo time TE: calculated signal intensities as a function of flow velocity *(V)* for TE 35 ms (curve *a*) and 70 ms (curve *b*) in SE technique. [After 116]

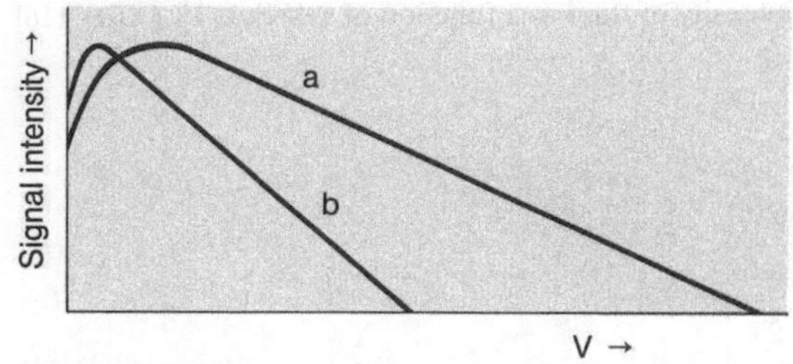

Fig. 1.38. Influence of slice thickness SL: calculated signal intensities as a function of flow velocity *(V)* for slice thickness of 6 mm (curve *a*) and 12 mm (curve *b*) in SE technique. [After 116]

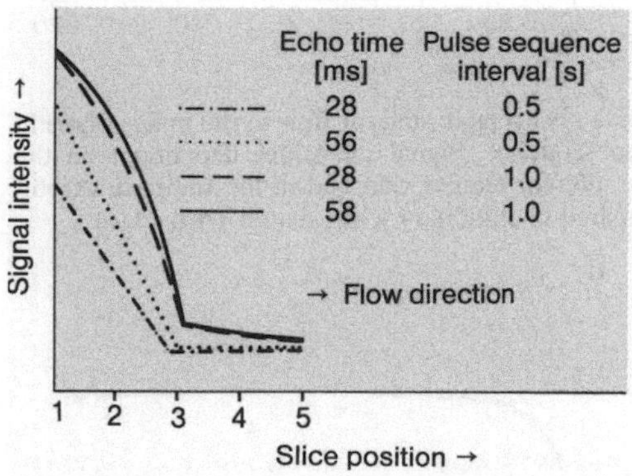

Fig. 1.39. Flow in a multislice sequence: signal intensities of perpendicularly flowing fluid in the parallel slices. [After 96]

flowing fluids. So far we have considered only the characteristics of the SE sequence.

In the *IR sequence,* blood flowing perpendicular to the image plane appears bright if it does not exceed the cutoff velocity. At higher flow velocities the signal becomes isointense with the background, and the vessel appears gray. Blood flowing in the image plane appears dark at a slow flow velocity and gray when the flow is rapid.

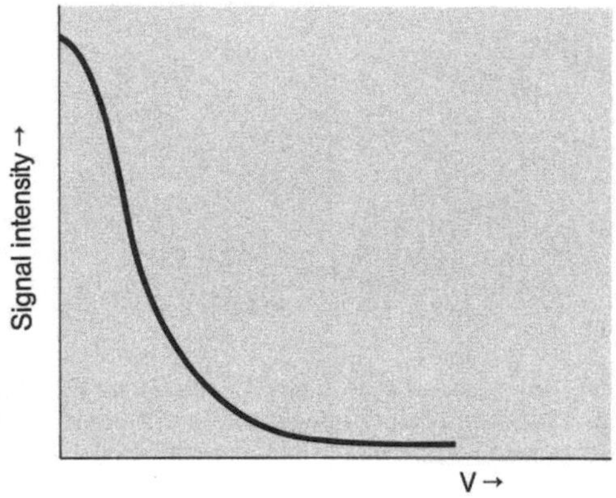

Fig. 1.40. Flow in the direction of the image plane: MR signal intensity of fluid as a function of velocity *(V)*. (After 116]

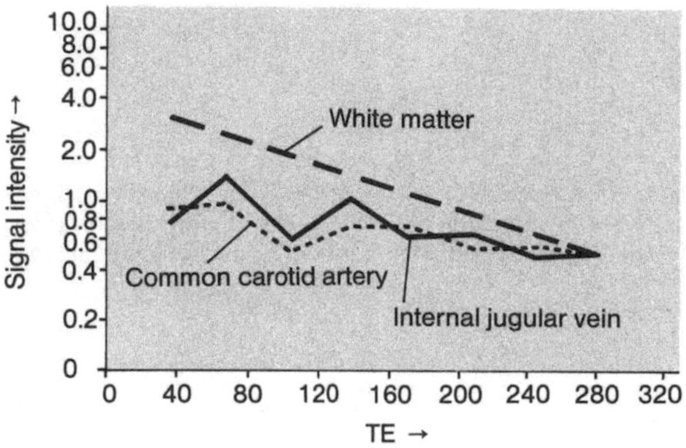

Fig. 1.41. Even-echo rephasing for flow in the image plane in a multiecho sequence. Signal intensities dependent on the echo in the internal jugular vein and in the common carotid artery compared to stationary white matter. [After 116]

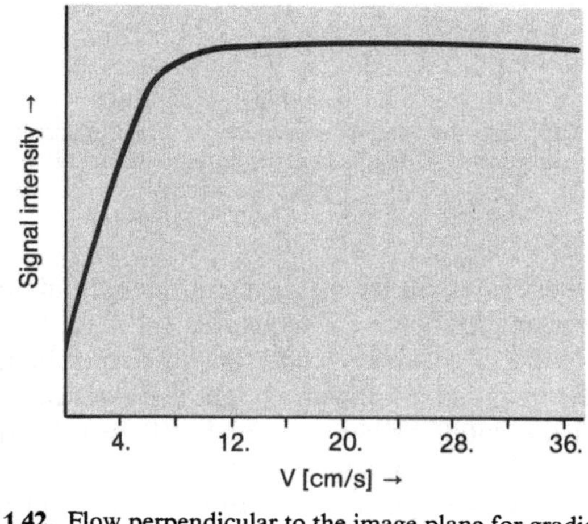

Fig. 1.42. Flow perpendicular to the image plane for gradient echo sequences. MR signal intensity of fluids as a function of velocity *(V)*: a cutoff velocity is not seen

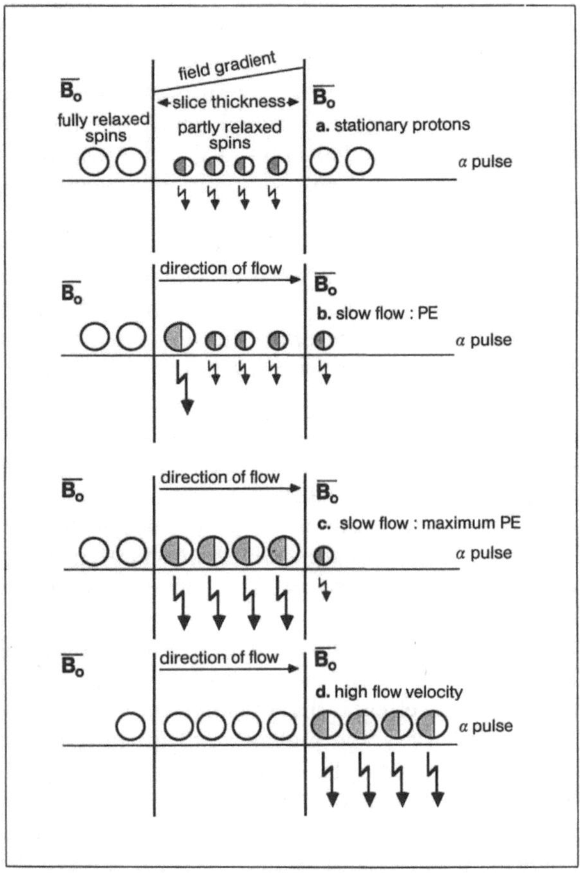

Fig. 1.43 a–d. Flow perpendicular to the image plane for gradient echo sequences. Diagram of tagged spins in the slice: all excited protons contribute to the signal, even if they have already left the section. **a** For stationary protons; **b, c** for slow flow; **d** for high flow velocity

The fast imaging sequences produce strong flow effects in the images, depending on the flip angle. With these sequences the rephasing of the spins is forced without the usual 180° pulse; therefore the signal of the bolus is not necessarily produced inside the image slice. It is also measured outside the slice provided that the spins are moving in the sensitive volume of the receiver coil. A cutoff velocity is not seen. The vessels give intense signals even with rapid flow (Fig. 1.42), because all excited protons contribute to the signal, even if they have already left the section (Fig. 1.43). With small pulse angles also stationary protons produce a higher signal so that the contrast to moving protons is lower. Flow on the image plane appears less dark than in the SE sequence, as dephasing of the spins is less pronounced due to the short echo times.

Flow and pulsations of the CSF represent a special case. The MR features of these phenomena have important clinical implications and are discussed in detail in Sect. 5.3.

1.3.5 Image Artifacts

W. SCHAJOR

As described in earlier sections of this chapter, the procedure of generating MR images involves steps to excite the spin system under investigation (normally the hydrogen atoms within the patient) and steps to receive the MR signal. In both, a variety of limitations of the system as well as patient-related phenomena can cause image artifacts.

The variety of image artifacts, their explanation and (if possible) guidelines to minimize their occurrence can be divided into three main categories:

1. Distortions of the magnetic and electromagnetic fields used in the MR imager
2. Distortions introduced by the receiver part of the MR imager
3. Artifacts introduced by the patient or by physical properties of the tissues or their components

An MRI artifact guide is given in Table 1.5.

Table 1.5. A guide to identification and avoidance of MR artifacts

Artifact	Image symptoms	Reasons	User action
Overfolding artifact (or aliasing artifact)			
Readout gradient direction	Image overfolding in read-out-direction	Field of view too small for anatomical area	Use extended matrix Increase field of view Use RF coil with smaller sensitive volume Use saturation pulses to suppress unwanted areas
Phase encoding gradient direction	Image overfolding in phase encoding direction	Field of view too small for anatomical area	Rotate gradients (if other direction has no aliasing) and use extended matrix Increase field of view Use RF coil with small sensitive volume Use saturation pulses to suppress unwanted areas
Edge definition artifacts			
Limited sampling (truncation artifact or Gibbs artifact)	Ringing of anatomical edges (repeated, fading out with the distance from the edge)	Limitations of Fourier transformation due to matrix acquisition	Use larger acquisition matrix or reduce field of view Use raw data filtering (e.g., Hanning filter)
Saturated gradient amplifier	Edge ringing artifacts similar to truncation artifacts, only in phase encoding direction	Bad raw data definition for high spatial frequences caused by saturated gradient amplifier	Check possibility of truncation artifacts (larger matrix) If persistent and severe, call service
Nonequidistant sampling raster	Edge ringing artifacts similar to truncation artifacts	Slice selection gradient or phase encoding gradient acts on readout interval Bad raw data definition for high spatial frequences	Check possibility of truncation artifacts (use larger acquisition matrix) If persistent and severe, call service (eddy current adjustment)
Nonequidistant sampling raster	Edge ringing artifacts similar to truncation artifacts Shading in readout direction	Readout gradient acts on read out interval Bad raw data definition for high spatial frequences	Check possibility of truncation artifacts (use larger acquisition matrix) Rotate gradients (artifact must react) If persistent and severe, call service (eddy current adjustment)
Chemical shift	Black rims between fat and water boundaries for gradient echo sequences, only in readout direction	Chemical shift causes in phase and opposed phase signal conditions in gradient echo sequences, depending on TE	Adapt TE to the desired signal behavior according to the field strength Rotate gradients in order to move artifacts to other anatomical areas

Table 1.5. (continued)

Artifact	Image symptoms	Reasons	User action
Zipper artifact (or central line artifact)			
Central zipper in phase encoding direction	Central zipperlike artifact in phase encoding direction	(Varying) transmitter leakage into the receiver channel	Call service
Central zipper in readout direction	Central zipperlike artifact in readout direction	Spurious FIDs due to imperfections of the 180° pulse Uncorrected ADC offset or ADC offset not constant	Use sequences with alternating RF pulses in order to move it to the image boundaries Call service
Zipper in readout direction, displaced to the boundaries of the image	Boundary zipper artifact in readout direction (displaced to the boundaries of the image)	Spurious FIDs due to imperfections of the 180° pulse	Usually not very severe (remainder of the previous artifact) If necessary use two acquisitions
Stripe Pattern			
Single digitization errors	Faint stripe pattern superimposed, orthogonal or incline	Single data point error in raw data matrix	Mostly a singular event: if frequent, call service
Singular failure of the phase encoding gradient	Severe stripe pattern superimposed, orthogonal or incline	Wrong raw data line due to a singular phase encoding gradient failure	Mostly a singular event: if frequent, call service
RF interference	Artifactual stripes in phase encoding direction, not related to anatomy	RF interference from environment picked up by the RF coil	Do not open RF shielding door during measurement Move cables additionally used from outside to inside the measurement cabin Check whether N_2 and He level measurement or patient table electronics are switched off during MR measurement
Stimulated echo ghost	Interference pattern in overlap zone		see "Ghost images"
Nonuniform signal			
ADC or preamplifier saturation	Inversion of signal intensity behavior in the image Bright background	Too high receiver gain causes an analog signal too large for the ADCs or for the preamplifier	Repeat receiver adjustment If not corrected, check coil parameters If not corrected, call application specialist or service
Tilted selected slice	Tilted slice orientation of the two RF pulses (spin-echo sequence) Signal shading in phase encoding direction, constant signal in readout direction	Phase encoding gradient acts on slice selection interval Turns slice orientation of the second selective RF pulse	Check with phantom and rotate gradients (artifact must react) Call service (eddy current adjustment)
Tilted selected slice	Tilted slice orientation of the two RF pulses (spin echo sequence) Signal shading in readout direction, constant signal in phase encoding direction	Readout gradient acts on slice selection interval Turns slice orientation of the second selective RF pulse	Check with phantom and rotate gradients (artifact must react) Call service (eddy current adjustment)
Receiver coil RF field non uniformity	Signal inhomogeneities in images	Inhomogeneous RF field of coil	Check coil with phantom Call service
RF penetration/skin effect	Diagonal shading in images	Skin effect (limited RF penetration into tissue); can be enhanced by improper RF pulse amplitudes	Use circular polarized RF resonators Repeat transmitter adjustment Use selective transmitter adjustment Check with application specialist Call service

Table 1.5. (continued)

Artifact	Image symptoms	Reasons	User action
Ghost images			
Off-slice MR signals	MR signals of another anatomical area superimposed (in slice selection direction) Ghost position depends on slice position Occurs for the 50-cm field of view and off-center slice positions	RF coil sensitive outside B_0 homogeneity volume Off-slice MR signal contributions from inhomogeneous magnetic field areas	Use coil with smaller sensitive volume, if possible Use thinner slices (increased selection gradient)
Improper slice selective RF pulse	Slice of another anatomical area superimposed (in slice selection direction)	Slice selection not unique due to imperfect single side band modulation of the RF pulse profile	Call service
Overfolding in slice selection direction	Slice of another anatomical area superimposed Occurs only in the first and last images of a 3D series	Object extends field of view in slice selection direction; overfolding occurs	3D acqusition: use larger 3D slice thickness
ADC bit defect	Faint edges visible as ghosts or severe but regular image distortions (contoured ghosts)	ADC loses digitized bits permanently	Check with phantom (exclusion of motion artifacts) Call service
One ADC failed	Same image with same intensity superimposed, mirrored around image center	One ADC fails permanently (single side band condition not fulfilled)	Check with asymmetrically positioned phantom Call service
Quadrature imbalance	Same image more or less faintly superimposed, mirrored around image center	Single side band condition for data acquisition not fulfilled due to imbalanced quadrature demodulator	Check with asymmetrically positioned phantom Call service
Inaccurate digitization of phase encoding gradient	Reproducible ghosting in phase encoding direction ("blurred images")	Bad raw data definition, caused by inaccurate DAC of phase encoding gradient	Check with phantom Call service
Motion artifacts (also magnetic field, shim gradient, or RF instabilities)	Nonperiodic ghosts ("blurred images")	Bad raw data definition caused by motion artifacts or magnetic field (magnet, shim or gradient) or RF instabilities	Use respiratory gating Use motion rephasing sequences Rotate gradients Increase number of acquisitions
Motion artifacts	Periodic ghosts (e.g., heart motion, blood flow, CSF flow)	Bad raw data definition caused by motion artifacts	Use ECG or pulse triggering Use motion rephasing sequences Rotate gradients Increase number of acquisitions
Ground loops in electrical circuits	Periodic or nonperiodic gosts (similar to motion artifacts)	Bad raw data definition caused by nonperiodic gradient or RF pulse distortions	Check with phantom Call service Increase number of acquisitions
Ferromagnetic materials	Strong motion artifacts involved with moving ferromagnetic material	E.g., patient with denture chewed during measurement	Remove ferromagnetic material, if possible
Incorrect signal alternation (or N/2-ghost)	Same image is more or less faintly superimposed, moved by half field of view in phase encoding direction	Incorrect RF pulse alternation or incorrect signal acquisition Occurs only with one acquisition	Check with asymmetrically positioned phantom Call service
Stimulated echo ghost	Ghost image superimposed, mirrored symmetrically around phase encoding direction, interference pattern in overlap zones of original and ghost images Can occur only in the second or higher echoes	Stimulated echos generated by slice selective RF pulses in multiple echo sequences	Use sequences with stimulated echo suppression (e.g., phase cycling techniques Use selective transmitter adjustment

Table 1.5. (continued)

Artifact	Image symptoms	Reasons	User action
Chemical shift	Fat and water images superimposed with spatial shift in readout direction	Chemical shift affects read out direction	Use normal bandwidth sequences Rotate gradients Use fat/water separation sequences
Spatial distortions			
B_0 inhomogeneity	Visible spatial distortions of anatomy	B_0 homogeneity out of specifications	Use normal bandwidth sequences Check with application specialist Call service
Chemical shift	Fat and water images belong to different slice positions	Chemical shift affects slice selection	Cant't be corrected
Gradient nonlinearity	Spatial disortions of anatomy	Gradient nonlinearity distorts spatial definition	Check with application specialist Call service
Eddy currents	Slice position and slice thickness incorrect	Slice selection gradient acts on slice selection interval	Check with phantom Call service (eddy current adjustment)
Incorrect gradient scaling	Elliptical distortion of circular structures	Gradient scaling is not adjusted	Check with phantom in all three orientations Call service
Local distortions			
Ferromagnetic materials	Local signal losses and signal increase beneath spatial distortions of anatomy	Local distortions of magnetic field homogeneity by ferromagnetic material in the body	Remove ferromagnetic material, if possible
Susceptibility	Local tissue signal losses above the sphenoidal sinus, or in the area of the intestines Occurs usually with gradient-echo or low bandwidth spin-echo sequences	Local distortions of the magnetic field at air/tissue boundaries, caused by the paramagnetic susceptibility of brain tissue	Use shorter TE Use spin-echo sequences Use thinner slices Use normal bandwidth sequences
Flow perpendicular to plane	Enhanced flow signal intensity in vessels perpendicular to the plane with slow flow velocities Reduced flow signal in vessels perpendicular to the plane with fast flow velocities	Unsaturated blood enters the selected slice during repetition Blood with prepared spins leaves the slice before echo readout	Can be reduced by longer TR ECG triggering, if needed Use sequences with presaturation techniques
In-plane flow ("flow artifacts")	Flow-induced signal loss in vessels with in-plane flow Signal disturbances caused by turbulent flow See also motion artifacts/periodic ghosts	Loss of the rephasing condition in the echo	If needed use flow/motion rephasing sequences for full flow signal and reduced flow artifacts
Noisy Images			
Application problems	Noisy images	Sequence parameters unsuitable	Discuss with application specialist
Spurious signal-to-noise ratio problems	Single events of low signal-to-noise ratio Overall signal losses Signal inhomogeneities in images Too high transmitter values	Adjustment incorrect RF tuning incorrect (may occur with extreme patient load due to weight or large metal implants)	Repeat adjustment Use selective transmitter adjustment Repeat tuning, check coil parameters Check with application specialist
Persistent signal-to-noise ratio problems	Sudden but persistent low signal-to-noise ratio in images	Various reasons in RF transmitter and receiver paths or gradient system possible	Is the problem coil specific or global? Check with phantom Check with application specialist Call service

Prepared by W. Hartl, Siemens Medical Engineering Group, Erlangen, FRG

Distortions of the Magnetic and Electromagnetic Fields

The homogeneity of the *static magnetic field* together with the linearity of the gradient field determines the amount of geometric distortions of the MR image. Geometric distortions can be measured with a specially designed phantom, which consists of a rectangular grid of plastic pins in a water-filled container (Fig. 1.44). The position of the pins in the MR image can be compared with the original pin positions in the phantom and give a description of the amount of geometric distortions [123]. Near the center of the magnet, distortions are less than the pixel size; at the border of the homogeneity volume the distortion can be up to several centimeters (Fig. 1.44a). For high-accuracy measurements, the distortions can be measured and the images can be corrected by software (Fig. 1.44b).

The stability of the static field with time is another important factor for image quality [80]. In cases where magnets with resistive coils are used, the stability of the magnet power supply is a very critical point in the design of an MR imager. With the state-of-the-art superconducting magnets, the stability is better than 0.1 ppm/h. This field drift is small enough to cause no problems during the imaging procedure. However, large magnetic objects such as vans or moving elevators can cause field variations and thus severe image distortions (Fig. 1.45).

Several image artifacts can be attributed to the nonideal behavior of the *linear field gradients* [10]. Most occur in cases where one of the three gradients does not work at all, either because of malfunction of the hardware (the gradient power supply) or due to the use of an inappropriate pulse sequence.

Measurements without the slice selection gradient result in a very thick slice (the actual thickness depending on the bandwidth of the exciting RF pulse) and thus in a signal overload and loss of spatial resolution in slice select direction (Fig. 1.46a). The two other gradients are used for the spatial resolution in the image plane. Their malfunction results in the coalescence of all signal components in a line perpendicular to the gradient axis (Fig. 1.46b). These images are in general unusable. The complete malfunction of one or more gradients results in very distinctive artifacts and can be detected easily.

The wrong gradient strength, again due either to the use of a nonsuitable sequence or to hardware

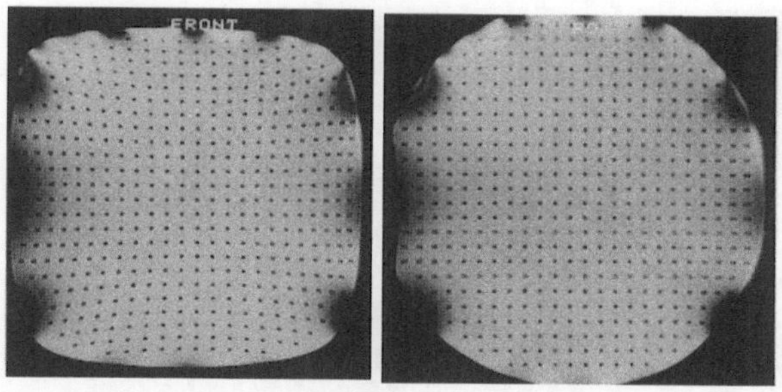

a, b

Fig. 1.44 a, b. Geometric distortion due to magnetic inhomogeneities of the static magnetic field: imaging of a rectangular pin grid phantom. **a** Image distortion at the border; **b** same image after software correction. [After 123]

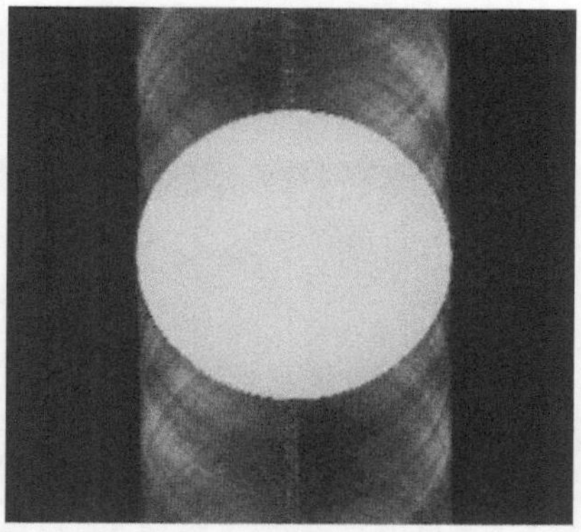

Fig. 1.45. Instabilities of the static field causing multiple ghost artifacts in phase encoding direction

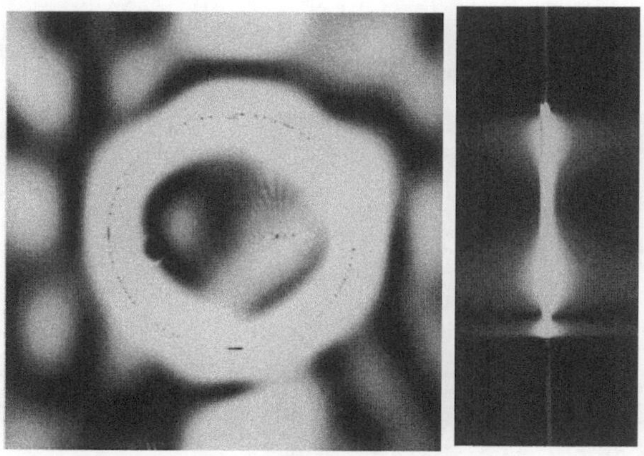

a, b

Fig. 1.46 a, b. Malfunction of magnetic field gradients. **a** No slice-selecting gradient, resulting in data overflow in the image. **b** No phase-encoding gradient, resulting in coalescence of signal to a single line

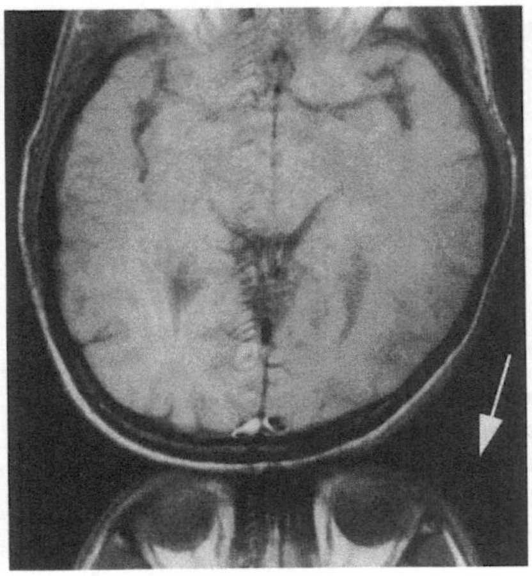

Fig. 1.47. Misadjustment of gradient strength: in-plane gradients too high (e.g., zoom) resulting in overfolding of image regions *(arrow)*

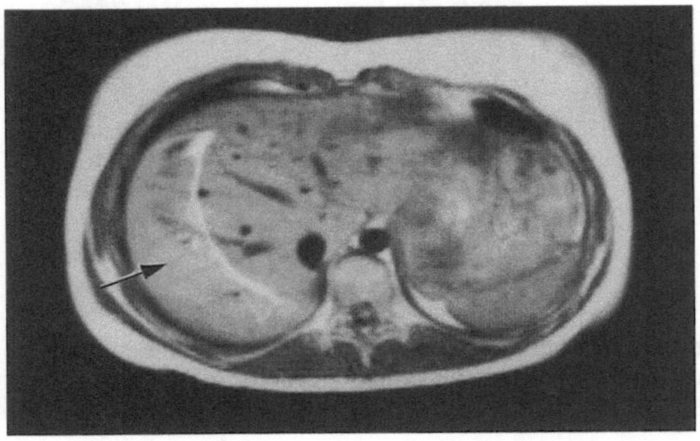

Fig. 1.48. Mis-selection artifacts: plane mis-selection results in additional signals from different planes of the object *(arrow)*

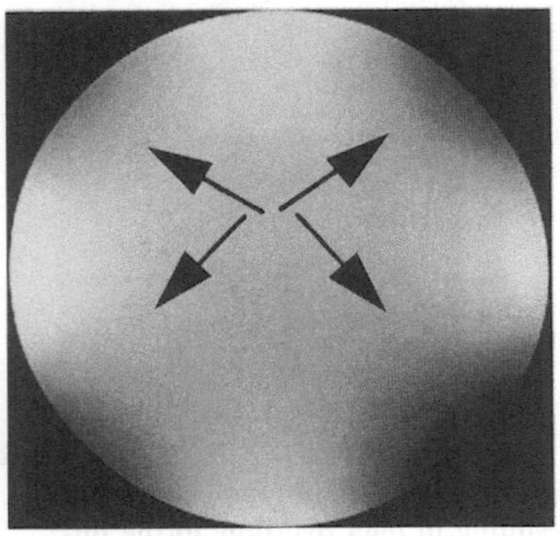

Fig. 1.49. Limited RF penetration: skin effect at high field strength in a phantom *(arrows)*

misadjustments, causes improper scaling of the respective gradient axis [112]. If the gradient strength is only slightly misadjusted, the MR images are compressed or expanded in the direction of the gradient. If the gradients are much too large, an overfolding of parts of the object which are normally outside the FOV into the image will occur. Images may still be useful as long as the interesting regions are not affected by the overfolding (Fig. 1.47).

The decrease of the static field outside the specified homogeneous volume can give rise to a mis-selection artifact (Fig. 1.48). This can be explained as follows: A rapid decay of the static field plus the linear increasing slice selection gradient will generate two surfaces of identical field strength, one at the desired position of the image plane, the second outside the imaging volume. If the RF system also excites the second, unwanted surface, these signals will be added to the plane of interest. To prevent this type of artifact, higher slice selection gradients must be used or a special sequence with different gradient signs for the 90° and 180° pulse can be applied.

The RF pulses are used to rotate the nuclear spins. The actual tip angle depends linearly on the *RF field* strength at the location of the spin. The exact determination of the pulse angles and equal pulse angles throughout the imaging volume are essential for good images.

If the distribution of pulse angles over the imaging region is not homogeneous, the intensity of the image will vary according to the pulse angles. With standard body and head coils, this can be avoided by a proper design of the coils. Surface coils, however, show a strong intensity profile along the coil axis (see Fig. 1.11).

The penetration of the RF fields into the objects to be imaged is limited. This is usually called the skin effect. In phantom studies the skin effect can be demonstrated most effectively at high frequencies (Fig. 1.49). In human imaging at fields up to 2 T, the skin effect can hardly be seen and is usually not a source of artifacts.

In a multislice sequence, several slices are examined in a single measurement. One slice is excited during the recovery time of all other slices. The RF pulses to excite the different slices usually do not have the desired ideal rectangular excitation profile. If the gap between adjacent slices is such that the excitation of one slice also affects the recovery of one or both neighboring slices, the signal of these slices is partially saturated. This "crosstalk" between slices reduces signal intensities compared to a single slice measurement. For quantitative measurements such as T1 and T2 tissue values, this may lead to incorrect results (see Sect. 1.4).

The partial volume effect is also due to the nonideal excitation profiles; signals of neighboring slices are added to the desired slice. However, this is not critical if the same tissue continues from one slice to the next.

The problems arising from the nonideal RF pulses can be minimized by choosing larger slice gaps, employing an "interleaved" measurement scheme (measuring slices 1-3-5 ... then 2-4-6 ..., instead of the 1-2-3-4-5-6 ... sequence), or by the design of optimized pulse profiles.

The RF pulses are usually modulated to get the proper shape of the pulse envelopes and to determine the phases of the different pulses. Many imaging systems use RF pulses with phases alternating from scan to scan. If the modulation process is different for positive and negative amplitudes, e.g., because of a mis-setting of the modulator unit, the resulting MR signal will vary from scan to scan in a systematic manner. This means a modulation of the data in phase encoding direction, and after the Fourier transform the object will reappear at a position shifted in the phase encoding direction by half the number of lines in the image. This is therefore called the $n/2$ artifact (Fig. 1.50). Proper adjustment of the modulator hardware or even numbers of acquisitions for averaging will suppress this kind of artifact.

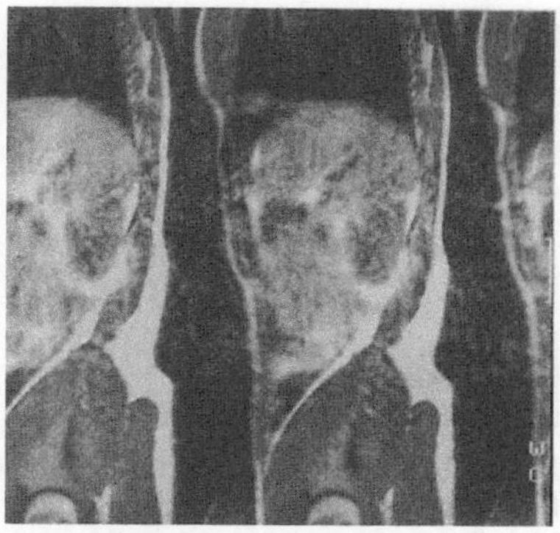

Fig. 1.50. Distortion of the RF field. The $n/2$ artifact: second appearance of the object at a distance of half the matrix size

Distortions of the RF Receiver Path

The *RF receiver path* amplifies and demodulates the RF signal coming from the excited spins. The demodulation process is normally done by a quadrature phase detector and results in two different output signals, the real and the imaginary. This is necessary to differentiate between positive and negative frequencies in the signal.

If the demodulator is unbalanced, e.g., if one channel has a different gain than the other, the ability of the system to differentiate between positive and negative frequencies is decreased or totally removed. This results in a ghost image, which is mirrored at the center of the image (Fig. 1.51 a). When the demodulated signals are converted to digital data, the offset of the AD converters must be measured and subtracted from the data. If the converter offset varies during the measurement or if the offset was measured incorrectly, a constant offset is added

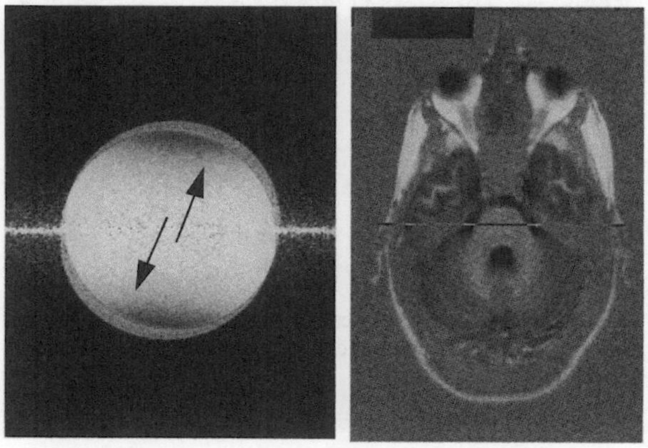

a, b

Fig. 1.51 a, b. Misadjustment of the receiver RF path. **a** Misfunction of one analog-digital converter channel (ADV) causes a mirrored image *(arrows)*. **b** Offset of the ADC results in an offset line at the center or the bottom of the image

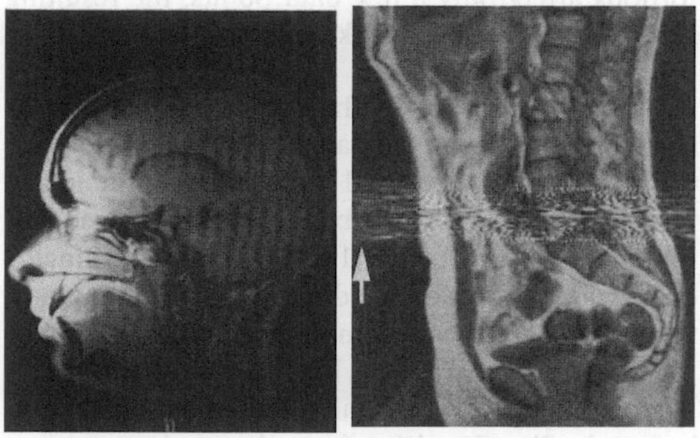

a, b

Fig. 1.52. a Sporadic distortion of the receiver signal causes a wavelike pattern in the image. **b** Continuing distortions of the receiver signal (e.g., from commercial radio stations) cause artifacts in phase encoding direction *(arrow)*

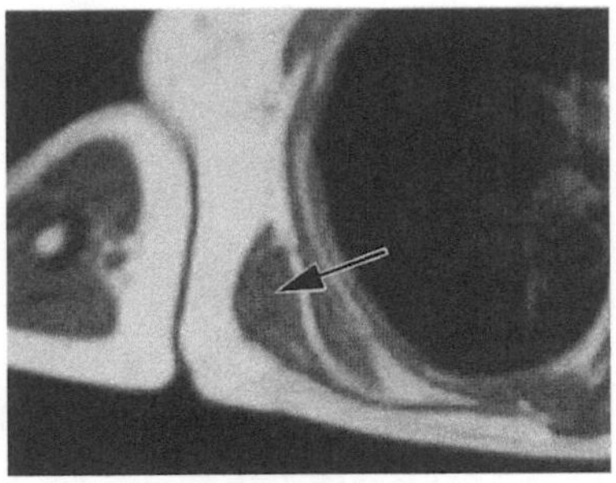

Fig. 1.53. Truncation artifact (Gibbs phenomenon) arising at high-contrast interfaces *(arrow)*. This artifact is caused by high-frequency components in the image

a, b

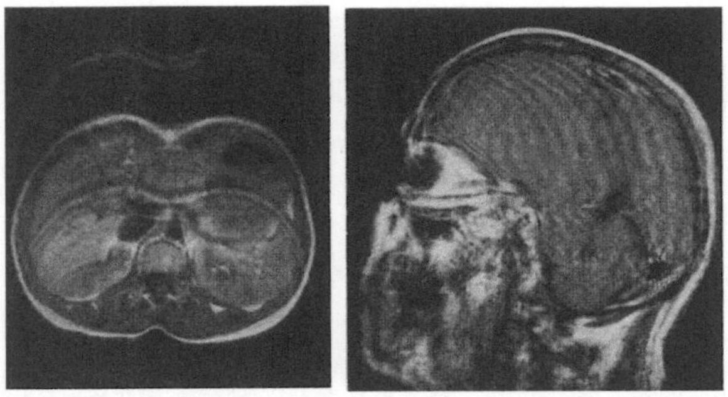

Fig. 1.54 a, b. Motion artifacts. **a** Breathing and **b** head motion during data acquisition cause "ghosting" in phase encoding direction

to the raw data. After the image reconstruction this will result in a bright point at the center of the image or a dashed line through the center (Fig. 1.51 b).

Sometimes sporadic spikes in receiver signal occur, induced by external noise sources. If these distortions affect only a few data points, the resulting image displays a wavelike pattern, as shown in Fig. 1.52 a.

If the distortions of the receiver signal appear continuously during the data acquisition period, for example from commercial radio stations, the image will show small stripes or bands in the phase encoding direction (Fig. 1.52 b) [10]. This kind of artifact is often related to bad shielding or grounding conditions of the electronic components.

The amount of time which can be spent in collecting a spin echo is usually limited to several milliseconds. Signals arising from sharp edges or steps with strong changes in the image intensity which have not yet decayed at the end of the sampling interval are thus truncated. Neglecting these signals leads to edge oscillations or ringing in the readout and phase encoding direction, called "truncation artifacts" (Fig. 1.53) The truncation artifact can be overcome by choosing a larger matrix (e.g., 512 × 512 instead of 256 × 256) or by the application of a filter function to the raw data. Filtering the raw data reduces the effects of the sharp truncation but reduces spatial resolution at the same time.

Patient-related Artifacts

The patient himself can be the cause of a variety of image artifacts. Due to the relatively long imaging times, patient motion is the most frequently encountered artifact.

Anatomical motion such as repositioning during the measurment or movements of the extremities, the head, the eyes, etc. can result in slightly distorted or totally unusable images. Certain movements, such as swallowing, coughing, breathing, the heartbeat, and peristaltic movement, however, cannot be completely controlled by the patient.

Motion not only produces a loss of resolution, but also induces phase changes, to which the 2 DFT image reconstruction (Sect. 1.2.5) is extremely sensitive. These phase changes lead to multiple ghost images in the phase encoding direction which overlap with the image, degrade contrast, and can affect quantitative measurements (Figs. 1.54, 2.45 b) [10, 112, 142].

There are several ways to lessen or eliminate motion artifacts. In general, signal averaging and smaller dimensions of the acquisition matrix reduce this kind of artifact. Since motion artifacts mostly represent low frequencies, nonuniform averaging instead of conventional averaging can be employed. In this technique, scans near the center of the hologram (raw data) (Sect. 1.2) are averaged more often than scans at the edges. With acceptable prolongation of scan time, this method can give satisfactory suppression of motion artifacts [53]. Another possibility involves modifications of the gradient waveforms. More complete refocusing of the transverse magnetization in the imaging plane is accomplished in order to zero the within-view random phase terms [109].

For motion artifacts appearing in the phase direction of the image, the interchange of the phase encoding and the readout gradient will rotate the artifacts by 90°. This method cannot eliminate these artifacts, but may still be useful in removing them from the region of interest.

The use of surface coils often removes motion artifacts because the limited sensitive volume of the coil can be restricted to nonmoving parts of the patient. An example is imaging of the thoracic spinal cord, which is less affected by cardiac and respiratory motion when a surface coil is used. Another technique uses selective RF pulses to saturate moving spins which are outside the imaging volume [53]. Special triggering and gating methods are able to remove artifacts from cardiac and respiratory motion. Cardiac triggering is a commonly applied method for studies of the heart. Gating the measurement with the respiratory cycle extends scan time by a factor of 2–4, but improves image quality significantly. More sophisticated methods like ROPE (respiratory ordered phase encoding) use a respiratory signal to determine in which order the rows of the data matrix are measured. The aim is to make the respiratory signal a slowly varying function of the time integral of the phase encoding gradient [8].

Beside several effects which are described in detail in Sect. 1.3.4, blood flow causes a special kind of motion artifact. Flow artifacts appear as a noisy band in the phase encoding direction crossing the blood vessel. This is often seen in coronal and axial slices of the brainstem and sellar region because of the basal arteries and veins as well as by the flowing and pulsating CSF (Figs. 1.55, 1.67). Special sequences with bipolar gradients are now available which at least partially compensate for flow effects.

A well-known artifact which occurs independently of static field homogeneity is the "fat-water" artifact [40]. The resonance frequencies of protons bound to water and protons bound to fatty tissue differ by approximately 3.5 ppm (the chemical shift; see Sects. 1.1.9, 1.4.4). In one spatial direction the MR signals are frequency encoded, i.e., their position is mapped to the image via the frequency emitted during the data acquisition. The system cannot tell the difference between frequency changes caused by chemical shift and those caused by different position of the protons. This means that signals coming from fat protons are shifted away from those from water protons, even though they occupy physically the same location in the body. Image interpretation can be affected in the presence of chemical shift artifacts [41] (Fig. 1.56). For example, the chemical shift at the border of the eyeball and the retro-orbital fatty tissue simulates a thickening of the sclera (Fig. 1.56a), or a straight signal void appears alone margin of a vertebral body and a disk (Fig. 156b). Chemical shift is more

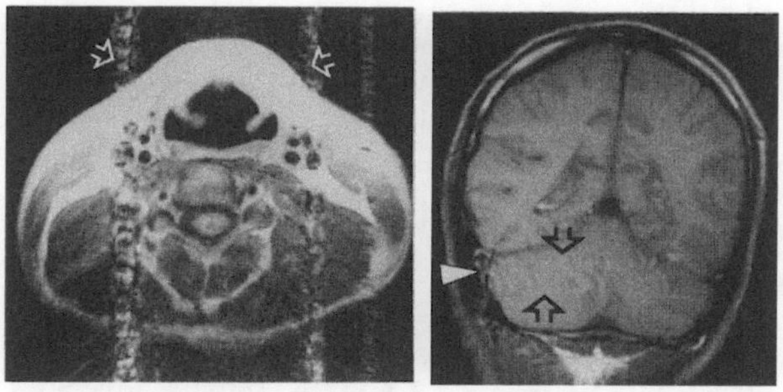

a, b

Fig. 1.55 a, b. Flow artifacts at the position of blood vessels extending in phase encoding direction *(open arrows);* **a** at the cervical vessels in an axial MR image; **b** at the venous sinus in a frontal MR image *(arrow head)*

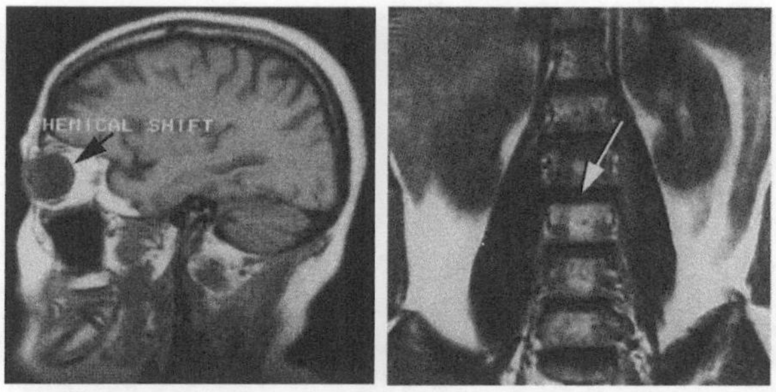

a, b

Fig. 1.56 a, b. Chemical shift artifacts. Doubling of contours in one direction (readout): **a** at the junction of the eye and the retroorbital fat; **b** at one end of each vertebral body *(arrow)*

pronounced with high static magnetic field. Higher gradients are required to keep the chemical shift within one pixel width. Alternatively, specially designed sequences [40, 46] are able to separate the signals form fat and water (see Sect. 1.4).

Metal objects inside the patient or on the surface of the patient's body have to be taken in account for two reasons: the potential hazard for the patient (see discussion of safety considerations in Chap. 3) and the image artifacts [102].

Metal implants include dental hardware, joint prostheses, surgical clips, wires, etc., ventricular shunt material and even microscopic filings from surgical instruments, for example in boreholes of the skull. The last can be completely occult in radiographic images. Metal objects produce local image distortions by local inhomogeneities of the B_0 field. The typical image artifact consists of a round zone of signal void bordered by a hyperintensive rim (Fig. 1.57). It looks as though all signals of the hole are pushed to the periphery. The size of the ar-

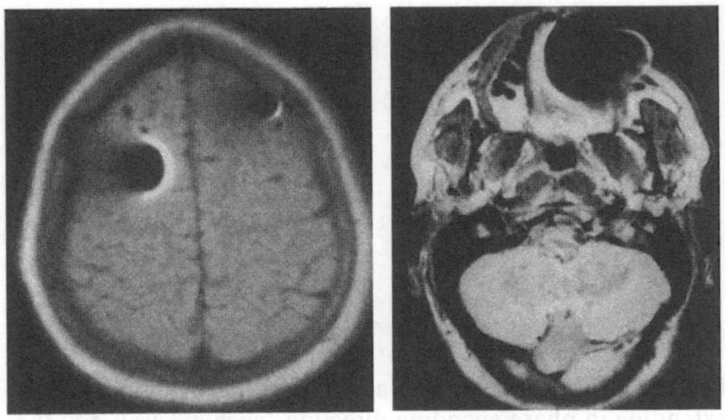

a, b

Fig. 1.57 a, b. Local image distortion by metal implants. **a** Ferromagnetic shunt material causes typical holes with high intensive walls. **b** Dental implants also made of nonferromagnetic metal produce similar artifacts by local eddy currents

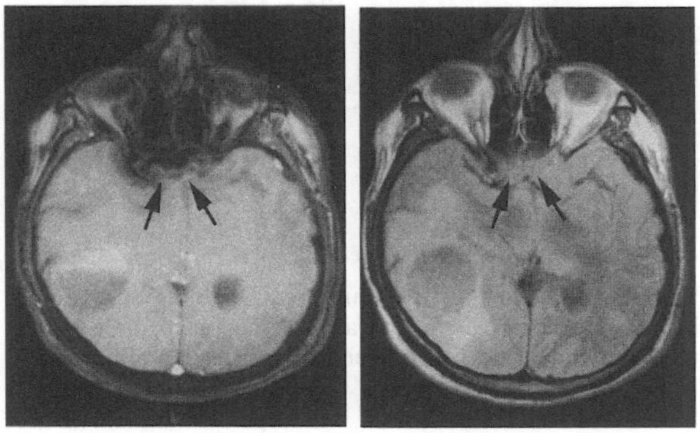

a, b

Fig. 1.58 a, b. Susceptibility artifacts in the head. **a** Axial slice with very short TR of 30 ms. Areas between the eyes appear with reduced intensity *(arrows)*. **b** Axial slice with TR of 3 s shows normal intensity in these areas *(arrows)*

tifact depends on the size of the object and the degree of its ferromagnetism. When the artifact is not located inside the image section it may be more discreet, leading to misinterpretation. Checking neighboring slices for artifacts is an important precaution in image interpretation. Also, metals in which no ferromagnetic properties can be measured cause similar, but less distinct effects in images. The rapid changes of the gradient field induce local eddy currents inside the conductor which in turn produce local field distortions.

All objects to be imaged become magnetized to a greater or lesser degree, in the static magnetic field if they are dia- or paramagnetic. Their magnetic susceptibility is a measure of the magnetic field inside the object. A positive susceptibility means a increase of the field, a negative one a decrease of the field. This leads to magnetic inhomogeneities in the object [81, 43]. For example, cavities in the human body manifest themselves as enhanced boundaries or bright spots. Imaging sequences using gradient echos (see Table 1.6) are very sensitive to field variations and to this kind of artifact (Fig. 1.58).

1.4 New Approaches in Clinical MR

The ability of MR tomography to differentiate among soft tissues with high sensitivity has gained MR imaging a solid position among the modalities used in neuroradiology. It is a unique feature of MR that image contrast between tissues can be optimized in various ways by the proper selection of pulse sequences to emphasize one of the three tissue parameters T1, T2, or proton density N(H) in the image. SE pulse sequences, particularly using saturation recovery, are routinely applied in diagnostic MR imaging (see Sect. 1.3.2).

MR offers many additional features, however, which are not yet used routinely, but which are being investigated for their potential to expand the present applications (Table 1.6). Fast imaging techniques, beyond their potential to reduce the total examination time, can be employed to evaluate dynamic functions. Imaging of the vessels, the representation of flow in the image, and the quantitative measurement of flow velocities are expected to complement existing angiographic procedures. The calculation of T1, T2, and N(H) parameter images can be considered a first step toward tissue characterization. Finally the analysis of metabolic functions may become feasible through MR spectroscopy.

Table 1.6. New topics in clinical MR

Fast imaging
MR angiography
Flow velocity
T1, T2, N(H) images
Synthetic images
Tissue characterization
Spectroscopy
Spectroscopic imaging
Sodium imaging

1.4.1 Fast Imaging

M. Deimling and R. Haerten

Many different approaches to speed up the process of data acquisition in MR have been reported in the literature (see Table 1.7). The rationale for the development of fast imaging techniques is twofold: The first aspect is the reduction of examination time in routine two-dimensional as well as three-dimensional diagnostic applications. The second is the visualization of rapid movement or change, such as blood flow in vessels, cardiac motion, and the uptake and washout of contrast material (Fig. 1.59). Half Fourier imaging (HFI) [87] and rapid acquisition with relaxation enhancement (RARE) [64] are techniques developed to address the economic aspect of routine imaging. For dynamic imaging, methods such as stimulated echo acquisition mode (STEAM) [47], echo planar imaging (EPI) [86], and fast gradient echo (GE) pulse sequences [61, 106] are being investigated.

Fast Imaging with Gradient Echo Techniques

In saturation recovery, the transverse magnetization needed to generate an echo signal can be recovered only if the interval TR between the SE pulses is long enough to allow for sufficient T1 relaxation. If TR is too short (e.g., <100 ms), the signal-to-noise ratio will be poor, and contrast between tissues will be lost. SE images with TR 100 ms, acquired in only 13 s with a matrix size of 128×128, are routinely used as quick or survey scans. They are not, however, suitable for diagnostic purposes.

GE pulse sequences have been developed to combine short TR (<100 ms) with good image contrast and high signal-to-noise ratio. For example, using TR 30 ms, a 128×128 matrix, and single-section acquisition, an image can be acquired in only 4 s per slice. An equilibrium between longitudinal and transverse magnetization is reached by applying a rapid sequence of RF pulses with a flip angle less than 90° (low angle). While the transverse component of the magnetization is used to generate an echo signal, a portion of the remaining longitudinal magnetization is used by the next pulse to restore the original transverse magnetization. In the equilibrium state, this portion is continuoulsy replaced because of relaxation. In contrast to conventional

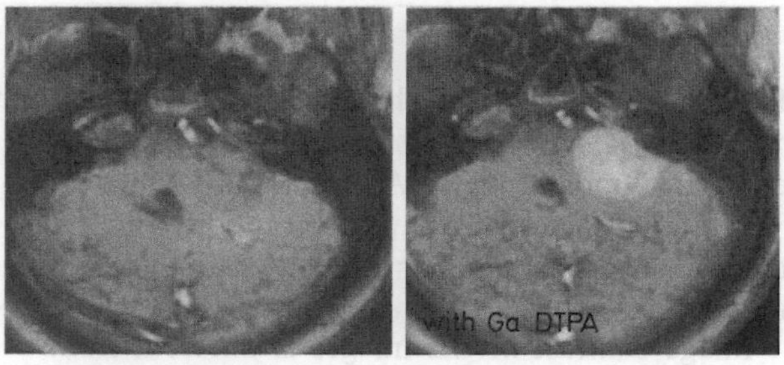

a, b

Fig. 1.59 a, b. Fast imaging: before **(a)** and after **(b)** uptake of contrast agent (gadolinium-DTPA)

Table 1.7. Fast imaging sequences

Acronym	Name	Manufacturer
Fast imaging		
Steady-state magnetization of longitudinal component		
FLASH	*F*ast *l*ow *a*ngle *sh*ot	Max-Planck-Institut, Göttingen [61] Siemens [136]
FFE	*F*ast *f*ield *e*cho	Philips [93]
FAST	*F*ourier *a*quired *s*teady-state *t*echnique (with spoiler gradient)	Picker [58]
GRASS	*G*radient *r*ecall *a*cquisition in a *s*teady-*s*tate mode (with spoiler gradient)	General Electric [134]
Contrast behavior: α low → T2* and N(H) weighted, (with medium TR and long TE more T2* weighted) α high → T1 dispersion high		
Steady-state magnetization of longitudinal and transverse components		
SSFP	*S*teady-*s*tate *f*ree *p*recession	Hinshaw [66]
FISP	*F*ast *i*maging with *s*teady *p*recession	Siemens [106]
FAST	*F*ourier *a*cquired *s*teady-*s*tate *t*echnique (without spoiler gradient)	Picker [58]
GRASS	*G*radient *r*ecall *a*cquisition in a *s*teady-*s*tate mode (without spoiler)	General Electric [134]
Contrast behavior: α low → T2* and N(H) weighted α high (ca. 80°) → strong T2* contrast, T1/T2 signal dependence		
DEFT	*D*riven *e*quilibrium *f*ourier *t*ransform	Philips [133]
GREED	*G*radient *re*versal *e*cho *e*quilibrium *d*riving	Technicare [125]
Contrast behavior: T2 weighted		
CE-FAST	*C*ontrast *e*nhanced FAST	Picker [57]
PSIF	Inverted FISP	Siemens [55]
Contrast behavior: Heavily T2 weighted, TR dependence		
FISPPSIF	Combination of FISP and PSIF	Siemens [55]
FADE	*F*ast *a*cquisition *d*ouble *e*cho	University of Aberdeen [115]
Very fast imaging		
EPI	*E*cho *p*lanar *i*maging	University of Nottingham [86]
INSTANT	Instant scan	Advanced NMR [120]
Miscellaneous		
RARE	*R*apid *a*cquisition with *r*elaxation *e*nhancement: multiecho sequence with different phase encoded echoes. Heavily T2 weighted, for very long T2 components only	Bruker [64]
FAME	*F*ast *a*cquisition with *m*ultiple *e*choes: half data acquisition in combination with RARE	Siemens [87]
HYBRID	Combination of 2DFT spin echo technique and EPI: spin echo contrast	Picker [60]
STEAM	*St*imulated *e*cho *a*cquisition *m*ode: T1-weighted echoes	Max-Planck-Institut, Göttingen [47]
STEP	*S*timulated *e*cho *p*rogressive	Picker [122]
FATE	*F*ast *l*ow *a*ngle spin *e*cho: T1, T2 spin echo contrast	University of Cleveland [132]

SE pulse sequences, GE techniques are used to generate the MR signal by a sudden inversion of the dephasing gradient field. A variety of sequences with different acronyms have been reported in the literature. The most familiar sequences are reviewed in Table 1.7.

Image contrast in GE images is different from the T1-weighted and T2-weighted images commonly used in routine diagnosis. We shall discuss briefly the contrast resulting from two different sequences, FLASH and FISP. While the FLASH technique yields images weighted toward T1, FISP produces images that are T1/T2 weighted. Signal intensity and image contrast are a function of the flip angle of the RF pulse. Optimum contrast between white matter and CSF is achieved at an angle of approximately 30° when using FLASH with TR 25 ms and TE 12 ms (Fig. 1.60), and of approximately 90° us-

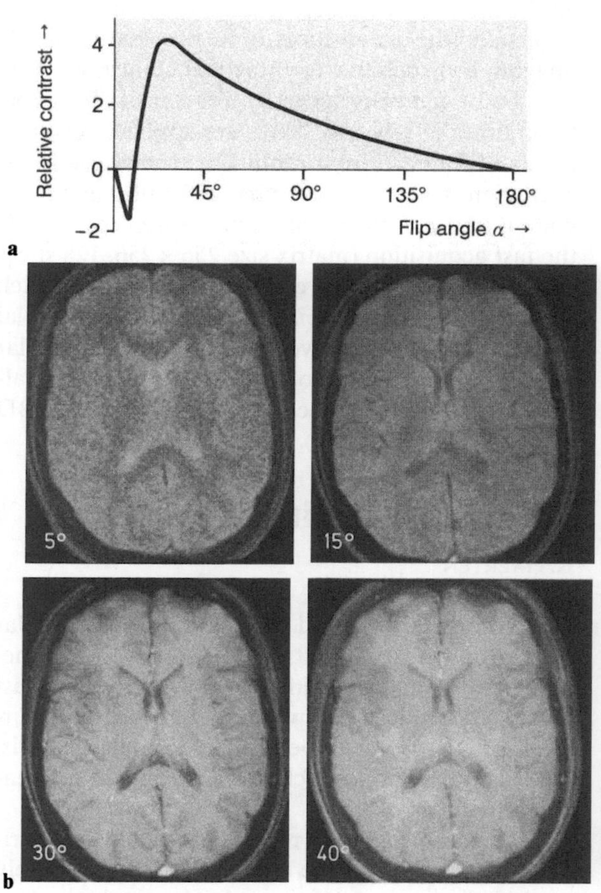

Fig. 1.60 a, b. Contrast between white matter and CSF **a** as a function of flip angle **b** in FLASH images (TR 25 ms, TE 12 ms)

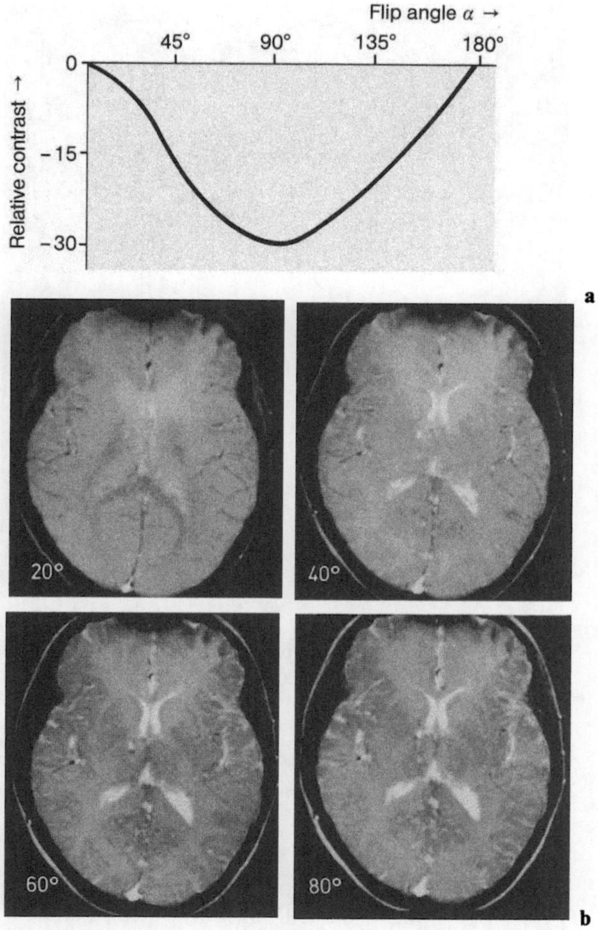

Fig. 1.61 a, b. Contrast between white matter and CSF **a** as a function of flip angle **b** in FISP images (TR 30 ms, TE 13 ms)

ing FISP with TR 30 ms and TE 13 ms (Fig. 1.61) [136]. Signal intensity is significantly higher than with standard SE sequences at TR <100 ms. Contrast between CSF and white matter is much more enhanced with FISP.

The fast imaging techniques can be applied in many ways. Besides their use for rapid surveying, they could substitute for conventional pulse sequences in situations where respiratory or cardiac motion effects or patient movement are a problem.

One of the most promising potential applications of GE sequences is in the area of dynamic imaging. With up to 32 images per cardiac cycle acquired in only 2-4 min, the function of the heart and vascular system can be evaluated, and irregularities of blood flow in the major arteries can be assessed (Fig. 1.62) [20, 71, 75, 76]. Bolus tracking of contrast agents also becomes feasible through the use of fast imaging (Fig. 1.59) [71].

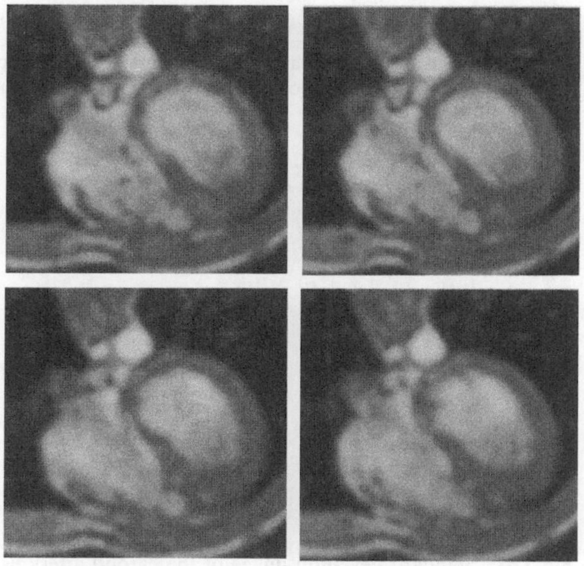

Fig. 1.62. Dynamic cardiac imaging with FLASH

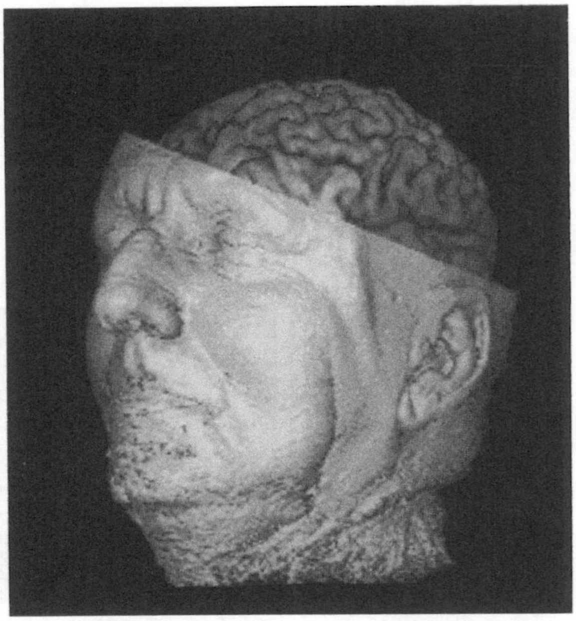

Fig. 1.63. 3 D image display of a set of FLASH images (Flip angle 40°, TR 40 ms, TE 9 ms, Matrix 256 × 256 × 128)

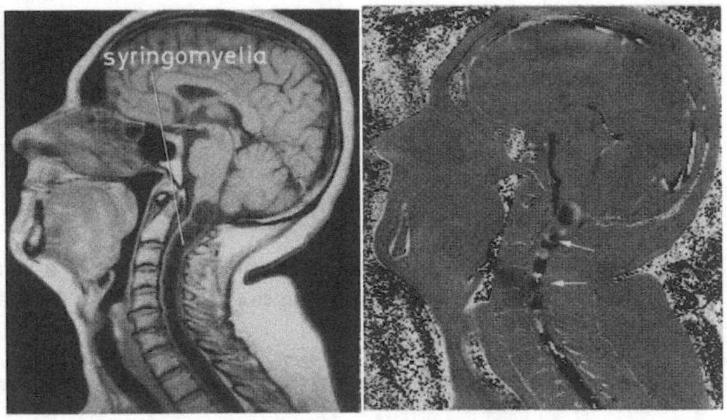

a, b

Fig. 1.64 a, b. Amplitude (**a**) and phase (**b**) images of the cervical spine: CSF flow phenomena associated with syringomyelia *(arrows)*

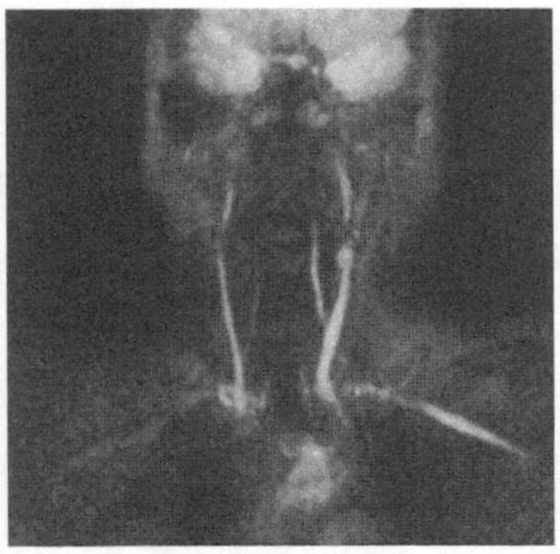

Fig. 1.65. Standard deviation image of the carotid artery using FLASH

Three-dimensional imaging is another attractive application of fast imaging [39]. With standard SE sequences the acquisition time necessary for 3D imaging is prohibitive for practical clinical application, but it can be reduced by a factor of 30 if repetition times of typically 20 ms are applied. A fundamental difference from multislice techniques is the excitation of the entire volume with subsequent encoding into *n* numbers of contiguous slices. Beside the fast acquisition (matrix size 256 × 256, 128 slices in 11 min) there are several other advantages, such as a higher signal-to-noise ratio, minimized partial volume effects due to very thin slices, rectangular slice profiles, and an isotropic resolution which allows for multiplanar reconstructions or even a 3D image display (Fig. 1.63).

1.4.2 Blood Flow and MR Angiography

R. HAERTEN

The MR signal of blood circulating in the vascular system depends upon its flow velocity. This phenomenon, combined with the high image contrast that can be achieved between blood vessels and surrounding tissues, may be utilized to image vessels, to visualize blood flow characteristics, and to measure flow rates.

The complex signal received in an MR experiment not only yields the amplitude image routinely used in diagnosis, but it can also be used to calculate a *phase image*. Phase images are highly sensitive to motion and are helpful in the assessment of blood flow characteristics [38] and of CSF flow phenomena, like those associated with syringomyelia (Fig. 1.64).

Various approaches exist for the imaging of arterial vessels *(MR angiography)*. One method is the gated acquisition of a systolic and diastolic image from a relatively thick slice. In the subtraction image, signal differences in the arteries due to the different flow rates during systole and diastole will result in an image of only those vessels, with stationary tissues disappearing.

Alternatively, *fast imaging* can be used to acquire a temporal series of images at various ECG trigger delay times within the cardiac cycle. The standard deviation of signal intensity, calculated from this series on a pixel-to-pixel basis, represents the angiographic image of arterial flow, stationary tissue being eliminated (Fig. 1.65). By using FLASH or FISP pulse sequences, it is possible to measure a series of 25–30 time-delayed frames per cardiac cycle in only a few minutes (see Sect. 1.4.1). The method is sensitive to pulsatile flow and can be employed for the angiographic representation of the carotid arteries. Fast 3D imaging has been demonstrated as a method for visualizing the carotid and cerebral arteries in an image representation that can be viewed from any direction [39, 76].

Yet another promising approach to MR angiography is the use of *bipolar gradient* techniques [75, 94]. Additional gradients applied symmetrically to the 180° pulse of a SE sequence will change the phase of spins moving at a constant velocity but will not affect the spins in stationary tissues. The additional gradients can be selected in such a way that all moving spins, regardless of their velocity, are rephased at the time of the spin echo. The result is a large signal contribution from material that is in motion. Reversal of the additional gradients, on the other hand, causes moving spins to be dephased, and their signal contribution will be low. Stationary tissue is eliminated in the subtraction image (Fig. 1.66). Because the two measurements are performed at the same ECG trigger delay time, the representation of vessels remains virtually unaffected by motion effects. When the bipolar gradient method is used, changes of signal intensity within the CSF of the cervical spine caused by pulsatile flow can also be documented and corrected to produce a more uniform signal intensity of the CSF (Fig. 1.67) [59].

A technique closely related to the bipolar gradient method can be used to measure the spatial distribution of the *diffusion coefficient* [131]. In diffusion images, tissue characterized by a high diffusion coefficient is represented with high intensity.

The *flow velocity* in vessels can be determined quantitatively from an ECG-gated multiecho experiment. Multiecho images are used to evaluate T2 relaxation times (see Sects. 1.3.2 and 1.4.3). In blood flowing perpendicularly across a slice, T2 is altered as a function of velocity [72, 98]. By utilizing this effect, it is possible to compute the flow velocities at different time intervals in the cardiac cycle and represent them as a plot of velocity versus time (Fig. 1.68). The same effect can be used to visualize *perfusion* in capillary systems [99].

1.4.3 Tissue Characterization

R. HAERTEN

MR images obtained with single-echo and multiecho pulse sequences are directly available for diag-

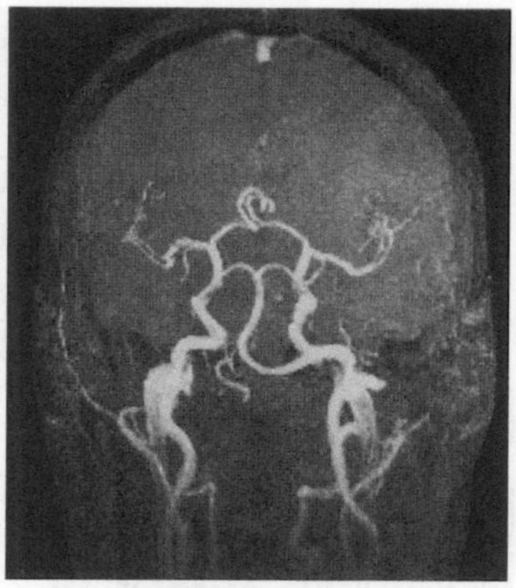

Fig. 1.66. Coronal MR-angiography (substraction image) in a 32-year old man with macroadenoma of the pituitary (FISP 20°, TR 0,04 s/TE 8 ms, 3D data acquisition)

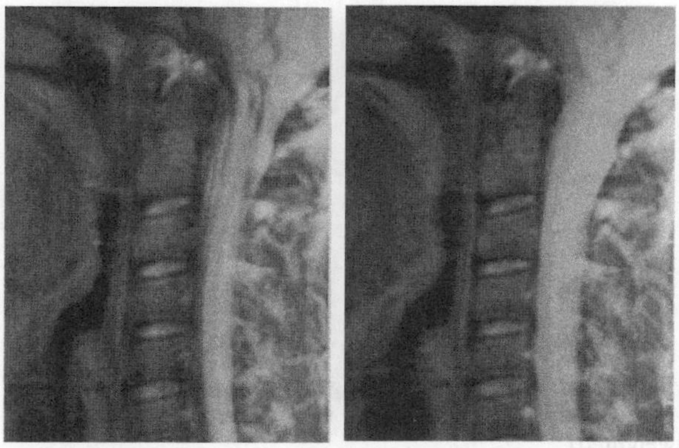

a, b

Fig. 1.67 a, b. CSF in the spine without (**a**) and with (**b**) flow compensation using bipolar gradients

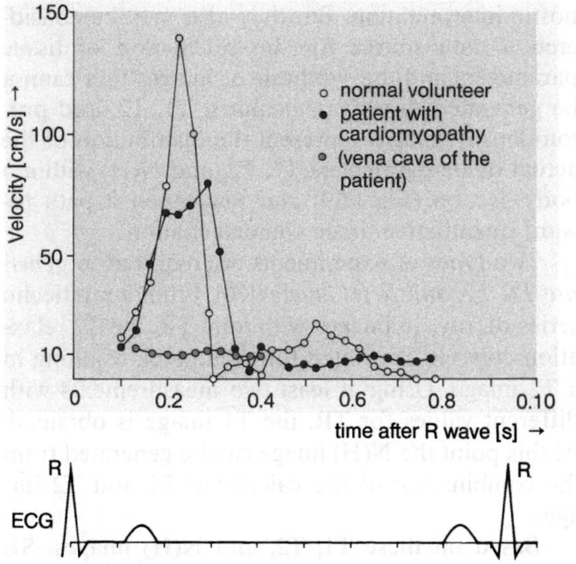

Fig. 1.68. Flow velocity in the abdominal aorta as a function of time

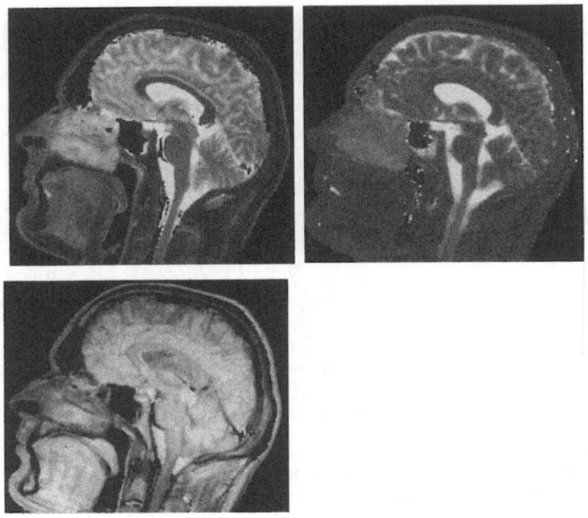

a, b

c

Fig. 1.69 a–c. Images of T1 (**a**), T2 (**b**), and N(H) (**c**)

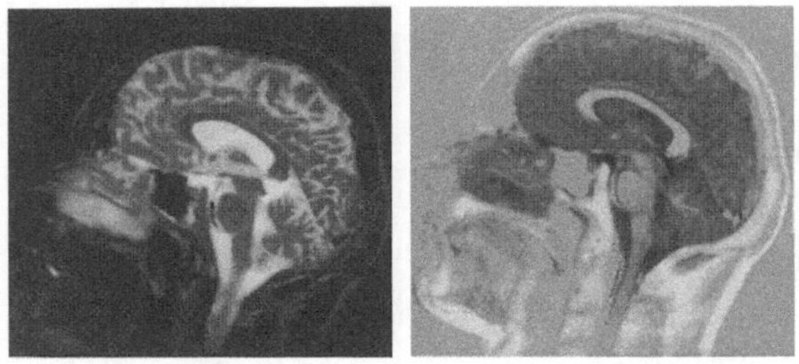

a, b

Fig. 1.70 a, b. Synthetic images in (**a**) saturation-recovery mode and (T2 weighted) (**b**) inversion-recovery mode (T1 weighted)

nostic interpretation. But they also may be considered a data source for the calculation of tissue parameters and the synthesis of images that cannot be generated directly. Calculated T1, T2, and proton-density images represent the distribution of the actual tissue parameters T1, T2, and N(H) within a body section (Fig. 1.69) and may open a path toward quantitative tissue characterization.

Two types of experiments are required to *generate T1, T2, and N(H) images* [70]. From a multiecho series of, say, 16 images with long TR, the T2 relaxation curve is calculated for each pixel, resulting in a T2 image. Using at least two measurements with different values for TR, the T1 image is obtained. At this point the N(H) image can be generated from the combination of the calculated T1 and T2 images.

Based on these T1, T2, and N(H) images, SE images with any TE or TR value may be generated by *image synthesis* [12, 17]. Synthetic images can be used as an educational tool to evaluate pulse-sequence parameters with respect to image contrast for specific diagnostic inquiries (Fig. 1.70).

The goal of *tissue characterization* in MR is to identify specific kinds of tissue, e.g. normal, benign, or malignant. Pattern recognition methods can be applied to approach this complex problem [70]. Based on a representative data base of case studies, including verified diagnoses and histologic findings, a mathematical "classifier" is created that can recognize tissues by their characteristic parameters. These parameters include T1, T2, and N(H), as well as morphologic features gleaned from the image data. As an example, the probabilities for edema, CSF, normal brain tissue, and tumor can be calculated and displayed in colors as an overlay to the actual image. A clinical example is shown in Fig. 5.35.

1.4.4 Spectroscopy and Chemical Shift Imaging

W. Heindel and W. Steinbrich

In a magnetic field, nuclei in different molecular environments experience slightly different local fields and therefore have slightly different resonance frequencies (Sect. 1.9). The difference in frequencies is called the chemical shift and amounts to only a few parts per million (ppm) relative to the resonance frequency of isolated nuclei. This constant and characteristic property is used in spectroscopy to identify molecular structures.

A spectrum represents a plot of signal intensities versus the chemical shift. The intensities indicate the concentrations of the observed molecules. Using a standard, the quantitative measurement of concentrations is possible and analysis of tissue metabolism can be performed. In combination with titration curves the tissue pH can be calculated from spectra. In addition, in vivo NMR spectroscopy using adequate techniques permits observation of normal and pathologic reaction rates of metabolic pathways.

Technical Requirements and Localization Techniques

The most promising clinical application for in vivo MR seems to be combined proton imaging and localized spectroscopy. MR imaging is used to define the volume of interest, MR spectroscopy to investigate the chemical composition and metabolism of that volume. Three basic difficulties must be overcome in this application of MR:

- The low concentrations of the nuclei of biologic interest
- The low MR sensitivity of many nuclei (see Table 1.8)
- The assignment of the spectra to a unique tissue volume

The sensitivity of the MR experiment increases with the field strength $B_0^{7/4}$ [5], and the spectral resolution also improves in higher fields. Therefore the main technical requirement is a superconducting magnet of adequate size with a minimum field strength of 1.5 T. Furthermore, the homogeneity of the magnetic field must be better than 10^{-7} (0.1 ppm) over the useful volume in order to resolve the chemical shifts of the different metabolites. This compares with a homogeneity requirement of only 10^{-5} (10 ppm) for simple imaging, where high field strength is not essential because of the high concentration of water protons in the body (about 100 mol/l)

The problem of spatial assignment of the spectra is solved most easily by the use of surface coils [2]. The coil is placed against the surface of the body region to be examined so that it receives only resonance signals from a typically hemispheric volume beneath the coil. More deeply situated organs are not accessible to this method (see also Sect. 1.2).

This disadvantage has been overcome by localization techniques that enable arbitrary and precise choice of the volume of interest. For example the *volume-selective excitation* (VSE) technique [6] has been proposed for proton spectroscopy. This kind of sequence is not suitable for phosphorus spectroscopy because of the short T2 times of the metabolites. This problem is countered by the *image-selected in vivo spectroscopy* (ISIS) technique [107], which we have used in a modified form [83]. Slice-selective inversion pulses in the *x, y* and *z* directions with accompanying gradient fields precede the 90° excition pulse. The signal is assigned to the desired volume by the addition and subtraction of eight acquired FIDs according to a predetermined scheme.

Another approach for studies of deeper tissues relies on a combination of imaging and spectroscopy (spectroscopic imaging or chemical shift imaging) that will show the spatial distribution of the chemical shifted resonances of a particular type of nucleus [11, 89].

Table 1.8. NMR properties of selected nuclei

Isotope	Natural prevalence (%)	Relative sensitivity	Resonance frequency at 1 T (MHz)
^{1}H	99.98	1.00	42.57
^{19}F	100.00	0.833	40.05
^{23}Na	100.00	0.0925	9.98
^{31}P	100.00	6.63×10^{-2}	17.23
^{13}C	1.11	1.59×10^{-2}	10.70
^{15}N	0.37	1.04×10^{-3}	4.31
^{14}N	99.63	1.01×10^{-3}	3.08

After [95]

Clinical Applications

The nuclei of biologic interest are listed in Table 1.8 in order of decreasing relative sensitivity, together with their resonance frequencies at 1T and their natural abundance. The sensitivity is based on the signal intensity that would be measurable for an equivalent number of water protons at constant field strength B_0.

^{23}Na Imaging and Spectroscopy

The clinical interest in the sodium nucleus originates in an observation made by energy-dispersive X-ray microanalysis: in fast-growing tumors a higher amount of intracellular sodium was detectable than in slow-growing tumors [28]. The data support the contentions that high intracellular sodium and chlorine concentrations are associated with mitogenesis and that even higher sodium and chlorine concentrations are associated with oncogenesis. Therefore a method for specific measurement of intracellular sodium is needed.

Despite the low tissue concentration, the low sensitivity (see Table 1.8) and the effect of quadrupolar interactions causing a very short T2 relaxation time, sodium imaging of the brain can be accomplished by specially formed sequences (gradient echos, volume acquisition, reduction of image matrix) [65]. By using a TR of 100 ms and a TE of 5.7 ms, it is possible to measure mainly the distribution of extracellular sodium. Figure 1.71 shows this in a patient with an astrocytoma.

Compared to imaging, spectroscopic methods with the aid of shift reagents seem to be more promising for the differentiation between intracellular and extracellular sodium. Shift reagents ideally do

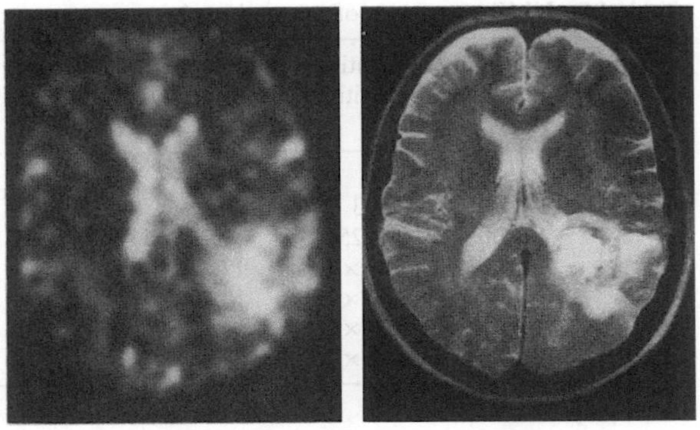

a, b

Fig. 1.71 a, b. ^{23}Na image (TR 100 ms, TE 5,7 ms) (**a**) and proton image (TR 1500 ms, TE 50 ms) (**b**) of a brain metastasis of a bronchial carcinoma

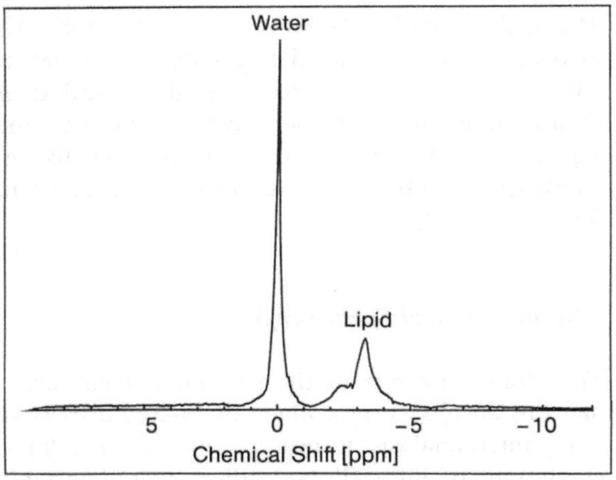

Fig. 1.72. Proton spectrum of a normal muscle obtained by a surface coil

not penetrate the cellular membrane and therefore shift the extracellular Na^+ resonance, whereas the intracellular Na^+ peak maintains its position. Up to now, this elegant method for selective detection of the intracellular and extracellular sodium portions has been employed only in animal experiments.

^{13}C MR Spectroscopy

The advantage of the carbon-13 nucleus is the large range of its chemical shift (200 ppm), which improves the resolution of the peaks and facilitates structural analysis. On the other hand, ^{13}C is a relatively rare isotope, with a natural abundance of only 1.11% (see Table 1.8). This limits MR observations to high-concentration components such as lipids and glycogen. An alternative would be to administer ^{13}C-labeled compounds so that the metabolism of the labeled compound could be selectively analyzed in vivo. Studies of this type in patients could be of great value in the diagnosis of enzyme deficiency diseases.

^{19}F MR Spectroscopy

Fluorine-19, like carbon-13, does not occur in large concentrations in the body. It has potential importance as a tracer for spectroscopic measurements, e.g. in the form of fluorinated blood substitutes or fluorinated sugars [90]. Experimental and clinical evidence suggests an even greater role in metabolic studies of patients being treated with the cytostatic drug 5-fluorouracil [141].

^{1}H MR Spectroscopy and Spectroscopic Imaging

Hydrogen MR images are generally based on the signals from tissue water and fat. The chemical shift of 3.5 ppm which is observed between water-bound and lipid-bound protons (Fig. 1.72) and which may be a source of chemical shift artifacts (see Sect. 1.3.5) can be utilized to selectively eliminate either the water or the fat component of the image (Fig. 1.73) [40, 46]. Its value in neuroradiologic MR, however, has yet to be established.

The goal of clincial hydrogen spectroscopy is the direct detection of metabolic products other than water and fat. Here suppression techniques must be used to ensure that the low-concentration metabolites can be observed in the presence of the intense water and fat signal. Additional problems result from the relatively small chemical shift range of about 10 ppm, which leads to an overlapping of different peaks. To improve the spectral resolution, a high static magnetic field is required.

Experiments in animals have demonstrated lactate formation during cerebral hypoxemia at field strengths less than 2T [9]. The chemical shift of *N*-acetylaspartate has been suggested as a means of determining temperatures within the brain [4]. Elevated histidine levels have been demonstrated in the brains of live mice with congenital histidinemia [51]. Recently it has been possible to observe the metabolites in a selected volume of human brain by applying a water suppression technique in combination with VSE [84]. Further studies of CNS diseases, especially in tumors and cerebrovascular diseases will be performed in the near future.

^{31}P MR Spectroscopy

Phosphorus-31 spectroscopy may acquire special importance for diagnostic applications, because the concentrations of phosphorus metabolites such as adenosine triphosphate (ATP), phosphocreatine (PCr), and inorganic phosphate (P_i), which determine the metabolic state of cells, can be directly demonstrated (Fig. 1.74). Thus, for example, ^{31}P MR spectroscopy can prove an energy deficit in cells by measurement of the PCr/P_i ratio.

Phosphorus-31 spectroscopy also permits noninvasive measurement of intracellular pH, as the chemical shift of the P_i depends on the hydrogen ion concentration. Because the dissociation reaction between $H_2PO_4^-$ and HPO_4^{2-} occurs at an extremely fast rate, rather than two separate peaks a single average peak is observed whose chemical shift depends on the relative concentration of the two dissociation steps. Usually the shift relative to the PCr signal is used to calculate the pH value after proper calibration.

Phosporus-31 MR spectroscopy has been applied for several years in studies of muscular pathophysiology [42, 114, 118] and more recently in the diagnosis of perinatal brain damage [27, 31].

Experiments in animals have shown that many tumors have ^{31}P spectra markedly different from those of normal tissues [56, 103], and that tumor therapies can lead to rapid changes in phosphorus metabolism which are detectable by spectroscopy [101, 103]. The spectra of tumor tissues often show a decreased intensity of the PCr peak compared to healthy muscle or brain, while the concentration of P_i is increased. These spectral differences have been attributed to an increased population of hypoxic cells caused by a deficiency blood supply. An informative review was published by Sostman et al. in 1984 [130].

Increased intensities of phosphomonoesters also can be demonstrated in tumor spectra. Most of these signals come from phosphorylethanolamine and to some degree from phosphorylcholine, both of which play a role in membrane synthesis as phospholipid precursors. A higher peak, therefore, could signify an increase in membrane synthesis. Another peak in the ^{31}P spectrum represents the phosphodiesters, which carry the signals of various phospholipids (e.g., lecithin).

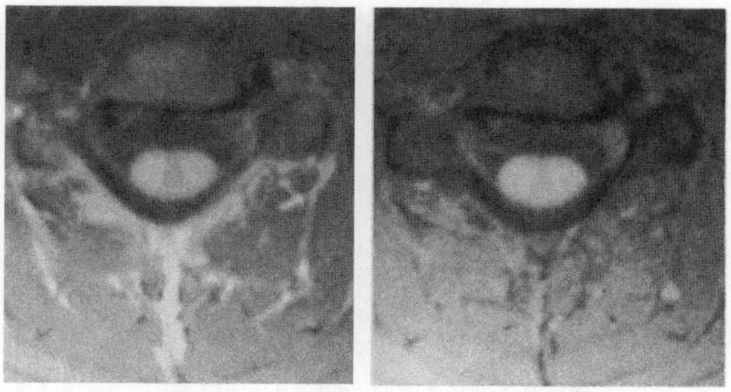

a, b

Fig. 1.73 a, b. Fat image (**a**) and water image (**b**) of the spine (Dixon method [40])

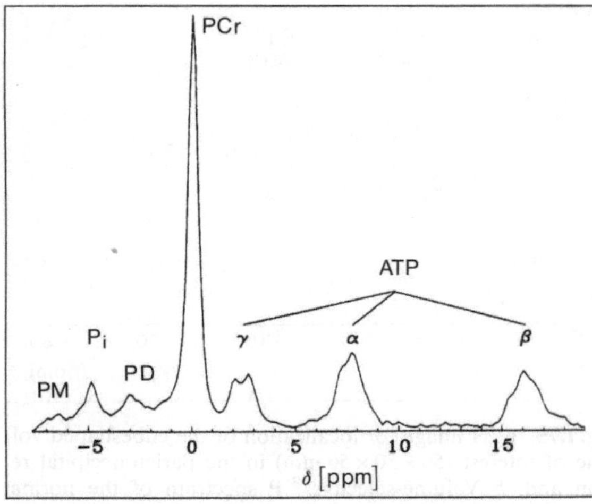

Fig. 1.74. ^{31}P spectrum of normal muscle at 1.5 T using a surface coil. *PM*, phosphomonoester; *P_i*, anorganic phosphate; *PD*, phosphodiester; *PCr*, phosphocreatine; *ATP*, adenosine triphosphates; *ADP*, adenosine diphosphate

So far, ^{31}P MR investigations of human tumors in situ have been limited to superficial growths [104, 105, 126]. For clinical applications in the brain, a technique is needed that will enable any volume of interest within the cranium to be precisely defined on the basis of sectional images [83].

Our initial experience with an image-based spectroscopic technique in patients with brain tumors has confirmed the spectral changes described above [63]. For comparison, analogous measurements were performed in healthy subjects (Fig. 1.75). The location of the cube-shaped volume of interest, with an edge length of 50 mm, is shown on a proton image. The observed resonances were identified according to the literature. The chemical shift is related to the PCr peak. The intracellular pH of healthy brain tissue was 7.01 ± 0.06 ($n = 30$).

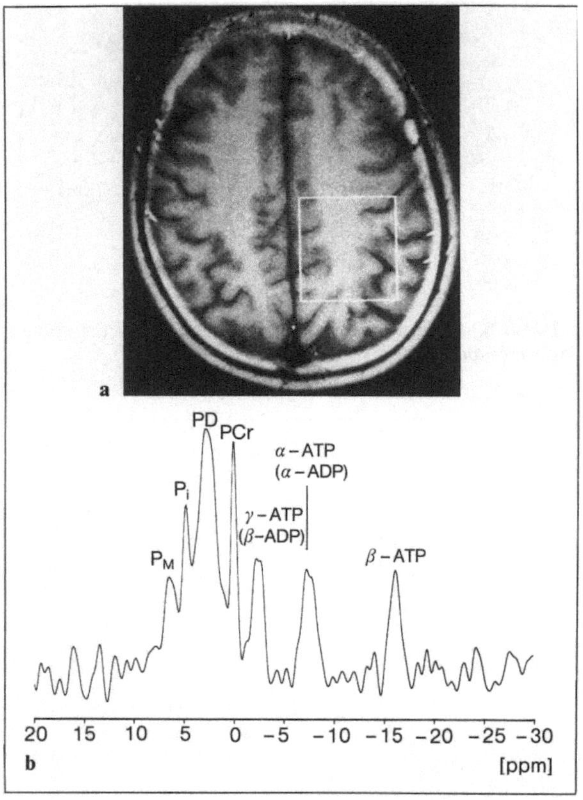

Fig. 1.75. **a** ^{1}H image for localization of the cubeshaped volume of interest (50 × 50 × 50 mm) in the parietooccipital region and **b** Volume-selective ^{31}P spectrum of the normal brain. Labels, see Fig. 1.74

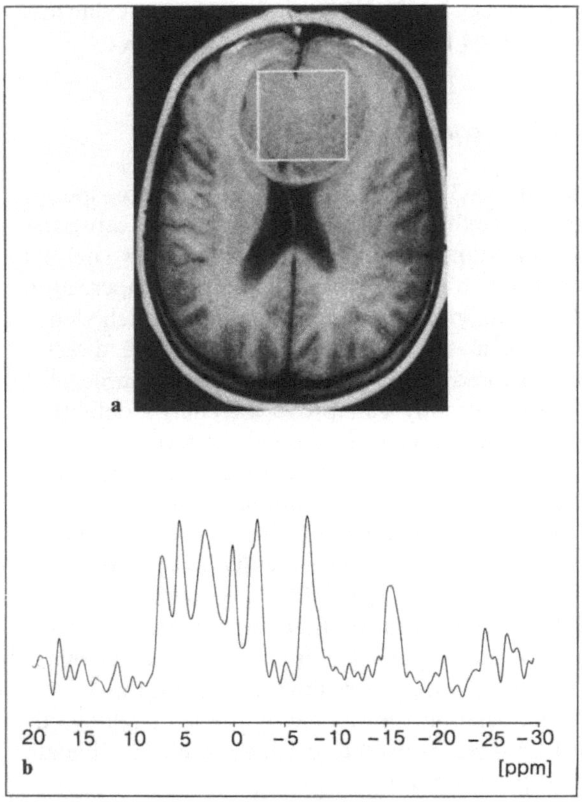

Fig. 1.76. **a** ^{1}H image for centering the volume of interest (40 × 40 × 40 mm) on the tumor and **b** localized ^{31}P spectrum of a large olfactory groove meningioma. The signal intensities of PCr and PD are significantly reduced compared to healthy brain tissue (see Fig. 1.75)

A broad resonance is superimposed over the brain spectrum and removed with the aid of a convolution difference filter function to obtain a straight baseline. The origin of this broad resonance with a half-width at half-maximum of about 30 ppm is not yet exactly known. It might stem from membrane-bound phosphorus atoms.

The ^{1}H image and ^{31}P spectrum of a large olfactory groove meningioma are shown in Fig. 1.76. Compared with the normal spectrum, the intensities of the phosphomonoester and P_i peaks are increased, while the PCr signal is diminished. The tissue pH of the tumor was 7.41, which is more alkaline than normal brain. Measurements in a patient with an inoperable oligodendroglioma (Fig. 1.77 a) disclosed similar abnormalities in the ^{31}P spectrum. In this tumor the pH did not differ from the value measured in normal brain. Similar spectral changes have been observed to varying degrees in other brain tumors, although it has not yet been possible to establish a histologic correlation.

Follow-up studies in patients undergoing radiotherapy have shown interesting spectral changes. In the oligodendroglioma tumor spectrum shown in Fig. 1.77, a marked rise of PCr intensity was noted following exposure to 10 Gy and 24 Gy (Fig. 1.77 b and c), even though there was no apparent gross change in the size or internal structure of the tumor. It is still too early to interpret these observations, but there is both clinical and experimental evidence that MR spectroscopy provides earlier detection of tumor response to radiation or chemotherapy than imaging procedures.

Summary

MR spectroscopy and spectroscopic imaging with nuclei other than protons can be performed with today's MR technology. In vivo spectroscopy is still in an early state of development, though investigations of cell suspensions and animal experiments

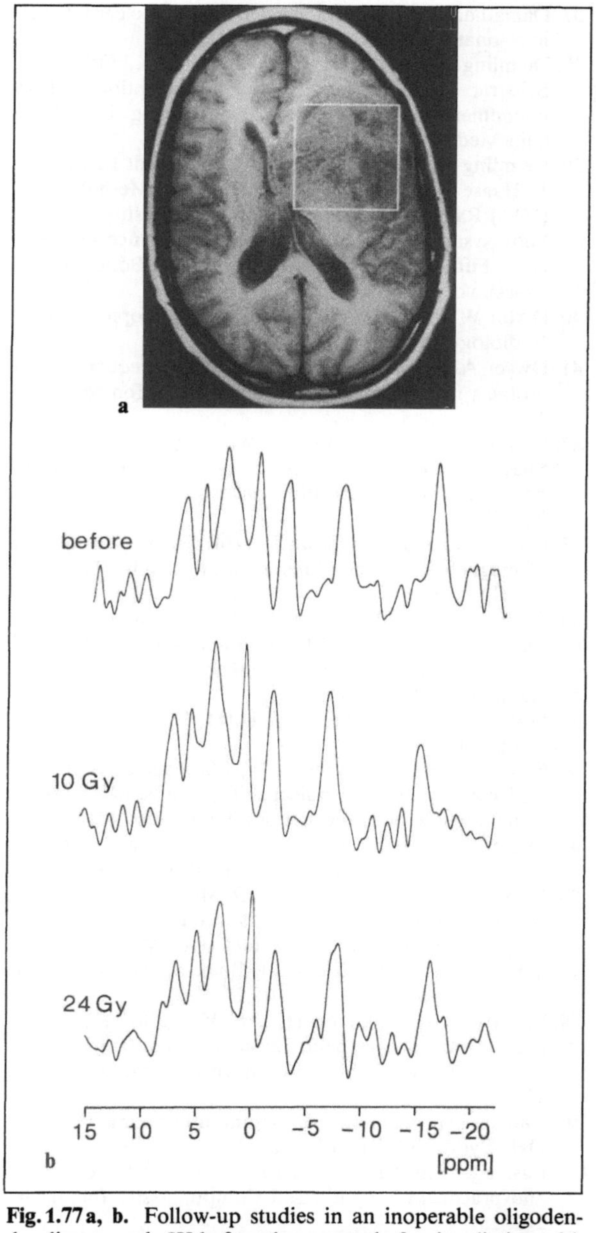

Fig. 1.77 a, b. Follow-up studies in an inoperable oligodendroglioma grade III before therapy and after irradiation with 10 Gy and 24 Gy. While proton imaging (**a**) did not show any changes, in localized ^{31}P MRS (**b**) a relative increase of the PCr intensity was observed

have clarified some fundamental principles. It will require continuing efforts in clinical research to establish these methods as tools for routine clinical diagnosis. The combination of imaging and localized spectroscopy of normal and pathologic tissue seems to be the most promising approach.

References

1. Abragam A (1961) The principles of nuclear magnetism. Clarendon Press, Oxford
2. Ackerman JJH, Grove TH, Wong GG, Gadian DG, Radda GK (1980) Mapping of metabolites in whole animals by ^{31}P NMR using surface coils. Nature 283: 167-170
3. American College of Radiology Commission in Magnetic Resonance (1987) Glossary of MR terms. American College of Radiology, Chicago
4. Arùs C, Chang Y-Ch, Barany M (1985) *N*-Acetylaspartate as an intrinsic thermometer for ^{1}H NMR of brain slices. J Mag Res 63: 376-379
5. Aue WP (1985) Nuclear magnetic resonance: tomography and in vivo spectroscopy. Swiss Chiropractors Association, Annals 8: 17-24
6. Aue WP, Müller S, Cross TA, Seelig J (1984) Volume-selective excitation: a novel approach to topical NMR. J Mag Res 56: 350-354
7. Axel L (1984) Blood flow effects in magnetic resonance imaging. AJR 143: 1157-1166
8. Bailes DR, Gilderdale DJ, Bydder GM, Collins AG, Firmin DN (1985) Respiratory ordered phase encoding (ROPE). J Comp Assist Tomogr 9 (4): 835-838
9. Behar KL, Rothman DL, Shulman RG, Petroff OAC, Prichard JW (1984) Detection of cerebral lactate in vivo during hypoxemia by ^{1}H NMR at relatively low field strength (1.9 T). Proc Natl Acad Sci USA 81: 2517-2519
10. Bellon EM, Haake EM, Coleman PE, Sacco DC, Steiger DA, Gangarosa RE (1986) MR artifacts: a review. AJR 147: 1271-1281
11. Bendel P, Lai CM, Lauterbur PC (1980) ^{31}P spectroscopic zeugmatography of phosphorus metabolites. J Mag Res 38: 343-356
12. Bielke G, Meves M, Meindl S, Brückner A, Seelen W von, Rinck PA, Pfannenstiel P (1984) A systematic approach to optimization of pulse sequences in NMR imaging by computer simulations. In: PD Esser and RE Johnston, Eds, Technology of nuclear magnetic resonance. Society of Nuclear Medicine, New York, p 109
13. Bilaniuk LT, Zimmerman RA, Wehrli FW, Goldberg HI, Grossman RI, Bottomley PA, Edelstein WA, Glover GH (1984) Cerebral magnetic resonance: comparison of high and low field strength imaging. Radiology 153: 409-414
14. Bloch F (1946) Nuclear induction. Phys Rev 70: 460-474
15. Bloch F, Hansen WW, Packard M (1946) Nuclear induction. Phys Rev 69: 127
16. Bloembergen N, Purcell EM, Pound RV (1948) Relaxation effects in nuclear magnetic resonance absorption. Phys Rev 73: 679-712
17. Bobman SA, Riederer SJ, Lee LN, Suddarth SA, Wang HZ, MacFall JR (1985) Synthesized MR images: comparison with acquired images. Radiology 155: 731-738
18. Boskamp EB (1985) Improved surface coil imaging in MR: decoupling of the excitation and receiver coils, Radiology 157: 449-452
19. Bottomley PA, Foster TH, Argsinger RE, Pfeifer LM (1984) A review of normal tissue hydrogen NMR relaxation time and relaxation mechanism from 1-100 MHz, dependence on tissue type, NMR frequency, temperature, species, exercise and age. Med Phys 11: 425-448
20. Bräckle G, Deimling M, Laub G, Weikl A, Bachus R, Reinhardt ER (1986) Vessel display with methods of fast

imaging techniques. Society of Magnetic Resonance in Medicine, Fifth Annual Meeting, Montreal, Book of Abstracts, vol 4, p 1097
21. Bradley WG, Waluch V, Lai K-S, Fernandez EJ, Spalter C (1984) The appearance of rapidly flowing blood on magnetic resonance images. AJR 143: 1167-1174
22. Brant-Zawadzki M, Norman D, Newton TH, Kelly WM, Kjos B, Mills CM, Dillon W, Sobel D, Crooks LE (1984) Magnetic resonance of the brain: the optimal screening technique. Radiology 152: 71-77
23. Brash RC (1983) Methods of contrast enhancement for NMR imaging and potential applications. Radiology 147: 781-788
24. Brenton DP, Garrod PJ, Krywawych S, Reynolds EOR, Bachelard HS, Cox DW, Morris PG (1983) Phosphoetholamine as major constituent of phosphomonoester peak detected by ^{31}P NMR in newborn brain. Lancet I: 115
25. Bydder GM, Young IR (1985) MR imaging: clinical use of the inversion recovery sequence. J Comp Ass Tomogr 9 (4): 659-675
26. Bydder GM, Steiner RE, Young IR, Hall AS, Thomas DJ, Marshall J, Pallis CA, Legg NJ (1982) Clinical NMR imaging of the brain: 140 cases. AJR 139: 215-236
27. Cady EB, Costello AM, Dawson MJ, Delpy DT, Hope PL, Reynolds EOR, Toft PS, Wilkie DR (1983) Non-invasive investigation of cerebral metabolism in newborn infants by phosphorus nuclear magnetic spectroscopy. Lancet I: 1059-1062
28. Cameron IL, Smith NKR, Pool TB, Sparks RL (1980) Intracellular concentration of sodium and other elements as related to mitogenesis and oncogenesis in vivo. Cancer Res 40: 1493-1500
29. Carr DH, Brown J, Bydder GM, Weinmann H-J, Speck U, Thomas DJ, Young IR (1984) Intravenous chelated gadolinium as a contrast agent in NMR imaging of cerebral tumors. Lancet 3: 484-486
30. Carr HY, Purcell EM (1954) Effects of diffusion on free precession in nuclear magnetic resonance experiments. Phys Rev 94: 630-638
31. Chance B, Younkin DP, Warnell R, Eleff S, Delivoria-Papadopoulos M (1983) ^{31}P NMR Spectroscopy of cortical oxidative metabolism in neonates. Ped Res 17: 397
32. Claussen C, Laniado M, Schörner W, Niendorf H-P, Weinmann H-J, Fiegler W, Felix R (1985) The use of gadolinium-DTPA in magnetic resonance imaging of glioblastomas and intracranial metastases. Am J Neuroradiol 6: 669-674
33. Condon B, Patterson J, Jenkins A, Wyper D, Hadley D, Grant R, Rowan J, Teasdale G (1987) MR relaxation times of cerebrospinal fluid. J Comp Assist Tomogr 11: 203-207
34. Crooks LE, Ortendahl DA, Kaufman L, Hoenninger JC, Arakwa M, Watts J, Cannon CN, Brant-Zawadzki M (1982) Clinical efficiency of nuclear magnetic resonance imaging. Radiology 142: 123-128
35. Crooks LE, Mills CM, Davis PL, Brant-Zawadzki M, Hoenninger J, Arakawa M, Watts J, Kaufman L (1982) Visualization of cerebral and vascular abnormalities by NMR imaging. The effect of imaging parameters on contrast. Radiology 144: 843-852
36. Crooks LE, Arakawa M, Hoenninger JC, McCarten B, Watts J, Kaufman L (1984) Magnetic resonance imaging: effects of magnetic field strength. Radiology 151: 127-133
37. Damadian R (1971) Tumor detection by nuclear magnetic resonance. Science 171: 1151-1153
38. Deimling M, Müller E, Lenz G, Barth K, Fritschy P, Seiderer M, Reinhardt ER (1986) Description of flow phenomena in magnetic resonance imaging. Diag Imag Clin Med 55: 37-51
39. Deimling M, Heubes P, Weber H, Reinhardt ER, Frahm J, Haase A, Matthaei D, Hänicke W, Merboldt KD (1986) Rapid three-dimensional imaging using a whole-body system. Society of Magnetic Resonance in Medicine, Fifth Annual Meeting, Montreal, Book of Abstracts, vol 3, p 663
40. Dixon WT (1984) Simple proton spectroscopic imaging. Radiology 153: 189-194
41. Dwyer AJ, Knop RH, Hoult DI (1985) Frequency shift artifacts in MR imaging. J Comp Assist Tomogr 9 (1): 16-18
42. Edwards RHT, Dawson MJ, Wilkie DR, Gordon RE, Shaw D (1982) Clinical use of nuclear magnetic resonance in the investigation of myopathy. Lancet I: 725-731
43. Faul D, Abart J, Margosian P (1984) Quick measurement of magnetic field variations within the body. Radiology 153 (P): 303
44. Feinberg DA, Mills CM, Posin JP, Ortendahl DA, Hylton NM, Crooks LE, Watts IC, Kaufman L, Arakawa M (1985) Multiple spin-echo magnetic resonance imaging. Radiology 155: 437-442
45. FONAR Ing., Melville, N.Y. 11741, USA. Manufacturer's brochure
46. Frahm J, Haase A, Hänicke W, Matthaei D, Bomsdorf H, Helzel T (1985) Chemical shift selective MR imaging using a whole-body magnet. Radiology 156: 441-444
47. Frahm J, Merboldt KD, Hänicke W, Haase A (1985) Stimulated echo imaging. J Mag Res 64: 81-93
48. Frahm J, Haase A, Merboldt KD, Matthaei D, Deimling M, Weber H (1986) Flow effects in rapid FLASH NMR imaging. Annual Meeting of Society of Magnetic Resonance in Medicine, Montreal, Book of Abstract, vol 3, p 967-968
49. Fullerton GD, Cameron IL, Ord VA (1984) Frequency dependence of magnetic resonance spin-lattice relaxation of protons in biological materials. Radiology 151: 135-138
50. Gadian DG, Clanton JA, Bryant DJ, Young IR, Carr DH, Bydder GM (1985) Gadolinium-DTPA as a contrast agent in NMR imaging - theoretical projections and practical observations. J Comput Assist Tumogr 9: 242-251
51. Gadian DG, Proctor E, Williams SR, Cady EB, Gardiners RM (1986) Neurometabolism effects of an inborn error of amino metabolism demonstrated in vivo by ^{1}H NMR. Mag Res Med 3: 150-156
52. George CR, Jacobs G, MacIntyre WJ, Lorig RJ, Go RT, Nose Y, Meaney TF (1984) Magnetic resonance signal intensity patterns obtained from continuous and pulsative flow models. Radiology 151: 421-428
53. Glover GH (1987) Flow artifact suppression in 2D and 3DFT MRI. Society of Magnetic Resonance in Medicine, Sixth Annual Meeting, New York, Book of Abstracts, vol 1, p 420
54. Goldman MR, Brady TJ, Pykett IL, Burt CT, Buonanno FS, Kistler JP, Newhouse JH, Hinshaw WS, Pohost FS (1982) Quantification of experimental myocardial infarction using nuclear magnetic resonance imaging and

paramagnetic ion contrast enhancement in excised canine hearts. Circulation 66: 1012-1016
55. Graumann R, Fischer H, Barfuss H, Bruder H, Oppelt A, Deimling M (1987) Contrast behaviour of steady state sequences in inhomogeneous fields. Society of Magnetic Resonance in Medicine, Sixth Annual Meeting, New York, Book of Abstracts, vol 1, p 444
56. Griffiths JR, Stevens AN, Iles RA, Gordon RE, Show D (1981) ^{31}P NMR investigation of solid tumours in the living rat. Biosci Rep 1: 319-325
57. Gyngell ML, Nayler GL, Paley M, Palmer N (1986) A comparison of fast acquisition modes in MRI. Mag Res Imag 4 (2): 101
58. Gyngell ML, Palmer ND, Eastwood LM (1986) The application of steady state free precession in 2D-FT MR imaging. Society of Magnetic Resonance in Medicine, Fifth Annual Meeting, Montreal, Book of Abstracts, vol 3, p 666
59. Haacke EM, Lenz G, Modic MT, Bachus R, Reinhardt ER (1986) Quantification of CSF flow and diffusion techniques. Society of Magnetic Resonance in Medicine, Fifth Annual Meeting, Montreal, Book of Abstracts, vol 3, p 1055
60. Haacke EM, Bearden FH, Clayton JR, Ling NR (1986) Reduction of MR imaging time by the HYBRID fast-scan technique. Radiology 158: 521-530
61. Haase A, Frahm J, Matthaei D, Hänicke W, Merboldt KD (1986) FLASH imaging. Rapid NMR imaging using low flip-angle pulses. J Mag Res 67: 258-266
62. Hahn EL (1950) Spin echoes. Phys Rev 80: 580-594
63. Heindel W, Bunke J, Steinbrich W (1987) Bildgesteuerte lokalisierte ^{31}P-NMR Spektroskopie des menschlichen Gehirns bei 1.5 Tesla. Fortschr Röntgenstr. 147: 374-378
64. Henning J, Nauerth A, Friedburg H (1986) RARE imaging: a fast imaging method for clincial MR. Mag Res Med 3: 823-833
65. Hilal SK, Maudsley AA, Ra JB, Simon HE, Roschmann P, Wittekoek S, Cho ZH, Mun SK (1985) In vivo NMR imaging of sodium-23 in the human head. J Comput Assist Tomogr 9: 1-7
66. Hinshaw W (1976) Image formation by nuclear magnetic resonance: the sensitive-point method. J Appl Phys 47: 3709-3721
67. Hoult DI, Chen C-N, Sank VJ (1986) The field dependence of NMR imaging. II. Arguments concerning optimal field strength. Mag Res Med 3: 730-746
68. Houndsfield G (1973) Computerized transverse axial scanning (tomography). Br J Radiology 46: 1016-1022
69. Johnson GA, Herfkens RJ, Brown MA (1985) Tissue relaxation time: in vivo field dependence. Radiology 156: 805-810
70. König HA, Bachus R, Reinhardt ER (1986) Pattern recognition for tissue characterization in magnetic resonance imaging. Health Care Instr 1 (6): 184-187
71. Kornmesser W, Laniado M, Deimling M, Felix R (1986) Dynamic MRI of intracranial and intraspinal tumors with fast imaging sequences and intravenous Gd-DTPA. Society of Magnetic Resonance in Medicine, Fifth Annual Meeting, Montreal, Book of Abstracts, vol 3, p 811-812
72. Kucharczyk W, Brant-Zawadzki M, Lemme-Plaghos L, Uske A, Kjos B, Feinberg DA, Norman D (1985) MR technology: effect of even-echo rephasing on calculated T2 values and T2 images. Radiology 157: 95-101
73. Kulkarni MV, Patton JA, Price RR (1986) Technical considerations for the use of surface coils in MRI. AJR 147: 373-378
74. Kumar A, Welti D, Ernst RR (1975) NMR Fourier zeugmatography. J Mag Res 18: 69-83
75. Laub G, Bräckle G, Bachus R, Reinhardt ER (1986) High resolution MR angiology with bipolar gradient pulses. Society of Magnetic Resonance in Medicine, Fifth Annual Meeting, Montreal, Book of Abstracts, vol. Add: 5-6
76. Laub G, Rossnick S, Bräckle G, Bachus R, Reinhardt ER (1986) 3-D representation of vessels by pixel classification. Society of Magnetic Resonance in Medicine, Fifth Annual Meeting, Montreal, Book of Abstracts, vol 2, p 508-509
77. Lauffer RB, Brady TJ, Brown RD, Baglin C, Koenig SH (1986) 1/T1 NMRD profiles of solutions of Mn^{2+} and Gd^{3+} protein-chelate conjugates. Mag Res Med 3: 541-548
78. Lauterbur PC (1973) Image formation by induced local interactions: examples employing nuclear magnetic resonance. Nature 242: 190-191
79. Lauterbur PC, Mendonca-Dias MH, Rudin AM (1978) Augmentation of tissue water protein spinlattice relaxation rates by in-vivo addition of paramagnetic ions. Front Biol Engin 1: 752-759
80. Lerski RA, Straughan K, Williams JL (1986) Practical aspects of ghosting in resistive NMR imaging systems. Phys Med Biol 31 (7): 721-735
81. Lüdeke KM, Röschmann P, Tischler R (1986) Susceptibility artifacts in NMR imaging. Mag Res Imag 3: 329-343
82. Luyten PR, den Hollander JA (1986) Observation of metabolites in the human brain by MR spectroscopy. Radiology 161: 795-798
83. Luyten PR, Groen JP, Arnold DA, Baleriaux D, den Hollander JA (1986) ^{31}P localized spectroscopy of the human brain in situ at 1.5 Tesla. Society of Magnetic Resonance in Medicine, Fifth Annual Meeting, Montreal, Book of Abstracts, vol 3, p 1083-1084
84. Luyten PR, Marien AJH, Sijtsma B et al. (1986) Solvent-suppressed spatially resolved spectroscopy: an approach to high resolution NMR on a whole body MR system. J Mag Res 67: 148-155
85. Mallard J, Hutchison JMS, Edelstein WA et al. (1980) In vivo NMR imaging in medicine: the Aberdeen approach, both physical and biological. Phil Trans R Soc London B 289: 519-533
86. Mansfield PM and Pykett IL (1978) Echo planar imaging: biological and medical imaging with NMR. J Mag Res 29: 373-395
87. Margosian P (1985) Faster imaging with half the data. Society of Magnetic Resonance in Medicine, Fourth Annual Meeting, London, Book of Abstracts, vol 2, p 1024
88. Margosian P, Schmitt F (1985) Faster MR imaging methods. Proceedings SPIE Cannes 593: 6
89. Maudsley AA, Hilal SK, Perman WH, Simon HE (1983) Spatially resolved high resolution spectroscopy by four-dimensional NMR. J Mag Res 51: 147-152
90. McFarland E, Koutcher JA, Rosen BR, Teicher B, Brady TJ (1985) In vivo ^{19}F NMR imaging. J Comp Assist Tomogr 9 (1): 8-15
91. Meiboom S, Gill D (1958) Modified spin-echo method for measuring nuclear relaxation times. Rev Sci Instrum 29: 688-691

92. Mendonca-Dias MH, Gaggelli E, Lauterbur PC (1983) Paramagnetic contrast agents in nuclear magnetic resonance medical imaging. Semin Nuclear Med 13: 364-376
93. van Meulen P, Groen JP, Cuppen JJ (1985) Very fast MR imaging by field echoes and small angle excitation. Mag Res Imag 3: 297-299
94. Meuli RA, Wedeen VJ, Geller SC, Edelman RR, Frank LR, Brady TJ, Rose BR (1986) MR gated substraction angiography: evaluation of lower extremities. Radiology 159: 411-418
95. Michel D (1981) Grundlagen und Methoden der kernmagnetischen Resonanz. Akademie Verlag, Berlin
96. Mills CM, Brant-Zawadzki M, Crooks LE, Kaufman L, Sheldon P, Norman D, Bank W, Newton TH (1984) Nuclear magnetic resonance: principles of blood flow imaging. AJR 142: 165-170
97. Morris PG, Nuclear resonance imaging in medicine and biology. Clarendon Press, Oxford 1986
98. Müller E, Deimling M, Reinhardt ER (1986) Analysis of T2 changes in ECG-gated multiecho experiments. Mag Res Med 3: 331-335
99. Müller E, Haacke EM, Lenz G, Nelson D, Stowe N, Reinhardt ER, Alfidi RJ (1986) Perfusion measurements of isolated kidneys with MRI. Society of Magnetic Resonance in Medicine, Fifth Annual Meeting, Montreal, Book of Abstracts, vol 1, p 80
100. Müller WH-G, Knüttel B (1983) Magnet choices for NMR tomography. Bruker Medical Report (1) 4
101. Naruse S, Hoikawa Y, Tabaka C, Tanaka C, Higuchi T, Ueda S, Hirakawa K, Nishikawa H, Watari H (1985) Observation of energy metabolism in neuroectodermal tumors using in vivo P-31 NMR. Mag Res Imag 3: 117-123
102. New PFJ, Rosen BR, Brady TJ, Buonanno FS, Kistler JP, Burt CT, Hinshaw WS, Newhouse JH, Pohost GM, Taveras JM (1983) Nuclear magnetic resonance. Potential hazards and artifacts of ferromagnetic and nonferromagnetic surgical and dental materials and devices in nuclear magnetic resonance imaging. Radiology 147: 139-148
103. Ng TC, Evanochko WT, Hiramoto RN, Ghanta VK, Lilly MB, Lawson AJ, Corbett TH, Durant JR, Glickson JD (1982) ^{31}P NMR spectroscopy of in vivo tumors. J Mag Res 49: 271-286
104. Ng TC, Majors AW, Meany TF (1986) In vivo MR spectroscopy of human subjects with a 1.4-T whole-body MR imager. Radiology 158: 517-520
105. Nidecker AC, Müller S, Aue WP, Seelig J, Fridrich R, Remagen W, Hartweg H, Benz UF (1985) Extremity bone tumors: evaluation by P-31 NMR spectroscopy. Radiology 157: 167-174
106. Oppelt A, Graumann R, Barfuß H, Fischer H, Hartl W, Schajor W (1986) FISP: eine neue schnelle Pulssequenz für die Kernspintomographie. Electromedica 1: 15-18
107. Ordidge RJ, Conelly A, Lohman JAB (1986) Image-selected in vivo spectroscopy (ISIS). A new technique for spatially selective NMR spectroscopy. J Mag Res 66: 283-294
108. Oxford Magnet Technology. Magnets in clinical use - site planning guide. Manufacturer's brochure, Oxford
109. Pattany PM, Phillips JJ, Chiu LC, Lipcamon JD, Duerk JL, McNally JM, Mohapatra SN (1987) Motion artifact suppression technique (MAST) for MR imaging. J Comp Assist Tomogr 11 (3): 369-377
110. Posin JP, Ortendahl DA, Hylton NM, Kaufman L, Watts JC, Crooks LE, Mills CM (1985) Variable magnetic resonance imaging parameters: effects on detection and characterization of lesions. Radiology 155: 719-725
111. Purcell EU, Torrey HC, Pound RV (1946) Resonance absorption by nuclear magnetic moments in a solid. Phys Rev 69: 37-38
112. Pursey E, Stark DD, Lufkin RB, Tarr RW, Brown RKJ, Hanafee WN, Solomon MA (1986) MRI artifacts: mechanism and clincial significance. Radio Graphics 6 (5): 891-909
113. Rabi II, Millman S, Kisch P, Zacharias JR (1939) The molecular beam resonance method for measuring nuclear magnetic moments. Phys Rev 55: 526-535
114. Radda GK, Bore PJ, Gadian DG, Ross BD, Styles P, Taylor D, Morgan-Hughes J (1982) ^{31}P NMR examination of two patients with NADH-CoQ reductase deficiency. Nature 295: 608-609
115. Redpath TW, Jones RA, Mallard JR (1987) FADE - a new fast imaging sequence. Society of Magnetic Resonance in Medicine, Sixth Annual Meeting, New York, Book of Abstracts, vol 1, p 228
116. Reuther G, Huk W, Deimling M (1985) Phänomenologie der kernspintomographischen Blutgefäßdarstellung: Aspekte und Perspektiven. Electromedica 53: 58-67
117. Rinck PA, Meindl S, Higer HP, Bieler EU, Pfannenstiel P (1985) Brain tumors: detection and typing by use of CPMG sequences and in vivo T2 measurements. Radiology 157: 103-106
118. Ross BD, Radda GK, Gadian DG, Rocker G, Esiri M, Falconer-Smith J (1981) Examination of a case of suspected McArdle's syndrome by P-31 nuclear magnetic resonance. N Engl J Med 304: 1338-1342
119. Runge VM, Clanton JA, Lukehart CM, Partain C, James AE (1983) Paramagnetic agents for contrast enhanced NMR imaging: a review. AJR 141: 1209-1215
120. Rzedzian RR, Pykett IL (1987) Instant images of the human heart using a new, whole-body MR imaging system. AJR 149: 245-250
121. Saini S, Hahn PF, Stark DD, Wittenberg J, Ferrucci JT (1986) Pulse sequence and dose considerations in MRI of liver cancer with ion oxide particles. Society of Magnetic Resonance in Medicine, Fifth Annual Meeting, Montreal, vol 4, p 1535-1536
122. Sattin W, Mareci TH, Scott KN (1985) Exploiting the stimulated echo in nuclear magnetic resonance imaging. II. Applications J Mag Res 65: 298-307
123. Schad L, Lott S, Schmitt F, Sturm V, Lorenz WJ (1987) Correction of spatial distortion in MR imaging: a prerequisite for accurate stereotaxy. J Comp Assist Tomogr 11 (3): 499-505
124. Schörner W, Felix R, Laniado M, et al. (1984) Prüfung des kernspintomographischen Kontrastmittels Gadolinium-DTPA am Menschen: Verträglichkeit, Kontrastbeeinflussung und erste klinische Ergebnisse. Fortschr Röntgenstr 140: 492-500
125. Sebok DA, Yeung HN (1986) Gradient-reversal echo, equilibrium-driving (GREED) - a new method of rapid imaging. Society of Magnetic Resonance in Medicine, Fifth Annual Meeting, Montreal, Book of Abstracts, vol 1, p 936-937
126. Semmler W, Gademann G, Bachert-Baumann P, Zabel H-J, Lorenz WJ, van Kaick G (1988) Monitoring of human tumor response to therapy by means of ^{31}P MR spectroscopy. Radiology 166: 533-539

127. Sepponen RE, Sipponen JT, Sivula A (1985) Low field (0.02) nuclear magnetic resonance imaging of the brain. J Comp Assist Tomography 9 (2): 237-241

128. Siemens Medical Engineering Group Manufacturer's brochure, Erlangen

129. Slichter CP (1978) Principles of magnetic resonance, 2nd edn. Springer, Berlin

130. Sostman HD, Armitage IM, Fisher JJ (1984) NMR in cancer. I. High resolution spectroscopy of tumors. Mag Res Imag 2: 265-278

131. Stejskal EO, Tanner JE (1965) Spin diffusion measurements: spin echo in the presence of a time-dependent field gradient. J Chem Phys 42: 288

132. Tkach JA, Haake EM (1987) Fast low angle spin echo imaging (abstract). Fast MRI Topical Conference, Cleveland, Ohio

133. van Uijen CMJ, den Boef JH (1984) Driven equilibrium radiofrequency pulses in NMR imaging. Mag Res Med 1: 502-507

134. Utz JA, Herfkens MD, Glover G, Pelc N (1986) Three second clinical NMR images using a gradient recall aquisition in a steady state mode (GRASS). Mag Res Imag 4: 106

135. Waluch V, Bradley WG (1984) NMR even echo rephasing in slow laminar flow. J Comp Assist Tomogr 8 (4): 594-598

136. Weber H, Purdy D, Deimling M, Oppelt A (1986) Contrast behaviour of the fast imaging sequences FLASH and FISP. Results from synthetic images. Society of Magnetic Resonance in Medicine. Fifth Annual Meeting, Montreal, Book of Abstracts. vol 3, p 957-958

137. Wehrli FW, MacFall JP, Newton TH (1983) Parameters determining the appearance of NMR imaging. In: Newton TH, Potts DG (ed) Advanced imaging techniques. Modern Neuroradiology, vol 2, p 81-117, San Anselmo (CA)

138. Wehrli FW, MacFall JR, Glover GH, Grigsby N, Haughton V, Johanson J (1984) The dependence of nuclear magnetic resonance image contrast on intrinsic and pulse sequence timing parameters. Mag Res Imag 2: 3-16

139. Weinmann H-J, Brash RC, Press W-R, Wesbey GE (1984) Characteristics of Gadolinium-DTPA complex, a potential NMR contrast agent. AJR 142: 619-624

140. Weinmann H-J, Laniado M, Mützel W (1984) Pharmakokinetics of GdDTPA/dimeglumine after intravenous injection into healthy volunteers. Physiol Chem Phys Med NMR 16: 167-172

141. Wolf W, Albright MJ, Silver MS, Weber H, Reichardt U, Sauer R (1987) Fluorine-19 spectroscopic studies of the metabolism of 5-fluorouracil in the liver of patients undergoing chemotherapy. Mag Res Imag 5 (3): 165-169

142. Wood ML, Henkelman RM (1986) The magnetic field dependence of the breathing artifact. Mag Res Imag 4: 387-392

143. Zimmermann BH, Löffler W, Makow L (1986) Influence of magnetic field strength on image contrasts. Diagn Imag Clin Med 55: 52-54

2 Normal Anatomy of the Central Nervous System

G. GADEMANN

2.1 Orientation

2.1.1 Organization of the Atlas

Because MR images are not confined to a specific plane as in CT, the atlas portion of the text does not follow a sectional format along the principal body axes, but is arranged more according to topographic and functional criteria. It covers the CNS in a descending hierarchy, beginning with the cerebral cortex and subcortical tracts and proceeding to the diencephalon, midbrain, the systems of the posterior fossa, and finally to the spinal cord (see midsagittal scan in Fig. 2.1). In this respect the atlas is organized more closely along the lines of an anatomy textbook than a clinical atlas. Brain areas are depicted in the sectional anatomy of different projections to provide a practice-oriented guide. Because the CSF spaces are important for orientation during diagnosis, they are dealt with in the introductory section.

Each section begins with a three-dimensional survey consisting of a midsagittal and an axial cut through a MR data cube [28] and accompanied by explanatory text. The anatomy of all important brain structures in the MR image is described, taking note of their clinical significance and contrast features. The illustrative MR scans were obtained using various techniques. Drawings of the principal functional tracts in the image are provided to illustrate neuroanatomic relationships and to aid in understanding the major neurologic symptoms presented in Chap. 4 [15, 39].

Most of the CNS images were made in a healthy 32-year-old male using a 1.0-T scanner. Unless otherwise stated, the slice thickness is 6 mm. The guidelines for positioning are outlined below and are explained in detail in Chap. 3. The imaging parameters are given for each scan, and data on the location of the scan are stated in terms of the coordinate system used. Atlases of topographic and sectional anatomy were used as references [19, 23, 33, 34, 42, 45, 48, 49, 54, 56, 61]. References to the figures within the text obviate the need for separate detailed legends.

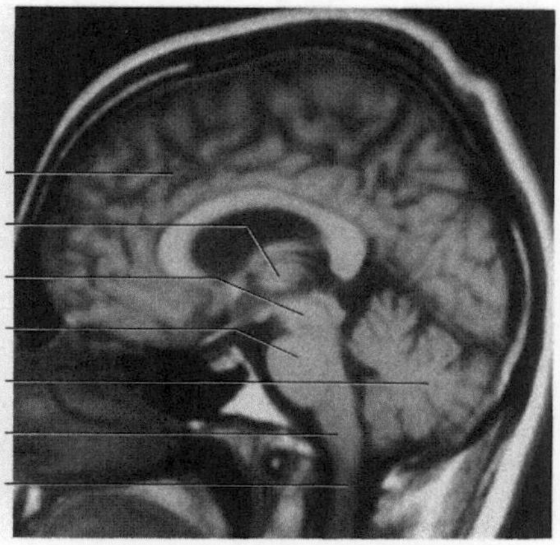

Fig. 2.1. Subdivision of the brain in a midsagittal MR image (SE, TR 0.6 s/TE 17 ms)

2.1.2 Coordinate Systems for the Central Nervous System

Any study of sectional anatomy requires the use of a reproducible orientation system. The ontogenic precursor of the CNS, the neural tube, displays a segmental arrangement which in itself provides a basis for orientation. Especially in a topographic sense, the vertebral bodies of the spinal column form the unit of reference for the nervous tissues of the spinal cord [47]. The sagittal section provides a general view that is not affected by the lordotic curvature of the lumbar spine or the kyphotic curvature of the thorax (Fig. 2.2). The orthogonal scan for evaluating the emerging nerves is made on the axial plane, parallel to the upper surfaces of the vertebral bodies. The functional-neurologic organization makes allowance for the ascent of the spinal cord with growth (see Sect. 2.9).

As the nervous system develops, the primitive neural tube becomes angled forward at its upper

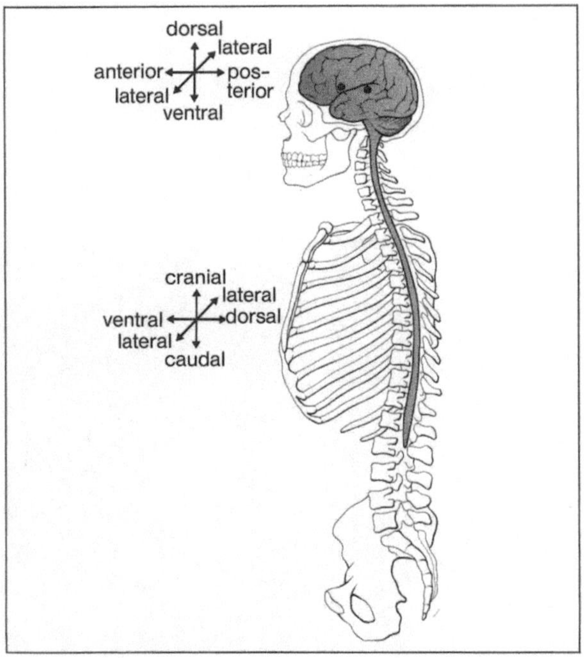

Fig. 2.2. Orientation systems of the spinal cord and the brain

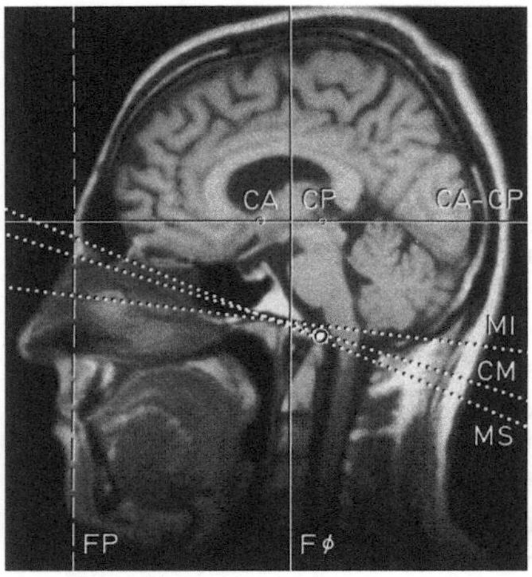

Fig. 2.3. Horizontal reference planes *(dotted lines)* and the basic reference planes of the CA-CP system in a midsagittal MR image (TR 0.6 s/TE 17 ms). *CA*, anterior commissure; *CP*, posterior commissure; *MI*, meatoinfraorbital plane; *CM*, canthomeatal plane; *MS*, meatosupraorbital plane; *FP*, facial plane

end, and so a separate coordinate system must bei applied to it (Fig. 2.2). The structures cranial to the midbrain no longer follow the craniocaudal direction, but assume an essentially anteroposterior (ventrodorsal) orientation. The brain lies posterocranial to the facial skull and is enclosed by the bony cranium, whose floor is formed by the three paired cranial fossae. The main directions of growth of the cerebrum - anteroposterior and lateral - reflect the fundamental importance of axial sections for diagnosis. Owing to the mobility of the head, however, we can define a great many axial planes of varying inclination. Traditionally, the bony structures of the skull have formed the basis for orientation, and the following reference planes have been widely used, especially in CT (Fig. 2.3) [34]:

1. The *meatosupraorbital* plane through the supraorbital margins and external auditory canals. Its course roughly parallels the skull base.
2. The *canthomeatal* plane through the canthi of the eyes and the external auditory canals. It is commonly used for positioning in CT and shows approximately 10° - 15° of dorsiflexion relative to the meatosupraorbital plane.
3. The *meatoinfraorbital* plane, called also Reid's plane or the Frankfurt horizontal. It corresponds most closely to the horizontal plane in the standing posture and has long played a part in anatomic studies of the brain [51].

MR imaging is the first soft tissue imaging modality that is capable of demonstrating very fine brain structures with high degrees of contrast. The reproducible visualization of such fine structures frequently enables the radiologist to make a more accurate diagnosis than with CT. However, this requires the use of a brain-based coordinate system which shows less interindividual variation than the orientation systems based on osseous structures [5, 20]. Brain-based reference systems of this kind have been used in stereotactic surgery for many years (see [51] for a brief historical review and further bibliographic references). Similar systems must be utilized in MR imaging.

The CA-CP-System

The stereotactic coordinate system upon which Schaltenbrand and Wahren based their stereotactic atlas of the brain [50] provides the orientation system for the MR images presented in this book. It is based on the position of the anterior commissure (CA) and the posterior commissure (CP). Both are small commissural tracts which cross the midsagittal plane at anatomically well-defined locations (Fig. 2.3). They are readily identified on T1-weighted midsagittal scans as rounded structures of high signal intensity. The anterior commissure passes caudal to the anterior (rostral) end of the genu of the corpus callosum, and the posterior commissure passes just cranial to the quadrigeminal plate. The line connecting the commissures, called the CA-CP line, lies on the midsagittal plane of the brain and also defines the axial plane perpendicular to the midsagittal, the intercommissural plane (Fig. 2.4). The inclination of that plane is usually between that of the canthomeatal and infraorbitomeatal planes. The coronal midcommissural plane bisects the CA-CP line and is oriented at right angles to the midsagittal and intercommissural planes. These three "basic reference planes," designated S0, F0, and H0, intersect at the origin of the coordinate system, which is the midpoint of the CA-CP line. Accordingly, the nomenclature for parallel planes of section uses the prefix "S" for sagittal, "F" for coronal (frontal), and "H" for axial (horizontal, transverse). Distances from the basic reference planes are stated in millimeters and are preceded by a lowercase letter: "l" denoting distance lateral to S0, "a" or "p" denoting distance anterior or posterior to F0, and "v" or "d" denoting distance ventral (caudal) or dorsal (cranial) to H0. Thus, for example, "F" p 16" designates the coronal plane located 16 mm posterior to the basic reference plane F0. The constancy of the coordinate system is greatest in the central brain regions. The variations in the coordinates of the major basal centers are listed in the appendix of the stereotactic atlas cited above [50]. Individual variations tend to be greatest in the region of the cerebral cortex.

2.1.3 Ventricular System

Imaging of the ventricular system permits the evaluation of circumscribed and diffuse areas of brain atrophy and gives information on space-occupying lesions and disturbances of CSF dynamics. Aside from minor individual variations, the internal CSF cavities of the brain show remarkable consistency in structure and thus provide useful primary landmarks for the positioning and localization of image planes [23]. Their general anatomic features are described below; details are given in the sections dealing with specific brain regions.

Each of the paired lateral ventricles is situated within a cerebral hemisphere, lateral to the arched corpus callosum. The frontal (anterior) horn projects forward into the frontal lobe and is continuous posteriorly with the central part of the ventricle and the trigone. From there the occipital (posterior)

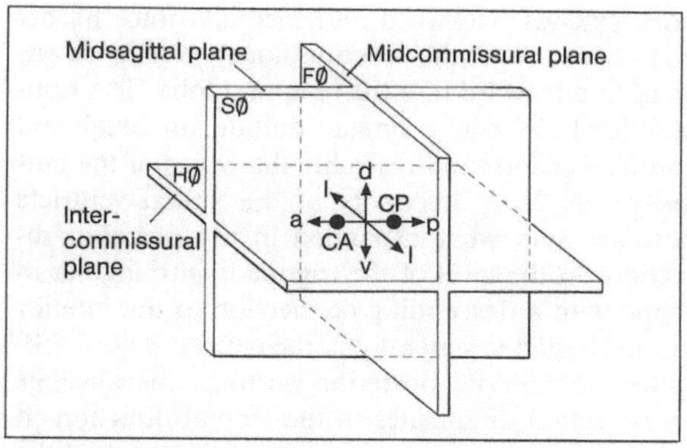

Fig. 2.4. Diagram of the CA-CP system: the three basic reference planes and their relation of the anterior *(CA)* and posterior *(CP)* commissures

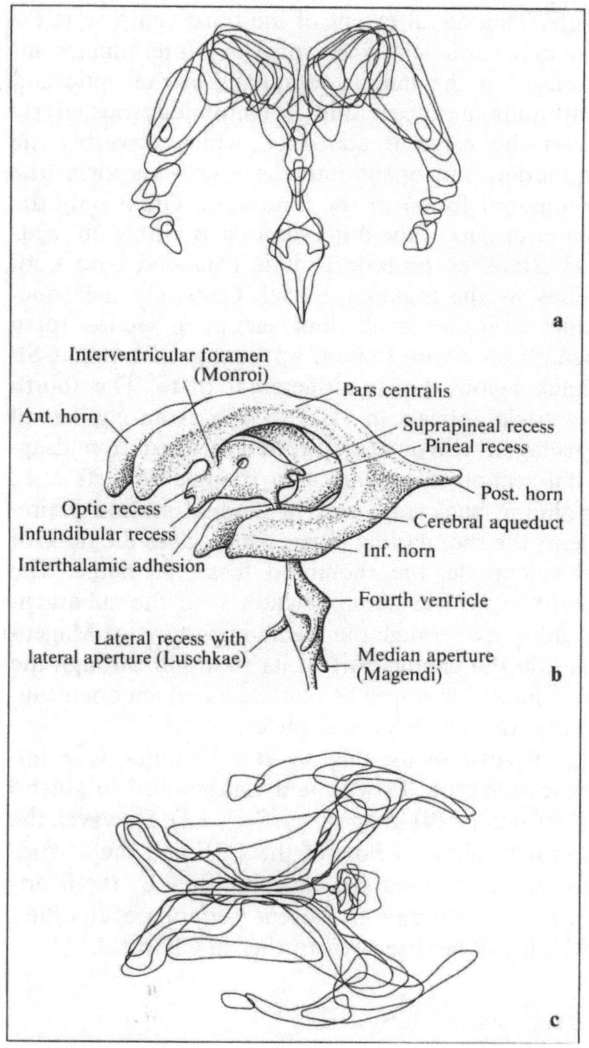

Fig. 2.5 a–c. The ventricular system: anatomic diagram (**b**), coronal (**a**) and axial (**c**) projections

horn extends backward and medially into the occipital lobe, and the inferior horn extends downward and forward into the temporal lobe. The frontal horns present a similar outline on axial and coronal sections and resemble the wings of the butterfly (Fig. 2.5). The cavity of the lateral ventricle becomes somewhat expanded in the posterior direction. At the level of the trigone it is triangular in shape with a descending connection to the inferior horn. The latter generally is recognizable as a CSF space only in its posterior portions, because its cross section diminishes in the frontal direction. It extends, however, into the region of the trunk of the parahippocampal gyrus. The lateral ventricles communicate with the unpaired third ventricle through the interventricular foramina (of Monro), which lies only a few millimeters above the anterior commissure. The lateral extent of the third ventricle is extremely variable (1.5–8.5 mm) [50]. It terminates anteriorly at the lamina terminalis in the optic and infundibular recess and is continuous posteriorly with the cerebral aqueduct, which traverses the midbrain and opens into the fourth ventricle (the rhomboid fossa) in the hindbrain. Often only the anterior part of the third ventricle is visible on sagittal scans, as posteriorly it is constricted on both sides by the thalamic nuclei. Generally the aqueduct is visible in all three planes of section for a length of about 15 mm, appearing as a thin CSF track below the quadrigeminal plate. The fourth ventricle appears in axial section as an equilateral pentagon with its apex directed forward. In midsagittal section it appears as a triangle with its apex pointing backward, and in coronal section it presents the rhomboidal shape which gives the floor of the ventricle, the rhomboid fossa, its name. The fourth ventricle communicates with the subarachnoid space through the median aperture (of Magendie) in the caudal part of its roof and through the two lateral apertures (of Luschka), which open caudal to the cerebellar peduncles.

Because of its long T1 and T2 times, CSF appears dark on T1-weighted images and bright on T2-weighted SE images (see Sect. 1.3). However, the caudally directed flow of the CSF and the to-and-fro movements imposed on that flow by the heartbeat and respiration present certain peculiarities, which will be discussed further in Chap. 5.3.

2.1.4 Functional Systems

An accurate knowledge of the neural pathways and major relay centers in the caudal and central portions of the brain can enhance our ability to recognize pathologic change. An important advantage of MR is its ability to demonstrate brain areas with high contrast and in topographically and functionally favorable projections in a way that no other modality can accomplish. A comparison of the major afferent and efferent systems on the one hand and their disease manifestations on the other should give us an appreciation of functional neuroanatomy that will enable us to examine selectively the presumptive site of disease on the basis of presenting symptoms [5]. Table 4.2 correlates symptoms with localizations and refers the reader to the corresponding sections on functional anatomy. To illustrate topographic relationships, we have indicated the major functional systems in different colors on representative IR images. Our principal source was the neuroanatomy text of Kretschmann [34] as well as the atlases named above. The following color coding system is employed:

- Red: pyramidal motor system
- Blue: sensory systems
- Violet: extrapyramidal system
- Yellow: optical system
- Green: acoustic system

The functional structure of the CNS is hierarchical, with phylogenetically younger areas monitoring and directing older ones. The spinal cord, which develops from the neural tube, consists mainly of long fiber tracts of dendrites, which conduct central nervous impulses to the periphery (motor activity) and carry peripheral information to the center (sensory activity). These tracts occupy the outer layers of the spinal cord and surround the cellular gray matter, which appears butterfly-shaped on axial section (Sect. 2.9).

The principal regions of the brain arise during embryonic development from the primary cerebral vesicles at the cranial end of the neural tube (see also Chap. 7) [47]. A proliferation of cells (gray matter) takes place in the medulla oblongata and pontine area. These cells constitute important relay centers and produce marked changes in the pattern of gray and white matter in relation to the cord (Sect. 2.5). In the midbrain the tracts again separate from the nuclei, with the cellular components (midbrain nuclei) moving more toward the periphery and the fiber tracts coursing medially (Sect. 2.4). This reversal in the disposition of gray and white matter finds its ultimate expression in the cerebral hemispheres (Sect. 2.2). MR can demonstrate with extreme clarity the cellular gray matter that lines the gyri, as well as the white matter tracts, which consist of ipsilateral association tracts and transverse commissural tracts. These white matter tracts are responsible for the internal communication among the various functional centers of the cerebrum (Sect. 2.2).

Long ascending and descending tracts, including the cranial nerves, establish contact between the sensory organs and motor systems, thus creating a link between the organism and its environment (Fig. 2.6). The farther peripheral a lesion is located, the more pronounced its neuropathologic correlate. Cortical or subcortical lesions are typically associated with whole symptom complexes, making topical diagnosis difficult.

Anatomically, the sensory and motor functional systems tend to follow the cardinal axes of the coordinate system. In coronal section F p 6 (and back to about F p 24), we recognize important fiber tracts of the pyramidal motor (red) and sensory (blue) systems. They can be traced bilaterally through the medulla oblongata, pons, and midbrain (see Sects. 2.4 and 2.5). All tracts enter the diencephalon through the cerebral crura (Sect. 2.3). While the sensory fibers pass first through thalamic relay nuclei and then through the internal capsule and corona radiata before reaching their projection areas in the postcentral gyrus, the pyramidal motor tracts project directly to the motor area in the precentral gyrus (Sect. 2.2).

The optical system (yellow) takes an anteroposterior course, which can be followed almost completely in an axial section at H v 6 inclined about 12°-15° from the horizontal (Sect. 2.6). These fibers, too, are relayed through an area in the posterior region of the thalamus, the lateral geniculate body.

The lateral course of the acoustic system (green) appears on coronal sections at about F p 12

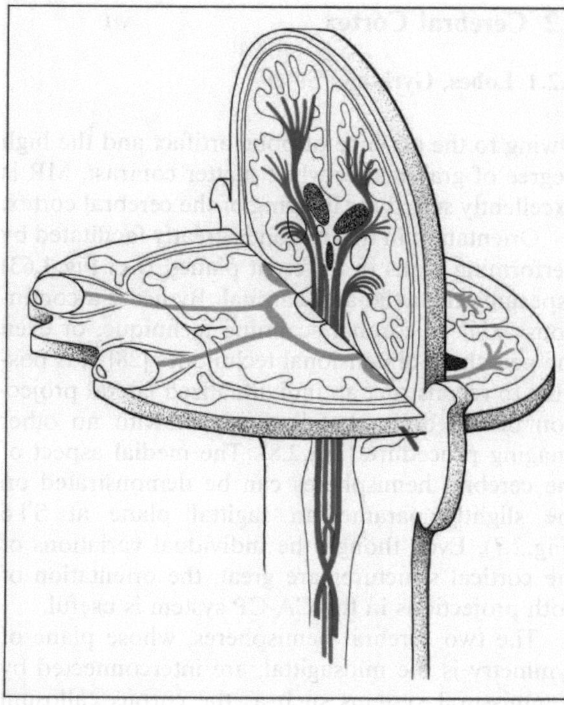

Fig. 2.6. Schematic axial and coronal sectional view of the main functional pathways: *red*, motoric; *blue*, sensoric; *yellow*, optic; *green*, acoustic

(Sect. 2.7). Again, the dendrites are relayed through a thalamic nucleus, the medial geniculate body, before reaching the primary acoustic center in the temporal lobe.

Thus, the thalamus represents an important relay station for all afferent pathways except the olfactory fibers. Its central location in the brain is consistent with this function, which is especially concerned with the filtering of incoming signals. The origin of the coordinate system is usually located in the anterior third of the thalamus.

2.2 Cerebral Cortex

2.2.1 Lobes, Gyri, and Sulci

Owing to the absence of bone artifact and the high degree of gray matter-white matter contrast, MR is excellently suited for imaging of the cerebral cortex.

Orientation in this region is greatly facilitated by performing scans in different planes, (i.e. Fig. 1.63) especially the axial and coronal. By using a continuous axial or coronal scanning technique, or even the new three-dimensional techniques [28], it is possible to reconstruct an individualized lateral projection of the brain that is available with no other imaging procedure (Fig. 2.8). The medial aspect of the cerebral hemispheres can be demonstrated on the slightly paramedian sagittal plane at S 16 (Fig. 2.7). Even though the individual variations of the cortical structures are great, the orientation of both projections in the CA-CP system is useful.

The two cerebral hemispheres, whose plane of symmetry is the midsagittal, are interconnected by commissural systems such as the corpus callosum and the anterior and posterior commissures. Each hemisphere is subdivided into four lobes, most of which are separated from one another by sulci that are consistently present from one individual to the next. The lobes are composed of "primary gyri" and "primary sulci," which differ from the secondary gyri and sulci in their relative constancy.

Frontal Lobe

The frontal lobe lies in the anterior fossa and consists mainly of three large frontal convolutions (frontal gyri) situated one above the other as well as orbital convolutions (orbital gyri) overlying the orbital roof. The frontal gyri course anterioposteriorly between the frontal pole and the precentral gyrus, which extends laterally downward as the primary projection area of the motor cortex (Fig. 2.9). The caudally situated inferior frontal gyrus contains its characteristic pars triangularis and pars opercularis, which flank the ascending ramus of the lateral sulcus. Because of the anteroposterior course of the frontal lobe gyri, the coronal plane of section is best suited for displaying the cortical structures. Axial scans are best for demonstrating the frontal pole.

Paracentral Region

Between the frontal lobe and parietal lobe, whose gyri are oriented along the brain axis, is an area called the paracentral lobule. It consists of two transverse gyri separated by the central sulcus. The precentral gyrus is assigned to the frontal lobe, and the postcentral gyrus to the parietal lobe. They are bounded anteriorly and posteriorly by the precentral sulcus and postcentral sulcus, respectively. Usually the precentral and postcentral sulci are

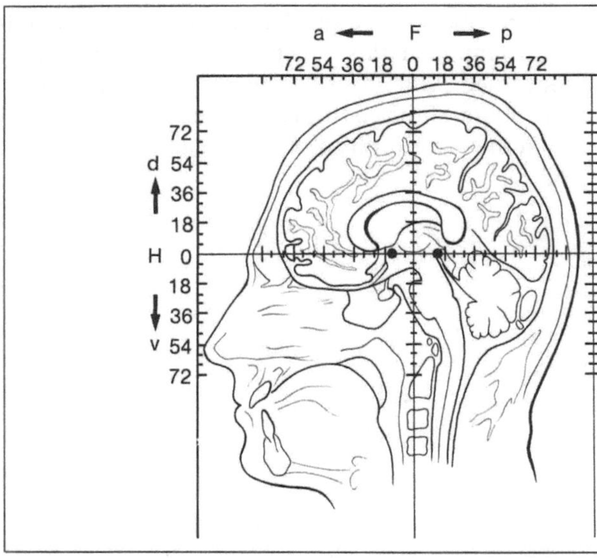

Fig. 2.7. Medial aspect of brain according to CA-CP system

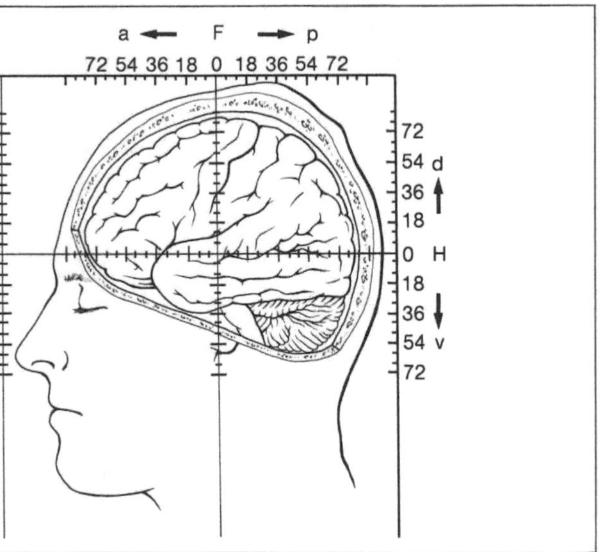

Fig. 2.8. Lateral aspect of cortex according to CA-CP system

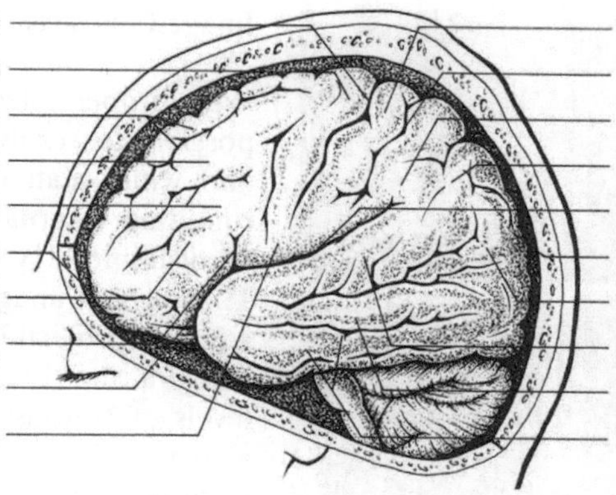

Fig. 2.9. Basic anatomy of lobes, gyri, and sulci in a reconstructed lateral view of the brain

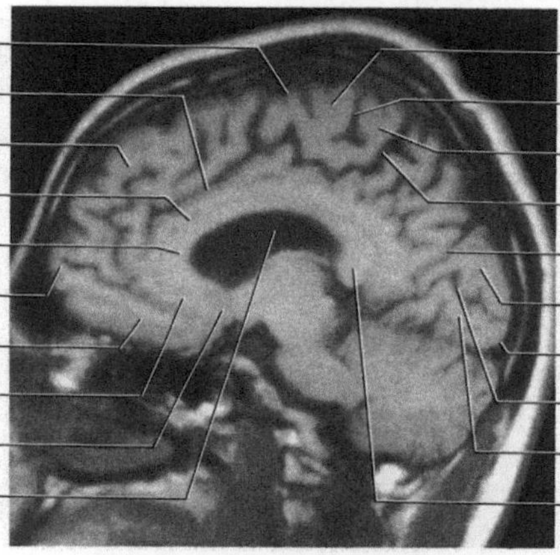

Fig. 2.10. Basic anatomy of lobes, gyri, and sulci in a sagittal MR image S l 6 (SE, TR 0.6 s/TE 17 ms)

much more conspicuous on midsagittal scans than the central sulcus itself. Often a connection is seen between the postcentral sulcus and the cingulate sulcus, which turns upward at about the level of the thalamus (pars marginalis of cingulate sulcus). The pars marginalis is posterior to the upper extremity of the central sulcus. The coronal basic reference plane F0 intersects the central sulcus about halfway up on a lateral projection of the brain (Fig. 2.8). Axial sections between the lateral sulcus and the middle of the central sulcus (from about H d 12 to H d 42) afford the best view of the precentral lobule.

Parietal and Occipital Lobes

The parietal and occipital lobes are separated by the parieto-occipital sulcus, which is best seen on the midsagittal plane (Fig. 2.10). This sulcus forms the boundary between the precuneus anteriorly and the cuneus posteriorly. The gyral pattern of the parietal and occipital lobes is less uniform than in the frontal lobe. However, one usually can recognize the intraparietal sulcus (Fig. 2.9) which extends posterioinferiorly across the parietal lobe, dividing it into superior and inferior lobules. An important landmark on the midsagittal section (Fig. 2.10) is the calcarine sulcus, which is surrounded by the primary visual cortex, the striate area. The calcarine sulcus extends forward from the occipital pole and, together with the parieto-occipital sulcus, forms the boundaries of the cuneus. The midsagittal section demonstrates this most clearly. The high parietal region is seen best on coronal scans, although it is usually difficult to distinguish the precentral and postcentral areas because of the relative obliquity of the scan. The occipital lobe and the posterior part of the parietal lobe are best evaluated on axial and coronal scans.

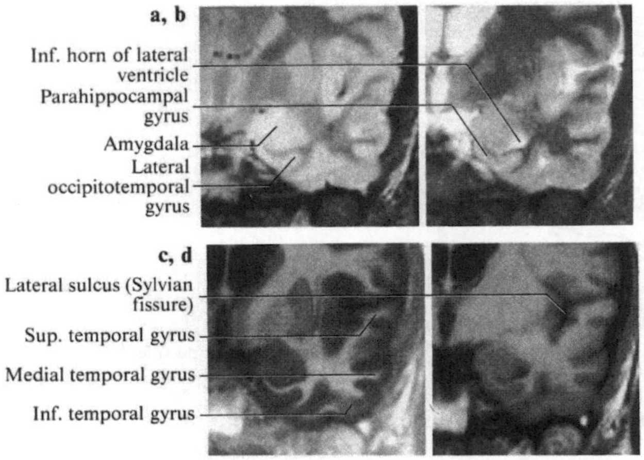

Fig. 2.11 a–d. Image contrast of cortical structures. Coronal section F a 6 of the temporal lobe. **a** N(H) weighted (SE, TR 2.4 s/TE 35 ms); **b** T2 weighted (SE, TR 2.4 s/TE 105 ms); **c** T1 weighted (IR, TR 1.5 s/TI 0.350 s); **d** T1 weighted (SE, TR 0.6 s/TE 17 ms)

Temporal Lobe

The formation of the temporal lobe through a reversal of growth from posterior to anterior is apparent in the supramarginal gyrus and adjacent angular gyrus at the junction of the temporal and parietal lobes. On the lateral projecton (Fig. 2.9) these gyri appear as strongly curved features at the posterior extremity of the lateral sulcus and superior temporal sulcus. The temporal lobe is divided into three large, lateral convolutions termed the superior, medial, and inferior temporal gyri, which are separated by the superior and inferior temporal sulci. The longitudinal gyral pattern is continued on the floor of the middle fossa. The lateral and medial occipitotemporal gyri are not visualized on the lateral projection; they and the parahippocampal gyrus that adjoins them medially are best appreciated on coronal sections (e.g., Fig. 2.11). A prominent feature in the dorsomedial part of the temporal pole is the amygdaloid body, which forms a conspicuous snail-like structure lateral to the uncus of the parahippocampal gyrus. Usually it appears in close relation to the flat inferior horn of the lateral ventricle. The junction of the temporal lobe with the frontal and parietal lobes is called the insula. Its whole extent is best appreciated on sagittal scans (e.g., S 1 42). As a rule, coronal scans are best for imaging the temporal lobe [40], with axial or sagittal scans added to evaluate the temporal pole.

Image Contrasts

With proper selection of the pulse sequence, it is possible to resolve the junction between the gray and white matter of the cerebral cortex, the surrounding external CSF spaces, and the numerous cortical blood vessels (see also Sect. 1.3). Slightly T2-weighted images are excellent for reconstructing a lateral projection and can be obtained quickly by using a multislice technique (Fig. 2.12b). Higher levels of contrast are seen on T1-weighted IR images (Fig. 2.11c), which closely resemble anatomic sections, and in SE sequences with a short repetition time TR and very short echo time TE (Fig. 2.11d). Spin-density SE images (Fig. 2.11a) provide good gray matter-white matter contrast and give a clear picture of superficial blood vessels (see Section 2.8). So far MR has not been useful for evaluating the laminar structure of the cortex (e.g., in congenital anomalies). There is reason to hope that progress can be made in this area through use of the IR technique and higher magnification, but the relatively long imaging times place limits on the overall visualization of the cerebral cortex with IR sequences.

2.2.2 Functional Anatomy

Functional System and Their Primary Projection Areas

A knowledge of the cerebral cortical structures and their exact location on MR images, made possible by the reconstruction of lateral views, has an important bearing on clinical topologic diagnosis as well as on research into functional relationships [46].

The cerebral cortex is at the top of the functional hierarchy of the CNS. It contains the primary projection centers for all sensory information and motor activity. A major sensory system can be assigned to each lobe. Impulses arising in the precentral gyrus of the frontal lobe are relayed through the pyramidal tracts to the peripheral *motor system* (the pyramidal system). These tracts and the frontal lobe are shown in red.

The postcentral gyrus of the parietal lobe is the primary projection area for almost all *sensations* (including the sense of taste), which are carried from the limbs, trunk, and head to the thalamus by the medial lemniscus or anterolateral system. These systems and the parietal lobe are shown in blue.

The most important of the human senses, *vision,* has as its projection area in the gray cells that surround the calcarine sulcus in the occipital lobe (the striate area). From there, association fibers branch to the neighboring secondary areas and finally to the temporal lobe. The optical system and the occipital lobe are shown in yellow.

The *acoustic system* terminates in a primary area located in the dorsal part of the superior temporal sulcus. This functional system is shown in green, as is the temporal lobe.

Secondary projection areas usually surround the primary areas in a concentric fashion, become intermingled, and form higher-order regions that unite several sensory modalites, such as the reading and writing center or the sensory and motor speech area. The commissural tracts and association tracts link these tertiary and quaternary areas with higher centers located in the superior temporal sulcus and the frontal lobe (Fig. 2.12). There, it is believed, originate the impulses for voluntary movement, which then are carried to the periphery through the adjacent motor cortex and pyramidal system. This completes the "circuit" of the central nervous control system. Generally one hemisphere is dominant (usually the left hemisphere, in right-handed persons), and injury to the dominant hemisphere will cause much more pronounced deficits than injury to the nondominant side.

The *sense of smell* occupies a special place among the human senses. The olfactory system in man has a very archaic structure. Its tracts bypass the thalamus and course directly to the limbic system, which includes central cortical areas such as portions of the subcallosal area, cingulate gyrus, indusium griseum, and hippocampal cortex, as well as the septum pellucidum, fornix, amygdaloid body, and nuclei of the hypothalamus and thalamus. Its functional significance is not fully understood. It is believed to be responsible for strongly emotional states of behavior that are accompanied by characteristic autonomic responses. The affective component of olfaction is well known and relates to its direct connection with the limbic system. The limbic system is also thought to be important for short-term memory. The MR features of the limbic system, like its anatomy, are not uniform. The structures are very closely related to the phylogenetically older diencephalon and will be discussed further in Sect. 2.3. Atlas et al. [2] and Naidich et al. [40, 41] present MR images illustrating the neuroanatomy of the limbic system.

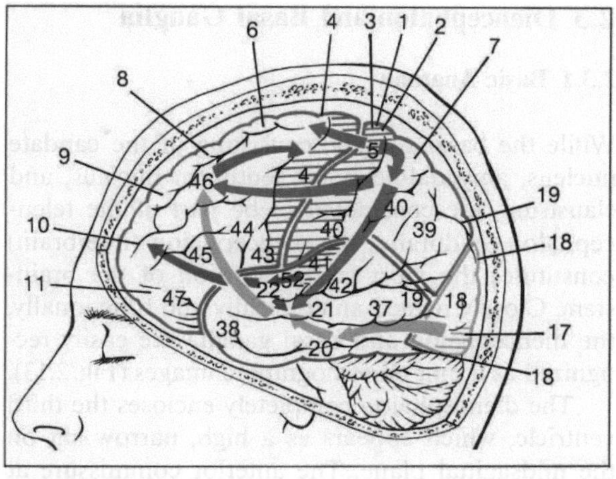

Fig. 2.12. Functional anatomy of the cortex. Brodmann areas and main association pathways in the lateral view

Brodmann Areas

As early as 1920, Brodmann (cited in [15]) found areas in the brain that exhibited diverse histologic structures, and he was able to assign different functions to them. The division into "Brodmann's areas," which are identified by arbitrary numbers, is still in use today. Figure 2.12 shows the location of the areas in medial and lateral projections of a cerebral hemisphere. The motor projection area belongs to Brodmann's area 4 in the precentral gyrus, and different parts of the body can be represented topically along its extent (motor homunculus). The lower limb is projected onto the vertex, while more proximal parts of the body are represented closer to the lateral sulcus. Brodmann's area 45, located in the pars triangularis of the inferior frontal gyrus, contains at least portions of the motor speech center (Broca's area). It lies in a tertiary area of the motor system close to the projection area for the tongue and adjacent to areas of the frontal lobe that are very closely related to thought. It projects approximately onto the coronal sections Fa 18–30 (cf. Fig. 2.7). The primary sensory region in the postcentral gyrus (Brodmann's areas 3, 1, 2) shows a similar pattern of somatotopic representation. The location of the sensory speech center (of Wernicke) in area 42 of the superior temporal sulcus indicates a close relation to facial sensation and to the primary acoustic cortex (41), thus giving it the function of a secondary acoustic center. Its approximate coordinates on the axial and coronal planes are H d 12 and F p 18. Table 4.2 shows the clinical symptoms that are associated with damage to specific Brodmann's areas.

2.3 Diencephalon and Basal Ganglia

2.3.1 Basic Anatomy

While the basal ganglia, consisting of the caudate nucleus, amygdaloid body, lentiform nucleus, and claustrum, are considered to be part of the telencephalon (endbrain), the diencephalon (interbrain) constitutes the most cranial portion of the brainstem. Closely related anatomically and functionally, the diencephalon and basal ganglia are easily recognized as a unit on tomographic images (Fig. 2.13).

The diencephalon completely encloses the third ventricle, which appears as a high, narrow slit on the midsagittal plane. The anterior commissure at its anterior end and the posterior commissure at its posterior end place it at the center of the coordinate system. The entire region extends anteroposteriorly from about F a 30 to F p 18, and ventrodorsally (craniocaudally) from H d 20 to H v 15. It is bounded anteriorly by the pituitary and behind by the pineal gland. The laterally situated basal ganglia project past these structures.

Midsagittal Section S0

The midsagittal section S0 (Fig. 2.14) is excellent for evaluating purely midline structures like the corpus callosum, third ventricle, pituitary, optic chiasm, and pineal gland. A thin section (<3 mm) will

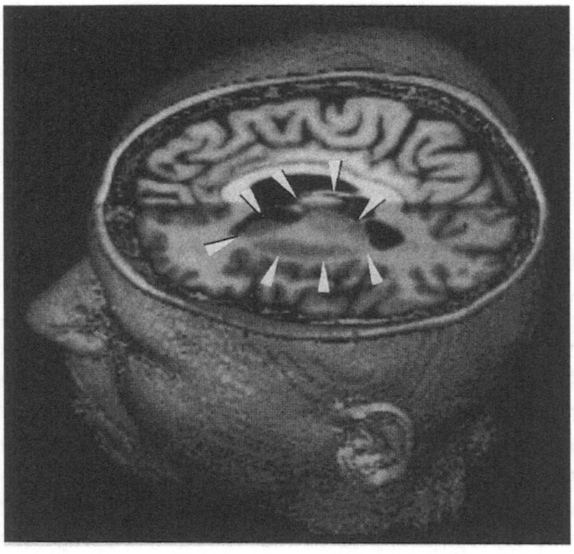

Fig. 2.13. Basic anatomy of the diencephalon and basal ganglia in a 3 D reconstruction (FLASH 40°)

demonstrate the recesses of the third ventricle without superimposing other structures (Fig. 2.17). These include the anterior infundibular and optic recesses, which point respectively in the direction of the pituitary stalk and the chiasm, and also the posterior suprapineal and pineal recesses. The third ventricle terminates at the inlet to the cerebral aqueduct. The corpus callosum, composed of white matter, forms the cranial (dorsal) boundary of the midbrain. It consists of a rostrum, genu, body, and posterior splenium. The width of the corpus callosum at its center is between 5 and 7.2 mm in healthy adults [55]. The septum pellucidum, which separates the frontal horns of the lateral ventricles, is visible in the anterior part of the diencephalon, but it usually exhibits partial volume effects with the ventricular cavities. The columns of the fornix appear to begin at the anterior commissure and pass over the centrally situated thalamus [41]. The posterior commissure is visible at the upper border of the quadrigeminal plate. The pineal gland often appears only as a faint structure in the quadrigeminal cistern, because the frequent calcifications give a low signal on MR images.

Axial Section H0

The axial basic reference plane H0 (Fig. 2.15) most clearly illustrates the topographic relations of the basal nuclei, the long tracts, and the ventricular system. The third ventricle presents medially as a slit-like cavity. The anterior commissure runs transversely in front of the columns of the fornix and the interventricular foramen (of Monro). The symmetrically arranged frontal horns are seen at this location. Posteriorly the third ventricle is separated from the quadrigeminal cistern in this plane by the posterior commissure and portions of the pineal gland. The thalamus adjoins the third ventricle on each side and restricts its lumen. Cranial (dorsal) nuclei of the hypothalamus appear in front of the thalamus. The internal capsule presents as a broad, V-shaped band of nerve fibers extending between the diencephalon and basal ganglia. Adjacent is the lens-shaped lentiform nucleus, which is divided into an internal part, the globus pallidus, and an external part, the putamen. Close relations exist between the putamen and the anteriorly situated caudate nucleus. The connection between them is interrupted only by the anterior limb of the internal capsule; the two areas are collectively termed the striatum. Analogous to the internal capsule, the fi-

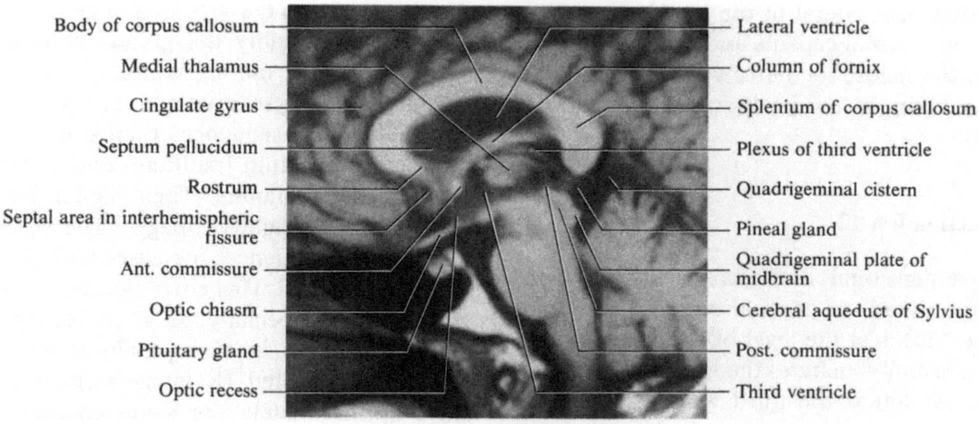

Fig. 2.14. Midsagittal section S0: diencephalic structures and basal ganglia (SE, TR 0.6 s/TE 17 ms)

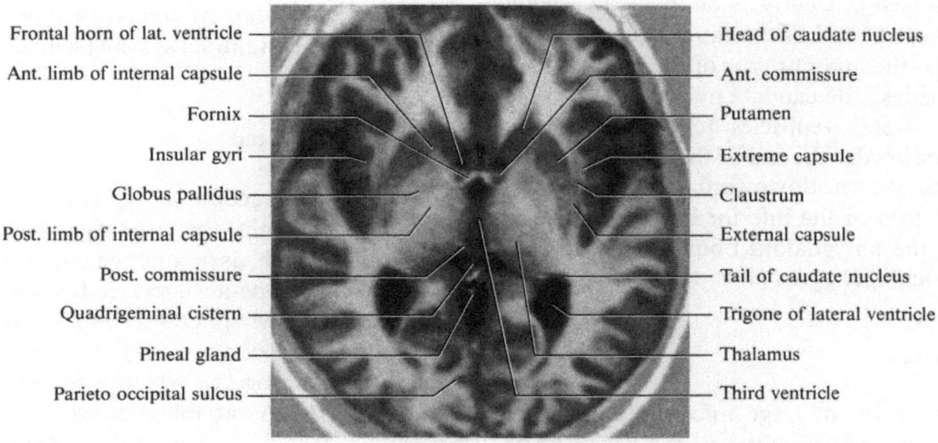

Fig. 2.15. Axial section H0 through the diencephalon and basal ganglia (IR, TR 1.5 s/TI 0.350 s)

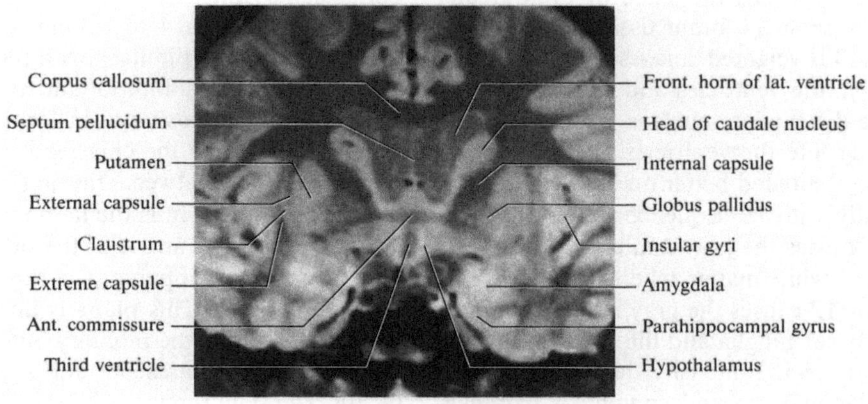

Fig. 2.16. Coronal section F a 12 through anterior portion of diencephalon and basal ganglia (SE, TR 2.4 s/TE 35 ms)

ber tracts that pass lateral to the lentiform nucleus are called the external capsule and extreme capsule, both of which enclose the narrow claustrum. At the site the basal ganglia are in direct contact with the insular gyri.

Coronal Section F a 12

The three-dimensional architecture of the region can be appreciated on coronal scans. The section F a 12 (Fig. 2.16) is at the level of the anterior commissure and usually includes the interventricular foramen. Below that is the third ventricle, which is surrounded in its anterior portions by hypothalamic nuclei. The internal capsule is displayed just anterior to its genu and forms a distinct medial boundary for the lentiform nucleus. The arrangement of the globus pallidus and putamen and their relation to the insula are seen as clearly as on the axial section H0 (Fig. 2.15). The head of the caudate nucleus presents medial to the anterior crus of the internal capsule on both sides. The caudate nucleus runs on the floor of the lateral ventricles to the trigone, at whose anterior border the tail of the nucleus can be seen (Fig. 2.15). It turns downward and forward and lies along the roof of the inferior horn, terminating bilaterally in the amygdaloid body at the hook of the parahippocampal gyrus [40].

Image Contrasts

The close proximity of large nuclei composed of gray matter of varying consistency, the broad white matter tracts, and the ventricular cavities gives excellent contrast when appropriate imaging sequences and parameters are employed. On spin-density images (e.g., Fig. 2.16) or heavily T2-weighted images, the CSF has the same or even greater signal intensity than the brain tissue. CSF gives a low signal on T1-weighted images (e.g., Fig. 2.14). Generally, then, the ventricles and closely adjacent structures like the caudate nucleus, as well as structures projecting into the ventricles like the choroid plexus, can be evaluated better on T1-weighted images. Especially with IR sequences (e.g., Fig. 2.15), T1 weighting causes the gray matter to appear less intense than the white matter, whereas weighting by spin density or T2 causes the gray matter to appear brighter. The basal ganglia and the thalamus do not show a uniform signal intensity due to differences in their cellular makeup and content of paramagnetic ions. A high iron concentration has been shown to exist in the gray matter of extrapyramidal nuclei, most notably the globus pallidus and the midbrain nuclei, the substantia nigra and the red nucleus [13]. These give a stronger signal in the T1-weighted IR sequences than other gray matter such as the striatum (pallidum and caudate nucleus) and the thalamus. Their signal intensity decreases in T2-weighted images. The signal loss on T2-weighted sequences increases with the magnetic field strength [14]. This corresponds to a shortening of the T1 and especially the T2 relaxation times due to local changes in susceptibilities (see Glossary) [22]. A T1-weighted IR image (e.g., Fig. 2.15) displays approximately the same contrasts of brain matter as one would find on anatomic sections. The T1-weighted SE sequence is markedly inferior in this regard to the IR sequence. The contrast between the basal ganglia and diencephalic nuclei provides a visual expression of the different stages of development and different functions that exist within the extrapyramidal system (see Sect. 2.3.5).

2.3.2 Pituitary Gland

The midsagittal section at S0 (Fig. 2.17) demonstrates the position of the pituitary gland within the sella turcica, which, as a bony structure, is not clearly imaged. The bone-air interface between the floor of the sella and the sphenoid sinus generally is not delineated. The dorsum sellae may yield a signal from the bone marrow, which also extends down along the clivus. A variable, flat area of high signal intensity is frequently seen on the sellar floor. Mark et al. [36] discussed whether this might represent fatty tissue; however, it is now believed to be the posterior lobe of the gland (see also Sect. 10.9). The pituitary gland appears as an oval structure of moderate signal intensity. The height of the normal gland ranges from 4 to 8.3 mm [36]. The narrow stalk connects the pituitary with the hypothalamus. The optic chiasm, an important structure in this region, is located above and in front of the pituitary stalk. It lies within the chiasmatic cistern. The fine connecting line between the anterior commissure and the optic chiasm is the lamina terminalis.

The cylindrical shape of the pituitary in the lateral direction is apparent on the coronal section F a 18 (Fig. 2.18). This plane is important not only for demonstrating the pituitary but also for evaluating the adjacent parasellar and suprasellar regions [9, 10]. The sella turcica is bounded laterally by the cavernous sinus and the internal carotid arteries;

lateral to the carotids and medial to Meckel's cavity are cranial nerves III–VI, which traverse the cavernous sinus at this level (see also Sect. 2.5). Thin-slice (<3 mm) high-resolution MR scans can delineate the oculomotor nerve (nerve III) lateral to the carotid artery, and below it the trochlear nerve (nerve IV) and the first division of the trigeminal (nerve V_1), which usually is indistinguishable from the abducens (nerve VI) [10]. A venous space of the cavernous sinus is usually visible between these nerves and nerve V_2. Proper angulation of the image plane will display the optic chiasm as a handle-shaped structure separated from the pituitary gland by the chiasmatic cistern. The diaphragma sellae appears as a thin plate of low signal intensity and normally presents a concave superior surface [31]. The pituitary stalk is generally demonstrated at this level and may even be imaged in its entirety. The close proximity of the vascular structures, CSF spaces, and cerebral soft tissues requires appropriate contrast, and this is best achieved on T1-weighted images [3]. Because the CSF gives a high signal on T2-weighted images, it is more difficult to distinguish from the soft tissue structures, although better contrast is seen relative to the blood vessels and bony structures.

2.3.3 Hypothalamus

The hypothalamic region (Fig. 2.19) is positioned anterior and caudal to the thalamus and is arranged symmetrically about the third ventricle. Generally it is superimposed over the third ventricle on sagittal sections, and the spatial arrangement of the structures is best appreciated on axial and coronal sections (Fig. 2.16). The hypothalamus extends forward to the anterior commissure, lamina terminalis, and optic chiasm. It is bounded laterally in part by the genu of the internal capsule. On axial section H v 6 (Fig. 2.19) the hypothalamus projects in front of the midbrain and is enclosed anteriorly by the optic tract [6]. The hypothalamic nuclei cannot be individually resolved with MR. The most anterior of the nuclei, the supraoptic and preoptic, are situated above the optic chiasm in the medial hypothalamic region. The mamillary bodies are the only hypothalamic nuclei that are clearly identifiable as separate structures in the sagittal plane (Fig. 2.17). They extend caudally into the basal cisterns and are considered part of the posterior and lateral nuclear groups. As in other regions, the IR technique appears to be the best for depicting the normal anatomy.

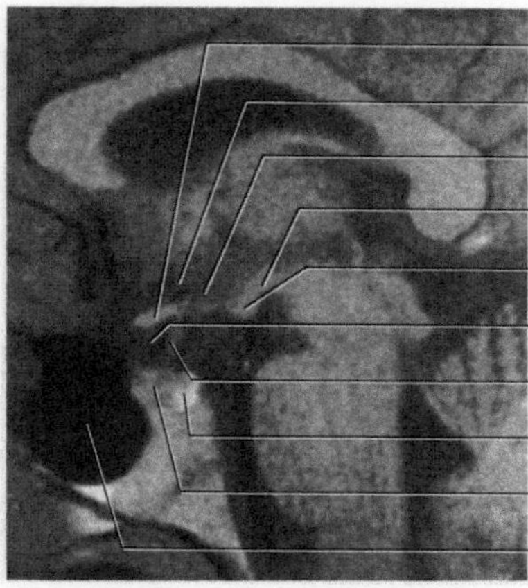

Fig. 2.17. Thin midsagittal section S0 through sella turcica (SE, TR 0.6 s/TE 10 ms, 3 mm)

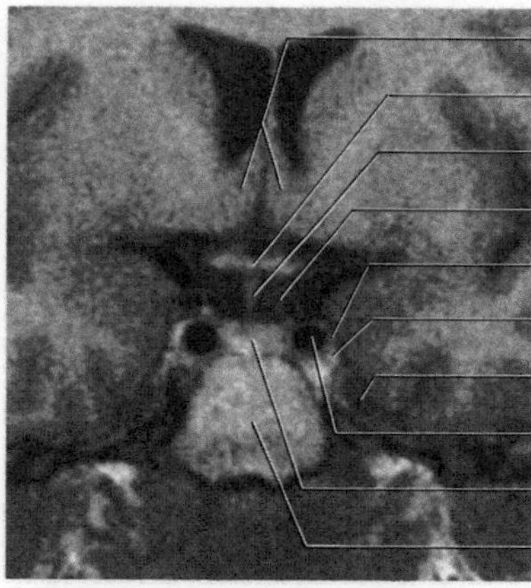

Fig. 2.18. Thin coronal section F a 18 through sella turcica (SE, TR 0.6 s/TE 10 ms, 3 mm)

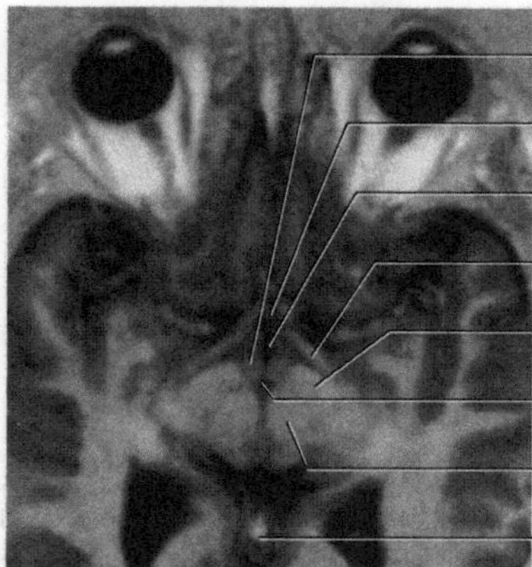

Fig. 2.19. Axial section H v 6 through hypothalamus (IR, TR 1.5 s/TI 0.350 s)

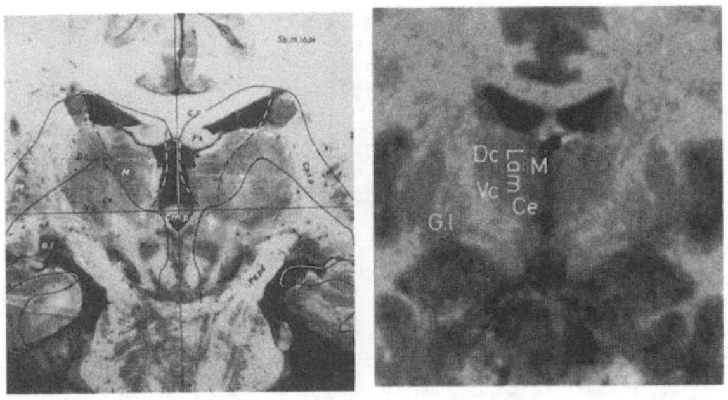

Fig. 2.20 a, b. Coronal section F a 6 through thalamus. **a** MR image (IR, TR 1.6 s/TI 400 ms, 4 mm); **b** anatomic section from stereotactical atlas of Schaltenbrand and Wahren [50]; *M*, medial nuclei; *Ce*, central nuclei; *Vc*, ventro caudal nuclei; *Dc*, posterior lateral nuclei; *Lam*, medial medullary lamella; *G.l*, lateral geniculate body

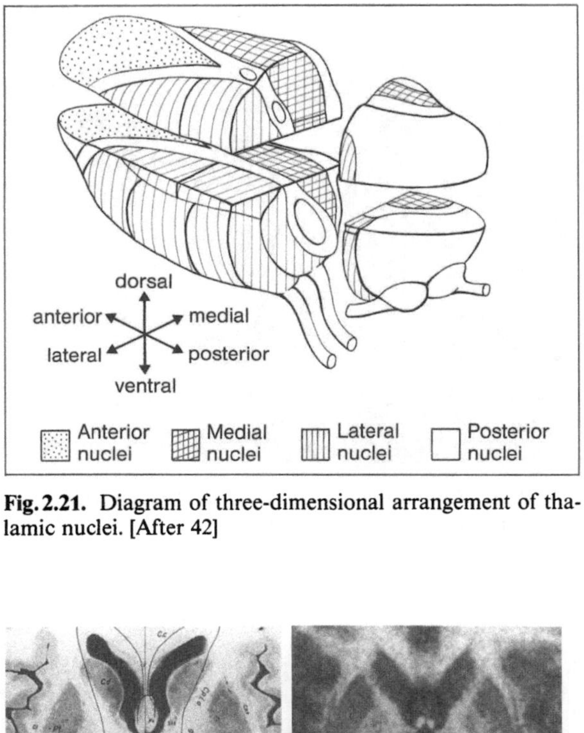

Fig. 2.21. Diagram of three-dimensional arrangement of thalamic nuclei. [After 42]

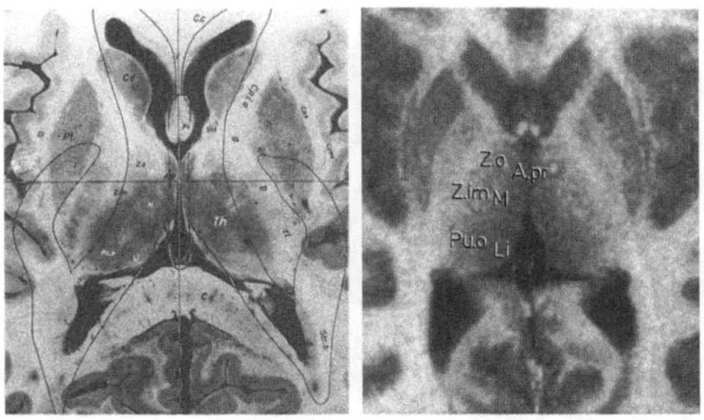

Fig. 2.22 a, b. Axial section H d 6 through thalamus **a** MR image (IR, TR 1.6 s/TI 400 ms, 4 mm); **b** anatomic section from stereotactical atlas of Schaltenbrand and Wahren [50]. *M*, medial nuclei; *Z.o*, centrolateral nucleus; *Z.im*, Intermediate centrolateral nucleus; *Pu.o*, oral pulvinar; *Li*, nucleus limitans; *A.pr*, anteroventral nucleus

2.3.4 Thalamus

The thalamus is the dominant structure of the interbrain. The paired, ovoid masses of the thalami flank the dorsal portion of the third ventricle, and usually are connected by a band called the interthalamic adhesion or "intermediate mass." The long axis of the thalamus is directed roughly parallel to the CA-CP line. The origin of the coordinate system lies within the thalamus, and hence the anatomy of this region is best appreciated on central coronal and axial sections (Figs. 2.20, 2.22). The spatial arrangement of the thalamic nuclei is shown diagramatically in Fig. 2.21 [after 42]. The anteroposterior extent of the thalamus is approximately 4 cm [42]. Being composed of gray matter, the nuclei of the thalamus contrast well with the tracts of the internal capsule. The internal medullary laminae of white matter also are easily recognized grossly and on high-resolution scans. The laminae divide the thalamus into three major parts - medial, lateral, and anterior corresponding to their position in the CA-CP system. These in turn are subdivided into many thalamic nuclei, which perform a variety of functions (Sect. 2.3.5). Scans usually will demonstrate the mamillothalamic tract, which passes upward to the anterior thalamic nuclei at the posterior border of the hypothalamus. High-resolution images are able to bring out the thalamic nuclei much as they appear in the stereotactic atlas [50]. Again, it is important to obtain thin sections that show good gray matter-white matter contrast. The best results are obtained with spin-density weighting or IR sequences.

2.3.5 Functional Anatomy

The basal ganglia and the diencephalon (interbrain) perform a variety of functional tasks in accordance with their central anatomic position. A knowledge of these functions is mainly useful in functional stereotaxy, and a detailed description would exceed the scope of this text. A good account may be found in the books by Netter [42], Duus [15], and Schaltenbrand [51].

The long fiber tracts of the motor system and of all sensory systems (except for the olfactory) pass through the *internal capsule*. The distribution of the individual fiber tract systems in the internal capsule can be appreciated on axial sections such as H0, which is pictured in Fig. 2.23. The corticonuclear (cranial nerves) tract (strippled red) and the corticospinal tract (red) course in the genu of the capsule and dorsal to it. Both tracts belong to the pyramidal system and present a somatotopic arrangement. Dorsal to them are the sensory fibers of the anterolateral and medial lemniscus systems (blue). Anterior and posterior to these sensorimotor pathways are the corticopontine tracts (violet) - the frontopontine tract anteriorly and the temporo-occipitopontine tract posteriorly. They have connections with the pons and medial parts of the cerebellum, their function being to coordinate and stabilize pyramidal and extrapyramidal motor activity. The acoustic radiation (green) and optic radiation (yellow) arise in the posterior end of the internal capsule and pass laterally and backward from it respectively. Portions of these long ascending and descending fiber tracts can be traced on the orthogonal coronal section F p 6 (Fig. 2.24), which gives an especially good view of the sensory thalamocortical tract (blue) ascending from the posterolateral ventral nucleus. Its primary field in the postcentral gyrus (areas 3, 1, 2) is projected below the corresponding motor (red) area (4).

The functions of the *thalamic nuclei* are diverse and closely interrelated, but the nuclei can be roughly classified as specific or nonspecific [15]. The anterior and medial nuclei are responsible for nonspecific tasks such as vigilance (medial nucleus and intralaminar nuclei), emotional behavior (paramedian regions), and short-term memory (anterior nucleus and dorsomedial nucleus). The lateral and posterior nuclei have specific functions as relay and filtering stations for all sensory and sensorimotor systems except for the olfactory pathways. All afferent tracts of the medial lemniscus and the anterolateral system are arranged somatotopically in the ventrolateral nuclei. That is the site of origin of the thalamocortical tract, which passes through the internal capsule into the postcentral gyrus (Fig. 2.24). Acoustic information is relayed in the medial geniculate body and carried by the acoustic radiation to the temporal lobe (Sect. 2.7). The lateral geniculate body is the thalamic relay station for optical information. The optic radiation passes from there to the primary visual areas in the occipital lobe (Sect. 2.6). The rest of the posterior nuclear region, consisting of the posterior lateral nucleus and the pulvinar, is associated with the functions of speech and vision, in accordance with its close proximity to the geniculate body.

The major cause of *thalamic symptoms* is cerebrovascular disease, most notably infarction [59] (see also Sect. 2.8). While a knowledge of thalamic functions is very important for certain stereotactic procedures [51], patients usually present clinically with a composite of various symptoms, since most lesions are not confined to individual nuclei [15]. Unilateral disorders of the anterior thalamic regions may be nonsymptomatic or may cause speech disturbances or impaired attentiveness. Akinesia can additionally result when bilateral lesions are present. Extrapyramidal symptoms like athetosis and chorea develop when the lesion spreads to involve the subthalamic region. Large or bilateral lesions of the medial thalamic nuclei can cause apathy or excitation, impaired wakefulness, or short-term memory loss. Lesions of the specific functional lateral thalamic regions are associated with sensory deficits, pain, and hemiataxia on the contralateral side. Lesions of the posterior region cause hemianesthesia, thalamic pain, and visual field defects.

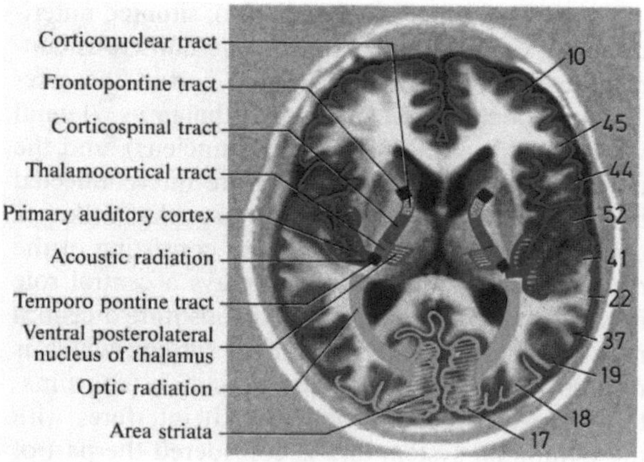

Fig. 2.23. Functional anatomy of diencephalon and basal ganglia in axial MR image H0 (IR, TR 1.5 s/TI 0.350 s)

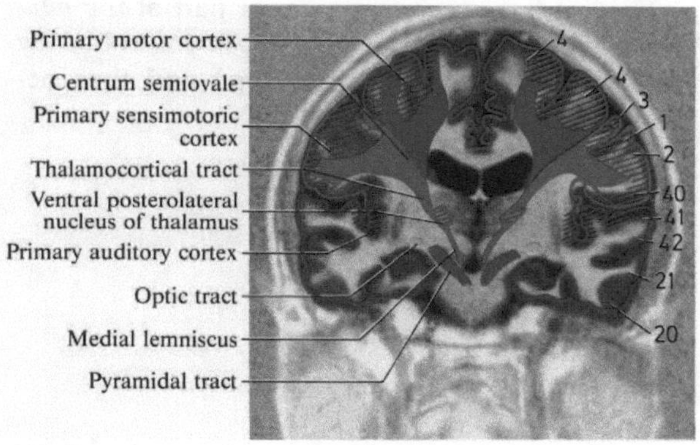

Fig. 2.24. Functional anatomy of diencephalon and basal ganglia in coronal MR image F p 6 (IR, TR 1.5 s/TI 0.350 s)

The *basal ganglia* (basal nuclei), situated anterior and lateral to the thalamus, have numerous connections with the motor endbrain cortex, the cerebellum (dentate nucleus), the thalamus (lateral ventral nucleus and intralaminar nucleus), and the midbrain nuclei. These regions are interconnected by several neuronal conduction arcs that follow a complicated course. The striatum, consisting of the caudate nucleus and putamen, plays a central role in this regard. The basal ganglia constitute a central relay point of the extrapyramidal system, which is responsible for the automatic execution (coordination) of learned motor activities. It interferes with the pyramidal system and is considered the part of the motor system that is chiefly controlled by the unconscious. Lesions of the basal ganglia are rarely discrete, and their effects are known collectively as "extrapyramidal symptoms" (see Tables 4.1, 4.2).

The hormone-secreting anterior part of the *pituitary gland,* the adenohypophysis, is controlled by neurotransmitters (releasing factors) and thus belongs to the endocrine system. The *neurohypophysis* and *hypothalamus,* on the other hand, form a very close neurologic functional unit. The hypothalamus sends connections to the midbrain (especially the posterior tegmentum), to the anteromedial thalamic region, and to the limbic system via the amygdaloid body. Equally important are its connections with the autonomic nuclei of the brainstem and spinal cord (e.g., the dorsal vagal nucleus). The hypothalamus is considered man's "internal clock," regulating a variety of circadian processes including the sleep-wake rhythm, the heat and water balance, and hunger and thirst.

Because of the smallness of the structures, hypothalamic symptoms usually occur in association with other deficits. Unilateral lesions are rarely symptomatic. Due to the age dependence of hypothalamic functions, lesions occurring at identical sites can produce different symptom complexes in different age groups. A list of hypothalamic symptoms is presented in Table 4.2.

2.4 Midbrain

2.4.1 Basic Anatomy

The midbrain (mesencephalon) is situated caudal (ventral) to the thalamus and caudal and posterior to the hypothalamus (Fig. 2.25). It is the smallest of the major brain divisions and can be imaged from about H0 to H v 18 from F0 to F p 24.

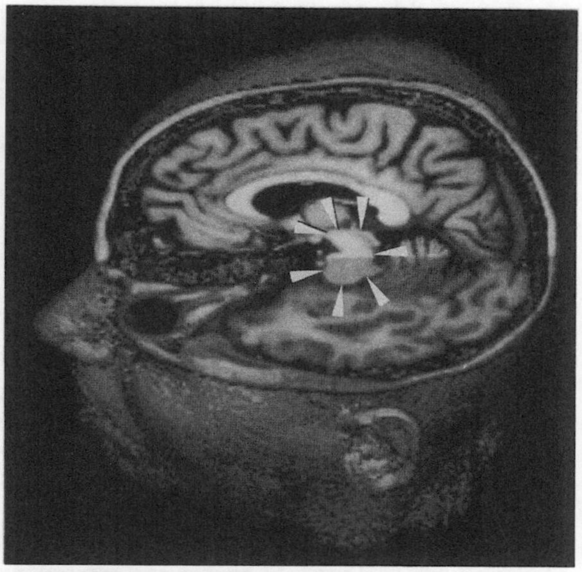

Fig. 2.25. Basic anatomy of midbrain in a 3D reconstruction (FLASH 40°)

Sagittal Section S l 6

The positional relationship of the midbrain to the diencephalic structures and the pons-medulla region can be appreciated on the parasagittal scan at S l 6 (Fig. 2.26). The narrow cerebral aqueduct separates the wide, anteriorly located tegmentum from the posteriorly situated quadrigeminal plate (tectum), from which arise the superior and inferior colliculi. These project into the quadrigeminal cistern, bordered from above by the posterior commissure, one of the basic reference points of the coordinate system, and caudally by the superior medullary velum. The parasagittal scan also demonstrates the midbrain nuclei, the red nucleus and substantia nigra. The oculomotor nerve is consistently visible within the interpeduncular cistern.

Axial Section H v 6

Several important tracts and nuclei can be identified on the axial midbrain scan. The upper scan should traverse the superior colliculi (at about H v 6), and the lower scan should pass through the inferior colliculi (at about H v 12). The red nuclei are clearly visible on H v 6 (Fig. 2.27) as a pair of round areas of low signal intensity flanking the midline. The substantia nigra presents as an elongated band coursing medial to the cerebral peduncles, which consist entirely of white matter. Generally the cerebral aqueduct is easy to identify despite its small extent. It is surrounded by gray matter. Also in that area are the nuclei of cranial nerves III and IV (oculomotor and trochlear). On the more caudal section H v 12 (Fig. 2.28), we see on that level the decussation of the superior cerebellar peduncles instead of the red nuclei.

Coronal Sections F p 12 and F p 18

Coronal section F p 12 (Fig. 2.29) passes approximately through the center of the midbrain and traverses the hippocampal region of the temporal lobe. The long pyramidal motor tracts extend from the pons through the cerebral peduncles, passing lateral to the midbrain nuclei. The red nuclei are situated medially at the level of the inferior horns of the lateral ventricles. They are bordered superiorly by the subthalamic nucleus, which also may be visualized. The T1-weighted coronal scan at F p 18 (Fig. 2.30) cuts the quadrigeminal plate. The midbrain is completely separated from the diencephalon and cerebrum at this level by the low-intensity ambient cisterns and quadrigeminal cistern, in which the pineal gland and great cerebral vein (of Galen) are visible.

Image Contrasts

The midbrain nuclei, composed of gray matter, give a lower signal than the white matter, especially on T2-weighted scans. Initially this was attributed to nerve fibers entering the nucleus from the superior cerebellar peduncle [18], but it may relate to an increased concentration of paramagnetic ions like that found in certain basal ganglia [13, 14] (see Sect. 2.3). It is believed that the T2 time is shortened by locally changing fields, and that this could ac-

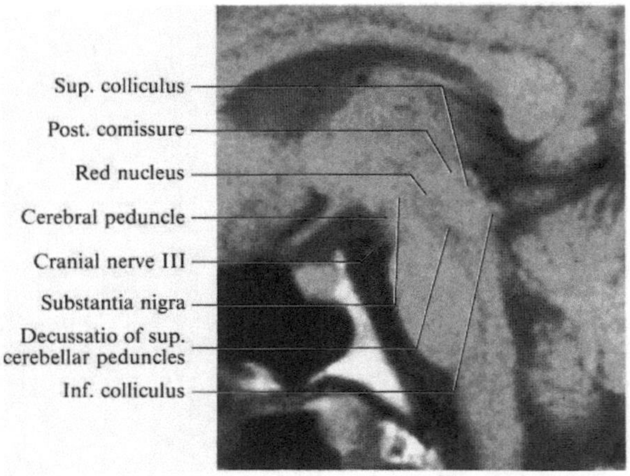

Fig. 2.26. Sagittal section S l 6 through midbrain (SE, TR 0.6 s/TE 17 ms)

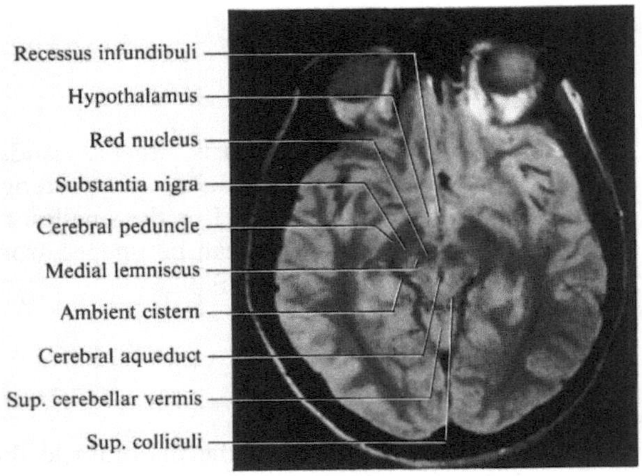

Fig. 2.27. Axial section H v 6 through superior colliculi of midbrain (SE, TR 2.4 s/TE 35 ms)

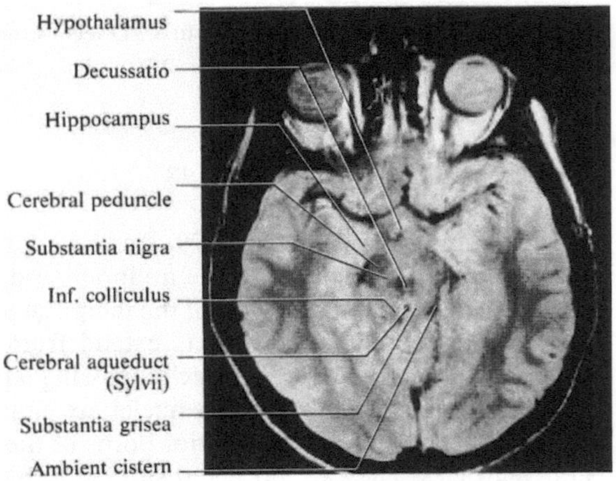

Fig. 2.28. Axial section H v 12 through inferior colliculi of midbrain (SE, TR 2.4 s/TE 35 ms)

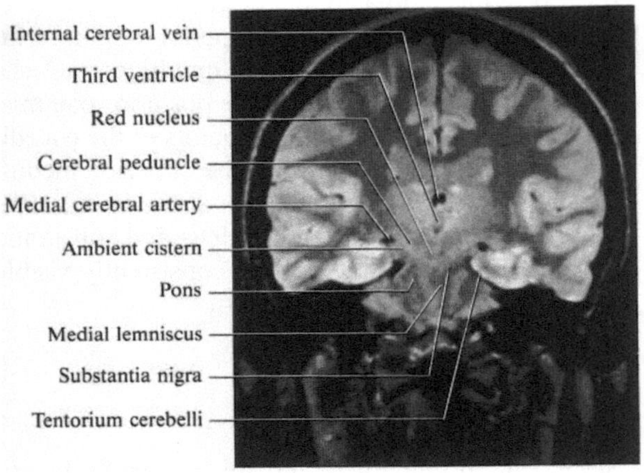

Fig. 2.29. Coronal section F p 12 through center of midbrain (SE, TR 2.4 s/TE 35 ms)

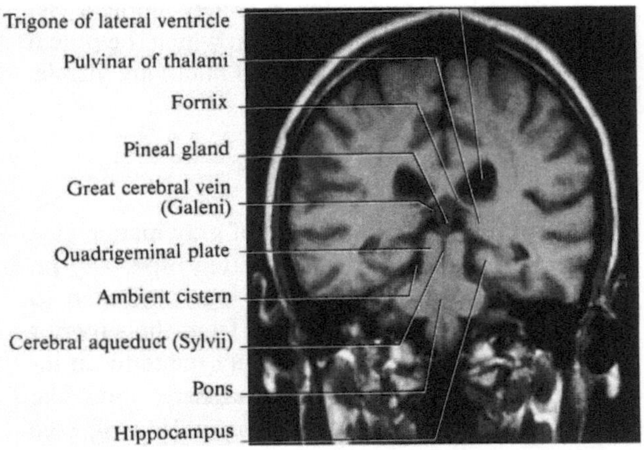

Fig. 2.30. Coronal section F p 18 through quadrigeminal plate (SE, TR 0.6 s/TE 17 ms)

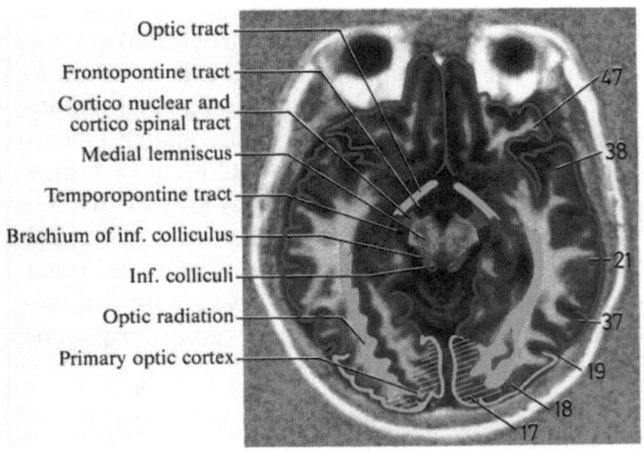

Fig. 2.31. Functional anatomy of midbrain in axial MR image H v 6 (IR, TR 1.5 s/TE 0.350 s)

count for the low signal intensity of these structures on T2-weighted sequences. The increase in this effect at higher field strengths is consistent with theory [22]. Because the spin-density weighted SE sequence (e.g., Figs. 2.27 and 2.28) gives contrasts comparable to the T2-weighted image but with a better signal-to-noise ratio, the former is preferred. The T1-weighted image is good for differentiating midbrain from the surrounding cisterns because of the low signal produced by CSF (Fig. 2.30).

2.4.2 Functional Anatomy

With its red nucleus and substantia nigra, the midbrain contains two major components of the *extrapyramidal system* (Fig. 2.31). The nuclei of the oculomotor (third cranial) and trochlear (fourth cranial) nerves lie at the center of the tegmentum. These nuclei regulate *eye movements*. (The functions and disorders of these areas are dicussed further in Sect. 2.6). The central gray matter and the reticular formation of the tegmentum are concerned with monitoring a variety of *autonomic* functions. The medial lemniscus (blue) gives an entire functional system its name; it conducts a major portion of the *sensory* fibers arriving from the periphery. The smaller, laterally situated lateral lemniscus (green) is extremely difficult to resolve with MR. It contains some fibers of the *acoustic system*. Both the *pyramidal* and the *extrapyramidal motor tracts* pass through the cerebral peduncles. As we saw in the internal capsule (Sect. 2.3.5), the corticopontine tracts (violet) course lateral to the pyramidal tract (red). A special function is associated with the quadrigeminal plate. The inferior colliculi are integrated into the *acoustic system*. They receive signals from the opposite side through the lateral lemniscus and in turn send fibers to the medial geniculate body, which belongs to the thalamus. The superior colliculi serve the *optical system*. They receive fibers from the optic tract (yellow) through which the reflexes of the internal and external ocular muscles are modulated.

Degeneration of the midbrain nuclei is manifested by extrapyramidal symptoms, most notably Parkinson disease associated with degeneration of the substantia nigra. Lesions occurring anteriorly, such as infarction or tumors, produce contralateral hemiplegia through damage to the corticospinal or corticobulbar pathways. Ipsilateral oculomotor pareses also are usually present (Weber's syndrome). Lesions at the center of the tegmentum likewise are associated with ipsilateral oculomotor pareses as well as contralateral extrapyramidal disturbances such as intention tremor, hemichorea, and hemiathetosis. The cause is damage to the red nuclei. Dorsal lesions, which generally are caused by hydrocephalus in the aqueductal region or by pineal neoplasms, result in disturbances of ocular motility (Parinaud's syndrome). A tabular description of symptoms is given in Table 4.2.

2.5 Posterior Fossa

2.5.1 Basic Anatomy

In the past, the portions of the brain occupying the posterior cranial fossa - the pons, medulla oblongata, and cerebellum - were not readily accessible to diagnostic radiology because of the thick bone surrounding the fossa. MR imaging provides an unobstructed view of this important region and thus has become the diagnostic modality of choice. The region of the posterior fossa is covered by the axial sections H v 18 to H v 66 and the coronal sections F0 to F p 72 (Fig. 2.32).

Midsagittal Section S0

The pons adjoins the caudal aspect of the midbrain, where the tentorium cerebelli forms the tentorial incisure (Fig. 2.33). The tentorium passes dorsal to the cerebellum at about a 45° angle to the horizontal plane and carries the straight sinus, which is clearly delineated at this level. The oval-shaped pars ventralis of the pons bulges ventrally and is always easily distinguished from the pars dorsalis. The caudal prolongation, the medulla oblongata, is the connecting link between the brainstem and spinal cord.

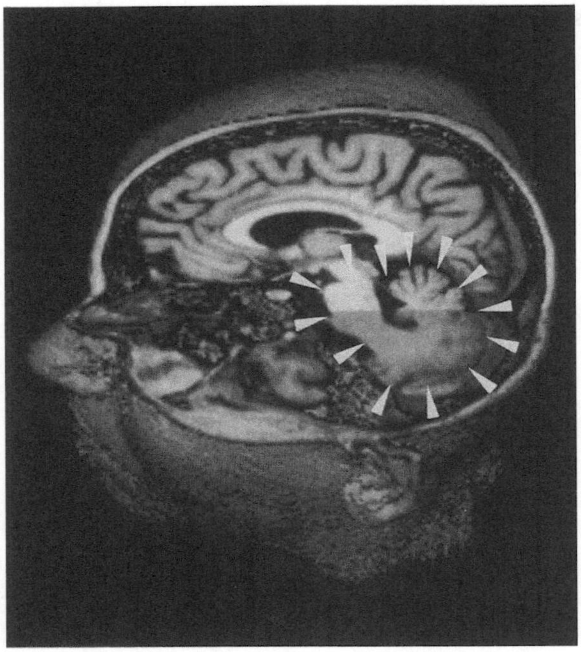

Fig. 2.32. Basic anatomy of posterior fossa in a 3D reconstruction (FLASH 40°)

On the midsagittal image the cerebellum appears to be connected to the midbrain behind the pons-medulla region by only the thin superior medullary velum, because only the vermis of the cerebellum is visualized. But shifting the image plane off the midline demonstrates the protruding cerebellar hemisphere with its broad connection to the pons, the medial cerebellar peduncle. The fourth ventricle lies between the cerebellum and the pons-medulla region. It is continuous superiorly with the cerebral aqueduct, and inferiorly it connects with the spinal canal. The fourth ventricle communicates with the subarachnoid space (cisterna magna) through three apertures - the two lateral foramina of Luschka and the dorsally opening foramen of Magendie at the lower edge of the inferior medullary velum, an area also known as the area postrema. The CSF space lying anterior to the pons, the pontine cistern, contains the basilar artery and is bordered anteriorly by the bony clivus, which usually contains marrow that gives a high-intensity signal.

Axial Section H v 42

The axial section H v 42 (Fig. 2.34) cuts the center of the rhomboid fossa (fourth ventricle), which presents centrally. It is bordered anteriorly by the tegmentum of the pons with its paired median eminences and median sulcus and is connected to the cerebellum by the wide medial cerebellar peduncles. The cerebellum clearly shows its hemispheric divisions and the medially situated vermis, which is continuous with the posterior cerebellar incisure. The scan cuts the petrous part of the temporal bone at its upper margin, and the basal portions of the temporal lobe are displayed in the middle fossa.

Coronal Section F p 6

The coronal section F p 6 (Fig. 2.35) traverses the posterior part of the fourth ventricle. The characteristic outline of the rhomboid fossa is seen only superiorly because of the obliquity of the scan. The foramina of Luschka are visible at its lateral recess. The three paired cerebellar peduncles appear as symmetrical, oval structures of white matter lateral to the rhomboid fossa. Their subdivision into superior, middle, and inferior peduncles is sometimes appreciated. The middle peduncle is the most massive of the three.

Image Contrasts

Because of the close proximity of brain tissue, CSF spaces, and bony structures in the posterior fossa, every MR sequence offers some advantage. T2-weighted SE images (Fig. 2.33) provide good differentiation of CSF from brain tissue and bone. Spin-density weighting (e.g. Fig. 2.37) gives the best signal-to-noise ratio and thus the best resolution of fine structures of the adjacent petrous bone or vessels. Subtracting the T2-weighted image from the associated first echo image of a double-echo sequence (Fig. 2.35) gives contrasts very similar to that of a spin-density image in terms of graymatter-white matter separation, but the CSF also is well displayed. The T1-enhanced SE image is recommended for evaluating the internal CSF spaces and the cranial nerve segments in the basal cisterns (Figs. 2.34, 236, 2.38), while IR images are best for visualizing the cerebellar gyri (Figs. 2.39, 2.40).

2.5.2 Pons and Medulla Oblongata

The subdivision of the pons into a pars ventralis and pars dorsalis is conspicuous on the midsagittal image (Fig. 2.33). The oval-shaped pars ventralis contains a complicated pattern of small nuclei and transverse and longitudinal fiber tracts, which are only faintly delineated on MR scans (Fig. 2.40). Sometimes the medial lemniscus can be identified as a long fiber tract at the posterior border. The dorsal part of the pons, which is directly connected to the midbrain and also to the cerebellum via the cerebellar peduncles, shows aggregations of gray matter on the floor of the rhomboid fossa which belong to the reticular formation and to the middle cranial nerve nuclei (Fig. 2.34).

The medulla oblongata extends caudally from the pons, appearing as a downward prolongation of its pars dorsalis. The pyramidal tract presents bilateral to the median anterior fissure on caudal axial scans. The more dorsally situated olivary nucleus also can be identified with some confidence on MR scans [25].

2.5.3 Cerebellum

The cerebellum consists of the paired hemispheres joined by an unpaired median strucure, the vermis. Clearly visible on the midsagittal section S0 (Figs. 2.33, 2.39), the vermis is subdivided into parts

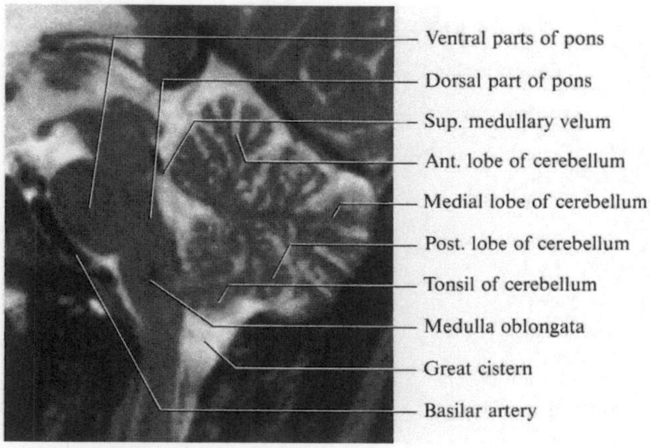

Fig. 2.33. Midsagittal section S0 through pons, medulla oblongata and cerebellum (SE, TR 2.4 s/TE 105 ms)

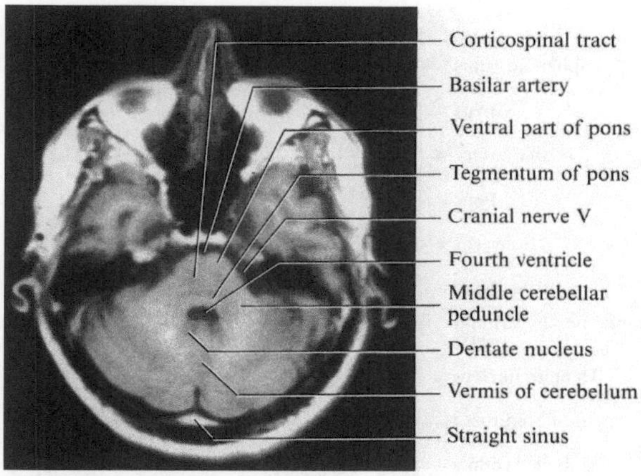

Fig. 2.34. Axial section H v 30 through posterior fossa (SE, TR 0.6 s/TE 17 ms)

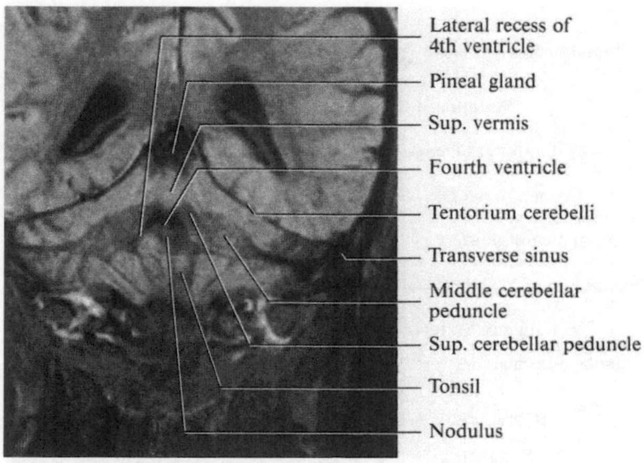

Fig. 2.35. Coronal section F p 6 through fourth ventricle (subtraction image SE, TR 2.4 s/TE 35 ms and TR 2.4 s/TE 105 ms)

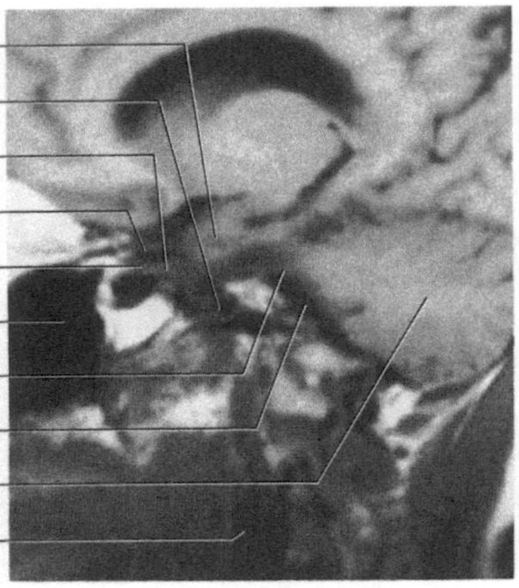

Fig. 2.36. Parasagittal section S l 15 through gasserian ganglion

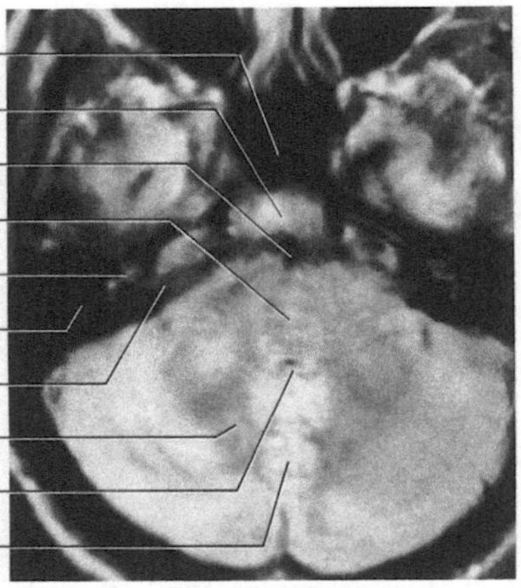

Fig. 2.37. Axial section H v 36 through internal auditory canal (SE, TR 2.4 s/TE 35 ms)

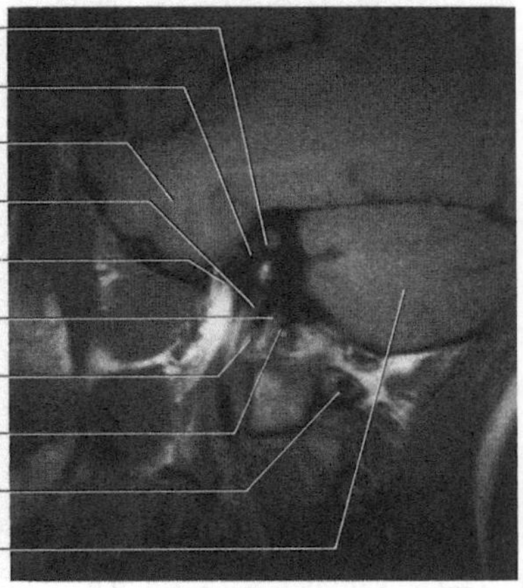

Fig. 2.38. Parasagittal section S l 27 through jugular foramen (SE, TR 0.6 s/TE 22 ms, 4 mm, surface coil)

which show a stellate arrangement and perform various functions (Sect. 2.5.5). The gross divisions of the anterior, middle, and posterior lobes can each be further subdivided into three lobules. This subdivision is partially continued into the two cerebellar hemispheres. The coronal section at F p 30 (Fig. 2.35), for example, demonstrates the cerebellar tonsil at the level of the uvula and shows some evidence of the flocculus, which is level with the nodule. The cerebellum, like the cerebral cortex, is composed of central white matter and a peripheral gray cortex. The gray matter of the cerebellum is substantially thinner than that of the cerebral cortex, and the gyral pattern is less pronounced. This is best appreciated on the axial IR image (Fig. 2.40). The cerebellar white matter contains several aggregations of gray matter, of which the dentate nucleus is most clearly visualized on scans (Fig. 2.37). The cerebellar peduncle is connected to the midbrain by the superior medullary velum and to the medulla oblongata by the inferior medullary velum (Fig. 2.39). It is connected to the brainstem by three symmetrical, laterally situated cerebellar peduncles (Fig. 2.35).

2.5.4 Basal Cranial Nerves

The cranial nerves of the cerebral cortex (nerve I, olfactory nerve, Sect. 2.2), the diencephalon (nerve II, optic nerve, Sect. 2.6), and the midbrain (nerves III and IV, oculomotor and trochlear nerves, Sects. 2.3, 2.4, 2.6) are discussed under the appropriate headings.

The remaining eight cranial nerves (V–XII) emerge laterally from the pons and medulla oblongata, pass ventrally or laterally, and leave the neurocranium through various apertures. Some of these nerves are readily seen on MR images, while others require special high-resolution techniques.

The various nuclei of the *trigeminal nerve* (cranial nerve V) are distributed via the posterior gray matter from the midbrain to the upper spinal cord. They cannot be delineated on MR scans, although the peripheral course of the nerve can consistently be traced on various image planes [12]. Its emergence from the pons is visible on the axial section H v 30 (Fig. 2.34), while its further course and the Gasserian ganglion are visible on the parasagittal section S l 15 (Fig. 2.36). From there three large nerve divisions are distributed (1) to the orbit through the superior orbital fissure (ophthalmic nerve, cranial nerve V_1); (2) to the maxilla and oral cavity through the foramen rotundum (maxillary nerve, cranial nerve V_2); and (3) to the mandible through the foramen ovale (mandibular nerve, cranial nerve V_3). A high-resolution coronal scan through the cavernous sinus at F a 18 (Fig. 2.18) can resolve the individual branches of the nerve [10].

The *abducens nerve* (cranial nerve VI) generally is too small to be visible as a separate structure on MR images (see also Sect. 2.3). It forms a bundle with the first division of the trigeminal nerve (V_1) within the cavernous sinus [10, 12].

MR displays very clearly the two nerves of the "facial group," the *facial nerve* and the *vestibulocochlear nerve* (cranial nerves VII and VIII) [7, 8, 32]. Both have their nuclei in the floor of the rhomboid fossa. The nerve fibers leave the caudal pons laterally at the level of the cerebellar peduncles and enter the bony internal acoustic canals. Only the intracanalicular segments are visible on the spin-density axial section H v 36. The nerve tissue contrasts sharply with the dark bone, appearing as an elongated band of high signal intensity. The orthogonal sagittal section S l 27 (Fig. 2.38) displays the nerves as rounded structures anterior to the cerebellum. Topographic aspects are discussed in some detail in Sect. 2.7, which deals with the acoustic system.

The *glossopharyngeal nerve* (cranial nerve IX), the *vagus nerve* (cranial nerve X), and the *accessory nerve* (cranial nerve XI) arise from common nuclei in the medulla oblongata, dorsal to the olive. They emerge on the dorsal surface of the brainstem, pass a short distance in the basal cisterns, and leave the cranial cavity jointly through the jugular foramen. They are not easily visualized with MR. Daniels [11] was best able to demonstrate the foramen and the extracranial course of the nerves on parasagittal scans using surface coils and 3-mm slices. Similar structures can be identified on the T1-weighted parasagittal section S l 27 (Fig. 2.38). With better resolution, it should be possible to evaluate this region with accuracy.

The *hypoglossal nerve* (cranial nerve XII) is the most caudal of the cranial nerves. It emerges from the medulla oblongata as a linear series of rootlets and passes laterally to exit from the neurocranium through the bony hypoglossal canal. This canal is displayed best on coronal scans [18].

2.5.5 Functional Anatomy

The functions of the *pons and medulla oblongata* can be divided into three main areas:

1. Conducting the long ascending and descending connections between the spinal cord, cerebellum, diencephalon, and cerebral cortex
2. Providing relay points for the neurons of the basal cranial nerves in the primary cranial nerve nuclei
3. Regulating autonomic processes such as respiration and circulation in the reticular formation

Only a few of these small structures can be resolved with MR. The corticospinal fibers (red) descend through the cerebral peduncles and enter the ventral part of the pons, where they become separated from one another by the transverse fibers of the pons (Fig. 2.39 and 2.40). They converge again on entering the pyramids of the medulla oblongata, which are consistently visualized. At the junction with the spinal cord, the majority of fibers cross the median plane at a site called the "decussation of the pyramids" and pass into the lateral funiculus of the cord as the lateral corticospinal tract (Sect. 2.9). The pyramidal tracts carry to the periphery the excitatory impulses for voluntary motor activity arising in the precentral region. Injury to the tracts above the decussation of the pyramids causes a contralateral spastic hemiparesis.

Dorsal and medial to the pyramids, the medial lemniscus (blue) passes to the thalamus (Fig. 2.40). It can be identified in the lower medulla oblongata as a narrow formation of white matter between the olivary nuclei [18]. It then passes transversely through the pars dorsalis of the pons and reenters the midbrain (Fig. 2.39). The medial lemniscus represents the continuation of the tracts of the posterior funiculus of the spinal cord (Sect. 2.9), which relay in the gracile and cuneate nuclei of the medulla oblongata. These nuclei lie dorsal and caudal to the olivary nucleus and cannot (yet) be individually resolved with MR. The tracts of the posterior funiculus and the medial lemniscus convey sensations of touch, posture, and vibration (superficial sensibility). The tracts cross before reaching the gracile and cuneate nuclei, so that lesions above the medulla oblongata lead to a contralateral reduction of these sensory qualities.

The anterolateral system, named for its position in the spinal cord, conveys somatic pain and thermal sensations to the thalamus (see also Sect. 2.9). It crosses to the opposite side in each cord segment and then passes as the uncrossed lateral spinothalamic tract (blue) through the medulla oblongata and the pars dorsalis of the pons. This tract passes lateral to the olive and medial lemniscus in its up-

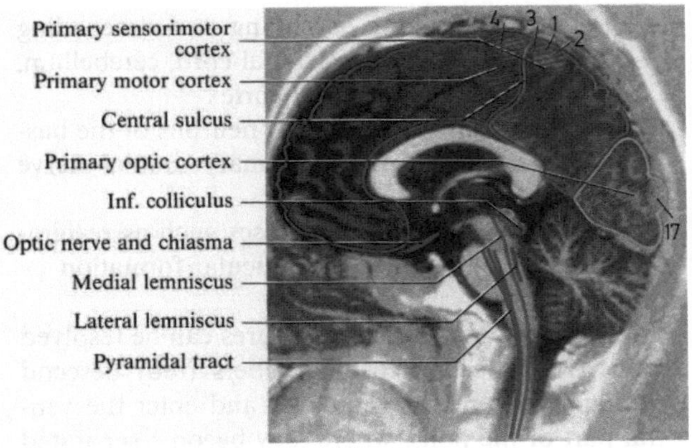

Fig. 2.39. Functional anatomy of medulla oblongata and pons in a midsagittal MR image (IR, TR 1.5 s/TI 0.350 s)

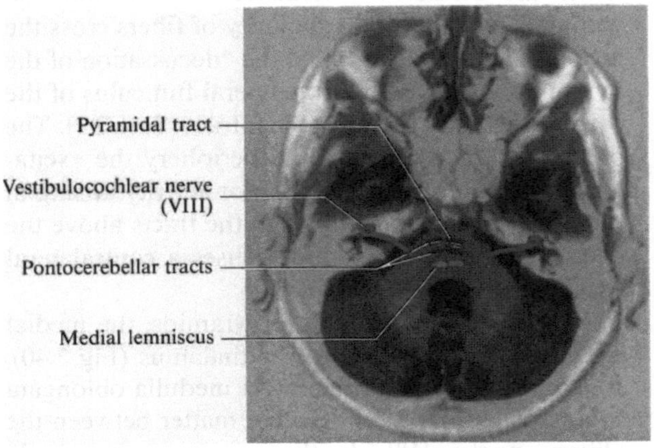

Fig. 2.40. Functional anatomy of pons in an axial MR image (IR, TR 15 s/TI 0.350 s)

ward aspect. Usually it is not visible on MR scans. Lesions of the lateral spinothalamic tract produce contralateral somatic analgesia and thermanesthesia.

The lateral lemniscus (green) arises from the middle rhomboid fossa and closely adjoins the medial lemniscus on the lateral side. It cannot (yet) be visualized with MR. It chiefly conveys the primary fibers of the acoustic system. The importance and anatomic course of the lateral lemniscus are discussed further in Sect. 2.7. Lesions are manifested by hypoacusis.

Other major tracts in the spinal cord, especially those leading to the cerebellum, cannot be discussed in the present context.

Most of the primary *cranial nerve nuclei* are located in the dorsal third of the pons and medulla oblongata. They are arranged in a cranial to caudal fashion and are numbered accordingly from V to XII. Lesions cause a variety of ipsilateral deficits, which are listed individually in Table 4.2. The location of the abducens nucleus in the floor of the rhomboid fossa is of diagnostic importance in this regard. With abducens paresis, it is imperative that the basal brainstem also be evaluated.

The *reticular formation* is a diffuse network of gray and white matter which performs a great variety of autonomic functions. It extends downward from the midbrain into the caudal medulla oblongata. A vomiting center has been identified in the area postrema at the inferior pole of the rhomboid fossa. Damage to the respiratory center in the region of the medulla oblongata may be manifested by hiccoughing when the lesion is limited in its extent. Symptoms vary with the level of the lesion and range from impaired consciousness to unconsciousness, cardiovascular disturbances, dysphagia, and autonomic symptoms.

The very position of the *cerebellum* - dorsal to the long motor tracts and separate from the cerebral cortex - reflects its function as a coordinating center which acts through complicated control pathways to assist in the maintenance of equilibrium, the regulation of muscle tone, and the purposeful execution of motor acts. It consists of several parts having different phylogenetic ages and different functional tasks, some closely linked to the extrapyramidal system. The oldest part of the cerebellum, called the archicerebellum, consists of the nodule of the vermis and the flocculus (Fig. 2.39). It has close connections with the vestibular nuclei via the inferior cerebellar peduncle and has special relevance to the maintenance of equilibrium. Lesions of its afferent and efferent pathways and of the archicerebellum itself lead to global truncal, standing, and gait ataxia. In contrast to posterior cord ataxia, the symptoms of cerebellar ataxia do not increase when the eyes are closed.

The anterior lobe, pyramid, and uvula of the vermis are collectively termed the paleocerebellum. These areas mainly receive spinal tracts, which accounts for their alternate name of "spinocerebellum." Their function is to sustain a muscle tone adequate to maintain balance during standing and walking. Each body half is supplied in that function by the ipsilateral cerebellar cortex. The function of the paleocerebellum is closely linked to that of the archicerebellum, and lesions of the former are similarly manifested by truncal ataxia, making it exceedingly difficult to pinpoint the localization of the deficits that are observed.

The phylogenetically youngest region of the cerebellum comprises the middle vermis and the hemispheres. It is termed the neocerebellum or "pontocerebellum" because of its very close relation to the pons and extrapyramidal system via the superior cerebellar peduncle. The corticopontine tracts pass in close proximity to the pyramidal tracts through the internal capsule and cerebral peduncles and unite the extrapyramidal system with the cerebellum. The cerebellum modifies and corrects the pyramidal and extrapyramidal motor processes so that all movements, whether voluntary or involuntary, are performed with precision. A continuous flow of information from the periphery enables the cerebellum to intervene in a corrective fashion when errors occur so that movements can be executed smoothly and purposefully. Lesions of the neocerebellum never cause a loss of voluntary movements, but they do interfere with their execution, leading to intention tremor, adiadochokinesia, dysmetria, scanning speech, or similar impairments.

2.6 Optical System

2.6.1 Basic Anatomy

The optical system may be subdivided into three topographic segments:

- The extracerebral sensory organ, the eye, which occupies the orbit together with its motor apparatus and the optic nerve.
- The pathways and nuclei located in the cerebrum and diencephalon, such as the optic chiasm, the optic tract, and the lateral geniculate body (Sect. 2.3)
- The cerebral cortical formations, consisting of the optic radiation, the primary visual cortex, and the secondary projection areas in the occipital lobe (Sect. 2.2).

The optical system extends chiefly in the anteroposterior direction but oriented at an angle to the CA-CP system. Its major parts are easily surveyed on a slightly tilted axial scan, as illustrated in Fig. 2.41). The topography of the intracerebral pathways has been previously reviewed (Sects. 2.3, 2.4), and the functional anatomy of the visual pathway is detailed in Sect. 2.6.2. The eccentric position of the sense organ may necessitate an examination technique different from that used for the rest of the CNS [53]. For more details see Chap. 3 and Chap. 12. Thus we shall direct our main attention in this section to the topography of the orbit.

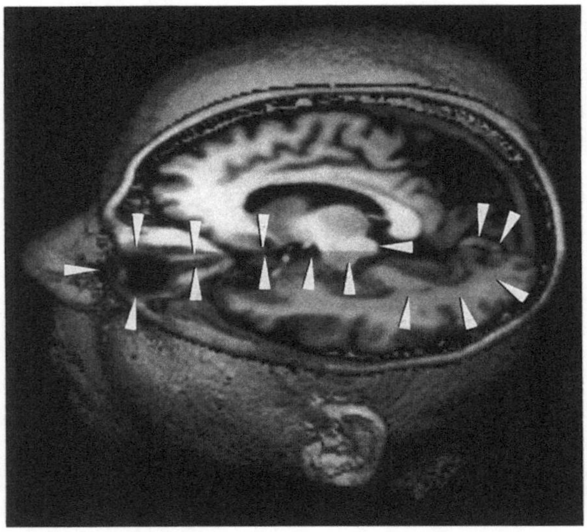

Fig. 2.41. Basic anatomy of optical system in a 3D reconstruction (FLASH 40°)

The orbit forms a four-sided pyramid whose apex is directed posteriorly. MR can demonstrate this region extremely well through the use of multidirectional scans [52]. Even very fine structures can be resolved when special surface coils are employed [4]. During examination of the orbit, the patient should fix his gaze on a point; otherwise motion artifacts will degrade the image and hamper the evaluation of ocular lesions. Different imaging techniques which have been developed to reduce these motion artifacts are discussed in Sect. 1.3.5.

Axial Section Through the Center of the Eye

The symmetrical imaging of both orbits in the supine patient is useful for comparing one side with the other (Fig. 2.42). The bony orbital walls are delicate and appear as thin zones of low signal. The medial bony lamina of the orbit normally cannot be differentiated from the air-filled nasal cavity or from the ethmoid cells. While the retro-orbital fat always gives a high signal, the lateral and medial rectus muscles and the often sinuous optic nerve yield a moderate signal [6]. SE images can demonstrate blood vessels very clearly as fine punctate or threadlike structures of low intensity in the orbital fat. The ophthalmic artery crosses the optic nerve in the posterior part of the orbital cavity. Blood vessels that may represent the posterior ciliary arteries, superior ophthalmic vein or vorticose vein can be seen just posterior to the globe. The globe itself presents a multilayered structure. The external sclera gives a less intense signal than the choroid and retinal layers. The fat-fluid interfaces can produce marked chemical-shift artifacts, especially in high-field imaging, which may mimic unilateral thickenings of the sclera (see Sect. 1.3.5).

Oblique Sagittal Section Through the Center of the Eye

The globe shows the same anatomy in sagittal section as in axial section, although its cranial and caudal poles and the adjacent orbital structures are displayed better on the sagittal scan. In the strictly sagittal section, the optic nerve leaves the image plane very quickly in the medial direction. An oblique sagittal scan is better for delineating the course of the nerve [29] (Fig. 2.43). It also gives a better picture of the superior and inferior rectus muscles and the levator palpebrae muscle, which courses just above the superior rectus. The scan cuts the inferior oblique muscle almost at right angles. Cranial to the orbit is the anterior fossa, which contains the frontal sinus in its anterior portion. Caudal to the orbit is the maxillary sinus.

Coronal Section Through the Posterior Part of the Orbit

Coronal sections are favorable for demonstrating the extraocular muscles. A section through the posterior third of the orbit (Fig. 2.44) displays the four rectus muscles (superior, inferior, medial, and lateral), which are arranged about the eye in diametrically opposed pairs and direct the gaze upward, downward, rightward, and leftward respectively. Of the superior and inferior oblique muscles, which control rotational movements of the eye, only the medially situated superior oblique muscle is visible on this section. Sometimes a signal contrasting with the orbital fat is seen above the superior rectus muscle. This presumably represents the frontal nerve (V_1), which arises from the ophthalmic division of the trigeminal nerve. The lacrimal gland is situated at the craniolateral pole of the orbit and is visible in more anterior coronal sections.

Image Contrasts

The cortical bone of the orbital walls, which gives no signal, the hyperintense retro-orbital fat, and the extraorbital muscles of moderate signal intensity present very similar contrasts on different types of image. At the same time, the vitreous body and the anterior chamber of the eye give low signals on T1-weighted images (Fig. 2.42) and gain in signal intensity with increasing proton density (Fig. 2.45a) and T2 weighting (Fig. 2.45b). The contrast of the lens is complementary to that of the vitreous body. It appears bright in heavily T1-weighted images (ie. IR images, Fig. 2.46) and dark on spin-density and T2-weighted sequences. Pathologic changes in the eye usually are apparent on the T1-weighted image [17]. T2-weighted sequences are recommended for differential diagnosis, e.g., distinguishing choroid melanoma from retinal detachment [4].

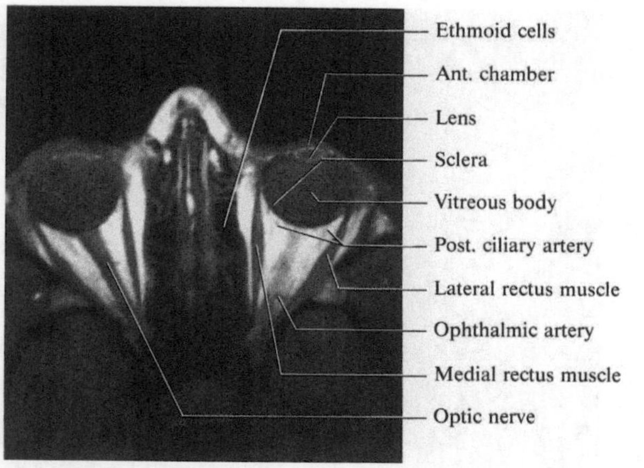

Fig. 2.42. Axial section through center of eyes (SE, TR 0.6 s/TE 22 ms, 3 mm, surface coil)

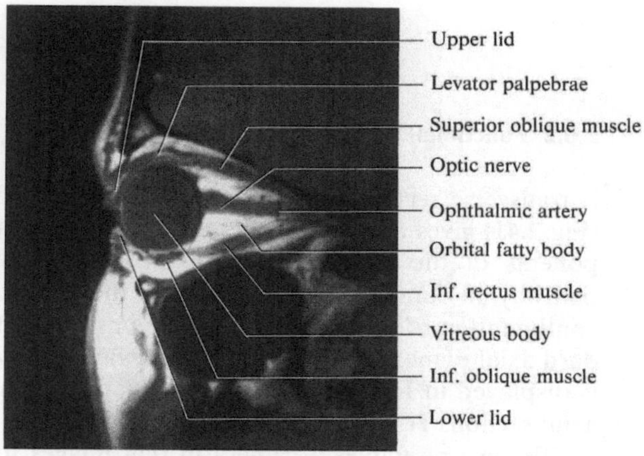

Fig. 2.43. Oblique sagittal section through center of eye (SE, TR 0.6 s/TE 24 ms, 3 mm, surface coil)

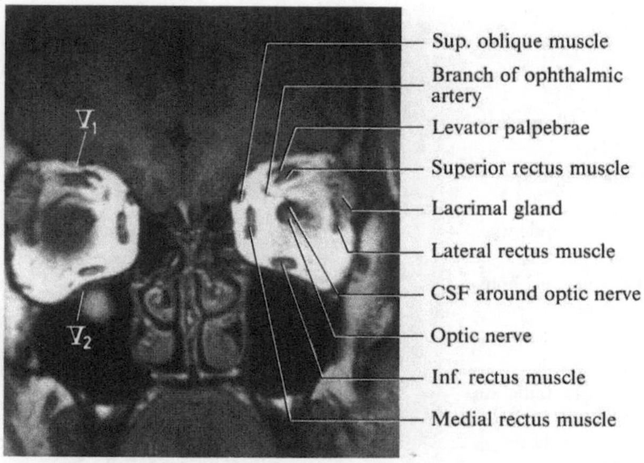

Fig. 2.44. Coronal section through center of eyes (SE, TR 06 s/TE 22 ms, 3 mm, surface coil). *V_1*, frontal nerve; *V_2*, infraorbital nerve (secondary finding: mucous polyp in the right maxillary sinus)

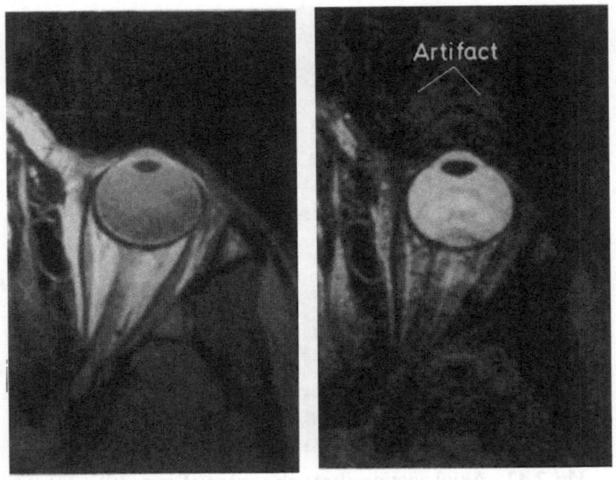

a, b

Fig. 2.45 a, b. Image contrasts of orbit. Axial sections: **a** N(H) weighted (SE, TR 2.4 s/TE 35 ms); **b** T2 weighted (SE, TR 2.4 s/TE 105 ms), *Artifact*, eye-blinking artifact

2.6.2 Functional Anatomy

A transverse section paraxial to the CA-CP system (Fig. 2.41) gives an overview of almost all the components of the optical system (called the visual pathway in functional anatomy), but the steplike configuration of the pathway favors the use of standard axial planes. Thus the visual pathway (yellow) is displayed in Fig. 2.46 using a combination of the axial sections H v 24, H v 12, H v 6, and H d 6.

The eye resembles a camera in that images focused onto the retina by the lens are uspide-down and reversed. Thus the lateral visual field is projected onto the medial portions of the retina, and vice versa. The afferent fiber bundles within the optic nerve retain their topologic arrangement (i.e., arrangement by site of origin). The medial portions, corresponding to the lateral visual field, cross to the opposite side in the optic chiasm, so that the nerve fibers of the right or left side of the retina become united in the optic tract. The tract extends backward from the optic chiasm, located anterior to the pituitary stalk, winds round the hypothalamic region, and terminates on both sides in the lateral geniculate bodies located at the caudal and lateral posterior border of the thalamus. As their function is related to the ventrodorsal thalamic nuclei, these bodies are known as the "thalamic relay centers" of the visual pathway.

A small portion of the optic nerve fibers course in front of the lateral geniculate body and enter the midbrain directly, passing especially to the superior colliculi. These fibers contribute to eye movements and particularly to the light reflex, i.e., the change in pupillary size. The ocular muscles are innervated by cranial nerves III, IV and VI. The oculomotor nerve (cranial nerve III) supplies the medial, superior, and inferior rectus muscles and the inferior oblique muscle; the trochlear nerve (cranial nerve IV) is the exclusive supplier of the superior oblique muscle; and the abducens nerve (cranial nerve VI) supplies the lateral rectus muscle. The nuclei of cranial nerves III and IV are closely adjacent and situated in the midbrain, while the abducens nerve has its nucleus deep in the rhomboid fossa (see Sect. 2.5). All three nerves converge peripherally in the cavernous sinus, from which they pass through the superior orbital fissure accompanied by the first division of the trigeminal nerve (cranial nerve V).

Damage to the nuclei of these cranial nerves causes defects of ocular motility resembling those observed in the case of peripheral nerve lesions, but typically occuring in association with other cranial nerve deficits. The most conspicuous sign of injury to the ocular muscles is double vision (diplopia). In most cases visual acuity is not impaired. An isolated lateral gaze palsy is highly suspicious of damage to the abducens nucleus and may indicate pontine disease. The most frequent causes are encephalitis, vascular disease, tumors, and multiple sclerosis. Peripheral oculomotor pareses are most commonly caused by meningitis, cavernous sinus thrombosis, internal carotid artery aneurysm, fractures, botulism, and tumors of the skull base or orbit.

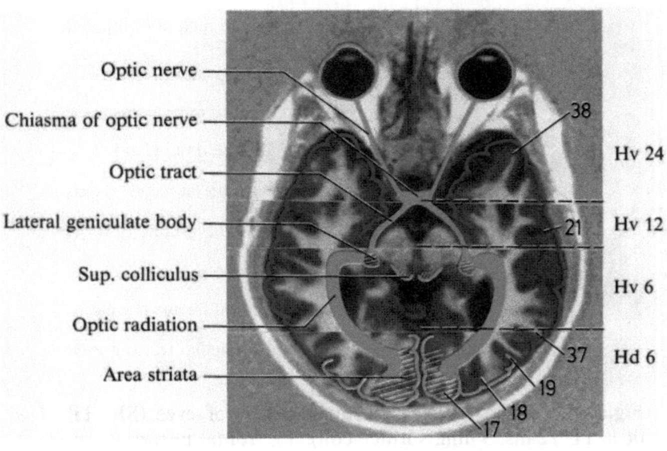

Fig. 2.46. Functional anatomy of visual pathway in axial MR images (IR, TR 1.5 s/TI 0.350 s)

The thalamocortical visual pathway is called the optic radiation. It begins at the lateral geniculate bodies, passes through the posterior limb of the internal capsule, and emerges as a wide band that winds around the inferior and occipital horns of the lateral ventricles. The primary visual cortex lies on the medial side of the occipital lobe, occupying both sides of the roughly horizontal calcarine sulcus. This is Brodmann's area 17, known also as the striate area (see Sect. 2.2). It is easily identified on the midsagittal section S0 and on the coronal section F p 60. The topical arrangement of the visual pathway can also be followed in the optic radiation and in the primary cortical area.

Damage to one optic nerve, as by an intraorbital lesion, causes impairment or loss of vision in the affected eye. Damage to the optic chiasm, as by a pituitary neoplasm, results in a heteronymous bitemporal hemianopia, for only the crossing pathways are destroyed. Homonymous hemianopia is seen with optic tract lesions and with diseases involving the geniculate body. Because the optic radiation forms a broad band as it sweeps backward, damage may be confined to discrete portions of it, resulting in a quadrantanopic form of visual defect. Lesions involving area 17, the primary visual cortex, also cause more or less circumscribed visual field defects, depending on their localization. Usually, the macular vision is maintained. Lesions involving the higher areas 18 and 19, which adjoin the striate area, can seriously disrupt the further processing of visual information. The patient is unable to recognize the shape, size, or contour of objects and manifests alexia or visual agnosia (see also Table 4.2).

2.7 Acoustic System

2.7.1 Basic Anatomy

The acoustic system is closely related topographically to the vestibular apparatus. The sensory organs of both systems are located in the petrous part of the temporal bone. The afferent fibers pass as separate fascicles of the vestibulocochlear nerve (cranial nerve VIII) through the internal auditory canal and enter the brainstem in the angle between the cerebellum, pons, and medulla oblongata. There the fibers are distributed to the various cranial nerve nuclei, which cannot be delineated with MR. The vestibular system has close connections with the spinal cord and cerebellum as well as with the oculomotor nuclei and the motor neurons of the cervical muscles. As these connections occur at a low hierarchic level, there is no well-defined pathway like that known from the acoustic system. The latter shows a course that is best appreciated in the coronal plane (Fig. 2.47). In the section on functional anatomy below (Sect. 2.7.2), we shall deal only with the acoustic system. The sensory organs of the inner ear located in the petrous bone are readily accessible to MR imaging and will be discussed separately.

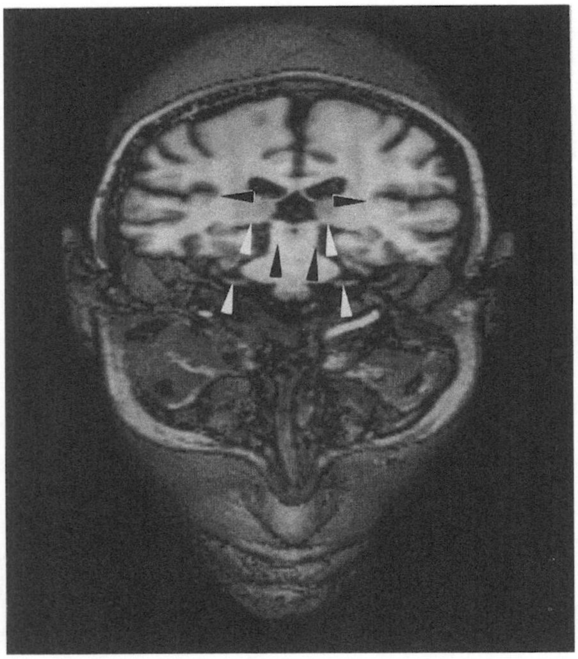

Fig. 2.47. Basic anatomy acoustic system in a 3D reconstruction (FLASH 40°)

Unlike CT scans, which can demonstrate bony structures [57], MR images display the soft tissues and the fluid-filled bony cavities of this region. The hard petrous bone, the mastoid air cells, and the large blood vessels do not produce a signal [8]. Thus, all larger foci of high signal intensity that cannot be assigned to the fine structures of the inner ear are considered pathologic and may signify inflammation, effusion, cholesteatoma, or other disease. Axial and coronal sections are suitable for demonstrating the auditory canals, which course lateroventrally and lie on a horizontal plane. Surface coils applied over the temporal area can provide high-resolution images of the inner ear region that rival CT images in their detail [32]. However, it is recommended that surface-coil images be supplemented with survey scans using the head coil so that the two sides can be compared (e.g., Fig. 2.37). Section thickness of 3 mm is desirable, but even 5-mm sections show good anatomic resolution [8] (see also Sect. 3.1).

Coronal Section

A coronal section at ca. F p 12 gives a good impression of the topographic relations of the statoacoustic organ (Fig. 2.48). It displays the gently upsloping external auditory canal, which terminates at the middle ear. Both of these give almost no signal in normal individuals, and the air-filled spaces show no contrast with the petrous bone or the ossicles of the middle ear. The three semicircular canals, which contain endolymph, appear as tiny loops at the center of the petrous bone.The anterior (superior) semicircular canal usually projects upward, while the posterior semicircular canal projects downward; the lateral semicircular canal is placed between them. Because the three canals are angled about 45° with respect to the CA-CP system, they appear foreshortened in all sections. They meet in the medially located vestibule, which is entered by cranial nerves VII and VIII. The cochlea lies several millimeters anterior to the semicircular canals. Sometimes the genu of the facial canal, which carries the facial nerve (cranial nerve VII) out of the cranium caudally through the stylomastoid foramen, can be identified lateral and cranial to the cochlea. The carotid artery and jugular vein pass ventrally, close to the inner ear, with only a thin lamina of bone separating them. The low signal of flowing blood on MR images makes it difficult to distinguish from bone. Cranial nerves VII and VIII take an approximately horizontal course as they traverse the internal auditory canal. The nerves enter the brainstem in the cerebellopontine angle, behind the inferior cerebellar peduncle.

Axial Section

An axial section at ca. H v 48 displays the lateral and usually slightly ventral course of cranial nerves VII and VIII in the auditory canal (Fig. 2.49). It is even possible to distinguish the individual nerve trunks on high-resolution scans. The segment within the basal cisterns is visible only on very heavily T1-weighted images, where the CSF-filled basal cistern appears dark. The vestibulocochlear nerve passes to the ventrally located cochlea and to the more laterally situated vestibule, from which the three semicircular canals arise. The lateral semicircular canal appears as an essentially closed circle and is bordered from behind by the posterior semicircular canal. The anterior semicircular canal projects above the vestibule. It is sometimes possible to identify the course of cranial nerve VII, which extends posteriorly between the cochlea and the spiral organ, and also the greater superficial petrosal nerve, which takes off anteriorly. The carotid artery appears as an elongated, transverse band whose close proximity to the cochlea is well displayed on this section.

Sagittal Section

The sagittal image plane is seldom used for otologic examinations, but it is excellent for demonstrating the site of emergence of the facial nerve from the skull base (Fig. 2.50). The nerve leaves the inner ear just below the semicircular canal, then turns downward and enters the stylomastoid foramen, which often is lined with bright fatty tissue. The middle ear (tympanic cavity) appears anterior to the foramen and is made visible by its mucosal lining, which has a relatively high signal.

Image Contrasts

Most investigations can be done using T1-weighted SE sequences, which can show early evidence of morphologic change owing to the excellent contrast of the soft tissues with the bone and air-filled spaces. T2-weighted images are used for the differentiation of tumors and effusions [43].

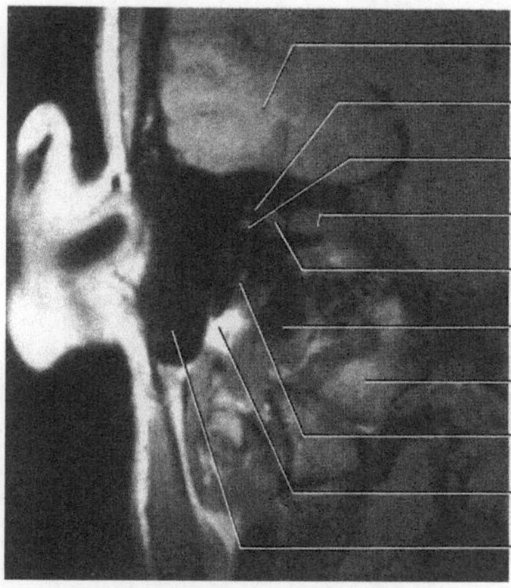

Fig. 2.48. Coronal section, ca. F p 12, through inner ear and internal auditory canal (SE, TR 0.6 s/TE 22 ms, 4 mm, surface coil)

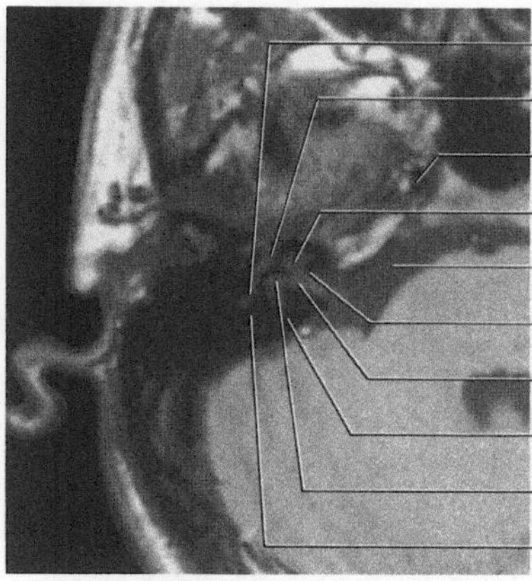

Fig. 2.49. Axial section, ca. H v 36, through inner ear and internal auditory canal (SE, TR 0.6 s/TE 22 ms, 4 mm)

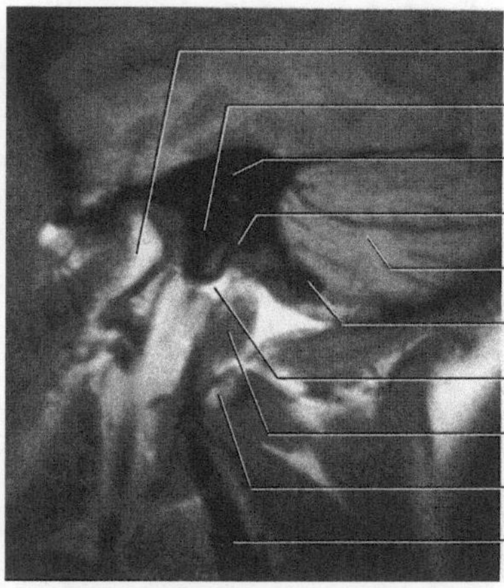

Fig. 2.50. Sagittal section through stylomastoid foramen (SE, TR 0.6 s/TE 22 ms, 4 mm, surface coil). See also neighboring slice (Fig. 2.38)

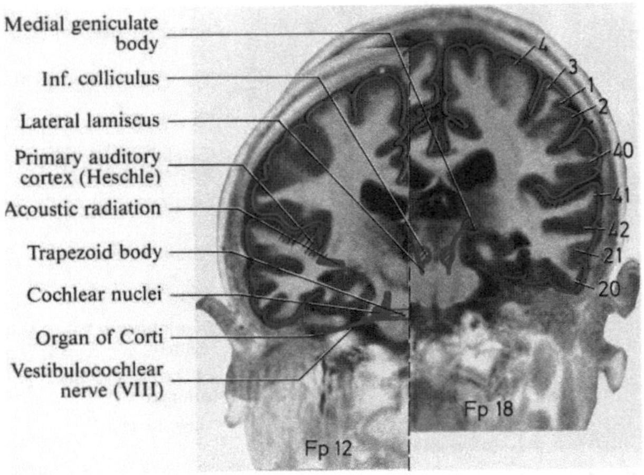

Fig. 2.51. Functional anatomy of auditory pathway in coronal MR images F p 12 and F p 18 (IR, TR 1.5 s/TI 0.350 s)

2.7.2 Functional Anatomy

Almost the entire auditory pathway is displayed on the coronal sections F p 6 to F p 18 (Fig. 2.51). Air pressure fluctuations transmitted to the inner ear by the external auditory canal and middle ear generate electrical action potentials by stimulating the hair cells of the spiral organ. These potentials are carried by the vestibular nerve to the ventral and dorsal vestibular nuclei situated lateral to the cerebellar peduncles. From there a portion of the fibers cross to the opposite side and join with the ipsilateral nerve fibers in the lateral lemniscus, which passes up to the midbrain through the pars dorsalis of the pons. The nerve cells relay in the inferior colliculi and pass via the brachium colliculi inferioris to the medial geniculate body of the posterior thalamus. Ultimately the fibers pass through the acoustic radiation, which runs closely adjacent to the optic radiation in the posterior limb of the internal capsule, to be distributed to the primary cortical projection area in the transverse temporal gyri, known also as Heschle's loop. The primary acoustic cortex is concentrated mainly in Brodmann's area 41. This adjoins secondary areas in which the acoustic signals are analyzed, identified, and compared with earlier acoustic memories. The major secondary areas are 42 (sensory speech center of Wernicke) and 22, both of which lie at the posterior end of the superior temporal gyrus (see Sect. 2.2).

Diseases of the middle ear such as inflammation, otosclerosis, and glomus tumors are within the domain of the otologist. Likewise, symptoms caused by vestibulocochlear nerve lesions should prompt otologic referral in most instances. Deficits involving the central auditory pathway, however, are the concern of the neurologist.

Sound conduction disturbances associated with diseases of the middle ear are manifested by hearing impairment for speech and low-pitched sounds. Inner ear disorders, on the other hand, tend to impair the hearing of high-pitched sounds. Damage to the cochlear nerve (e.g., by an acoustic neuroma) may lead to unilateral tinnitus, progressive hearing loss, and impaired directional hearing. As the lesion enlarges, additional symptoms appear due to involvement of the parallel facial and vestibular nerve fibers and a mass effect in the cerebellopontine angle. These symptoms can include peripheral facial paralysis, a nystagmus toward the side of the lesion, and impairment of balance, as well as brain compression symptoms caused by displacement of the caudal ventricles with CSF stasis and corresponding dilatation of the higher ventricles. Unilateral lesions of the ascending auditory pathway in the pons and midbrain region and of the relay centers in the inferior colliculi and medial geniculate bodies usually cause no more than a general reduction of hearing (hypoacusis) due to the bilateral course of the pathways. A bilateral disruption of the auditory pathway must be present in order for bilateral deafness to occur. Temporal lobe epilepsies may be associated with an acoustic aura. Lesions involving adjacent areas of the temporal lobe result in sensory aphasia, or the inability to recognize acoustic perceptions (see also Table 4.2).

2.8 Cerebral Blood Supply

2.8.1 Basic Anatomy

The brain receives most of its blood supply from the paired carotid and vertebral arteries (Fig. 2.52). Ventral to the midbrain, at the skull base, these vessels interanatomose through small communicating arteries in the circle of Willis (circulus arteriosus). The blood supply to the cerebrum is arranged in three parts. The anterior cerebral arteries arising from the internal carotids pass forward along the medial surfaces of the frontal lobes. The middle cerebral arteries, which form direct prolongations of the carotids, run laterally in the lateral cerebral sulci and from there are distributed to the temporal lobes and portions of the parietal lobes. The posterior cerebral arteries arise from the basilar artery. They run posteriorly on the tentorium and supply the posterior portions of the brain. The cerebellum receives its major supply from the superior and inferior cerebellar arteries and from several paramedian arteries.

Venous drainage is effected by the superficial veins, which empty mainly into the superior sagittal sinus, petrosal sinus, and transverse sinus, and by the deep veins, which drain the white matter and basal ganglia. These are collected in the great cerebral vein and finally drain into the straight sinus (Fig. 2.53). The sinuses are not blood vessels in the true sense, but spaces formed by septa between the periosteal and meningeal layers of the dura. The superior sagittal sinus runs along the vertex between the two cerebral hemispheres and joins with the straight sinus and occipital sinus at the confluence of sinuses. From there blood is carried by the transverse sinus along the attached margin of the tentorium and around the posterior fossa to the sigmoid sinus, which finally opens into the internal jugular vein. A small portion of the blood leaves the intracranial space through diploic and emissary veins, which drain into the cranial bone and scalp. Blood is also carried from the cranium by the ophthalmic vein.

Image Contrasts

The MR contrast features of flowing blood differ from those of stationary tissue. Generally the blood does not produce a signal, because the excited protons are washed out of the image slice before the MR signal can be received or phase distortions reduce the spin echo. However, blood flow can produce a variety of MR effects depending on the direction and velocity of the flow and on the pulse sequence (see Sect. 1.3.4 and Sect. 5.3). Blood vessels may contrast very strongly with brain tissue on spin-density-weighted images because of their low signal. Usually only very short segments of the vessels are visualized unless they run exactly parallel to the image plane. With slice thicknesses of 1.5–3 cm, however, it may be possible to follow the vessels out to their small peripheral branches. The technique of MR angiography is still in the initial stages of development (see Sect. 1.4) and will not be discussed

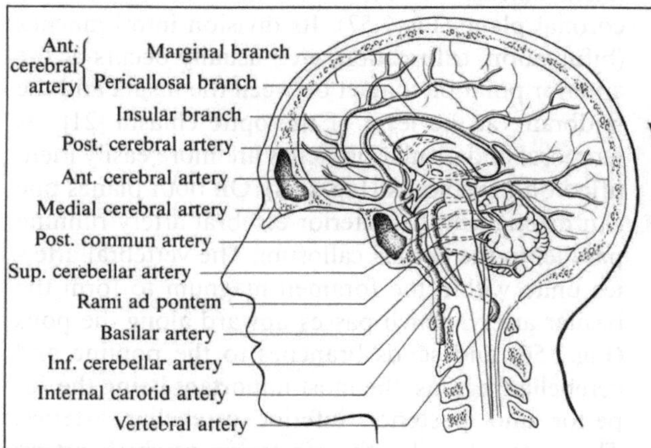

Fig. 2.52. Basic anatomy of cerebral arterial system

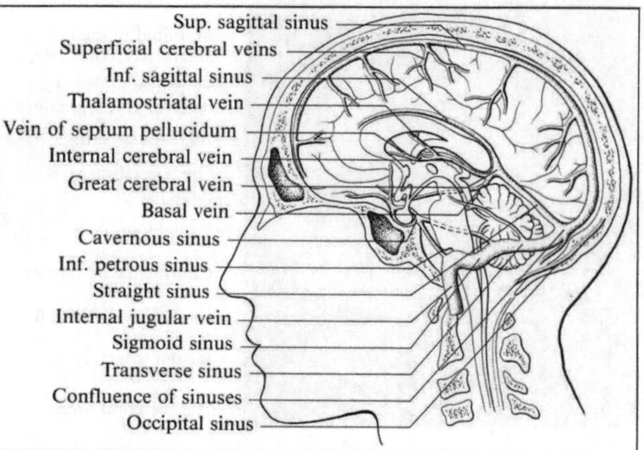

Fig. 2.53. Basic anatomy of cerebral venous system

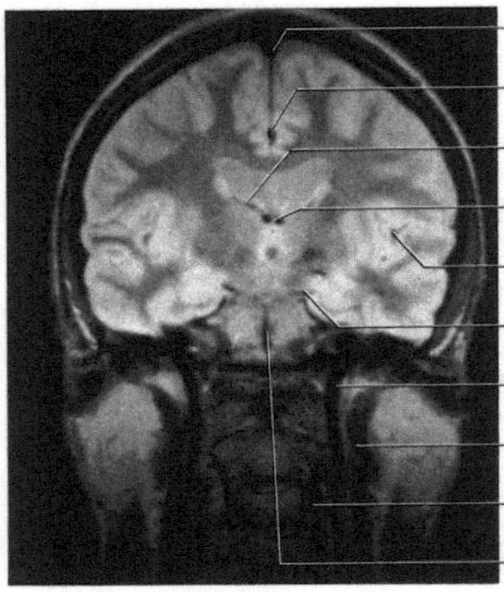

Fig. 2.54. Coronal section F0 along major supply vessels of brain (SE, TR 2.4 s/TE 35 ms, 6 mm)

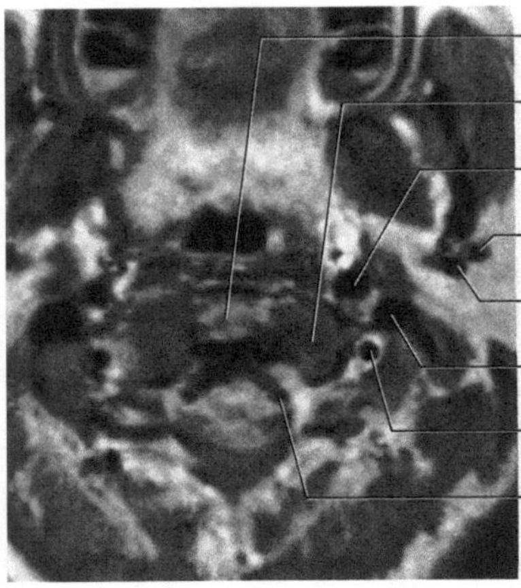

Fig. 2.55. Axial section (H v 72) at level of axis (C2) showing major supply vessels of brain (SE, TR 2.4 s/TE 35 ms, 6 mm)

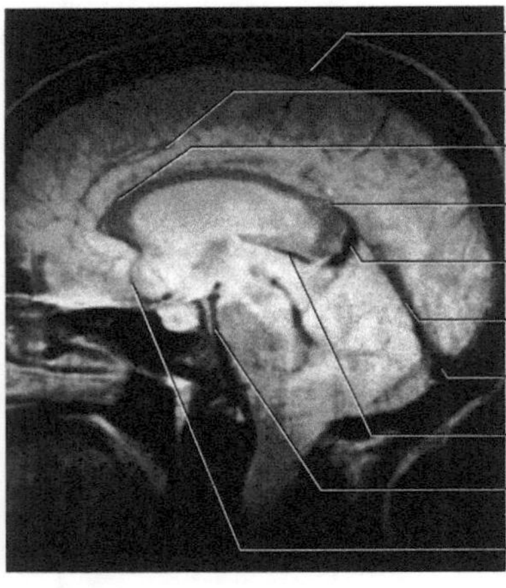

Fig. 2.56. Midsagittal section S0 (SE, TR 2.4 s/TE 35 ms, 15 mm): medial arteries and veins

here. It is important and helpful to know the sectional anatomy of the cerebral blood vessels, and we shall examine this in some detail.

2.8.2 Arterial System

The major arteries supplying the brain - the carotid and the vertebral - can be traced in their ascending course on coronal scans centered at about the level F0 (Fig. 2.54). The same section cuts the unpaired basilar artery, which gives rise to the posterior cerebral arteries. An axial section in the cervical region clearly demonstrates the major vessels situated paravertebrally, posterolateral to the pharynx (Fig. 2.55). The most medial vessel is the internal carotid, with the internal jugular vein situated behind and lateral to it. The vertebral artery appears within the transverse foramen of the cervical vertebra. The anterior spinal artery, supplied by both vertebral arteries, is still bipartite at this level. A sagittal scan at S0 (Fig. 2.56) with spin-density weighting and slice thickness >1 cm shows the course of the anterior cerebral artery, which arises directly from the carotid bifurcation on each side of the sella turcica. Usually two branches pass along the sulcus corporis callosi and the cingulate sulcus, first running forward and then turning backward. The uppermost branch of the artery is called the marginal branch, and the branch running along the corpus callosum is called the pericallosal branch. This midsagittal scan shows portions of the circle of Willis, such as the anterior communicating artery that unites the two anterior cerebral arteries, as well as the origins of the middle cerebral artery and posterior cerebral artery. The middle cerebral artery arises directly from the internal carotid and runs laterally in the lateral sulcus, where it is most easily followed in the coronal plane (Fig. 2.57). Its division into branches (bifurcation, trifurcation, etc.) usually occurs at the anterior point of contact between the insula and the midbrain, at the level of the optic chiasm [21]. Its temporal and insular branches are more easily identified on axial scans (Fig. 2.58). On both planes one can distinguish the anterior cerebral artery running parallel to the corpus callosum. The vertebral arteries unite within the foramen magnum to form the basilar artery, which passes upward along the pons (Fig. 2.56) and sends branches to the pontine and cerebellar regions, the most important being the superior and posterior inferior cerebellar arteries. These vessels, like the posterior cerebral artery, course within the tentorial incisure. Sometimes this can be appreciated on coronal sections (e.g. F p 30 in Fig. 2.35). The division of the posterior cerebral artery into branches supplying the occipital lobe is rarely displayed.

2.8.3 Venous System

The intracerebral veins and arteries cannot be differentiated on ordinary MR scans. The superficial veins and arteries usually take a parallel course in the cerebral gyri, the veins then emptying directly into the large dural sinuses. The emissary veins, which establish communications between the venous sinuses and the veins of the scalp, and the diploic veins to the cranial bone are consistently visible on T1-weighted SE images as bright punctate or linear features on the bony cranium (Fig. 2.59). Individual deep cerebral veins can be recognized from their locations. The thalamostriate vein, which runs forward and laterally toward the head of the caudate nucleus, can usually be identified on axial and coronal scans at the level of the thalamus and basal ganglia (Figs 2.54 and 2.58). It opens into the relatively large-caliber, paired internal cerebral veins, which in turn unite to form the great cerebral vein (of Galen). This vessel is easily traced on a midsagittal image (Fig. 2.56). The length of the great cerebral vein is variable (ca. 1 cm), and often it is seen to unite directly with the straight sinus [21]. The basal vein passes backward from the midbrain region and terminates in the great cerebral vein near the confluence of the internal cerebral veins. The straight sinus occurs at the junction of the falx cerebri and tentorium cerebelli, and its shape is maintained by those structures. Besides the great cerebral vein, it receives blood from the inferior sagittal sinus in the inferior margin of the falx cerebri. Most of the venous sinuses run adjacent to the calvarium as duplications of the dura. A midsagittal section displays the entire course of the superior sagittal sinus and the confluence of the sinuses at the internal occipital protuberance of the occipital squama. T1-weighted images with a short TR demonstrate flow effects from the slow venous blood flow which cause the sinuses to appear bright (paradoxical enhancement). Posterior coronal sections (Fig. 2.59) give an especially good view of the superior sagittal sinus, the transverse sinuses coursing along the attached tentorial margins, and the junctions of the transverse sinuses with the sigmoid sinuses.

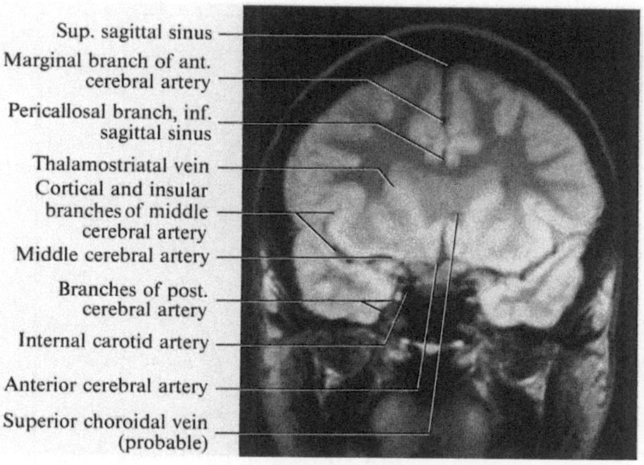

Fig. 2.57. Coronal section F a 21 (SE, TR 2.4 s/TE 35 ms, 12 mm): branches of medial cerebral artery

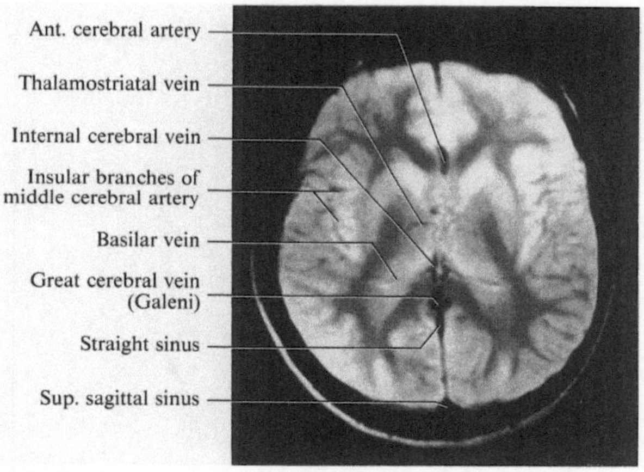

Fig. 2.58. Axial section H d 12 (SE, TR 2.4 s/TE 35 ms, 18 mm): insular branches of medial cerebral artery and central veins

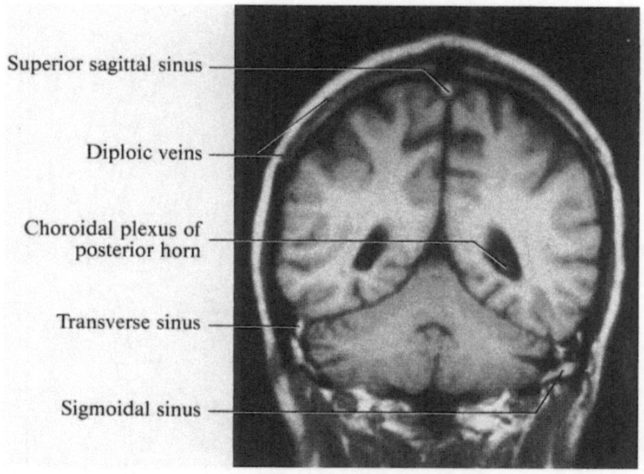

Fig. 2.59. Coronal section F p 30 (SE TR 0.6 s/TE 17): venous sinuses

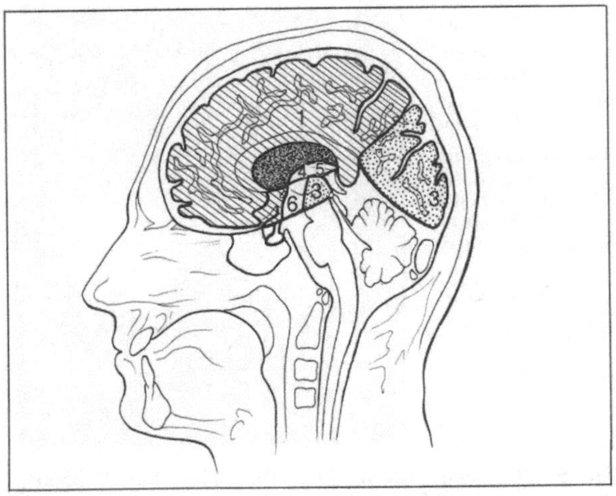

Fig. 2.60. Circulation areas of medial brain structures: *1* anterior cerebral artery; *2* medial cerebral artery; *3* posterior cerebral artery; *4* anterior choroidal artery; *5* posterior choroidal artery; *6* posterior communicans artery

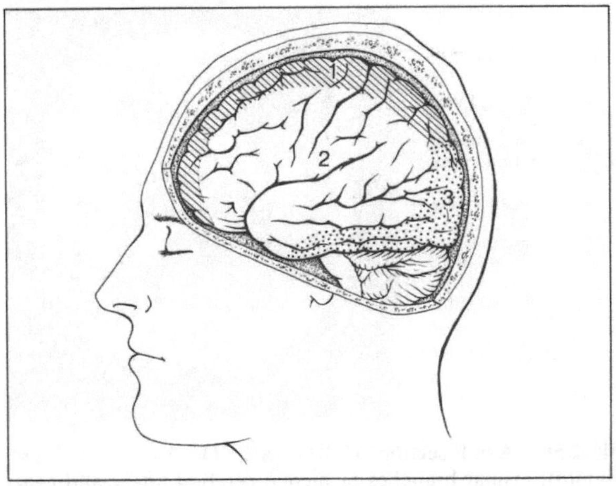

Fig. 2.61. Circulation areas of lateral cortex (see Fig. 2.60)

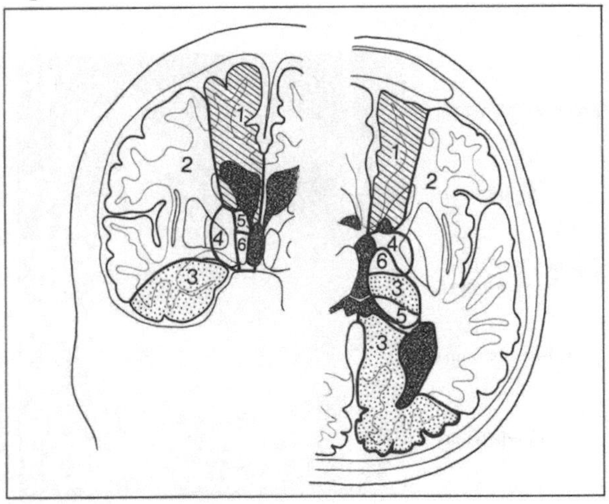

Fig. 2.62. Circulation areas of basal ganglia and interbrain in a coronal and axial diagram (see Fig. 2.60)

2.8.4 Supply Areas of the Cerebral Arteries

The cerebral cortex, basal ganglia, and midbrain are supplied by the three paired cerebral arteries - anterior, middle, and posterior. However, the areas supplied by the individual arteries are extremely variable from one person to the next and are additionally influenced by anastomoses among the areas and with dural vessels (Heubner's anastomoses) [21]. Thus, the distribution pattern described below is intended only as an illustration. The anterior cerebral artery supplies the anterior two-thirds of the medial cerebral hemispheres, including the paracentral lobule and almost the entire corpus callosum (Fig. 2.60). On the lateral aspect, this artery supplies only the cortical structures on the convexity (Fig. 2.61). The middle cerebral artery mainly supplies the lateral part of the brain, including the cortical portions of the lateral frontal lobe and temporal lobe. It also supplies the primary and secondary cortical areas of the acoustic and motor system, especially the motor and sensory speech center (Broca and Wernicke, see also Sects. 2.2, 2.7). The occipital region and the basal surface of the brain, including large areas of the temporal lobe, are supplied by the posterior cerebral artery. This includes the visual centers and portions of the limbic system (Sects. 2.2 and 2.6).

The vessels supplying the basal ganglia form a roughly stellate pattern on the sagittal section with the interthalamic adhesion at the center (Fig. 2.62) [21]. The optic chiasm, the ventral portions of the hypothalamus, and the pituitary gland may be supplied directly by the internal carotid artery or by basal branches of the anterior cerebral artery. The blood supply of the basal ganglia and thalamus is well displayed on an axial scan at H0 (Fig. 2.62). The anterior striate vessels supply the basal ganglia, the lentiform nucleus, and the caudate nucleus [58]. They usually arise from the anterior and middle cerebral arteries. The thalamus is supplied by thalamic arterial groups, small vessels which arise from the posterior communicating artery or posterior cerebral artery and pass posteriorly into the midbrain region [59].

Special consideration is given to the fenestrating vessels in the region of the plexus, pineal gland, pituitary gland, and sites about the rhomboid fossa (median eminence, tuber cinereum, area postrema). The high degree of uptake of contrast medium (i.e. gadolinium-DTPA) in these areas is due to the absence of a true blood-brain barrier and should not be considered pathologic [27].

Foci of infarction are readily identified on MR images in various planes. By identifying the supply area, it is possible to establish the affected blood vessel, and the resulting neurologic symptoms can be inferred from the localization. This is discussed further in the appropriate sections. A summary of the disorders affecting the cerebral cortex is presented in Table 4.2.

2.9 Spinal Cord

2.9.1 Basic Anatomy

We must apply the coordinate system of the trunk to the spinal cord, and so the terms "ventral" and "dorsal" regain their original meaning (see Sect. 2.1). The anatomic unit of the bony vertebral column and spinal cord is demonstrated most clearly in the sagittal section (Fig. 2.63). With correct positioning, the T1-weighted image displays the spinal cord as a bright band within the dark subarachnoid space. Ventral to the cord are the bright vertebral bodies, separated by the intervertebral discs. Points along the craniocaudal axis of the spine are designated according to the vertebral bodies. The spinal column consists of seven cervical vertebrae (C), 12 thoracic vertebrae (T), five lumbar vertebrae (L), the sacrum (S), and the coccyx (Co). While C1 (the atlas) appears only as a punctate feature ventral and dorsal to the foramen magnum, C2 (the axis), presents a conspicuous, upward-projecting bony process, the dens. C7 has an especially prominent spinous process (a feature usually shared by the first-thoracic vertebra) and is thus sometimes referred to as the vertebra prominens. T11 is approximately level with the junction of the thoracic cavity and the abdomen in the sagittal projection. An important landmark is the promontory at the pelvic inlet, which marks the boundary between the lumbar spine and the sacral spine. Landmarks of the ventral body surface which are useful for correct positioning are shown in Fig. 2.63.

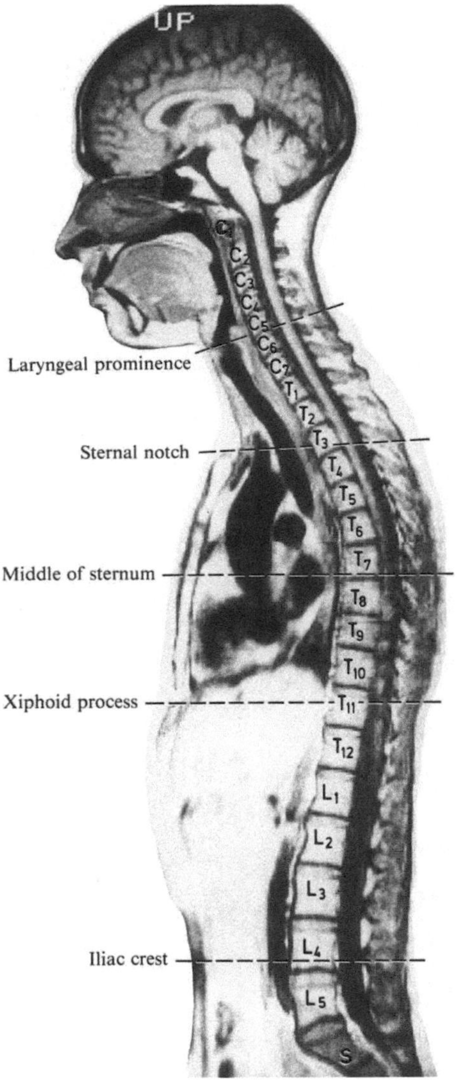

Fig. 2.63. Basic anatomy of spinal cord in a midsagittal MR section (SE, TR 0.6/TE 17 ms, 10 mm)

The spinal cord begins at the foramen magnum of the skull base and in adults terminates at about the level of L1. This most caudal part of the spinal cord is called the conus medullaris. From there the nerves of all roots caudal to L2 pass through the low-signal subarachnoid space and leave the spinal column through the corresponding intervertebral foramina. The dural sheath terminates in the sacral region, usually at the level of the second sacral segment. Nonspecific fatty and connective tissue continues caudally from the dural sheath; the sacral and coccygeal nerves pass through this tissue to their sites of emergence.

Image Contrasts

The MR examination of the spinal cord ordinarily begins with a relatively thick sagittal scan of the region of interest (section thickness about 1 cm). In all cases, imaging of the spinal cord should start with a heavily T1-weighted SE sequence (see also Sect. 3.2 and Chap. 17), which will give marked contrast between the cord (light) and the surrounding subarachnoid space (dark). Artifact problems caused by pulsations of the CSF may necessitate ECG triggering or special pulse sequences. This is discussed in Chap. 5. The IR technique is not advantageous for spinal imaging [37]. The heavily T2-weighted image shows a reversal of contrast in the vertebral canal, so that disc protrusions, for example, appear as dark voids in the bright CSF. A very heavily T2-weighted imaging technique is used for MR myelography [26]. Fast imaging sequences are gaining more and more importance. The contrast can be switched from T1 weighting by FLASH (Fig. 2.70) to T2 weighting using FISP sequences (Fig. 2.71).

2.9.2 Cervical Cord

In most MR systems, good images of the cervical cord can be obtained with use of the head coil, although surface coils contoured to the neck are also employed (e.g., the Helmholtz arrangement). A coil of this type was used to make Fig. 2.64.

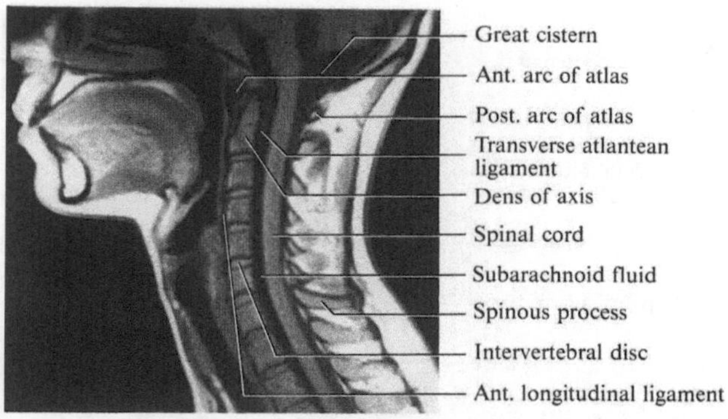

Fig. 2.64. Sagittal section of cervical spine and cord (SE, TR 0.6 s/TE 22 ms, 5 mm, Helmholtz coil)

Midsagittal Section

Every sagittal scan of the cervical cord should include as much of the brain as is necessary to display the craniocervical junction from the medulla oblongata to the cervical cord (Fig. 2.64) [35]. The cisterna magna fills the posterior part of the foramen magnum and the funnel-shaped upper cervical dural sac. The cervical cord is well delineated and presents a slight physiologic enlargement, the intumescentia cervicalis between C3 and T2. The most conspicuous vertebra is C2, the atlas, with its dens projecting upward through the anterior part of the atlas. Together with the condyles of the occipital squama, these structures form the craniovertebral articulations. The ligamentous system of the atlanto-occipital and atlantoaxial joints is integrated into the dark bony contours and cannot be resolved. C5 and C6 are projected behind the larynx. C7 is also called the vertebra prominens because of its long spinous process - a feature usually shared by the first thoracic vertebra.

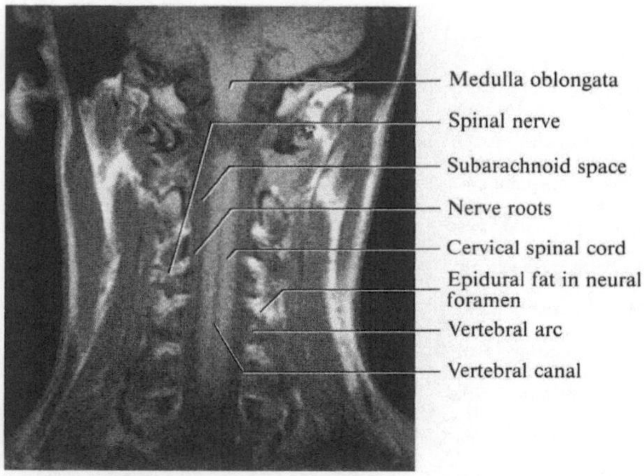

Fig. 2.65. Coronal section of cervical spine and cord (SE, TR 0.6 s/TE 24 ms, 5 mm, surface coil)

Coronal Sections

Because of the lordotic curvature of the cervical spine, coronal imaging often requires placing the patient in an uncomfortable position or using an oblique image plane. Coronal sections (Fig. 2.65) are useful for comparing the nerve roots on both sides of the cord and for verifying a fusiform swelling noted in the sagittal scan. It is important to keep in mind the intumescentia cervicalis between C3 and T2, which is more distinct in the coronal view than in the sagittal. It is caused by the brachial plexus. While the ventrodorsal diameter of the spi-

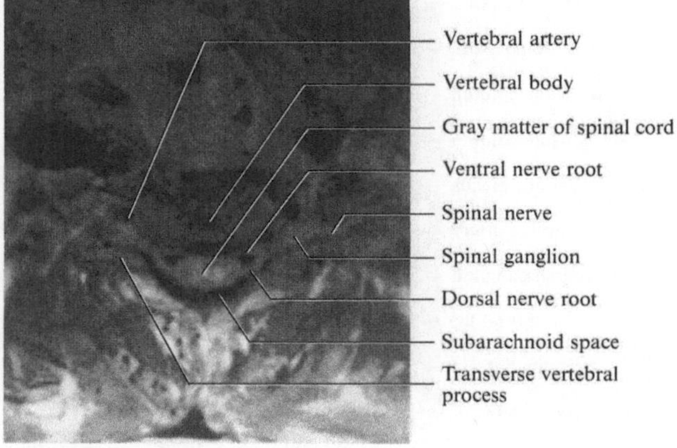

Fig. 2.66. Axial section at level of intervertebral foramina C2/C3 (SE, TR 1.8 s/TE 22 ms 5 mm, surface coil)

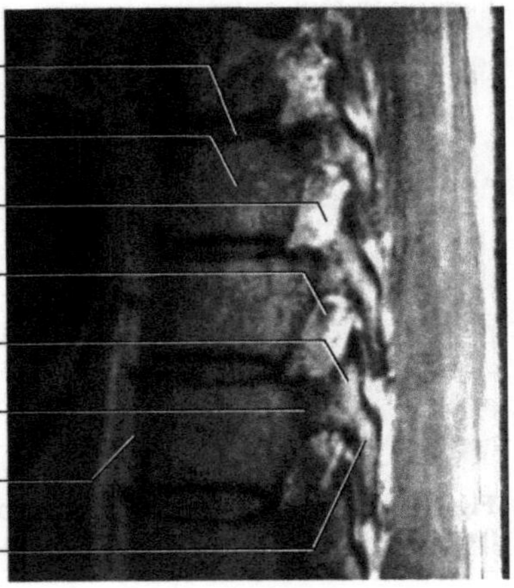

Fig. 2.67. Parasagittal section of thoracic spine ca. 10 mm lateral to midline (SE, TR 0.6 s/TE 22 ms, 3 mm, surface coil)

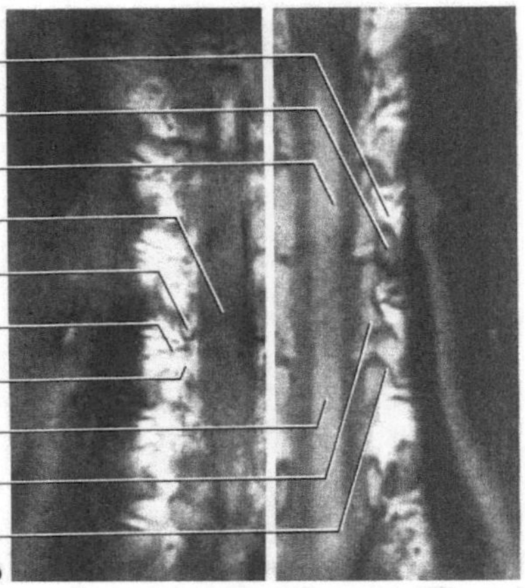

Fig. 2.68. Coronal sections through dorsal vertebral canal (**a**) and thoracic spine (**b**) (SE, TR 0.6 s/TE 22 ms, 3 mm, surface coil)

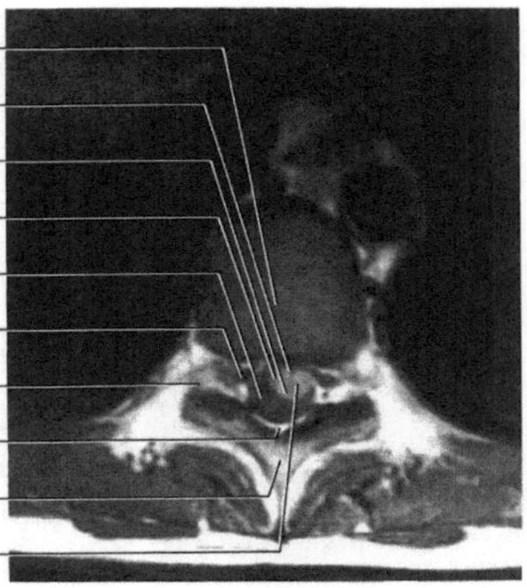

Fig. 2.69. Axial section through middle thoracic spine (SE, TR 0.6 s/TE 30 ms, 5 mm, surface coil)

nal cord varies from about 6 to 7 mm, the transverse width can increase from 7 mm at the level of C1 to 12 mm at C7 [42]. The spinal nerves, formed by the union of the dorsal and ventral roots in the intervertebral foramina, still show an essentially horizontal course in the cervical cord. Enclosed by nonspecific fatty tissue, the spinal nerves pass through the foramina and leave the image section very soon afterward in the anterolateral direction. Yenerich and Haughton [62] recommend a longitudinal scan angled 45° to the coronal or sagittal plane for imaging the intervertebral foramina. Anteriorly placed coronal scans are good for evaluating the dens of the axis and the contours of the craniovertebral articulations.

Axial Sections

As MR resolution has improved through the use of surface coils, axial images have assumed increasing importance in the cervical cord (Fig. 2.66). Generally the standard axial plane as defined by the instrument coordinates is sufficient. T1-weighted SE images display the bright spinal cord within its dark subarachnoid space, surrounded in turn by a venous plexus, fibrofatty tissue, and cortical bone. The axial section displays the anterior median fissure of the cord and may even show the "butterfly" outline of the central gray matter, which is especially pronounced in the cervical region. The dorsal and ventral roots pass laterally and unite in the spinal ganglion, which lies in the intervertebral foramen [44]. The vertebral artery and vein present lateral to the cervical vertebrae and just anterior to the spinal ganglion. The scan may demonstrate the peripheral course of the spinal nerves including the sympathetic trunk, but this is unusual.

2.9.3 Thoracic Cord

The thoracic part of the spinal cord is the most difficult to image because of cardiac and respiratory movements. On the other hand, the kyphotic curvature in this region is well suited for imaging with flat surface coils placed beneath the supine patient (see Sec. 3.1). The use of these coils can largely suppress motion artifacts originating from the anterior aspect. Even so, multiple averaging of the images or even ECG triggering is recommended for examinations of the thoracic cord.

Sagittal Sections

In sagittal sections the thoracic cord appears as a band of uniform thickness extending downward through the spinal sac. Frequently it shows anterior displacement. With oblique positioning of the patient, the scan often will cut the lateral vertebral arches and intervertebral joints, which produce areas of moderate signal intensity that can mimic an intraspinal tumor. This is illustrated in the parasagittal section in Fig. 2.67 ca. 1 cm lateral to the midline. The dark bony structures outline the intervertebral foramen, which is traversed by the spinal nerve. The nerve gives a low signal that contrasts well with the surrounding fibrofatty tissue and demonstrates the relative roominess of the aperture [16, 54].

Coronal Sections

The best coronal scans of the thoracic cord are obtained by lowering the head and elevating the legs of the patient to straighten the thoracic spine (Sect. 3.1) (Fig. 2.68). As in the cervical cord, coronal sections permit bilateral comparison of the emerging nerve roots, and they aid in the diagnosis of asymmetrical mass lesions and fusiform thickenings of the cord by intramedullary processes. The physiologic enlargement between T9 and L2 produced by the emerging thoracolumbar plexus (intumescentia lumbalis) is less pronounced than its counterpart in the cervical region. Usually the central canal, which is superimposed on the anterior median fissure, is visible as a central stripe of low signal. The spinal nerves passing laterally downward from the cord and their sites of emergence through the intervertebral foramina are depicted to some degree. Coronal scans made through the dorsal part of the vertebral canal demonstrate the emerging branches of the spinal nerves.

Axial Sections

The axial section of the vertebral canal in the thoracic region is almost circular (Fig. 2.69). The spinal cord may be centered within the canal or may be eccentrically positioned if postural deformity exists. The diameter of the cord in this region is approximately 6-7 mm. An image of sufficiently high resolution will show the characteristic butterfly shape of the central gray matter. Due to the relative shortening of the cord with respect to the vertebral column, the spinal nerves at this level no longer pass straight from the cord into the intervertebral foramen, but must pass laterally downward before exiting from the vertebral column. As a result, the ventral and dorsal roots can no longer be individually resolved. The spinal ganglion presents in the intervertebral foramen as a structure of moderate intensity that is separate from the cord. The blood vessels of the spinal cord are more easily recognized than in the cervical region.

2.9.4 Lumbosacral Region

Surface coils placed dorsally beneath the patient are excellent for imaging the lumbar cord. The legs should be well elevated to straighten the lumbar spine (Sect. 3.1).

Sagittal Section

The spinal cord terminates caudally in the conus medullaris at about the level of L1. From there the spinal nerves pass as the cauda equina to their individual sites of emergence. The conus medullaris is usually well displayed in sagittal images, whereas the roots of the cauda equina are not always visualized because of their predominantly lateral, fanlike expansion from the apex of the cord (Fig. 2.70). The water-rich intervertebral discs of the lumbar region give an intense signal on T2-weighted images, with the central nucleus pulposus appearing brighter than the surrounding annulus fibrosus [37, 38]. With increasing age and loading of the vertebral column, this signal pattern dwindles as a result of degenerative changes [30]. After about 30 years of age, a cleft of decreased signal intensity is often seen at the center of the disc; this feature represents ingrowth of connective tissue [1]. Degenerating discs may give almost no signal in T2-weighted SE sequences. Thus, an initial sagittal survey scan can direct the examiner's attention to the affected region, which can then be scrutinized using thinner sections in an oblique axial plane [16, 29].

Axial Sections

As in CT examinations, lateral disc protrusions are seen best on axial scans directed parallel to the end plates of the vertebral bodies [60]. Optimum contrast with CSF is obtained on heavily T1-weighted images and especially on the T2-weighted scan

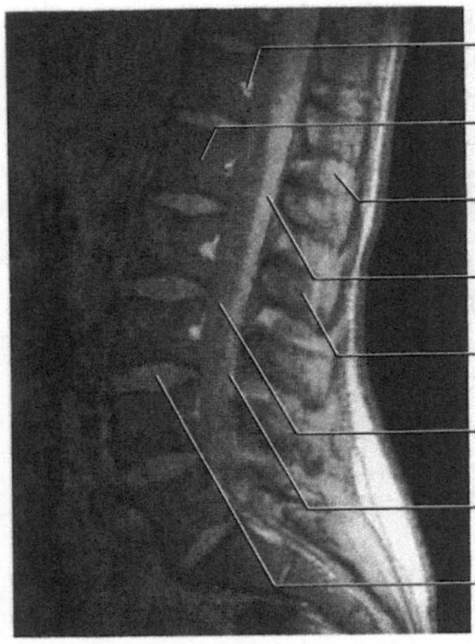

Fig. 2.70. Midsagittal section of lumbosacral region (FLASH 40°, 5 mm, surface coil)

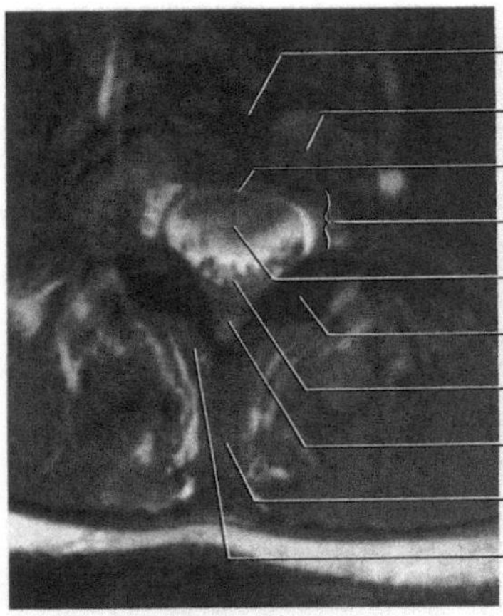

Fig. 2.71. Axial section through middle lumbar spine, T2 weighted (FISP 90°, 5 mm surface coil)

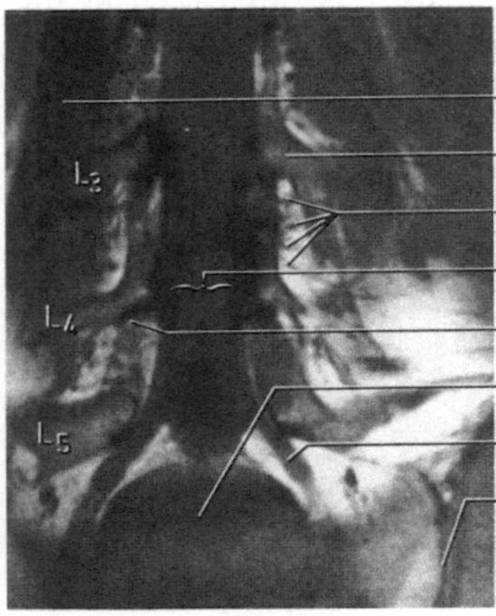

Fig. 2.72. Coronal section through middle lumbar spine and cord (SE, TR 0.6 s/TE 22 ms)

(Fig. 2.71). Here the mass presents as an area of low signal in the bright CSF of the spinal sac. The nerve fibers coursing in the dural sac appear as conspicuous voids in the bright fluid.

Coronal Sections

It is almost impossible to demonstrate the entire lumbar dural sheath on standard coronal sections because of the strong lordotic curvature of the lumbar spine. As a rule, only the region between L3 and L4 lies on the standard coronal plane of the MR imager (Fig. 2.72). The oblique, dorsally angled scan can at least display the intradural structures from L1 to L3 on one image. Bright fatty tissue is seen in the intervertebral foramina, through which the spinal nerves pass caudally as thin structures of low signal. In contrast to the thoracic spine, the spinal nerves of this region can be traced outside the vertebral column for several centimeters as they course parallel to the psoas major muscle.

2.9.5 Functional Anatomy

All motor and sensory fibers that travel from the brain to the periphery or in the reverse direction unite in the spinal cord. Spinal nerves leave the cord on the right and left sides and pass through the intervertebral foramina to their target organs. The segmentation of the spinal column (subdivision into vertebrae) is reflected in the spinal cord, although there it is not morphologically apparent (Fig. 2.73). In early childhood the longitudinal growth of the spinal cord starts to lag behind that of the vertebral skeleton (ascent of the cord). Thus, the cord extends to the sacral region only in the first months of life; by the age of 3 years it extends to the level of L3 or L4, and by adulthood it extends only to L1 or L2.

The relative shortening of the spinal cord in relation to the vertebral column results in a proximal displacement of the cord segments - a fact that must be considered when establishing the level of spinal lesions (Fig. 2.73). While there are seven cervical vertebrae, there are eight spinal cord segments in the cervical region. Their roots pass through the intervertebral foramina located *above* the corresponding cervical vertebrae. Thus the spinal nerve of the eight cervical cord segment exits the vertebral canal between C7 and T1. The 12 roots of the thoracic cord, the five roots of the lumbar cord, and the five roots of the sacral cord all emerge *below* the corresponding vertebra or sacral segment. The eight cervical cord segment is approximately at the level of the C7 vertebra, while the twelfth thoracic segment is level with the T10 vertebra and the fifth lumbar segment is level with the L1 vertebra. The five sacral segments of the cord span only about 1½ vertebral bodies (L1–L2).

The spinal nerves converge in the plexuses to form the peripheral nerve trunks, which no longer have a segmental arrangement. But this segmentation reoccurs in the periphery with the appearance of the dermatomes (Fig. 2.73). The dermatomes are an important guide for the neurologist in determining the level of spinal lesions. Unless stated otherwise, the neurologist's report will refer to the involved spinal cord segment, and not to the vertebra itself. This must be kept in mind when the MR examination is performed. In patients with root compression relating, say, to cauda equina syndrome caused by a herniated lumbar disc, the level of the lesion will be designated according to the bony segments of the vertebral column.

Continual improvements in the resolution of the spinal cord on axial sections by the use of surface coils, with the capability for gray-white matter differentiation, may give MR imaging an important role in patients with partial impairments of individual cord functions. The gray matter of the spinal cord consists of cells that form an H-shaped or butterfly pattern at the center of the cord. This is surrounded by the white matter, which contains the long ascending and descending fiber tracts (Fig. 2.74). The "butterfly" is formed by the ventral horns, which contain motor cells, the sensory dorsal horns, and the intermediate substance. The ventral and dorsal nerve roots emerge from the ventral and dorsal horns, respectively, and unite in the spinal ganglion. The white matter is divided into a right and left posterior funiculus, lateral funiculus, and anterior funiculus. The posterior funiculus contains ascending sensory tracts (the fasciculi gracilis and cuneatus) which convey proprioceptive sensation. The lateral funiculus contains the pyramidal or lateral corticospinal tract, which carries in part the efferents of the precentral area. The lateral funiculus also conveys sensory tracts (temperature, pain, etc.) which, together with the tracts in the anterior funiculus, comprise the "anterolateral system". The anterior funiculus in particular contains several pathways of the extrapyramidal system as well as the anterior corticospinal tract formed by the uncrossed pyramidal fibers.

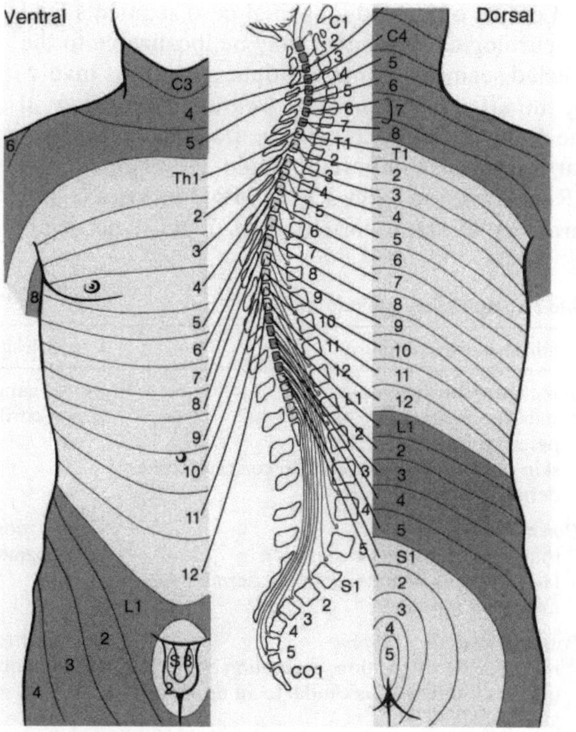

Fig. 2.73. Functional anatomy of spinal cord along its axis: segmental arrangement of spine and cord, ventral and dorsal dermatomes

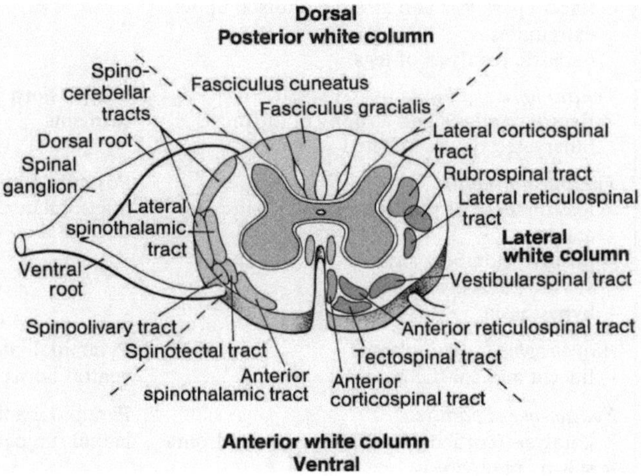

Fig. 2.74. Functional anatomy of spinal cord in an axial diagram: long fiber tracts, gray matter ("butterfly"), and nerve roots

Lesions of individual spinal cord segments lead to neurologic deficits that may be localizable to the affected segment or may produce symptoms involving the affected segment as well as those below it. The level indicated by the neurologist is the primary and most important guide for planning the MR examination (Sect. 3.1). If MRI discloses an abnormality at the indicated level, it must be determined whether the MR finding is consistent with the neurologic syndrome described. Thus, a knowledge of the various spinal cord syndromes can be of great value to the examiner. A detailed treatment of this topic would exceed the scope of this text. Tables 2.1 gives an overview of the cord syndromes associated with damage to individual pathways or nuclei.

Table 2.1. Spinal cord syndromes

Syndrome, symptoms	Site of lesion	Cause
Spinal ganglion syndrome - stabbing pains - paresthesias - skin reddening and vesicles in corresponding dermatome, unilateral	Spinal ganglion of corresponding spinal cord segments, ipsilateral	Inflammation (virus, e.g., zoster)
Dorsal root syndrome - total or partial loss of sensation - lancing pains in corresponding dermatome - muscular hypotonia	Dorsal root of corresponding spinal cord segments, ipsilateral	Inflammation (e.g., tabes dorsalis)
Posterior funiculi syndrome - loss of sense of position, perception of vibration, and stereognosis caudal to an upper margin, ipsilateral - positive Romberg test - ataxia with eyes closed	Posterior funiculus at upper margin of symptoms	Inflammation Spinal funicular disease Friedreich's ataxia Trauma Extramedullary tumor
Dorsal horn syndrome - segmental pains and defects of temperature perception (dissociated defects of perception) in affected segment	Dorsal horn of affected spinal cord	Syringomelia Hematomyelia Intramedullary tumor
Gray matter syndrome - analgesia and thermanalgesia in affected area, bilateral - flaccid paralysis and atrophy of distal upper extremities (-spastic paralysis of legs)	Center of gray matter	Syringomelia or Hematomyelia (usually in the cervical cord) Intramedullary tumor
Ventral horn syndrome - flaccid paralysis and atrophy of the muscles innervated by the affected segments	Ventral horn of affected spinal cord segments	Acute poliomyelitis Chronic progressive spinal muscular dystrophy
Funicular myelosis - loss of sense of position of lower extremity - ataxia - positive Romberg sign - spastic paraparesis - hypesthesia	Posterior funiculi and pyramidal tracts, bilateral	Pernicious anemia Nutritional deficiencies
Amyotrophic lateral sclerosis - flaccid and spastic pareses	Pyramidal lateral funiculus and ventral horns	Degenerative
Spastic spinal paralysis - paralysis (corticospinal) pathways syndrome - spastic paraparesis	Pyramidal anterior funiculus and lateral funiculus	Degenerative
Brown-Sequard syndrome - ipsilateral: spastic paralysis, loss of perception of position and of vibration, hyperesthesia below the lesion - contralateral: analgesia, thermanalgesia below the lesion	Pyramidal tract, posterior funiculi, ventral horns, ventral root, spinothalamic tracts in segment of upper sensitive margin, ipsilateral	Multiple sclerosis Tumor Trauma Radiomyelopathy

References

1. Aguila LA, Piraino DW, Modic MT, Dudley AW, Duchesneau PM, Weinstein MA (1985) The intranuclear cleft of the intervertebral disk: magnetic resoncance imaging. Radiology 155: 155-158
2. Atlas SW, Zimmerman RA, Bilaniuk LT, Rorke L, Hackney DB, Goldberg HI, Grossman RI (1986) Corpus callosum and limbic system: neuroanatomic MR evaluation of developmental anomalies. Radiology 160: 355-362
3. Bilaniuk LT, Zimmerman RA, Wehrli FW, Snyder PJ, Goldberg HI, Grossman RI, Bottomley PA, Edelstein WA (1984) Magnetic resonance imaging of pituitary lesions using 1.0 to 1.5 T field strength. Radiology 153: 415-418
4. Bilaniuk LT, Schenck JF, Zimmerman RA, Hart HR, Foster TH, Edelstein WA, Goldberg HI, Grossman RI (1985) Ocular and orbital lesions: surface coil MR imaging. Radiology 156: 674-699
5. Biller J, Graff-Radford NR, Smoker WRK, Adams HP, Johnston P (1986) MR imaging in "lacunar" hemiballismus. J Comp Assist Tomogr 10 (5): 793-797
6. Daniels DL, Herfkins R, Gager WE, Meyer GA, Koehler PR, Williams AL, Haughton VM (1984) Magnetic resonance imaging of the optic nerves and chiasm. Radiology 152: 79-83
7. Daniels DL, Herfkins R, Koehler PR, Millen SJ, Shaffer KA, Williams AL, Haughton VM (1984) Magnetic resonance imaging of the internal auditory canal. Radiology 151: 195-208
8. Daniels DL, Pech P, Haughton VM (1984) Magnetic resonance imaging of the temporal bone. General Electric Company, Milwaukee, Wisconsin
9. Daniels DL, Pojunas KW, Pech P, Haughton VM (1984) Magnetic resonance imaging of the sella and juxtasellar region. General Electric Company Milwaukee, Wisconsin
10. Daniels DL, Pech P, Mark L, Pojunas K, Williams AL, Haughton VM (1985) Magnetic resonance imaging of the cavernous sinus. AJR 144: 1009-1014
11. Daniels DL, Schenck JF, Foster T, Hart H, Millen SJ, Meyer GA, Pech P, Haughton VM (1985) Magnetic resonance imaging of the jugular foramen. AJNR 6: 699-703
12. Daniels DL, Pech P, Pojunas KW, Kilgore DP, Williams AL, Haughton VM (1986) Trigeminal nerve: anatomic correlation with MR imaging. Radiology 159: 577-583
13. Drayer B, Burger P, Darwin R, Riederer S, Herfkens R, Johnson GA (1986) MRI of brain iron. AJR 174: 103-110
14. Drayer BP, Olanow W, Burger P, Johnson GA, Herfkens R, Riederer S (1986) Parkinson plus syndrome: Diagnosis using high field MR imaging of brain iron. Radiology 159: 493-498
15. Duus P (1983) Neurologisch topische Diagnostik, 3. Auflage, Georg Thieme Verlag Stuttgart
16. Edelman RR, Shoukimas GM, Stark DD, Davis KR, New PFJ, Saini S, Rosenthal DI, Wismer GL, Brady TJ (1985) High-resolution surface-coil imaging of lumbar disk disease. AJR 144: 1123-1129
17. Edwards JH, Hyman RA, Vacirca SJ, Boxer MA, Packer S, Kaufman IH, Stein HL (1985) 0.6 T magnetic resonance imaging of the orbit. AJR 144: 1015-1020
18. Flannigan BD, Bradley WG, Mazziotta JC, Raschning W, Bentson JR, Lufkin RB, Hieshima GB (1985) Magnetic resonance imaging of the brainstem: normal structure and basic functional anatomy. Radiology 154: 375-383
19. Gademann G (1984) NMR tomography of the normal brain. Springer, Berlin, Heidelberg
20. Gademann G (1985) Normal cerebral anatomy in the NMR tomogram as basis of therapeutic intervention. Röntgen-Bl 38: 137-142
21. Gänshirt H (1972) (Editor), Der Hirnkreislauf. Georg Thieme Verlag Stuttgart
22. Gomori JM, Grossman RI, Goldberg HI, Zimmerman RA, Bilaniuk LT (1985) Intracranial hematomas: imaging by high-field MR. Radiology 157: 87-93
23. de Groot J (1984) Correlative neuroanatomy of computed tomography and magnetic resonance imaging. Lea & Febiger, Philadelphia
24. Han JS, Kaufman B, El Yousef SJ, Benson JE, Bonstelle CT, Alfidi RJ, Haaga JR, Yeung H, Huss RG (1983) NMR imaging of the spine. AJR 141: 1137-1145
25. Han JS, Bonstelle CT, Kaufman B, Benson JE, Alfidi RJ, Clampitt M, Van Dyke C, Huss RG (1984) Magnetic resonance imaging in the evaluation of the brainstem. Radiology 150: 705-712
26. Hennig J, Friedburg H, Ströbel B (1986) Rapid nontomographic approach to MR myelography without contrast agents. J Comp Assist Tomogr 10: 375-378
27. Hirano A (1981) A guide to neuropathology. New York, Tokyo, Igaku-Shoin
28. Höhne K-H, Witte G, Heller M, Riemer M (1986) Three dimensional investigation of tomography volumes (CT and MR imaging) 72nd scientific assembly and annual meeting of the Radiological Society of North America, Nov 30-Dec 5, 1986. Book of Abstracts p 378
29. Huber DJ, Mueller E, Heubes P (1985) Oblique magnetic resonance imaging of normal structures. AJR 145: 843-846
30. Jenkins JPR, Hickey DS, Zhu XP, Machin M, Isherwood I (1985) MR imaging of the intervertebral disk: a quantitative study. Br J Radiol 58: 705-709
31. Kaufman B (1984) Magnetic resonance imaging of the pituitary gland. Radiologic Clinics of North America 22 (4): 795-803
32. Koenig H, Lenz M, Sauter R (1986) Temporal bone region: High-resolution MR imaging using surface coils. Radiology 159: 191-194
33. Koritke JG, Sick H (1982) Atlas anatomischer Schnittbilder des Menschen, 1. Band: Kopf, Hals, Brust. Urban & Schwarzenberg, München, Wien, Baltimore
34. Kretschmann H-J, Weinrich W (1984) Neuroanatomie der kraniellen Computertomographie. Georg Thieme Verlag Stuttgart, New York
35. Lee BCP, Deck MDF, Kneeland JB, Cahill DT (1985) MR imaging of the craniocervical junction. AJNR 6: 209-213
36. Mark L, Pech P, Daniels D, Charles C, Williams A, Haughton V (1984) The pituitary fossa: a correlative anatomic and MR study. Radiology 153: 453-457
37. Modic MT, Weinstein MA, Pavlicek W, Boumphrey F, Starnes D, Duchesneau PM (1983) Magnetic resonance imaging of the cervical spine: technical and clinical observations. AJR 141: 1129-1139
38. Modic MT, Pavlicek W, Weinstein MA, Boumphrey F, Ngo F, Hardy R, Duchesneau PM (1984) Magnetic resonance imaging of intervertebral disk disease. Radiology 152: 103-111
39. Mumenthaler M (1982) Neurologie. 7. Auflage, Georg Thieme Verlag Stuttgart
40. Naidich TP, Daniels DL, Haughton VM, Williams A, Po-

junas K, Palacios E (1987) Hippocampal formations and related structures of the limbic lobe: anatomic-MR correlation. Part I. Surface features and coronal sections. Radiology 162: 747-754
41. Naidich TP, Daniels DL, Haughton VM, Pech P, Williams A, Pojunas K, Palacios E (1987) Hippocampal formations and related structures of the limbic lobe: anatomical-MR correlation. Part II. Sagittal sections. Radiology 162: 755-761
42. Netter FH (1983) The Ciba collection of medial illustrations. Vol I: Nervous system. Part I: Anatomy and physiology. CIBA Pharmaceutical Company West Caldwell
43. New PFJ, Bachow TB, Wismer GL, Rosen BR, Brady TJ (1985) MR imaging of the acoustic nerves and small acoustic neuromas at 0.6 T: prospective study. AJR 144: 1021-1026
44. Pech P, Daniels DL, Williams AL, Haughton VM (1985) The cervical neural foramina: correlation of microtomy and CT anatomy. Radiology 155: 143-146
45. Pernkopf E, Ferner H (1980) Atlas der topographischen und angewandten Anatomie des Menschen. Bd I: Kopf und Hals. Urban & Schwarzenberg München
46. Popper KR, Eccles JC (1977) The self and its brain - an argument for interactionism. Springer Verlag Heidelberg, Berlin, London, New York
47. Rohen JW (1975) Funktionelle Anatomie des Nervensystems, FK Schattauer Verlag Stuttgart, New York
48. Rohen JW, Yokochi C (1982) Anatomie des Menschen. Band I: Kopf, Hals, Rumpf. FK Schattauer Verlag Stuttgart, New York
49. Salamon G, Huang YP (1980) Computed tomography of the brain. Springer Verlag Berlin Heidelberg New York
50. Schaltenbrand G, Wahren W (1977) Atlas for stereotaxy of the human brain. Georg Thieme Verlag Stuttgart
51. Schaltenbrand G, Walker AE (1982) Stereotaxy of the human brain. Georg Thieme Verlag Stuttgart, New York
52. Schenck JF, Zimmerman RA, Bilaniuk LT (1984) Magnetic resonance imaging of the orbit. General Electric Company, Milwaukee, Wisconsin
53. Schenck JF, Hart HR, Foster TH, Edelstein WA, Bottomley PA, Redington RW, Hardy CJ, Zimmerman RA, Bilaniuk LT (1985) Improved MR imaging of the orbit at 1.5 T with surface coils. AJR 144: 1033-1036
54. Schnitzlein HN, Murtagh FR, Clarke LP, Jones JD, Arrington JA, Silbiger ML (1985) Imaging anatomy of the head and spine. Urban & Schwarzenberg Medical Publishers Baltimore, Munich
55. Simon JH, Holtas SL, Schiffer RB, Rudick RA, Herndon RM, Kido DK, Utz R (1986) Corpus callosum and subcallosal-periventricular lesions in multiple sclerosis: detection with MR. Radiology 169: 363-367
56. Sobotta J, Ferner H, Staubesand J (1982) Atlas der Anatomie des Menschen Bd I: Kopf, Hals, obere Extremitäten. Urban & Schwarzenberg, München, Berlin, Wien
57. Swartz JD (1984) The facial nerve canal: CT analysis of the protruding typanic segment. Radiology 153: 443-447
58. Takahashi S, Goto K, Fukasawa H, Kawata Y, Uemura K, Suzuki K (1985) Computed tomography of cerebral infarction along the distribution of the basal perforation arteries. Part I: Striate arterial group. Radiology 155: 107-118
59. Takahashi S, Goto K, Fukasawa H, Kawata Y, Uemura K, Yaguchi K (1985) Computer tomography of cerebral infarction along the distribution of the basal perforation arteries. Part II: Thalamic arterial group. Radiology 155: 119-130
60. Thurn P, Friedmann G (1983) Computertomographie der Wirbelsäule und des Spinalkanals. Ferdinand Enke Verlag Stuttgart
61. Update, Magnetic resonance tomographic imaging of the head and spine. General Electric Company, Milwaukee, Wisconsin 1983
62. Yenerich DO, Haughton VM (1986) Oblique plane MR imaging of the cervical spine. J Comp Assist Tomogr 10 (5): 823-826

3 Practical Aspects of the MR Examination

3.1 Preparations

W. J. Huk, G. Gademann, and G. Friedmann

3.1.1 Explaining the Procedure to the Patient

The fear that many patients have of the imaging equipment can be relieved by explaining to them in simple language how the scanner operates and how the examination will proceed. MR imaging is not known to be associated with any lasting injurious effects when the unit is operated at the field strengths recommended by the manufacturer. However, the static magnetic field, the changing gradient fields, and the RF pulses can interfere with the function of cardiac pacemakers and neurostimulators and can cause metallic implants to become displaced. It is necessary, therefore, that the patient be asked several questions prior to the examination so that risk factors can be identified. The standard question list is shown in Table 3.1, and absolute and relative contraindications are listed in Table 3.2. In patients whose vital functions are unstable, the examination should either be withheld or conducted with suitable precautionary measures; these are listed in Table 3.3. Risks and side effects are discussed at the end of this chapter (Sect. 3.4).

Before the patient enters the magnet room, he should be divested of all loose metallic objects that could be attracted by the magnet (keys, glasses, watch, coin purse, pocket knife, hair clips, hairpins, etc.). Credit cards are removed, since the magnetic data can be erased by the magnetic field. One must remember to remove objects like dentures, necklaces, and earrings before examinations of the head.

3.1.2 Positioning

The patient should be positioned as comfortably as possible. This may involve placing pads beneath the knees, for example, or covering the patient with a light blanket.

Table 3.1. Questions to be asked candidates for MR examination

- "Do you wear a cardiac pacemaker or other active implant like an insulin pump, etc.?" The magnetic field can interfere with the proper function of these devices.
- "Do you have any metal objects in your body such as an artificial hip, surgical clips, shrapnel, or bone pins?" Metallic objects of this kind may become heated or displaced by the magnetic field.
- "Is there a chance you are pregnant?" So far there is no evidence that the examination can harm the embryo or fetus, but for safety it is best to postpone examinations in pregnant women until after the first trimester.
- "Do you have any allergies?" This question is chiefly of interest if the use of contrast agents is proposed (see also Chap. 5).

Table 3.2. Contraindications to MR examination

1. Cardiac pacemaker or other neurostimulating device that is apt to malfunction in the magnetic field.
2. Intracranial vascular clips that are magnetic or whose magnetic properties are unknown.
3. First trimester of pregnancy. At present this is only a precautionary measure, since MR is not known to have any adverse effects on the embryo or fetus.
4. Unstable vital functions in cases where instrument monitoring is unavailable.

Table 3.3. Precautionary measures

1. Continuous monitoring of patients:
   a) with seizure disorder, by means of a video camera or an observer in close attendance. Patients with a seizure disorder should not discontinue their antiepileptic medication before the examination.
   b) with unstable cardiovascular function on ECG.
   c) with a tracheostomy or impaired swallowing and cough reflex (e.g., secondary to brainstem lesion or cranial neuropathy).
2. Rapid access to the patient and means for immediate removal of the patient from the scanner for emergency care in the event of a seizure, cardiac arrest, respiratory distress, or other incident. A nonferromagnetic stretcher should be available for transporting the patient.
3. An emergency kit that is equipped for all contingencies and whose contents are regularly checked. The instruments should have no ferromagnetic parts so that they can be handled in proximity to the magnet.

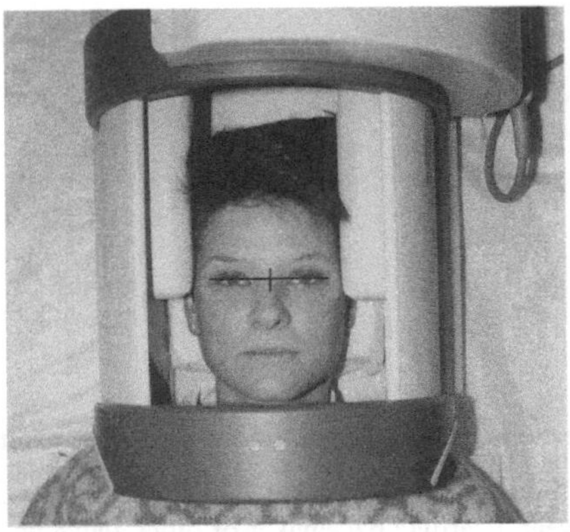

Fig. 3.1. Positioning of patient in head coil

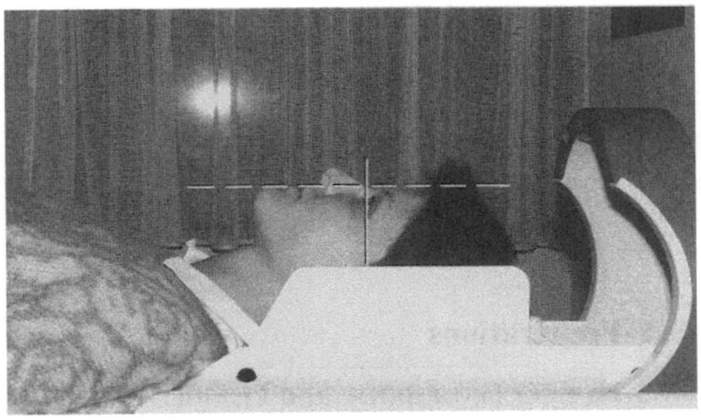

Fig. 3.2. Approximate positioning relative to the CA-CP system: "facial plane" *(dashed line)* along the *z* axis (see also Fig. 2.3)

For examinations of the *head,* the patient's head is centered in the head coil and oriented at right angles to it. The indicator light should be centered on the root of the nose, with the edges of the beam evenly touching the lateral canthi of the eyes (Fig. 3.1). For reproducibility of image planes, it is best to use a constant inclination of the head. This can be achieved by referral to the "facial plane" extending from the chin to the superior orbital margin, which closely approximates the coronal plane of the CA-CP system (see Fig. 3.2 and Sect. 2.1). The head is held in place with a foam-rubber rest and side cushions.

For examinations of the *vertebral column,* the spine should be as straight as possible (correct for thoracic kyphosis, lumbar lordosis, and lateral curvatures) so that a significant length of spine can be visualized on a given sagittal or coronal plane. The cervical cord is imaged most effectively by moving the head coil caudally or by using a Helmholtz coil configuration (Fig. 3.3). When surface coils are used, care must be taken that the region of interest is positioned at the center of the coil, where image quality is best. In thoracic spine imaging, artifacts from cardiac motion can be reduced by the use of ECG triggering or by changing the direction of the phase gradient (see also Sect. 1.3.5 and Chap. 17).

For studies of the *orbital region,* it is best to image both orbits concurrently with the head in the exact sagittal position (see also Chap. 12). This allows comparison of the orbits and can be achieved by the use of oval or eyeglass-shaped surface coils (Fig. 3.4).

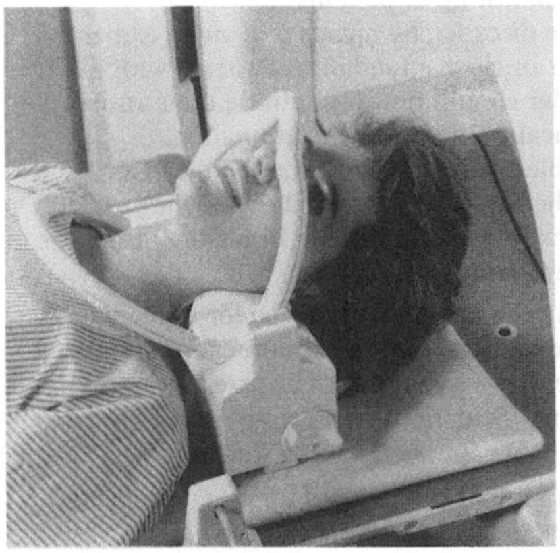

Fig. 3.3. Examination of cervical spine and cord using a Helmholtz coil configuration. (Photograph from Siemens)

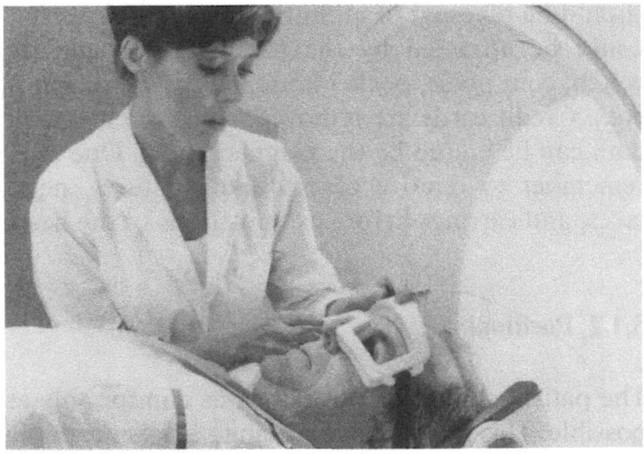

Fig. 3.4. Examination of both orbits using a special orbit coil. (Photograph from Picker International)

High-resolution images of the *petrous bone* in patients with middle ear disease or cranial neuropathy (cranial nerves VII and VIII) are obtained by using a round surface coil approximately 10 cm in diameter that is centered over the external auditory meatus (Fig. 3.5). Because the images made with this setup are strictly unilateral, it is recommended that head-coil images also be obtained so that the two sides can be compared.

Details on examinations using *contrast agents* are given in Sect. 5.5.

Newborns and small infants will fit comfortably within a standard head coil, resulting in images with excellent anatomic detail. Special methods for immobilization are described in Sect. 3.3 and Chap. 6.

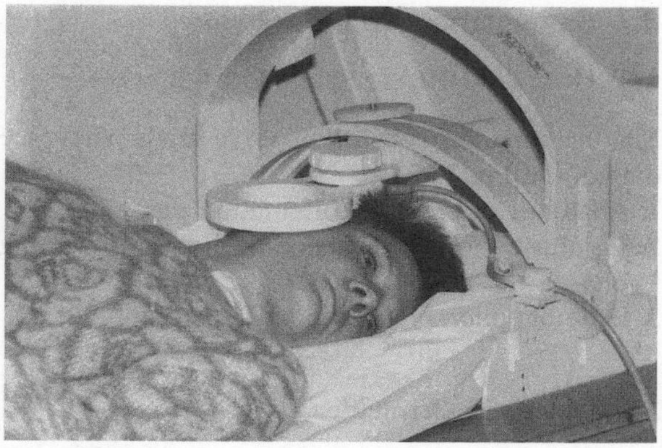

Fig. 3.5. Examination of temporal region using a plane circular surface coil

3.2 Examination Procedure

W.J. HUK, G. GADEMANN, and G. FRIEDMANN

The examination consists of three main parts (see diagram in Fig. 3.6):

1. Anatomic orientation (orientation phase)
2. Demonstration or exclusion of disease (screening phase)
3. Differentiation of disease (differentiation phase).

3.2.1 Anatomic Orientation

The purpose of the orientation scan is twofold: to confirm that the patient is correctly positioned, and to locate the region of diagnostic interest. This part of the examination is analogous to the topogram or "scout view" of the CT examination. We prefer for orientation a T1-weighted SE sequence with short TR and short TE, perhaps using a reduced matrix of 128 × 128. Fast imaging also may be used for this part of the examination.

Since axial and coronal images are preferred for lesions not located on the midsagittal line, the midsagittal plane is considered ideal for orientation, analogous to the lateral tomogram in CT. The midsagittal image accurately displays the position of the anterior and posterior commissures, making it possible to apply the anatomic orientation system described in Sect. 2.1.

For lesions that are presumed to lie on the midsagittal plane, it is reasonable to begin the orientation with an axial scan. This makes it possible to confirm an exact vertical position of the head so that an accurate midsagittal plane can be established.

Fast axial scans are used for spinal cord orientation, again for the purpose of accurately establishing the important midsagittal plane.

3.2.2 Demonstration or Exclusion of Disease

In the screening phase an optimum signal-to-noise ratio is necessary for maximum anatomic detail, and high contrast is required for the detection of disease. The SE sequence with a long TR and a short and long TE (spin-density and T2 weighted) satisfies these requirements. Usually the whole region of interest in the brain can be screened using a series of 8-mm slices.

A region of interest in the spinal cord can generally be screened with a T1-weighted sagittal image (e.g., TR 250–600 ms, TE <30 ms).

3.2.3 Differentiation of Disease

The differentiation phase provides information on the extent, characteristics, and location of the disease focus as a prelude to therapeutic planning. Figure 3.7 illustrates the contrasts of different normal and pathologic tissues on SE images made with different types of weighting and without contrast agents. Even the screening phase, with its combination of spin-density and T2 weighting, can provide some tissue differentiation and, depending on the diagnostic problem, may be of sufficient quality to obviate the need for a separate differentiation phase. If a tumor is suspected, a multiecho sequence can be of further help in differentiating edema, necrosis, and tumor. Vascular malformations can be accurately differentiated with T1-weighted images or mixed images using the double-echo technique (a symmetrical echo sequence is preferred because of the flow phenomenon of even-echo rephasing; see Sect. 1.3 and Chap. 5). T1-weighted images are suitable for detecting subacute and chronic hemorrhages, demonstrating fatty tissue, and defining the boundaries of the brain owing to the high level of contrast between brain tissue and the dark CSF. The contrast between CSF and bone is low in these sequences but is higher in the T2-weighted scan. Gray matter - white matter contrast is expecially high in the IR sequence. Repeating the measurement of a series of slices using a modified pulse sequence (e.g., a multiecho image of a selected slice combined with a heavily T1-weighted image) permits the calculation of T1, T2, and N(H) images and the construction of synthetic images (see Sect. 1.4).

In the present context we can deal only with fairly general imaging strategies. Each case must be considered individually on the basis of clinical and other findings so that an appropriate diagnostic program can be devised. Additional recommendations on the use of the various pulse sequences may be found in [2, 12, 29].

An important concern besides the tissue differentiation of a lesion is its location, which usually is more easily assessed in a separate orthogonal scan. Thus, the differentiation sequence should be performed with the same imaging technique but on a plane corresponding to the anatomic site of the lesion (see Sects. 2.2–2.6).

The use of contrast agents (gadolinium-DTPA) greatly enhances the appearance of many CNS lesions and will confirm a disruption of the blood-brain barrier in brain diseases (see also Chap. 5).

	Brain: Periphery – Section	Brain: Periphery – Sequence	Brain: Midline – Section	Brain: Midline – Sequence	Spine – Section	Spine – Sequence
Orientation-phase	Sagittal	"Fast" SE: T1	Axial	"Fast" SE: T1	Axial	"Fast" SE: T1
Screeningphase	Axial	SE: N(H) and T2	Sagittal	SE: T1	Sagittal	SE: T1 bipolar (flow!)
Differentiation-phase	Axial	SE: T1 IR: T1 Multiecho	Sagittal	SE: N(H), T2 IR	Sagittal	SE: N(H), T2
	Coronal	SE: T1, T2, N(H) IR	Coronal	SE: T1 N(H), T2 IR	Coronal	SE: T1, T2
	Sagittal	SE: T1, T2, N(H) IR	Axial	SE: T1 N(H), T2 IR	Axial	SE: T1, T2

Fig. 3.6. Diagram of an examination procedure

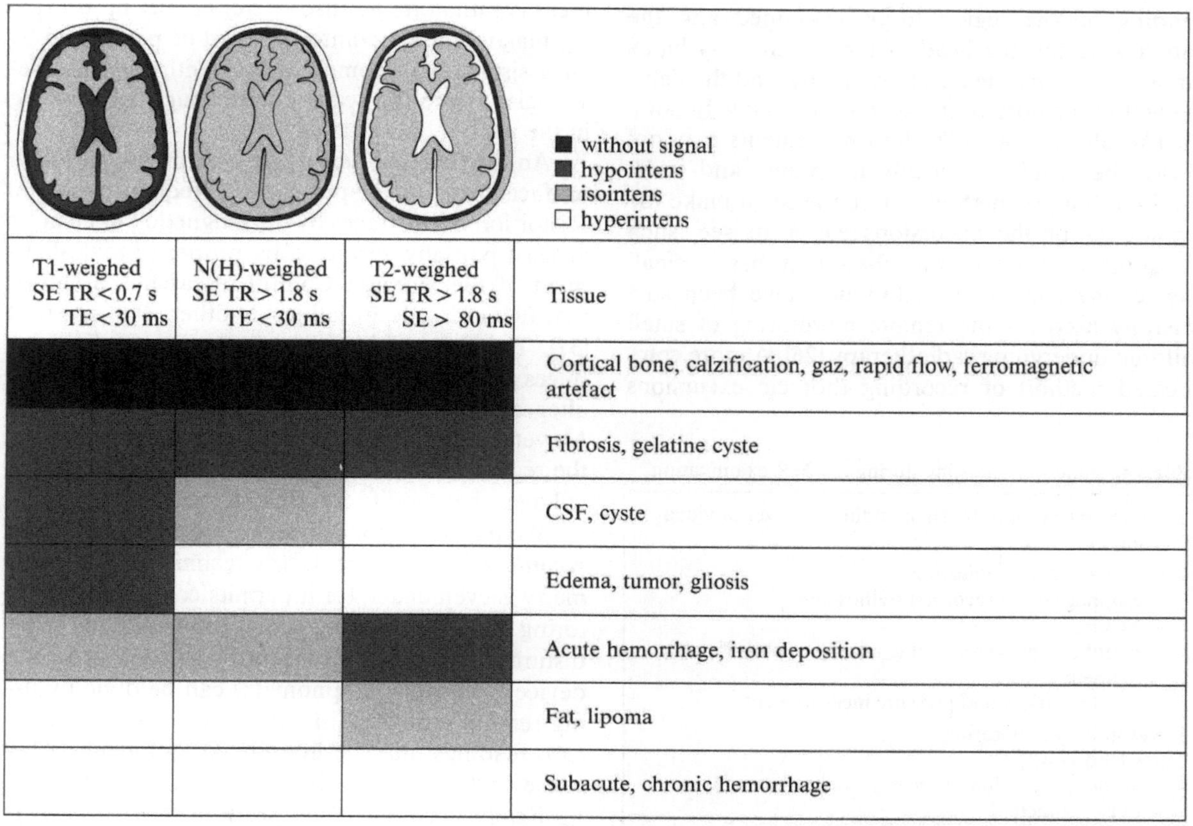

Fig. 3.7. Contrasts in the native MR image (SE) and their corresponding normal or pathologic tissue

3.3 Sedation, Anesthesia, and Anesthesiologic Monitoring During MR Examinations

TH. PASCH, H. GÖTZ, and E. KRAUS

The duties of the anesthesiologist in MR examinations are basically the same as in CT examinations [1]. In uncooperative or seriously ill patients, suitable means must be employed for the monitoring of vital cardiovascular and respiratory functions. Besides the maintenance of these vital functions, adequate immobilization may be necessary to ensure that a proper MR examination can be carried out.

3.3.1 **Monitoring** (Table 3.4)

Given the peculiarities of the MR imaging technique, *traditional routine monitoring procedures* either are not applicable or can be used only with restrictions [22,25]. If the examination is performed under general anesthesia or heavy sedation, an anesthesiologist must be present in the magnet room throughout the procedure so that he can observe the patient directly. Of course, the opportunities for direct clinical observation are limited. Depending on the region to be examined and the patient's height, the head of the patient may be as far as 2.5 m from the anesthesiologist, and the lighting within the bore of the scanner is relatively poor. As a result, the patient's chest movements may not always be visible, especially in infants and small children. Simple methods can be used to make the amplitudes of the excursions easier to see, such as taping a straw to the chest that has a small flag at one end. Such techniques have been successfully used for the remote monitoring of small children undergoing radiotherapy [26]. A more complicated method of recording thoracic excursions involves the use of a rubber pneumatic bellows [25].

Table 3.4. Patient monitoring during the MR examination

1. Direct observation (by an attending observer or video camera)
2. Cardiovascular monitoring
   - esophageal or precordial stethoscope
   - ECG
   - peripheral pulse recording, usually as part of pulse oximetry
   - oscillometric blood pressure measurement
3. Respiratory monitoring
   - stethoscope
   - visual observation of chest excursions
   - pulse oximetry
   - capnometry

For the reasons stated above, an esophageal stethoscope is preferable to a precordial stethoscope for auscultation of the anesthetized patient. Long connective tubing is needed for this purpose. Metal connectors should not be used.

We are unable to give detailed guidelines on *monitoring with electronic instruments,* because so far there has been little experience on what procedures can be used with what MR scanners without interfering with signal acquisition. A basic rule is that monitors should be set up outside the shielded area. Cathode ray tubes do not make the best monitoring screens, and liquid crystal displays (LCD) are preferred. Digital LED readouts also are reliable.

In MR systems with external shielding, leads as long as 6–8 m must be used to connect the sensors on the patient to the monitoring equipment. The possibility of image degradation should always be considered during placement of the wires. Loops of wire from monitoring equipment can degrade the RF pulses and the reception of the MR signals; also, spurious signals can be induced in the monitoring transducers [22]. If monitors and other equipment (ventilators, perfusors, etc) are set up outside the magnet room, monitoring must be performed by an assistant who communicates with the anesthesiologist inside the scan room through an opening in the wall.

An *ECG record* can usually be made, although artifacts from the RF pulses are a frequent problem. Distortion of the traces by the magnetic field can be at least partially corrected by proper spatial alignment of the monitor. Careful research has shown that ECG records are subject to other effects as well [31]. The flow of blood in the magnetic field induces a voltage through the Hall effect, and this can alter a number of ECG components (P, ST, T). Movements of electrodes and cables, especially in the region of the limbs or cardiac apex, also induce voltages that modify the ECG trace.

We have had good results with peripheral *pulse recording* by the photoelectric technique. Pulse oximetry is even better, for it permits concurrent monitoring of the respiration. It may, however, markedly disturb the imaging procedure (depending on the device employed). Capnometry can be done by using remote sampling, in which case end-expiratory CO_2 readings must be interpreted with caution because of the length of the sampling tube [22].

Really accurate *blood pressure measurement* is not possible directly or by the cuff method. The connections between the intra-arterial cannula or cuff and the actual monitor are so long that they cannot transmit pressure data accurately. Thus, as in capnography, we are able to monitor trends, but we cannot obtain true absolute readings. Nevertheless, it is worthwhile to monitor the blood pressure with an oscillometric instrument, which likewise is set up outside the shielded area. As with all tubing and connections (e.g., on the endotracheal tube), metallic connectors should be replaced by plastic connectors.

3.3.2 Sedation

All patients who must be heavily sedated or anesthetized require an i.v. line. The bottle can be suspended from a hook mounted at the head end of the scanner, where the anesthesiologist is seated. The standard tubes must be lengthened to about 2-3 m. Three-way stopcocks for administering medication should be installed close to the patient but still within easy reach. All valves and connectors must be made of plastic. Syringes containing the necessary medications are laid out close to the stopcocks. Patients who are sedated but breathing spontaneously are given oxygen supplied through a line from a source outside the magnet room. The oxygen line is secured inside the nose or attached to an oral tube.

Varying degrees of *sedation* will be required for children and for adults not cooperative enough to lie still during the imaging procedure. Recommendations for pediatric sedation are given in Table 3.5. It should be noted that the use of *chlorprothixene drops,* while very effective, is also problematic because at least 60 min are needed for the drug to take effect, and the duration of effect is so long that outpatient use is impractical. The therapeutic range of this drug is limited, and it is contraindicated in patients with heart problems. Prolonged supervision is also necessary following the use of *flunitrazepam drops.*

The rectal use of *diazepam* or *chloral hydrate* would seem attractive, but the absorption and thus the effect of these drugs is difficult to predict, and their sedative action may be inadequate.

If immobilization for the duration of the imaging procedure cannot be confidently expected - and this tends not be the case in infants and small children - general anesthesia by endotracheal intubation should be planned. This has been done successfully in spontaneously breathing patients [11], but we always use relaxation and controlled ventilation for safety and to facilitate monitoring.

Table 3.5. Sedation of children

1. Midazolam 0.1-0.2 mg/kg body weight sublingually (using a flavored preparation) 0.5 mg/kg body weight rectally
2. Flunitrazepam 0.05-0.1 mg/kg body weight sublingually (max. dose 2 mg) Prolonged effect contraindicates outpatient use! Benzodiazepine injection solutions are given sublingually or rectally.
3. Chlorprothixene 0.5-1 mg/kg body weight in oral drops. Onset of action in 60-90 min, duration of action several hours. Not for outpatient use, therefore.

3.3.3 General Anesthesia

Anesthetic Equipment

Ventilation during general anesthesia should be carried out in semi-open systems if possible. The simplest device for manual ventilation is the Ambu-bag, to which oxygen is delivered from a remote source. The nonrebreathing valve must be installed close to the patient, i.e., connected directly to the endotracheal tube. We have had good results with an original Ambu-valve made of plastic [16]. It should be noted that at least 2 m of connecting hose is needed between the Ambu-bag and the Ambu-valve. This hose should have the smallest possible compressible volume, meaning a low compliance of the wall material. A compromise must be found for the hose caliber so that the gas volume in the hose is not too large, but the flow resistance is not too high.

If general anesthesia only is rarely induced for MR imaging, simple transportable devices may be used as ventilators, such as the Oxylog unit manufactured by Draeger [16]. This unit is only oxygen driven. By connecting the air intakes of the Oxylog unit to a nitrous oxide source, O_2/N_2O ventilation is possible. Generally, the ventilator must be placed outside the magnet room next to the monitors and deliver the gas mixture to the oral tube through a 6-8 m length of hose. These hoses should also have a small compressible volume with minimum flow resistance. Because the induction of anesthesia is always performed outside the magnet room, the long hoses and all other components of the ventila-

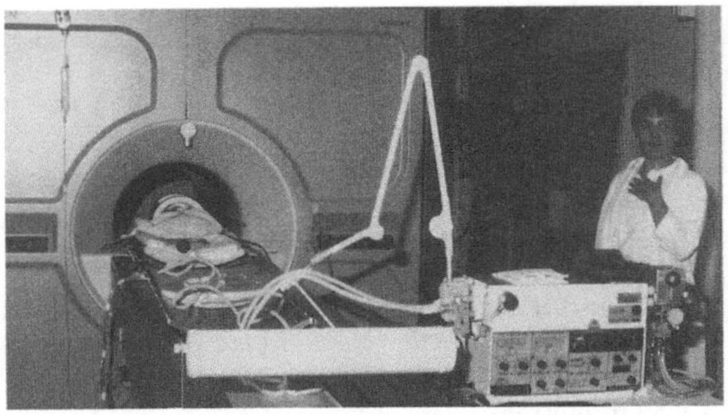

Fig. 3.8. Arrangement of ventilation equipment in magnet room

tion system can be thoroughly tested before the patient is wheeled into the room and moved into the scanner. The system may include facilities for volumetry, pulse oximetry, capnometry, and blood gas analysis. Of course other types of anesthetic and ventilation equipment also may be used, taking care that appropriate gas reservoirs are provided.

Frequent use of general anesthesia, as well as a sophisticated ventilation regimen in patients with pulmonary insufficiency, demands the installation of the ventilation system as close as possible to the patient inside the magnet room. We therefore installed, in cooperation with Siemens, a model 900 D anesthetic servoventilator with appropriate magnetic shielding of the metering valve in proximity to the tube (see Fig. 3.8). If necessary, a volatile anesthetic may be administered by vaporizer. The built-in monitoring systems for pressures, flows, volumes, and oxygen concentration can be fully utilized with this setup. The position of the ventilator and its exact alignment in the magnetic field depends on several factors, for example the strength of the magnetic field. In a field strength of 1.5 T the ventilating equipment installed on a wooden table, stands on firm ground at a distance of 3 m from the scanner. Without moving more than a very small distance it is possible to measure and determine the differences between analog and digital readouts. It has been shown that digital readouts are affected only little by the magnetic field. Analog instruments are strongly influenced by the magnetic field; even with optimum equipment placement they do not function reliably. In the knowledge of these differences and of the compressible volume of the no more than 3–4 m breathing hoses, it is possible to carry out adequate, safe, and sophisticated ventilation and general anesthesia with volatile anesthetics. If the ventilator is suitably aligned in the magnetic field, no interference with the imaging procedure will occur.

Table 3.6. Recommended dose of intravenous anesthetics for MR examination (especially in infants and small children)

1. Methohexital	
Bolus:	2 mg/kg
Maintenance:	2 mg/kg/h by perfusor
2. Vecuronium	
Bolus:	0.1 mg/kg
After 10 min:	0.2 mg/kg/h by perfusor
3. Ventilation usually with air/O_2 or N_2O/O_2	

Induction of Anesthesia

The goal of anesthesia is to immobilize the patient during the examination, which is totally painless. Loss of consciousness and relaxation are sufficient, therefore analgesia is not required. By operating an anesthetic ventilator inside the magnet room it is possible to induce anesthesia with volatile anesthetics (e.g., isoflurane) and relaxation with vecuronium. If the use of volatile anesthetics is contraindicated, i.v. anesthesia has to be carried out. To ensure a uniform depth of anesthesia and prevent intermittent motion artifacts, which will prolong the examination, we recommend that the standard induction be followed by a continuous infusion.

The perfusors are placed near the monitors outside the restricted area and operated by an assistant. The lines for the various medications are bundled together near the patient. Recommendations for the use and dosage of i.v. anesthetics are given in Table 3.6. The doses of both drugs listed, *methohexital* and *vecuronium,* were selected to ensure that the patient will not wake prematurely and that he will awake 15–20 min after the perfusor is turned off [14, 21]. For safety, we always antagonize the effect of the relaxant. Of course other kinds of anesthetics and relaxants also may be used, such as *benzodiazepines, pancuronium,* or the drugs *propofol* and *atracurium,* which are not yet available commercially [15, 17]. The choice depends upon the experience of the anesthetist, the presumed length of the examination, the condition of the patient, the possibilities of postanesthetic monitoring and nursing, and on whether the patient is a small child or an adult. For termination of anesthesia, the patient is removed from the scanner and the magnet room so that all the customary equipment will be available, as it was during induction.

Many problems of monitoring and anesthesia during MR imaging remain unsolved. Thus, the statements made in this chapter are tentative in nature and cannot apply equally to all types of equipment. It is hoped that the manufacturers of MR imagers will gain a clearer appreciation of anesthesiologic requirements and find design solutions that will enable these requirements to be met with greater efficiency.

3.4 Side Effects and Contraindications

W. J. HUK, K. GADEMANN, and G. FRIEDMANN

3.4.1 Biological Effects

It is conceivable that MR tomography could produce undesired side effects from the three types of electromagnetic fields that act upon the patient during imaging (Sect. 1.2.). To date, these fields have not been found to have any lasting adverse effects on the patient or examiner [28]. However, observation times have been relatively short, and long-term data on significant numbers of exposed patients are not yet available. In 1981 the British National Radiological Protection Board [18, 19] established guidelines for the operation of MR units, and similar guidelines were adopted 1 year later by the U.S. Bureau of Radiological Health (BRH) [7]. However, these guidelines are only temporary recommendations and are somewhat arbitrary. Similar recommendations have been issued by agencies in other countries, such as the Federal Board of Health [6] in the Federal Republic of Germany (see Table 3.7).

We shall now examine the effects of the three different fields on physiologic parameters in organisms [after 5].

It is known that *static magnetic fields* (0.02–2 T) can influence electromagnetic processes in organisms. These processes include impulse conduction in the heart (ECG trace), the velocity of nerve conduction, and membrane potentials. Flowing blood, which contains moving charge carriers in the form of dissociated salts, induces an electric voltage when placed in a magnetic field, and this voltage can have effects on the environment. ECG studies in rats have shown an increase in the T-wave amplitude while the animals were in the magnetic field. This effect can also be explained by a superposition of voltages induced by blood flow in the large vessels on the ECG tracing. Field strengths above 5 T have been shown to cause reversible changes in nerve conduction velocity in primates.

Previous studies on potential mutagenic effects and effects on hematopoietic and other fast-growing tissues have demonstrated no reproducible side effects [23, 27, 32].

Static fields could conceivably affect molecules whose magnetic properties vary with direction. The field could reorient these molecules and change their position in larger molecular aggregates [10]. This could lead to changes in enzyme kinetics.

Rapidly *changing gradient fields,* whose strengths range from 3 to 12 mT/m depending on the MR unit, are used to produce sectional images. These time-varying fields can induce electric currents that affect physiologic processes. These currents are estimated to be on the order of 1–5 μA/cm². Time-varying fields are known to induce light flashes, called phosphenes, when the rate of change of field intensity is 2–5 T/s. This phenomenon is caused by a direct stimulation of the optic nerves or retina but has no lasting injurious effects.

Radiofrequency pulses are used to excite the protons in tissues and elicit MR signals. Absorption of

Table 3.7. Recommended limits of exposure to MR imaging

	NRPB (1981, 1983)	BRH (1981)	BGA (1983)
Static magnetic field	2.5 T (whole and partial body)	2 T (whole and partial body)	2 T (whole and partial body)
Changing magnetic fields	20 T/s for SP 10 ms and longer; $(\frac{a\beta}{at})^2\, t < 4$ for SP shorter than 10 ms	3 T/s (whole and partial body)	Max. 3 μA/cm² or 3 mV/cm for SP 10 ms and longer; 30/τ μA/cm² or 30/τ μV/cm for SP shorter than 10 ms (τ in ms)
Radiofrequency fields	1 °C increase of body temperature SAR = 0.4 W/kg (whole body), SAR = 4 W/kg (av¹)	SAR = 0.4 W/kg (whole body); SAR = 2 W/kg (av¹)	SAR = 1 W/kg (whole body); SAR = 5 W/kg (partial body for every 1 kg of tissue excl. eye)

SP, switching period; *SAR*, specific absorption rate; av¹, averaged over any 1 g of tissue the high-frequency energy within the body leads to tissue heating, which increases with the frequency of the radiation [4, 8]. Also, the amount of energy that is dissipated as heat increases with the ionization of biochemical substances in the tissues. It is conceivable, then, that "hot spots" could develop within the nonhomogeneous human tissue, and so the RF energy should be kept as low as possible. So far, even high fields have been unable to raise tissue temperatures by more than about 1 °C [30]. The RF energy transmitted to the body during MR imaging is on the order of several W/kg (BRH: 0.4 W/kg averaged over the whole body, 2 W/kg averaged over any 1 g of tissue). By comparison, 10–15 W/kg of energy is transmitted by high-frequency (shortwave) therapy. Some risk is associated with the use of special coils, which usually are used strictly for receiving. Unfavorable coupling of the transmitter and receiver coils due to switching errors or faulty positioning can amplify the RF field in the area of the coil, causing substantially higher energies to be released to the adjacent tissues [3]. This can be particularly damaging in the orbital region due to the danger of cataract formation in lenses heated to 43 °C or above.

In summary, though, it may be said that clinical experience and scientific research to date have demonstrated no irreversible injury of either a somatic or genetic nature in association with MR imaging. This does not justify unnecessary or high-risk experimentation, however. Strict criteria should be applied to the selection of women during the early months of pregnancy.

3.4.2 Practical Effects

MR units pose a hazard to patients wearing cardiac pacemakers or other neurostimulators [24, 33]. The static magnetic field and RF pulses can interfere with the demand function of cardiac pacemakers. Time-varying fields can induce voltages in pacemakers which stimulate cardiac activity and thus can cause a failure of cardiac excitation to go undetected. Finally, the static magnetic field can exert a twisting force on the pacemaker beneath the skin, causing the leads to become damaged or dislodged. Because of these potential dangers, cardiac pacemakers are considered an absolute contraindication to MR imaging. Patients with cardiac pacemakers should remain outside the 5-gauss ($5 \cdot 10^{-4}$-T) line of the fringe field around the magnet. This line should be indicated around all MR units.

A serious danger is posed by loose metal objects (keys, pens, screwdrivers, scissors, etc.), which will be drawn at high velocity into the bore of the magnet. This can be avoided by having all persons pass through a metal detector gate before entering the magnet room [9].

Small metallic implants such as hemostatic clips or aneurysm clips that have a high nickel content can experience a torque when the patient is moved into the magnet [13, 20]. Patients with intracranial implants of this type should be excluded from examination. This restriction does not apply to patients whose clips were tested before the operation and were definitely found to be nonmagnetic. Any other information on the magnetic properties of the implants is unreliable. Surgical clips in body regions other than the brain, like the retroperitoneum, generally can be examined without danger if at least 14 days have passed between the operation and the MR examination. Because the forces acting on metal implants are field-dependent, implants are a particularly great concern during high-field imaging at 1 T or above.

Larger metal objects embedded in tissues, like shrapnel or prosthetic implants (artificial hips, dentures), can absorb considerable RF energy during long imaging sequences because of the high conductivity of the metal and can undergo significant heating [8]. Also, materials with ferromagnetic properties can exert forces within the body that may cause unpleasant sensations. However, these effects have proved to be less limiting in clinical practice than was once believed, and they represent only a relative contraindication that must be assessed case by case.

References

1. Andrews IC (1984) Anesthetic management for neuroradiologic diagnostic procedures. In: Frost EAM (ed) Clinical anesthesia in neurosurgery. Butterworth, Boston London Sydney Wellington Durban Toronto, p 95
2. Arbeitsgemeinschaft Kernspintomographie der Deutschen Röntgengesellschaft (1986) Empfehlungen für einen optimierten diagnostischen Einsatz der Kernspintomographie
3. Boskamp EB (1985) Improved surface coil imaging in MR: decoupling of the excitation and receiver coils. Radiology 157: 449–452
4. Bottommley PA, Redington PW, Edelstein WA, Schenk JF (1985) Estimating radiofrequency power deposition in body MR imaging. Mag Res Med 2 (4): 336–349
5. Budinger TF (1981) Nuclear magnetic resonance (NMR) in vivo studies: known thresholds for health effects. J Comp Assist Tomogr 5: 800–811

6. Bundesgesundheitsamt (1984) Empfehlungen zur Vermeidung gesundheitlicher Risiken, verursacht durch magnetische und hochfrequente elektromagnetische Felder bei der NMR-Tomographie und In-vivo-NMR-Spektroskopie. Bundesgesundheitsblatt 27 (3): 92-96
7. Bureau of Radiological Health (1982) Guidelines for evaluating electromagnetic risk for trials of clinical NMR systems. Food and Drug Administration, Rockville, MD 20857
8. Davis PL, Crooks L, Arakawa M, Mcree R, Kaufman L, Margulis AR (1981) Potential hazards in NMR imaging: heating effects of changing magnetic fields and RF fields on small metallic implants. AJR 137: 857-860
9. Finn EJ, Di Chiro G, Brooks RA, Sato S (1985) Ferromagnetic materials in patients: detection before MR imaging. Radiology 156: 139-141
10. Fullerton GD, Cameron IL, Ord VA (1985) Orientation of tendons in the magnetic field and its effect on T2 relaxation times. Radiology 155: 433-435
11. Geiger RS, Cascorbi HF (1984) Anesthesia in a NMR scanner. Anesth Analg 63: 622-623
12. Heiken JP, Glazer HS, Lee JKT, Murphy WA, Gado M (1986) Manual of clinical magnetic resonance imaging. Raven Press, New York
13. Laakman RW, Kaufman B, Han JS, Nelson AD, Clampitt M, O'Block AM, Haaga JR, Alfifi RJ (1985) MR imaging in patients with metallic implants, Radiology 157: 711-714
14. Laumer R, Brandl M, Härtl L, Meusel E (1986) Longterm sedation of neurosurgical intensive care patients with methohexitane. Intens Care Med 12 [Suppl]: 261
15. Mackenzie N, Grant IS (1985) Propofol ("Diprivan") for continuous intravenous anasthesia: a comparison with methohexitone. Postgrad Med J 1985 [Suppl 3]: 70-75
16. Meierhofer JN, Herb L (1988) Intravenöse Narkose zur Kernspintomographie. Anaesthesiol 205: 521-529
17. Meretoja DA, Kalli I (1986) Atacurium infusion in paediatric patients. Br J Anaesth 58 [Suppl 1]: 108
18. National Radiological Protection Board United Kingdom (1981) Exposure to nuclear magnetic resonance, clinical imaging. Radiography 47: 258-260
19. National Radiological Protection Board, United Kingdom (1983) Revised guidance on acceptable limits of exposure during nuclear magnetic resonance clinical imaging. Br J Radiology 56: 974-977
20. New PFJ, Rosen BR, Brady TJ, Buonanno FS, Kistler JP, Burt CT, Hinshaw WS, Newhouse JH, Pohost GM, Taveras JM (1983) Nuclear magnetic resonance. Potential hazards and artifacts of ferromagnetic and nonferromagnetic surgical and dental materials and devices in nuclear magnetic resonance imaging. Radiology 147: 139-148
21. Nightingale DA (1986) Neuromuscular blocking drugs in paediatric anesthesia. In: Proceedings of the 1st European Congress of Paediatric Anaesthesia, Rotterdam, p 48
22. Nixon C, Hirsch NP, Ormerod IEC, Johnson G (1986) Nuclear magnetic resonance, its application for the anaesthesist. Anaesthesia 41: 131-137
23. Osbakken, Griffith J, Taczanowsky P (1986) A cross morphologic, hematologic, and blood chemistry study of adult and neonatal mice chronically exposed to high magnetic fields. Mag Res 3 (4): 502-517
24. Pavlicek W, Geisinger M, Castle L, Borkomski GP, Meaney TF, Bream BL, Gallagher JH (1983) The effect of nuclear magnetic resonance on patients with cardiac pacemakers. Radiology 147: 149-153
25. Roth JL, Nugent M, Gray JE, Julsrud PR, Berquist TH, Sill JC, Kispert DB (1985) Patient monitoring during magnetic resonance imaging. Anaesthesiology 62: 80-83
26. Saunders RJ, Humphrey M (1981) A simple device for remote monitoring of respiration. Anaesthesiology 55: 609
27. Schwartz JL, Crooks LE (1982) NMR imaging produces no observable mutations or cytotoxicity in mammalian cells. AJR 139: 583-585
28. Shellock F (1987) Biological effects of MRI: a clean safety record so far. Diagn Imag Feb: 96-101, 177
29. Siemens Medical Systems (1986) Clinical sequence protocol catalog and image quality guidelines for magnetic resonance imaging. Iselin, New Jersey 08830, USA
30. Vogl Th (1986) Biologische Effekte und gesundheitliche Risiken. In: Lissner J, Seiderer M (Hrsg) Klinische Kernspintomographie. Enke, Stuttgart
31. Weikl A, Hentschel D, Schittenhelm R (1988) EKG-Veränderungen bei der Kernspintomographie. Anaesthesiol Intensivmed 205: 506-514
32. Wolff S, James T, Young GB, Margulis AR, Bodycote J, Afzal V (1985) Magnetic resonance imaging: absence of in vitro cytogenetic damage. Radiology 155: 163-165
33. Zimmermann BH, Faul DD (1984) Artifacts and hazards in NMR imaging due to metal implants and cardiac pacemakers. Diagn Imag Clin Med 53 (1): 53-56

4 Symptoms and Pathologic Anatomy: A Tabular Listing

G. Gademann and W. J. Huk

The following tabular listing of symptoms and functionally associated anatomic regions (Tables 4.1, 4.2) is not intended as a substitute for a basic knowledge of the pathomorphology of the CNS. Its purpose is to direct the examiner who is not a specialist in neurology to the possible seat of a disease so that he can give special attention to the region in question.

Table 4.2 includes references to the sections in Chap. 2 of this book so that the reader can refresh his knowledge of the normal anatomy of the CNS. The alphabetized index of symptoms in Table 4.1 will help the reader locate the part of Table 4.2 where a specific symptom may be found.

Table 4.1. Index of symptoms

Symptom	Number of symptom group in Table 4.2
Abducens paresis	4, 12
Agnosia	
- acoustic	14
- olfactory	2c
- tactile	2b
- visual	2d
Agraphia	2b
Acalculia	2b
Accommodation disturbance	12
Acromegaly	8
Amaurosis	
- total	11
- unilateral	11
Anal reflex, absence of	17
Analgesia	5
Anarthria	16
Anesthesia	17
- saddle-block	17
Anisocoria	1
Anosmia	15
Aphasia	
- motor	3
- sensory	2c, 3
Apraxia	
- constructional	2b
- motor	2b
Ataxia	
- truncal	9
Athetosis	10
Ballistic syndrome	10
Behavioral change	2a
Bladder disturbance	17
Bulbar brain syndrome	16
Bulbar paralysis	
- progressive	16
- pseudo	16
Cauda equina syndrome	17
Cerebellar symptoms	9
Cerebral compression symptoms	1
Choked disk	1
Chorea	10
Compulsive	
- crying	16
- laughter	16
Consciousness, disturbance of	6
Conus medullaris syndrome	17
Convergence, disturbance of	12
Cortical blindness	11
Cranial neuropathies, other	15
Déjà vu experience	2c
Diabetes insipidus	7
Diplopia	12
Disease	
- Cushing's	8
- Parkinson's	10
Dysarthria	16
Dysdiadochokinesis	9
Dysmetria	9
Dysphagia	16
Dystonic syndrome	10
Electrolyte disorders	7
Extrapyramidal symptoms	10
Facial pain	15
Facial paralysis	15

Table 4.1 (continued)

Symptom	Number of symptom group in Table 4.2
Facial paresis	4, 16
- central	15
- peripheral	15
Fasciculations	16
Fever	
- central	7
Finger agnosia	2b
Frontal brain syndrome	2a
Gaze paresis	13
- horizontal (lateral)	13
- vertical	13
Gradenigo's syndrome	15
Headache	1
Hearing defects	14
Hemianopsia	
- binasal	11
- bitemporal	11
- heteronymous	11
- homonymous	2d, 11
Hemiballism	10
Hemiparesis	
- flaccid	4
- spastic	4
Hemiplegia	
- alternans	4
- cruciate	4
- flaccid	4
- spastic	4
Horner's syndrome	16
Hypoacusis	14
Hypoesthesia	5, 15
Hyperpathia	5
Hyperprolactinemia	8
Hypoglossal paresis	4
Hyposmia	15
Hypothalamic symptoms	7
Impotence	17
Intention tremor	9
Ischialgia	17
Korsakoff's syndrome	3
Labyrinthine deafness	14
Masseter reflex	15
Masticatory muscles, paralysis of	15
Memory	3
Motor disturbances	4, 17
Mydriasis	12
Nausea	1
Neglect syndrome	2b
Nerve	
- abducens	15
- sciatic	17
- trigeminal	16

Symptom	Number of symptom group in Table 4.2
Nuchal pain	1
Nystagmus	9, 15, 16
Occipital lobe syndrome	2d
Oculomotor paresis	4, 12
Olfactory hallucinations	2c
Papilledema	1
Paralysis	
- crossed (cruciate)	4
- flaccid	4, 17
- spastic	4
Paraplegia	17
Performance, diminished	1
Personality change	1, 2a
Pituitary disorder	8
Postural sense	5
Proprioception	5
Pubertas praecox	7
Pupils, unequal	1
Rectal disturbance	17
Respiratory difficulties	6
Right-left disturbance	2b
Saddle-block anesthesia	17
Seizures	
- complex partial	2c
Sensory disturbances	5, 17
Sleep-wake rhythm	7
Space sense, disturbance of	2b
Speech	
- scanning	9
Speech comprehension, disturbance of	2c
Spinal cord symptoms	17
Swallowing difficulties	6, 16
Tactile sensation	5
Temporal lobe syndrome	2c
Thermal hypoesthesia or anesthesia	5
Tongue	
- atrophy	16
- fasciculations	16
Torsion dystonia	10
Torticollis	10
Trigeminal nerve	
- neuralgia	5
Trophic disturbances	17
Truncal ataxia	9
Unconsciousness	6
Vertigo	15
Vibratory sensation	5
Visual disturbances	11
Vomiting	1
- central	6
- morning	1
Word deafness	14

Table 4.2. Relating symptoms to anatomic regions

Symptoms	Localization	Section in Chap. 2
1. General symptoms		
Cerebral compression symptoms [headache, nausea and vomiting (morning!), diminished performance, personality change, papilledema, nuchal pain, unequal pupils]	Space-occupying lesion: tumor, hemorrhage, abscess, inflammation, CSF stasis (ventricular dilatation) Whole-head screening!	2.1
2. Cerebral cortical symptoms		
2a) Frontal brain syndrome Personality and behavior change	Frontal brain, especially the basal areas (Brodmann areas 9, 10, 11, 46, 47)	2.2
2b) Parietal brain syndrome Right-left disturbance, neglect syndrome, finger agnosia, agraphia, acalculia	Angular gyrus (area 39), supramarginal gyrus (area 40) in dominant hemisphere	2.2
Motor apraxia	Left parietal, bilateral frontal	2.2
Constructional apraxia and disturbance of space sense	Bilateral parietal, often with right predominance	2.2
Tactile agnosia	Superior and inferior parietal lobes (areas 5,6)	2.2
2c) Temporal lobe syndrome		
Complex partial seizures (aura, deja vu experience)	Temporal lobe, amygdala, hippocampus	2.2
Disturbance of speech comprehension	Superior temporal gyrus (pars posterior, area 22a)	2.2
Olfactory agnosia, olfactory hallucinations	Parahippocampal gyrus, uncus (areas 34, 38)	2.2
2d) Occipital lobe syndrome		
Visual agnosia	Cuneus, bilateral occipital gyri (areas 18, 19)	2.2, 2.6
Homonymous hemianopsia	Occipital lobe contralateral to visual field defect	2.2, 2.6
3. Aphasias		
Sensory	Superior temporal gyrus pars posterior (Wernicke) (area 22a)	2.2, 2.7
Motor	Inferior frontal gyrus, pars triangularis (Broca) (area 44)	2.2
Short-term memory loss (Korsakoff's syndrome)	Mamillary bodies, fornix, hippocampus	2.2, 2.3
4. Motor disturbances		
Flaccid paralysis of a muscle group	Peripheral nerve	–
Flaccid paralysis of individual body parts	Contralateral precentral gyrus (area 4)	2.2
Flaccid hemiparesis	Contralateral pyramidal tract, medulla oblongata	2.5
Spastic hemiplegia with ipsilateral facial or hypoglossal paresis	Contralateral internal capsule	2.3
Spastic hemiplegia with contralateral oculomotor paresis	Cerebral peduncle of opposite side, midbrain	2.4
Spastic hemiplegia with contralateral abducens or facial paralysis	Contralateral pons	2.5
Crossed paralysis (cruciate hemiplegia = paresis of a lower limb and contralateral upper limb)	Lateral decussation of pyramid on same side, lower medulla oblongata	2.5
Hemiplegia alternans (cranial nerve deficit on side of lesion, disturbances of contralateral long tracts)	Brainstem	2.3-2.5
5. Sensory disturbances		
Hemihypoesthesia of trunk and face	Posterolateral thalamus, contralateral	2.3
Decreased sensation (mainly proprioception), hyperpathia	Posterolateral thalamus	2.3
Sensory disturbances in face, trigeminal neuralgia	Trigeminal nerve (brainstem, cerebellopontine angle, Meckel's cavity)	2.3, 2.5
Disturbance of tactile, postural, and vibratory sense, spinal ataxia (posterior funiculus)	Medial lemniscus, medulla oblongata, pons and midbrain, contralateral	2.4, 2.5
Analgesia and thermal anesthesia of trunk with level of sensation	Spinal cord above level of sensation	2.9

Table 4.2 (continued)

Symptoms	Localization	Section in Chap. 2
6. Disturbances of consciousness		
Unconsciousness, impaired consciousness	General: rise of intracranial pressure, subarachnoid hemorrhage, intoxication, metabolic coma	2.1
	Local: reticular formation of midbrain, pons	2.4, 2.5
Respiratory difficulties	Reticular formation of medulla oblongata, intoxication	2.5
Central dysphagia	Caudal rhomboid fossa	2.5
Central vomiting	Area postrema of medulla oblongata	2.5
7. Hypothalamic symptoms		
Diabetes insipidus, electrolyte disorders, central fever, disturbances of sleep-wake rhythm, pubertas praecox	Hypothalamus, third ventricle	2.3
8. Pituitary disorders		
Hyperprolactinemia, Cushing's disease, acromegaly	Sella turcica, pituitary	2.3
9. Cerebellar symptoms		
Truncal ataxia, nystagmus	Nodulus, flocculus, superior and inferior vermis (archicerebellum)	2.5
Limb ataxia with tendency to fall toward the lesion side, dysmetria, dysdiadochokinesia, intention tremor, scanning speech	Ipsilateral cerebellar hemisphere (neocerebellum)	2.5
10. Extrapyramidal symptoms		
Parkinson's disease	Substantia nigra of midbrain, caudate nucleus	2.4
Athetosis	Putamen, caudate nucleus	2.3
Chorea	Striatum	2.3
Dystonic syndrome (spastic torticollis, torsion dystonia)	Putamen, centromedian nucleus, VA nuclei of thalamus	2.3
Ballistic syndrome, hemiballismus	Subthalamic nucleus, connection to outer pallidum	2.3, 2.4
11. Visual disturbance		
Unilateral amaurosis	Optic nerve	2.6
Heteronymous, bitemporal hemianopsia (chiasmal syndrome from pituitary neoplasm)	Center of optic chiasm	2.3, 2.6
Heteronymous, binasal hemianopsia	Lateral chiasm, bilateral	2.3, 2.6
Homonymous hemianopsia	Optic tract	2.6
Incomplete, homonymous hemianopsia	Optic radiation	2.2, 2.6
Homonymous hemianopsia with preservation of central vision	Contralateral occipital lobe (area 17)	2.2, 2.6
Total amaurosis (cortical blindness)	Bilateral occipital lobes	2.2, 2.6
12. Oculomotor paresis (motor disturbance in one eye)		
Diplopia, mydriasis, disturbance of convergence and accommodation	Oculomotor nerve, trochlear nerve, abducens nerve; basal cisterns, superior orbital fissure, cavernous sinus	2.3, 2.4
13. Gaze paresis (conjugate motor disturbance in both eyes without diplopia)		
Oculomotor paralysis with midbrain syndrome Vertical gaze paresis (Parinaud's syndrome)	Central gray matter of midbrain, bilateral mesodiencephalic reticular formation (rostromedial to red nucleus = prerubral area)	2.4
Horizontal or lateral gaze paresis	Nucleus of abducens nerve or paramedian pontine reticular formation, ipsilateral	2.5

Table 4.2 (continued)

Symptoms	Localization	Section in Chap. 2
14. Hearing defects		
Laryrinthine deafness	Spiral organ in petrous bone	2.7
Hypoacusis	Cochlear nucleus of pons, lateral lemniscus, inferior colliculus of midbrain, lateral geniculate body	
Acoustic agnosia (word deafness)	Superior temporal gyrus, pars posterior (area 41)	2.2, 2.7
15. Other cranial neuropathies		
Hyposmia, anosmia	Olfactory filaments, frontal base	2.2
Vertigo, spontaneous nystagmus	Vestibular apparatus of inner ear	2.7
	Vestibular nerve in porus acusticus, vestibular nerve nuclei in rhomboid fossa	2.7, 2.5
Paralysis and atrophy of masticatory muscles; absence of masseter reflex	Motor part of trigeminal nerve, Gasserian ganglion, motor trigeminal nucleus in lateral tegmentum of pons	2.3, 2.5
Hypoesthesia in portions of the face	Peripheral trigeminal branches, Gasserian ganglion	2.3, 2.5
General facial hypoesthesia, facial pain	Ipsilateral: Gasserian ganglion, basal cisterns, dorsal midbrain nuclei, dorsolateral tegmentum of pons, medulla oblongata	2.3, 2.5 2.4, 2.5
	Contralateral: medial lemniscus, midbrain	2.4
	Posteromedial ventral nucleus of thalamus	2.3
	Internal capsule, postcentral gyrus	2.2
Gradenigo's syndrome (paresis of abducens nerve, trigeminal nerve irritation and deficits, mainly involving nerve V_1)	Apex of petrous pyramid	2.7
Facial paralysis not involving the forehead (central facial paresis)	Contralateral precentral gyrus, pars opercularis (area 4), corona radiata, contralateral internal capsule and medial cerebral peduncle	2.2–2.4
Facial paralysis involving the forehead (peripheral facial paresis)	Ipsilateral nuclear and peripheral facial nerve, lateral rhomboid fossa, porus acusticus, stylomastoid foramen, parotid gland	2.5, 2.7
16. Bulbar brain symptoms		
Progressive bulbar paralysis - dysarthria to anarthria - dysphagia - atrophy and fasciculations of the tongue - nystagmus, Horner's syndrome - facial paresis	Motor nuclei of cranial nerves IX–XII (VII), medulla oblongata, inferior pons	2.5
Pseudobulbar paralysis - dysarthria - dysphagia - tendency toward compulsive laughter and crying	Bilateral damage to corticonuclear tract in pons and midbrain	2.4, 2.5
17. Spinal cord symptoms		
Paraplegia (total cord lesion) - sensory and motor losses - bladder and rectal disturbance - trophic disturbances	Spinal cord above upper limit of sensory deficits to T12	2.9
Conus medullaris syndrome - saddle-block anesthesia - loss of anal reflex - bladder paralysis, fecal incontinence, impotence (- no lower limb paralysis)	Spinal cord (conus medullaris) at L1/2, sensory level past S3	
Cauda equina syndrome - pain and sensory deficits in sciatic nerve distribution - bladder and rectal incontinence - flaccid paralysis of lower limbs with loss of reflexes	Cauda equina from L2 to sacrum	

5 General Aspects of the MR Signal Pattern of Certain Normal and Pathologic Structures

5.1 Brain Edema

W. J. Huk

Edema is the primary response of the brain tissue to a variety of insults. In explaining and describing brain edema, we recognize the existence of three types: vasogenic edema, cytotoxic edema, and interstitial edema [2].

Vasogenic edema, the most common type, is associated with a disruption of the blood-brain barrier and the escape of plasma filtrates into the extracellular space. Vasogenic edema spreads chiefly in the white matter of the brain, sparing the more tightly integrated cortical gray matter [4]. This accounts for the typical fingerlike configuration of this type of edema (Fig. 5.1). It is seen in association with various conditions: tumors, hemorrhages, infarctions, inflammations, contusions.

Cytotoxic edema is caused by ischemia. A significant oxygen deficit leads to failure of the Na/K pump, allowing sodium and water to pass into the cells. With expansion of the intracellular volume, the extracellular space dwindles. Although the function of the cell is disordered, its structure remains intact, and the insult is considered reversible when the oxygen supply is restored [5]. Cytotoxic edema affects gray and white matter equally and also occurs at the periphery of infarcted areas. Vasogenic edema at the center of the infarction is kept from spreading freely by the constricted extracellular spaces of the peripheral cytotoxic zone.

Interstitial edema occurs when a rise of intraventricular pressure causes a transependymal influx of CSF into the periventricular white matter (Fig. 5.2).

MR Findings

Vasogenic edema has a high content of free, interstitial water, known as bulk phase water, which has very long T1 and T2 relaxation times. When increased proteins are present in the edematous fluid, a portion of the bulk phase water becomes bound in "hydration layers" around the large protein molecules. Hydration layer water has natural frequencies closer to the Larmor frequency and therefore has a shorter T1 relaxation time than bulk phase water. Indeed, a linear relationship has been shown to exist between protein concentration and the relaxation rate 1/T1 [1, 3].

Incipient edema may show up as an area of increased signal intensity on T2-weighted sequences before it can be seen on CT scans. The edema appears correspondingly dark on T1-weighted images. Thus, associated edema can serve to indicate the presence of an underlying tumor at a very early stage. However, because the tumor tissue itself usually shows edematous expansion, edema may mask the tumor on T2-weighted scans. The differentiation of edema and tumor can be improved by using very long TE times or multiecho sequences, but often (as in metastasis) it will be necessary to use paramagnetic contrast agents such as gadolinium chelate. Low-grade gliomas show no contrast uptake and can be most difficult to distinguish from edema. If mass effects are absent as well, it is necessary to consider inflammatory, demyelinating, and other processes in the differential diagnosis.

Cytotoxic edema: There is no appreciable difference between the MR features of vasogenic and cytotoxic edema.

Interstitial edema appears as a high-signal border of periventricular white matter on T2-weighted images, although the contrast with intraventricular CSF is very slight. On proton-density images, however, the edematous border clearly gives a higher signal than the CSF (Fig. 5.2). This may result from the hydration effect of protons in the interstitial space, leading to a shortening of T1 (see above), or from the pulsatile movement of the free intraventricular CSF, which decreases the signal through an increased dephasing of the protons. It may be impossible in older patients to distinguish interstitial edema from similar changes associated with white matter disease of vascular etiology (normal pressure hydrocephalus) without also taking into account clinical manifestations.

The three types of edema cannot be distinguished from one another by their signal intensities. Localization and water distribution provide the best clues. Vasogenic edema tends to spread in the white matter, while cytotoxic edema involves both the cortex and the white matter and may show a relation to vascular distributions. Interstitial edema displays a characteristic periventricular pattern of spread. Vasogenic and cytotoxic edema contribute concurrently to post-traumatic brain edema, which is based on mechanical as well as hypoxic-ischemic causes.

5.2 Intracranial Hemorrhage and Iron Metabolism

W. Steinbrich and W. J. Huk

Intracranial Hemorrhage

In many diseases of the central nervous system (CNS), hemorrhage is both a potentially grave complication and a valuable aid to differential diagnosis. The detection of intracranial hemorrhage, therefore, is one of the primary tasks of diagnostic imaging.

Hemorrhages may be epidural or subdural, subarachnoid, intraparenchymatous, or intraventricular, depending on the underlying condition (trauma, degenerative vasopathy, vascular malformation, inflammation). *Hemorrhages into CSF spaces* disperse relatively quickly, and even large amounts of blood in the ventricles may leave no traces (on CT) after 1-2 weeks. *Subependymal* hemorrhages, which can mimic intraventricular hemorrhage, and especially *intraparenchymatous* hemorrhages take much longer to resolve. Evidence of a larger hemorrhage may still be visible several months after its occurrence.

As extravasated blood undergoes liquefaction and absorption, changes occur in its CT density and MR signal intensity. Because the breakdown process follows general laws regardless of the cause or location of the hemorrhage, we may give a common description of its effects on MR image contrasts for all disease types and thus avoid repetition later on. For both MR and CT one can separate an acute stage of hemorrhage (0-2 days) from a subacute stage (3-14 days) and a chronic stage ($>$ 14 days).

CT Findings

The CT features of intracranial hemorrhages are well known (Fig. 5.3): The conspicuous hyperdense phase of the acute hematoma is followed by an isodense phase, which progresses to the hypodense lesion of the old, liquefied hemorrhage. In intracerebral hemorrhages this process of liquefaction can be seen to proceed from the periphery of the hemorrhage toward its center, accompanied by the spread of a hypodense perifocal edema that is not easily distinguished from liquefaction. When finally the entire hemorrhagic cavity becomes hypodense, it can no longer be determined how far absorption has progressed, whether a residual hematoma cavity still exists, or even whether a different type of hypodense lesion is present (Fig. 5.4a). With use of an i.v. contrast agent, the hyperemic margin of the hematoma cavity shows a sustained, moderate enhancement that may resemble a malignant glioma. Very small hemorrhages (e.g., hemorrhagic infiltrations secondary to contusion) can become isodense or hypodense in only a few hours or days through edematous influx and can no longer be identified as hemorrhages. With large intracerebral hemorrhages, on the other hand, hypodense mass lesions remain visible for a period of weeks or even months.

MR Findings

The biochemical processes that take place in hemorrhages and their effects on MR image parameters are not yet fully understood. This is indicated by the diversity of presentations and interpretations in the literature concerning intracranial hemorrhages. The following description is based on our current understanding of these processes:

Flowing blood is rich in oxyhemoglobin; after giving up its oxygen, the blood contains the deoxyhemoglobin (both Fe^{2+}) [20]. In contrast to methemoglobin, the paramagnetic effect of both oxy- and deoxyhemoglobin is only weak because of the great distance between the iron and the hydrogen molecules due to the architecture of the surrounding porphyrin ring. When the iron in the hemoglobin is oxidized to the trivalent state, $Hb(Fe^{3+})OH$ methemoglobin is formed, which can no longer bind oxygen. In intact red cells the methemoglobin is continuously reduced back to hemoglobin [17]. This reduction is energy-dependent and cannot occur in coagulated blood.

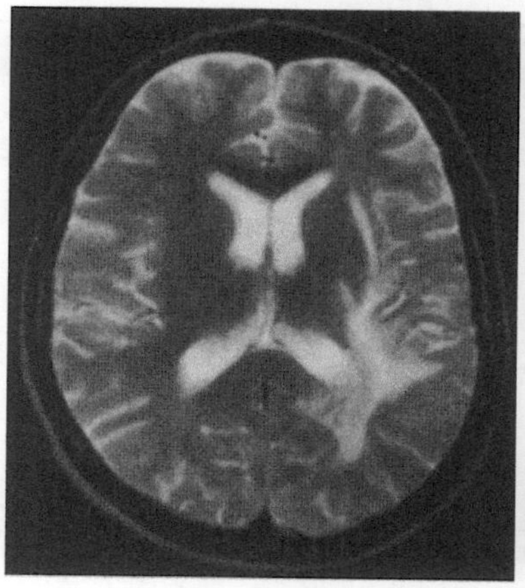

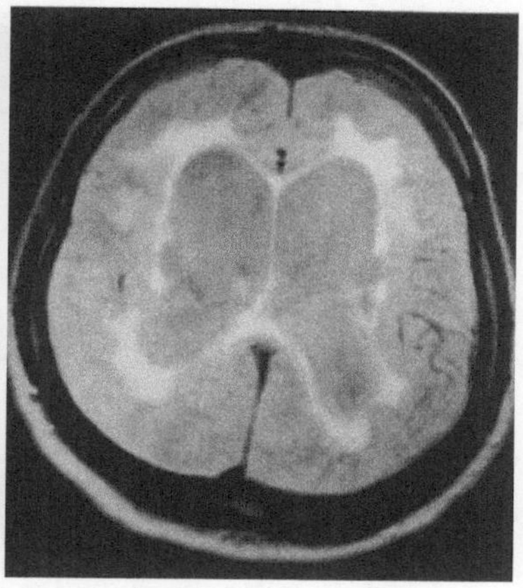

5.1 5.2

Fig. 5.1. Vasogenic edema associated with a right temporobasal tumor. Typical fingerlike distribution. Axial scan: SE 3.0 s/120 ms (1.0 T)

Fig. 5.2. Interstitial edema in a case of occlusive hydrocephalus. Axial scan at level of pars centralis. SE 3.0 s/45 ms (1.0 T)

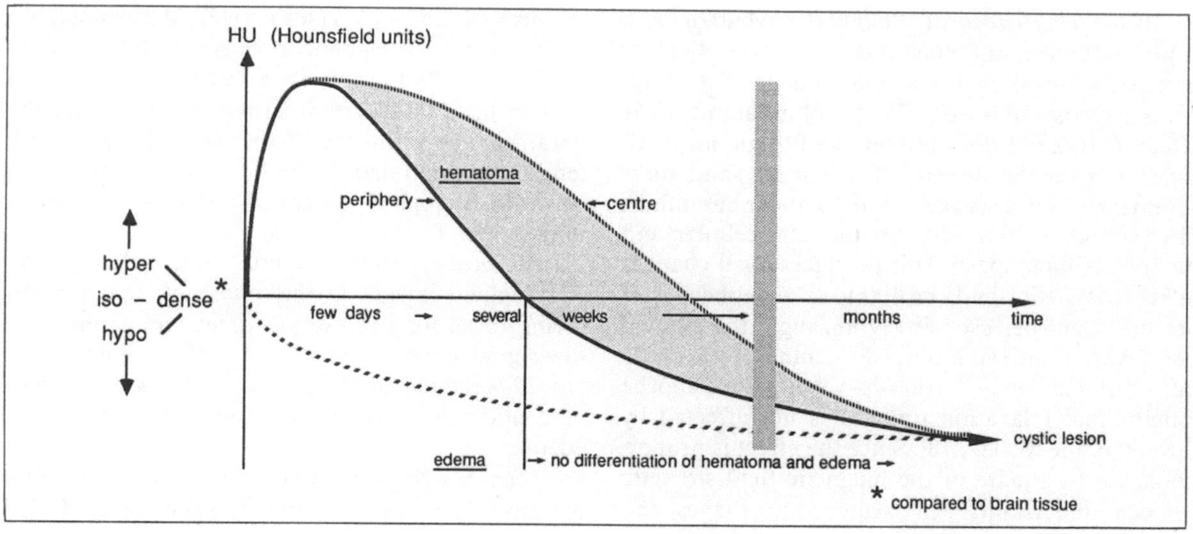

Fig. 5.3. (see text on page 116)

Fig. 5.4 a, b. Intracerebral hemorrhage, chronic stage. CT (**a**) and MRI (**b**) 40 days after the acute event. In CT, an unspecific hypodense lesion is seen; in MRI it appears more characteristic as a hyperintense area (methemoglobin) with dark rim (hemosiderin deposits). Axial scan (**b**) SE 2.0 s/45 ms (1.5 T)

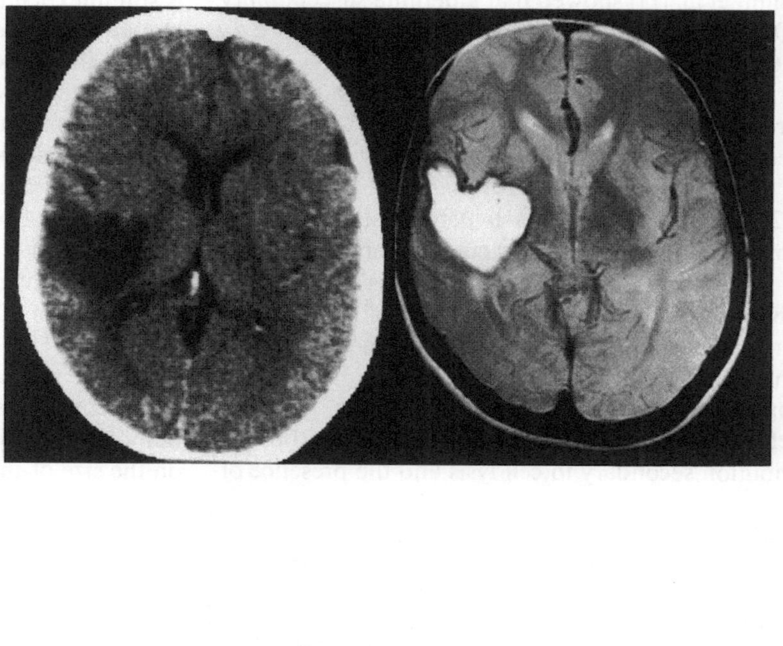

a b

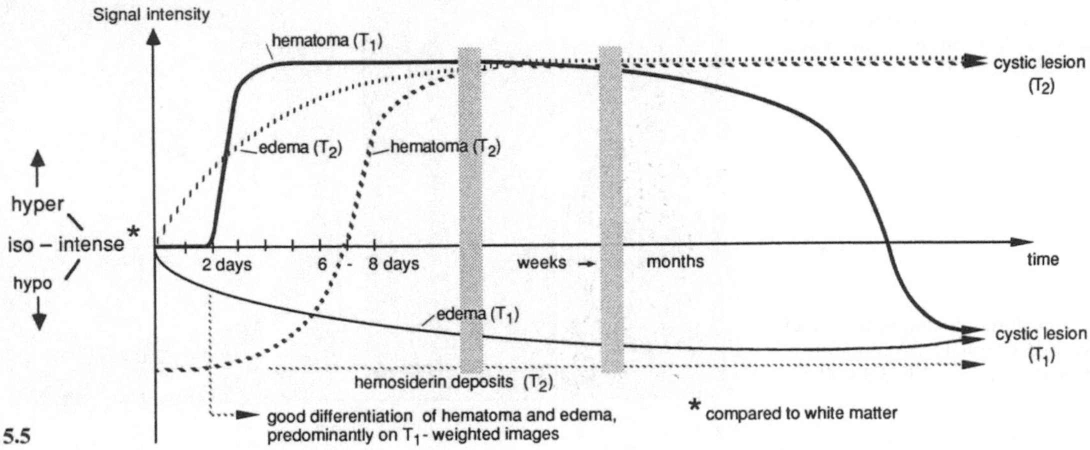

Fig. 5.5

In *acutely extravasated blood* deoxyhemoglobin is present in the still intact red cells, and it displays a very low signal on T2-weighted images (i.e., it appears dark; see Fig. 5.6). This is not a paramagnetic effect. It results from differences of tissue magnetization ("magnetic susceptibility") in the same measurement volume (voxel) due to the nonuniform distribution of iron between the extracellular and the intracellular space. This produces local changes in the magnetic field, resulting in a dephasing of protons that perfuse slowly through the altered field, with a corresponding shortening of T2 and a fall of signal intensity on T2-weighted scans. The longitudinal relaxation time T1 is not affected by this phenomenon [12, 18]. Since the effect is proportional to the square of the magnetic field strength, we can understand why acute hemorrhages and hemosiderin deposits (e.g., in angiographically occult vascular malformations) are difficult to identify in low fields [10] (see Fig. 14.38). However, Edelmann et al. [11] showed that a definite susceptibility effect can be observed even in lower fields (e.g., 0.6 T) by using gradient echo techniques.

Because the signal loss is a T2 effect, acute hemorrhage usually cannot be identified in T1-weighted sequences (see Fig. 16.11).

An incipient *perifocal edema* appears on T2-weighted images as a hyperintense border surrounding the hypointense acute hemorrhage.

The acute phase of hemorrhage is followed on about the 3rd day by an abrupt rise of signal intensity (subacute stage), which becomes apparent somewhat earlier in short-TR/TE scans than in long-TR/TE scans [21]. This high signal intensity reflects both the loss of inhomogeneity of iron distribution secondary to cell lysis and the presence of methemoglobin (Fe^{3+}) (see above). Methemoglobin is strongly paramagnetic because of the covalent binding of a OH group. By a fast exchange of protons to this OH group, hydrogen comes under the paramagnetic influence of the iron [8]. This effect tends to shorten mainly the T1 relaxation time, because in biological systems T1 is generally much longer than T2 (Figs. 5.7–5.8).

Perifocal edema glands out clearly on T1-weighted images in this phase of denaturation owing to its long relaxation times, appearing as a low-signal border around the bright hemorrhage. On T2-weighted images there is a progressive loss of contrast between hemorrhage and surrounding edema.

After 6–8 days there is again a gradual prolongation of the relaxation times, especially of T2, so that the hemorrhage gives an intense signal on both T1-weighted and T2-weighted scans [8] (Figs. 5.4, 5.7). DiChiro et al. [8] reports that this phenomenon is still unexplained, because oxidation of the hemoglobin to methemoglobin plays only a negligible role at this time. In the later subacute and early chronic stage, lysis of red cells proceeds from the periphery of the hemorrhage toward its center [8] due to lytic activity of macrophages.

So with time the appearance of hemorrhage changes on T1-weighted images from a ring of high signal intensity to a homogeneous area of bright signal. The image shown in this stage, especially the width of the ring, also depends on the imaging parameters (TR and TE) because of the contrary effect of the magnetic susceptibility and the paramagnetic activity to signal intensity. The time at which a homogeneous signal is obtained differs depending on the size of the hemorrhage.

Fig. 5.6 a, b. Pontine hemorrhage in the acute stage in a 49-year-old man. **a** Initial rim of hyperintense methemoglobin (SE 0.6 s/15 ms). **b** With T2 weighting the entire hematoma still appears hypointense; SE 2.9 s/90 ms; (1.5 t)

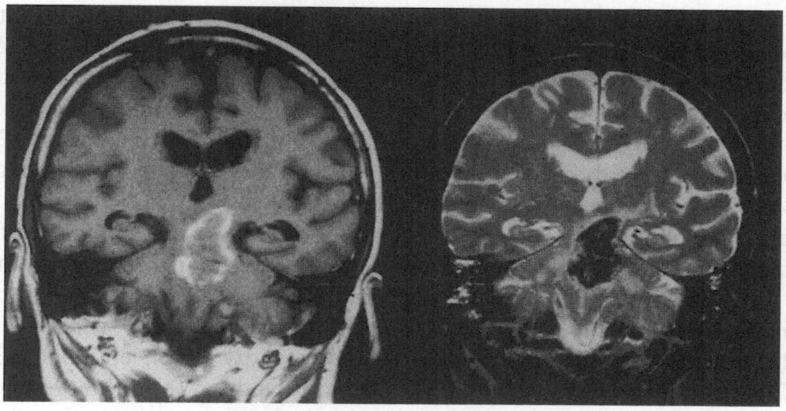

a b

Fig. 5.7 a, b. Intracerebral hemorrhage in a 42-year-old-woman. **a** About 5 weeks after the acute event the hematoma displays short T1 and long T2. In the center the hematoma still appeared isointense to white matter. In **a** a dark rim of hemosiderin contrasts with the slight peripheral edema **b** Six months after the acute event: irregular area of low signal due to hemosiderin deposits. The hyperintensity of the surrounding brain tissue reflects demyelination, axial scans: **a** SE 2.5 s/120 ms, **b** SE 3.0 s/120 ms (1.0 T)

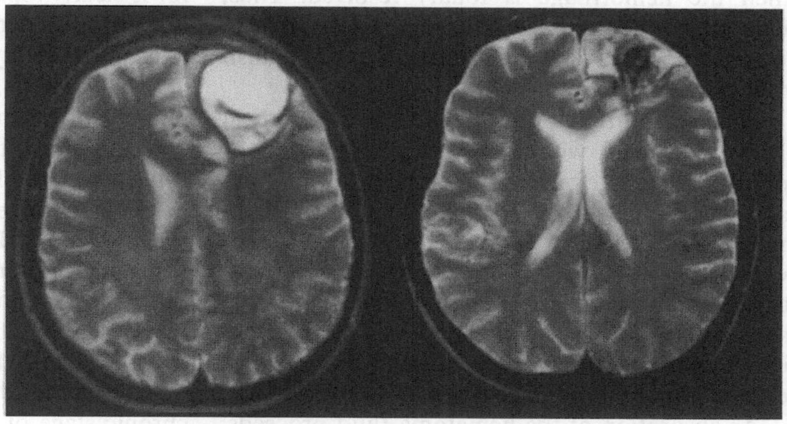

a b

Fig. 5.8. A 21-day-old hemorrhage in a 55-year-old woman during anticoagulant therapy. Hyperintense rim of methemoglobin *(small arrows)* and perifocal adema *(large arrows)*. Axial scan: SE 1.35 s/50 ms, (1.5 T)

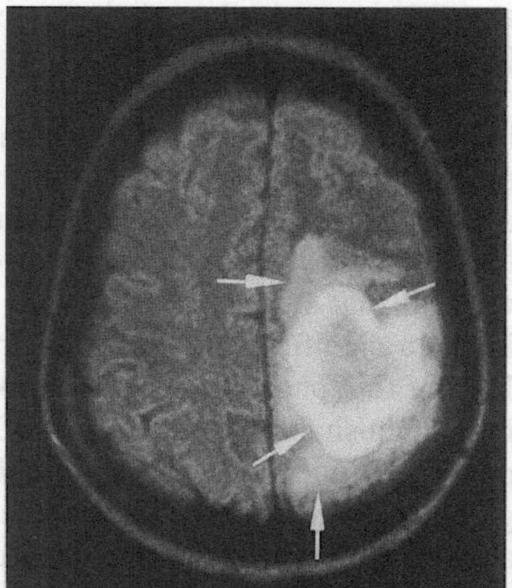

The period of *high signal intensity* of extravasated blood on MR images lasts considerably longer than the period of high radioabsorption on CT scans. Hematomas that already appear completely hypodense on CT, and thus have a nonspecific appearance, can still be clearly identified as blood on MR images (Fig. 5.4). As in CT, contrast agents (e.g., gadolinium chelate) can be useful for enhancement of the hyperemic border.

At the end of the subacute stage, and more distinctly in the chronic stage, a dark ring appears at the periphery of the zone of high signal intensity. This phenomenon results from hemosiderin deposits in macrophages again causing signal loss due to inhomogeneity of tissue magnetization. As known from pathology, hemosiderin deposits persist even when the hemorrhage is totally resolved. Thus, years after a hemorrhage MR may still be able to demonstrate small dark areas difficult to distinguish from calcifications.

Small hemorrhagic foci, and especially cortical bleeds associated with hemorrhagic infarction or contusion, do not form the hyperintense ring typically seen in the subacute stage. Proper T1 weighting demonstrates the foci directly as intense, homogeneous areas, often with a somewhat irregular structure. In other respects these lesions display the same progression of signal changes as more extensive hemorrhagic foci, except that absorption proceeds at a more rapid pace (see Fig. 16.13).

As absorption of the hematoma fluid proceeds, the hemorrhagic cavity decreases in size, often leaving behind a relatively small *tissue defect*. The liquefied contents of the cavity exhibit prolonged T1 and T2 times. A pure glial scar is rarely observed (Fig. 5.7).

In *subarachnoid hemorrhages*, the extravasated blood mixes with the CSF, which retards coagulation. Also, the phospholipase in the CSF [6] effects a rapid lysis of the red cells, leading to an early release of deoxyhemoglobin. As a result of cell lysis, we find that susceptibility-related shortening of T2 is not a significant factor, even in the acute stage. During this phase the subarachnoid hemorrhage is indistinguishable from normal CSF, because the paramagnetic effect of the dissolved deoxyhemoglobin is slight due to its molecular structure (see above). However, oxidative denaturation of the deoxyhemoglobin to methemoglobin leads quickly (within 24–48 h) to a marked shortening of T1 with a corresponding rise of signal on T1-weighted images [7, 15]. In contrast to intracerebral hematomas (bright ring, dark center), the signal increase affects the whole extent of the hemorrhage, and it persists for weeks (Figs. 5.9, 5.10; see also Fig. 16.14).

In practice, then, acute hemorrhages like those occurring in the first hours after trauma appear as dark areas on T2-weighted sequences obtained with a high-field imager. However, these areas are not as pathognomonic for intracranial hemorrhage as are the hyperdense foci on CT scans, which is why CT is preferred in the early period after trauma.

At *lower field strengths,* acute hemorrhages generally cannot be directly demonstrated with the conventional SE sequence and must be inferred from the presence of perifocal edema. Direct diagnosis requires the use of gradient echo sequences.

In the long subacute and chronic phases that follow, MR is superior to CT at all field strengths, for it clearly separates the hemorrhagic cavity from its perifocal edema and also characterizes the contents of the cavity as old blood.

Hemosiderin deposits are a consistent feature of intracerebral hemorrhages. The brain tissue is unable to remove the macrophages that have phagocytized the old blood, and consequently hemosiderin deposits linger at the periphery of the hemorrhagic cavity. The ferritin iron present in the hemosiderin granules in the macrophages shortens the T2 relaxation time through the susceptibility effect described above, causing the ferritin to give a low MR signal (Fig. 5.7; see Figs. 14.25, 16.16).

The hemosiderin deposits that are seen in the chronic stage of even smaller hemorrhages usually extend well beyond the original boundaries of the hemorrhagic focus (see Fig. 14.25 c). With the passage of time, the hemosiderin ring tends to lose its sharp margins and may appear fragmented.

Differentiation is required from dense calcium deposits and from flow voids in blood vessels, which likewise give a low signal on T1- and T2-weighted sequences. Gomori et al. [13] present several criteria for differential diagnosis using a high-field imager:

- Calcium deposits occur preferentially at the center of lesions. They display a constant, moderate signal reduction and constant extent on T1- and T2-weighted images and have irregular borders. Also, calcifications are easy to recognize on CT scans.
- Hemosiderin deposits give even lower signals and appear more extensive on T2-weighted images than on T1-weighted scans. They occur at the periphery of lesions like shells and have relatively smooth margins. High-field MR is more

Fig. 5.9. Circumscribed subarachnoid bleeding surrounding the division of the right middle cerebral artery in a 59-year-old man 6 days after acute onset of aphasia and disturbance of left hand coordination. Axial scan SE 1.5 s/100 ms; *arrow,* aneurysm.

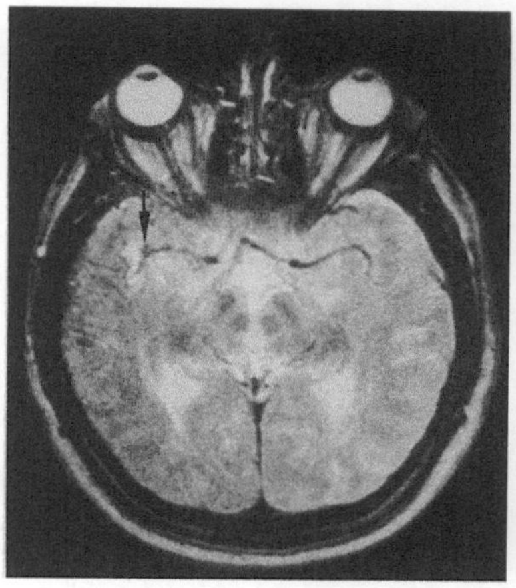

5.9

Fig. 5.10. Subarachnoid hemorrhage from a ruptured aneurysm of the internal carotid artery in a 64-year-old woman 5 days after the bleeding. Axial scan, SE 0.5 s/30 ms (1.5 T)

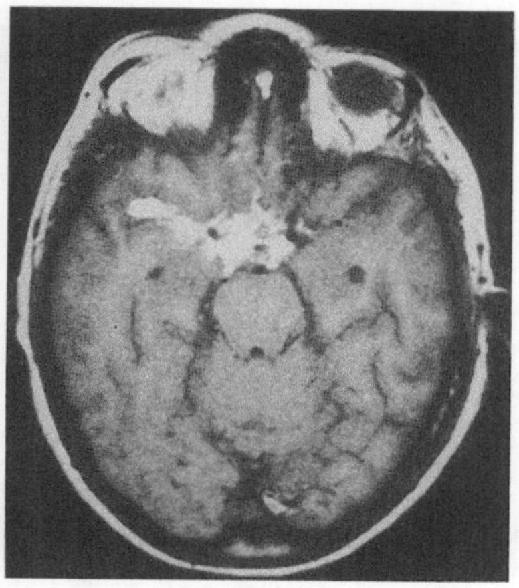

5.10

sensitive than CT in its ability to display hemosiderin.

- Flow voids are distinguished from hemosiderin by their branching, vessel-like pattern and by the presence of flow effects, which produce paradoxical enhancement on T1-weighted images and appear as even-echo rephasing or direct phase maps in fast or T2-weighted sequences.

Iron Metabolism of the CNS

A number of CNS diseases are associated with an increased deposition of iron in central brain tissues.

Iron is absorbed from the food in the small intestine. It is incorporated into protein in the form of heme (hemoglobin, myoglobin, etc.), and stored chiefly as ferritin, from which it can be rapidly mobilized [9]. Iron also is a constituent of iron enzymes, which play a major role in the oxidation reaction [16]. Further details on iron metabolism may be found in the specialized literature.

High-field imaging with T2-weighted sequences demonstrates areas of reduced signal in the globus pallidus, red nucleus, pars reticularis of the substantia nigra, subthalamic nucleus of Luys, dentate nucleus, and, to a lesser degree, in the putamen. This signal pattern corresponds closely to the sites of predilection for iron deposition in the brain as confirmed by pathologic studies (Fig. 5.11). A similar correlation is not seen with any other stored substance (calcium, melanin, lipofuscin). The caudate nucleus and thalamus have been found to contain smaller amounts of iron than any of the nuclear structures listed above. Iron contents are lowest in the gray and white matter of the cerebral and cerebellar hemispheres. Iron is somewhat more abundant in the subcortical U fibers of the temporal lobe, and the frontal white matter contains more iron than the occipital white matter [14]. No iron has been found in the extreme posterior limb of the internal capsule or in the optic radiation.

Studies on the *age dependence* of the iron content of the human brain have shown that iron is absent in the neonatal brain. Iron can be detected in the globus pallidus at about 6 months, in the substantia nigra at 9–12 months, in the red nucleus at 18–24 months, and in the dentate nucleus at 3–7 years [10, 14].

A high ferritin content produces an isolated shortening of T2 with no change in T1. The ferritin molecule contains up to 4000 iron ions and is surrounded by a protein shell 2.5 nm thick. As described above, this stored intracellular iron possesses a high magnetic susceptibility. Because the susceptibility effect is suppressed by conventional SE sequences, the iron concentrations of normal brain tissue are not displayed well in low fields and are clearly demonstrated only at higher field strengths (see above).

This biochemical characterization by proton MR gives useful information on *diseases of the CNS* that are associated with changes in iron metabolism. These include a number of degenerative, demyelinating, and vascular disorders [10]:

- Neuroaxonal dystrophy (Hallervorden-Spatz) (see p. 215)
- Huntington's disease (iron deposits in the caudate nucleus and putamen)

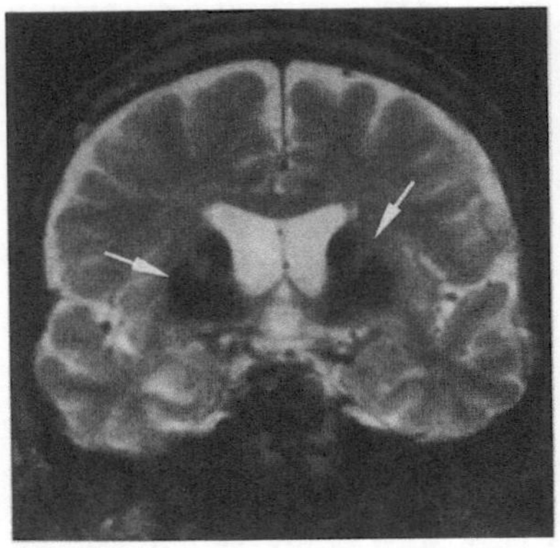

5.11

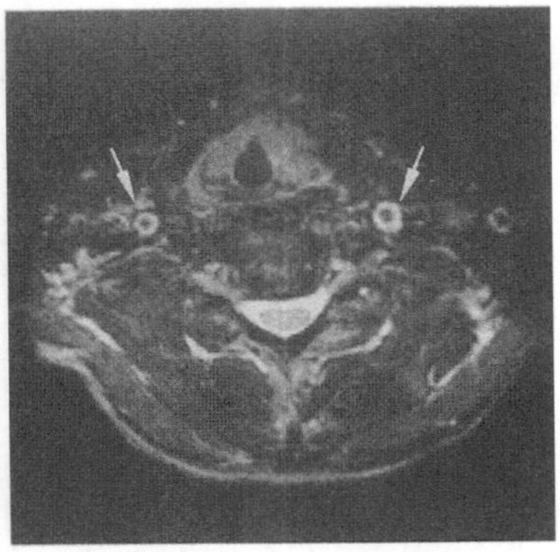

5.12

Fig. 5.11. Striking hypointensity in the central gray structures suggesting increased amount of iron deposits *(arrows)*. Incidental finding in a 58-year-old man without clinical signs relevant to iron metabolism. Coronal scan: SE 2.5 s/120 ms (1.0 T)

Fig. 5.12. Axial section of the neck showing a bull's-eye pattern in the major vessels *(arrows)*. Axial scan, SE 3.0 s/90 ms (1.5 T)

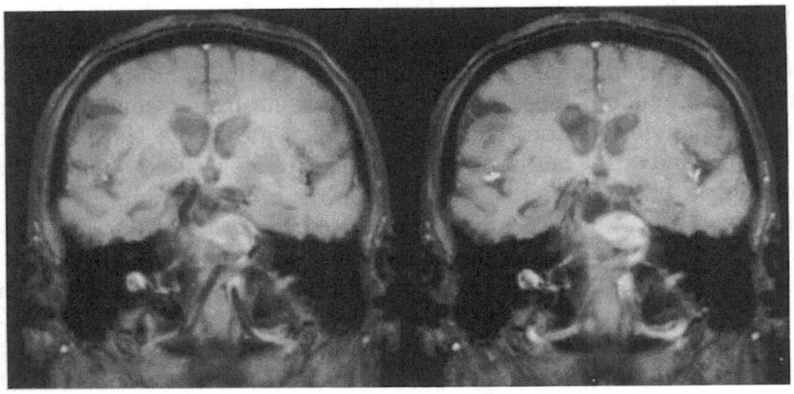

a b

Fig. 5.13 a, b. Large aneurysm of the basilar artery: incidental finding in a 64-year-old man with frontal brain tumor. Coronal scans with cine mode, FLASH 50°/0.66 s/10 ms (1.5 T): **a** 115 ms and **b** 461 ms after the R wave (ECG). Note the changing signal intensity in the vertebral, basilar and middle cerebral arteries, and the changing flow pattern within the aneurysm and the ventricles in relation to the different phases of the cardiac cycle

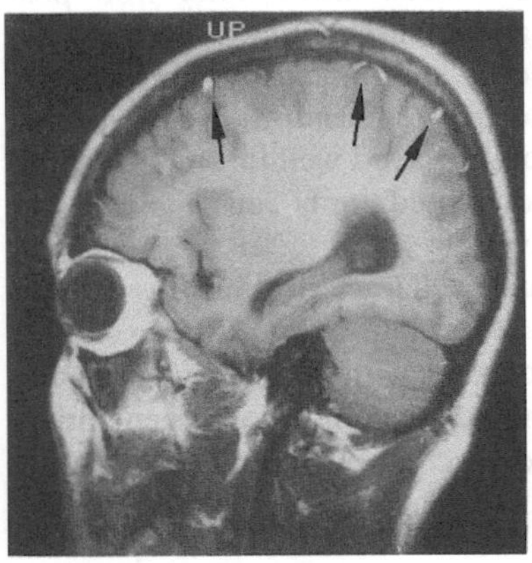

Fig. 5.14. Slow flow perpendicular to the image plane creates high signal intensity (paradoxical enhancement) in bridging veins *(arrows)* when T1-weighted SE sequences are used. Sagittal scan, SE 0.6 s/15 ms (1.5 T)

- Parkinson's disease and multisystem atrophy variants (iron deposits in the putamen, globus pallidus)
- Alzheimer's disease (iron deposits in the cerebral cortex)
- Multiple sclerosis (iron deposits adjacent to MS plaques)
- Radiation effects (iron deposits in vascular endothelium)
- Chronic hemorrhagic cerebral infarction (ferrugination)
- Intracerebral hematoma, periphery (macrophage-laden ferritin and hemosiderin accumulation occurring within 24 h)

Neuroaxonal dystrophy, Huntington's disease, Parkinson's disease, and other diseases involving the extrapyramidal motor system are associated with different kinds of movement disorders, such as tremor, chorea, and athetosis. In a larger number of patients with such movement disorders, Rutledge et al. [19] describe complex patterns of atrophy, regions of signal void on T2-weighted images, and areas of increased signal in the various extrapyramidal nuclei. With further experience, these initial results will enable closer correlations between morphological and signal changes, functional disturbances, and concentrations of trace metal deposits.

5.3 Practical Aspects of Blood and CSF Flow

W. J. Huk

The physical principles underlying the appearance of flowing fluids on MR images have been discussed in Sects. 1.3 and 1.4. Here we shall consider some general practical aspects of blood and CSF flow as they relate to MR imaging of the central nervous system.

General Aspects of Blood Flow

When blood is flowing perpendicular to the image plane, slow flow produces a high signal in the conventional SE sequence, while rapid flow produces no signal. When findings deviate from this pattern, it can be difficult to distinguish between stationary and moving protons, i.e., slow flow and thrombosis.

Slow flow is frequently laminar with a parabolic profile, meaning that the flow velocity decreases from the center of the vessel to its periphery, with the velocity falling to zero in the "boundary layer" at the vessel wall [25]. This accounts for the „bull's-eye" pattern occasionally seen in blood vessels with MR (Fig. 5.12). Usually, however, the tortuosity and wall irregularities of the vessels and the pulsatile movements of the blood produce flow components directed across the long axis of the vessel, resulting in turbulence. In vivo, then, it is usual for laminar and turbulent flows to coexist and to alternate. *Turbulence* causes a dephasing of the spins and a loss of coherence, resulting in a low signal; hence turbulent flows, even when slow-moving, appear dark on MR images.

In larger arteries, whose *rapid* systolic *flow* appears dark, an increased intraluminal signal can be seen when the section is imaged during the slow flow of diastole. This effect can be used to advantage by performing ECG-triggered measurements in different phases of the cardiac cycle. When there is chance synchronization of the heart action and MR sequence (e.g., for a pulse of 60/min and a TR of 1 s), the phenomenon of *diastolic pseudogating* can occur: because of the time shift in the sequences, certain sections in a multislice series are acquired during systole, while others are acquired during diastole [24]. Selective ECG triggering can be employed for differentiation between thrombus and slow-flowing blood (see below). With *cine studies* (see below) the correlation between the phase of the cardiac cycle and the signal intensity of moving blood can be analysed in detail (Figs. 5.13, 5.29, 5.30). In examinations of the CNS, the foregoing phenomena can have practical significance in evaluation of the venous sinuses, the bridging veins (Fig. 5.14), the large arteries, angiomas, and aneurysms.

In the *arteries,* a high signal on SE images is strongly suggestive of thrombosis, provided a chance effect like pseudogating can be excluded (Figs. 5.15-5.16). When "fast imaging" is used, even rapid flow perpendicular to the imaging plane can produce a high-intensity signal; a lower signal is seen with thrombi (Fig. 5.17). With rephasing sequences, rapid flow parallel to the imaging plane also appears hyperintense (see Sect. 1.4) (Fig. 5.23b).

In the *veins,* a high signal (on SE sequences) signifies slow blood flow perpendicular to the image plane (e.g., bridging veins in sagittal mages or transverse sinus in coronal images; see Sect. 2.8). A thrombus cannot be reliably distinguished from slow flow on this plane. Slow flow parallel to the image plane appears dark because of phase effects (e.g., sagittal sinus and straight sinus on midsagittal scans). Thrombi are easily recognized on this plane by their intense signal (Fig. 5.18).

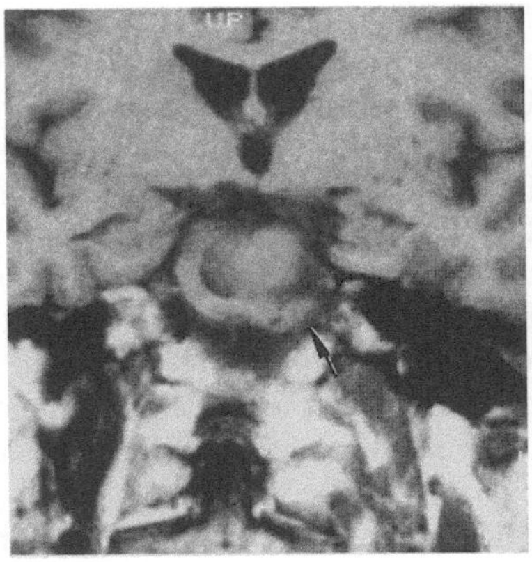

5.15

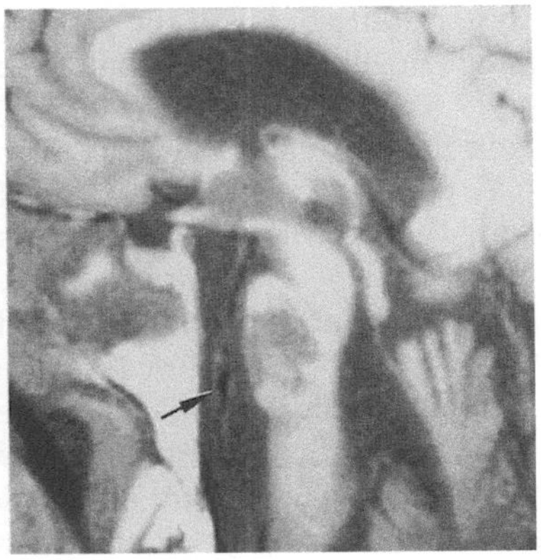

5.16

Fig. 5.15. Megadolichobasilaris with thrombosis in a 62-year-old man with rapidly developing locked-in syndrome. On angiography the contrast medium only reached the left lateral lower portion of the vessel *(arrow)* and did not show the true configuration of the artery. Hyperintense signal of the basilar artery is caused by stationary protons of thrombus. Coronal scan, SE 0.45 s/15 ms (1.5 T)

Fig. 5.16. Recanalization of thrombosis of the basilar artery *(arrow)* in a 59-year-old woman with tetraparesis following infarction of the pons. Midsagittal scan, SE 0.6 s/15 ms (1.5 T).

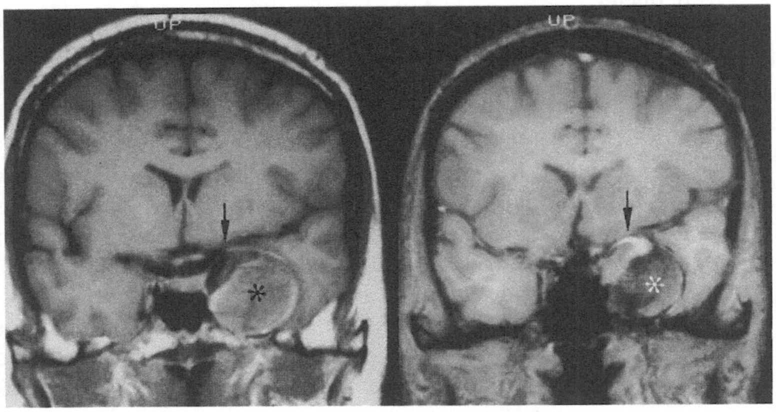

a b

Fig. 5.17 a, b. Partial thrombosis of infraclinoidal carotid aneurysm. Coronal scans of same section: **a** SE 0.6 s/15 ms, **b** FLASH 50°/0.1 s/10 ms (1.5 T). Rapid flow *(arrows)* within the aneurym appears dark in **a** and hyperintense in **b**. The thrombus *(asterisk)* is isointense in **a** and hypointense in **b**

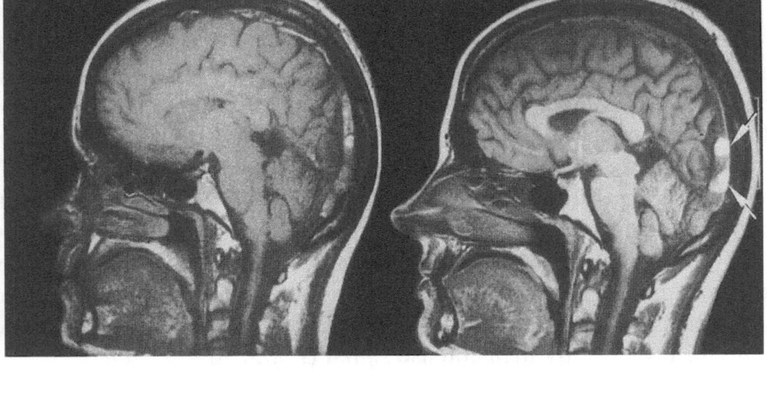

a b

Fig. 5.18 a, b. Thrombosis of sagittal and transverse sinus in a 36-year-old woman complaining of persistent headache. **a** Before treatment; **b** months later: no recanalization of the sinus, two small hyperintense areas indicating methemoglobin *(arrows)*. **a** Sagittal scan, SE 0.6 s/22 ms; **b** sagittal scan, SE 0.6 s/15 ms (1.5 T)

Fig. 5.19 a, b. Same section *(vertical arrows: 2* in **a**, *1* in **b**) examined in two multislice acquisitions in different positions with respect to the adjacent sections. With subtraction of *2* from *1* only the signal of moving spins is clearly seen. *Horizontal arrows,* direction of flow. [From 45]

Fig. 5.20. Subtraction image of popliteal vessels made from images of the same section in different positions in two consecutive multislice sequences (position 1 minus position 3). Blood flow within the vessels *(arrows)* appears hyperintense. Axial scan, T1 weighted. [From 45]

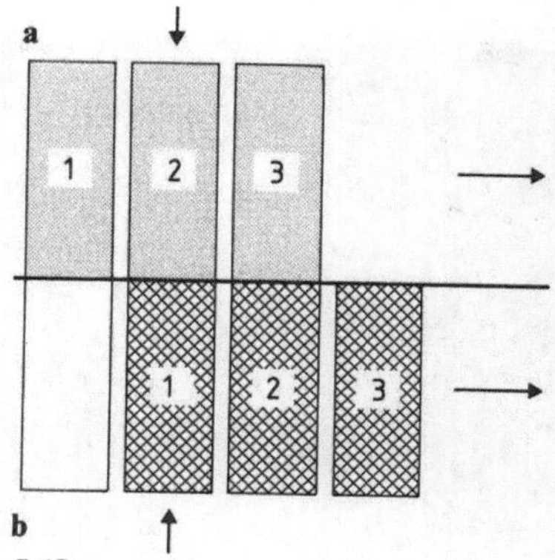

5.19

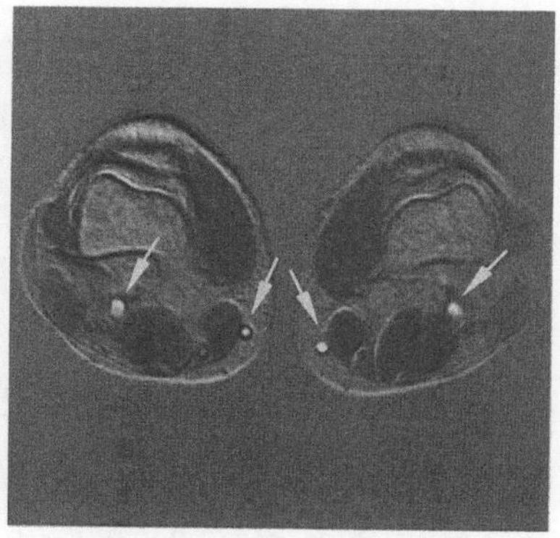

5.20

The following means are available for *distinguishing between moving and stationary blood* (45):

- Repeating the scan in a second projection perpendicular to the first.
- Subtraction of time-shift images made in the axial plane. The section of interest is examined in two multislice acquisitions in different positions with respect to the adjacent sections, using identical image parameters. Subtracting the images of the same section will give a clear picture of moving structures (Figs. 5.19, 5.20). In longitudinal scans of vessels, it is helpful to subtract an odd-numbered echo from an even-numbered echo, preferably the first from the second (even-echo rephasing, see Sect. 1.4) (Fig. 5.21).
- ECG gating in different phases of the cardiac cycle does not change the MR signal in the presence of a thrombus.
- Direct visualization of the phase angle (phase mapping). Because phase and velocity are roughly proportional for the reasons stated above, a spatially resolved flow measurement can be achieved by direct measurement of the phase angle. Stationary tissues appear uniformly gray, while flow in one direction appears bright (positive phase angle), and flow in the opposite direction appears dark (negative phase angle). The gray level correlates with the velocity of the flow. This phase analysis is possible as long as excited spins are still available in the image section for signal acquisition (see Sect. 1.4) (Fig. 5.22; see also Fig. 14.17).
- When images of the same section obtained with dephasing and rephasing sequences are subtracted, only the signal of moving protons is visualized (Fig. 5.23).

The *differentiation between rapid and slow flow* is possible in angiomatous masses and in highly vascular tumors. Because the area of interest (lesion) is usually displayed at the center of the image volume in the multislice technique, it shows very little flow-related enhancement (see above). Thus, a single-slice acquisition is best for the estimation of flow velocity, because a single section is an entry section to blood flowing from either direction perpendicular to the image plane, and so maximum paradoxical enhancement is obtained [37]. The effect can be further optimized by matching the section thickness, repetition time TR, and echo time TE (as short as possible) to the flow velocity according to the guidelines in Table 5.1 [37]. Bright intraluminal areas indicate slow flow, while dark areas indicate rapidly flowing and/or turbulent blood. Similar information can be obtained by using a partial-saturation sequence and gradient echo [27] or by the use of fast sequences (see Sect. 1.4).

Blood flow artifacts: The physical aspects of flow artifacts are discussed in Sect. 1.3. The artifacts

Table 5.1. Maximum flow-related enhancement velocity (cm/s) with variable TR and section thickness

TR (s)	Section thickness (cm)		
	0.3	0.5	1.0
0.150	2.00	3.33	6.67
0.200	1.50	2.50	5.00
0.300	1.00	1.67	3.33
0.400	0.75	1.25	2.50
0.500	0.60	1.00	2.00
0.600	0.50	0.83	1.67
0.800	0.38	0.63	1.25
1.00	0.33	0.50	1.00

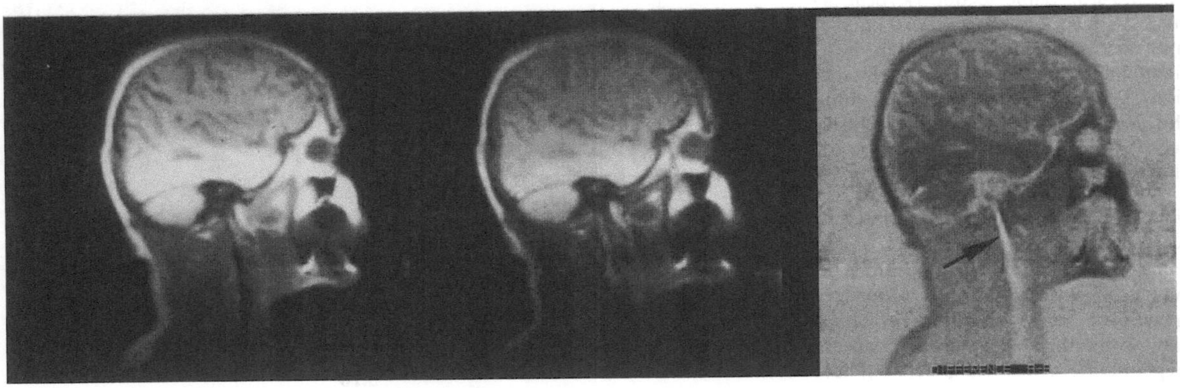

a b c

▲ **Fig. 5.21 a–c.** Subtraction image (**c**) of the jugular vein *(arrow)* made by subtracting an odd-numbered (first) echo from an even-numbered (second) echo. Sagittal scans, multiecho SE sequence (0.5 T). [From 45]

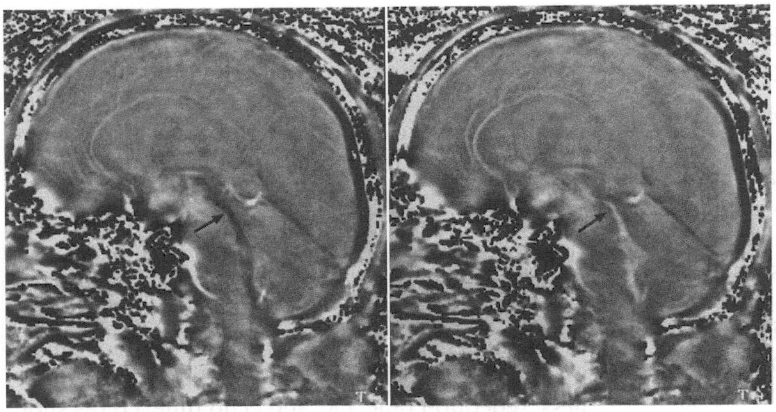

a b

Fig. 5.22. Phase images of the central portions of the ventricular system, obtained **a** 153 ms, and **b** 468 ms after the R wave (ECG). The aqueduct *(arrow)* appears dark in **a**, during systole. Sagittal scans, FLASH 40°/0.073 s/10 ms

that emanate from larger blood vessels along the phase encoding axis can be troublesome for image interpretation. These artifacts are most commonly caused by the parasellar portions of the internal carotid arteries, from which a succession of streak-like ghost images spread in the posterior (axial scans) or temporal (coronal scans) direction. The latter type is especially troublesome in evaluations of temporal lobe epilepsy. The basilar artery, sigmoid sinus, superior sagittal sinus, and the bulbs also give rise to ghost images, which are more pronounced on T2-weighted scans than with T1 weighting or proton-density weighting. With gradient motion refocusing (GMR) sequences, these artifacts can be reduced or eliminated.

MR Imaging of CSF and CSF Flow Effects

The MR appearance of CSF differs in several respects from its CT counterpart. Whereas CSF always appears hypodense on CT scans, its MR signal intensity, and thus its degree of contrast with adjacent structures, depends on the choice of imaging parameters. CSF has very long T1 and T2 relaxation times. Consequently it appears dark on T1-weighted scans (e.g., SE with short TR and TE, inversion recovery) and contrasts poorly with the surrounding cortical bone, paranasal sinus air (low proton density), and blood vessels (flow void). On the other hand, CSF gives a very high signal on T2-weighted images (e.g., SE with a long TR and TE). This greatly increases its contrast with neighboring bony structures, which is advantageous in the skull base region and spinal canal. CSF shows less contrast, however, with lesions that also have long relaxation times (gliomas, cysts, MS plaques, etc.) and with periventricular edema. These cases are best evaluated by proton-density images with an intermediate TR (e.g., 1.5–2.0 s), which cause the lesions to appear brighter than brain tissue, and by images with a short TE (e.g., 30 ms), which cause

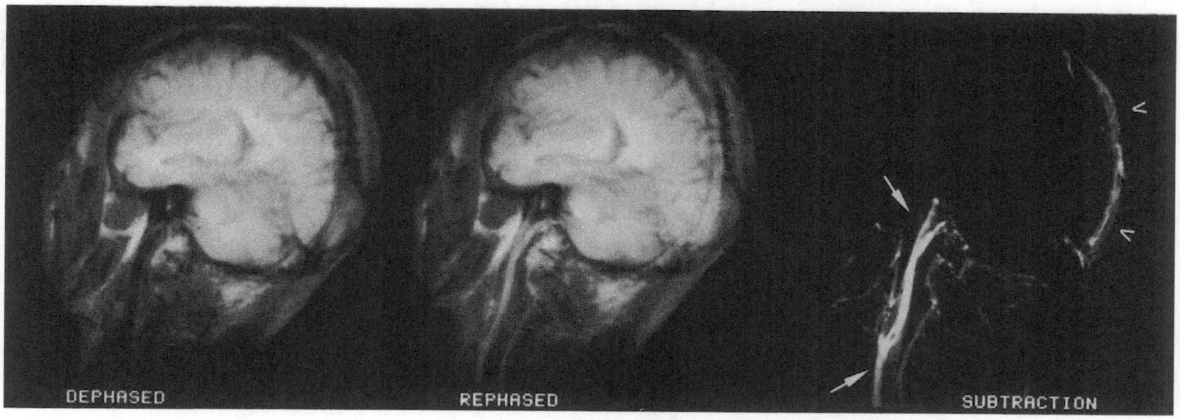

a b c

▲ **Fig. 5.23 a–c.** When the dephased image (**a**) is subtracted from the rephased image (**b**), only the signal of moving protons is depicted (**c**). *Arrows,* corotid artery; *arrowheads,* sagittal sinus

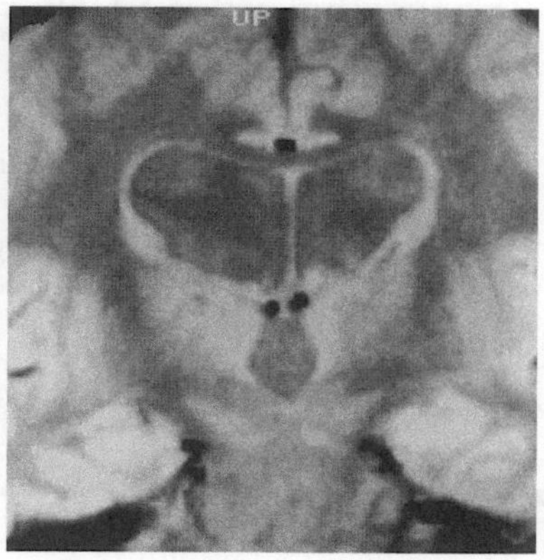

Fig. 5.24. CSF flow pattern in a patient with hydrocephalus. Coronal scan SE 3.0 s/35 ms (1.0 T)

lesions and brain tissue to appear brighter than the CSF [26, 39, 44], for example in cases of multiple sclerosis or interstitial edema (see Fig. 5.2).

But other signal changes are seen with MR that cannot be explained by the long relaxation times of CSF (Fig. 5.24). These changes relate more to the flow of CSF from sites of formation to sites of absorption, a flow that is further modulated by pulse waves associated with cardiac and respiratory activity. As already mentioned in the description of blood flow, the movement of protons has effects on signal intensity, which in turn depends on the image sequence.

The average *CSF volume* in adults is about 135 ml, 35 ml of which are intraventricular. In its physical and chemical properties, CSF closely resembles an ultrafiltrate of plasma [46]. The present view is that CSF is formed by the choroid plexus of the lateral ventricles (0.4 ml/min according to Cutler et al. [28]) and the fourth ventricle, and also by the ventricular ependyma [41]. From the lateral ventricles, CSF flows into the third ventricle through the slitlike foramina of Monro, and into the fourth ventricle through the aqueduct of Sylvius (see Sect. 2.1). It passes from the fourth ventricle into the posterior fossa cisterns through the midline foramen of Magendie and lateral foramina of Luschka, bathes the surface of the brain, and finally is returned to the blood across the arachnoid villi.

Factors which influence the movement of CSF are as follows:

1. The quantity of CSF that moves from sites of formation to sites of absorption per unit time. This volume is decreased or increased by inflammatory diseases, hydrocephalus, etc.
2. The ependymal ciliary activity [41, 46].
3. The pulsations of the brain, which match the frequency of the heart rate and lead to rhythmic displacements and accelerations of the CSF with to-and-fro movements in the foramina of Monro, the aqueduct, and the third and fourth ventricles.

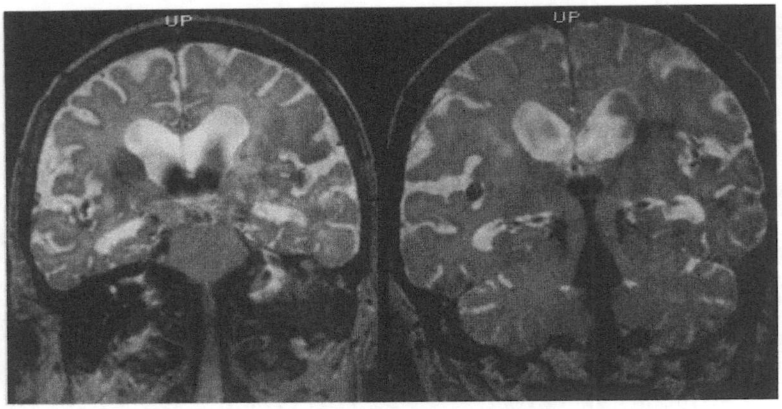

a b

Fig. 5.25 a, b. CSF flow at the foramen of Monro (**a**) and the aqueduct (**b**). Coronal scans (**a, b**) FISP 40°/0.03 s/10 ms (1.5 T). Moving CSF appears dark also in the ambient and insular cisterns (**a, b**)

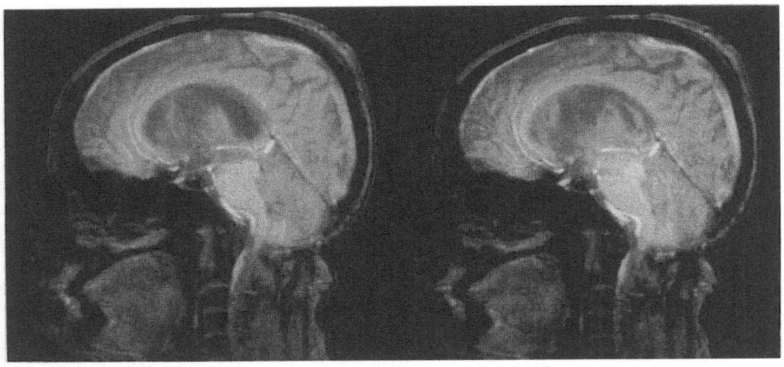

a b

Fig. 5.26 a, b. Flow effects of the lateral ventricles in a case of stenosis of the aqueduct: 38-year-old man with hydrocephalus. Midsagittal scans. FISP 40°/0.05 s/12 ms, 107 ms (**a**) and 592 ms (**b**) after the R wave (ECG) (1.5 T). Note also the high signal intensity of vessels in the image plane

The direction of the flow is antegrade during systole and retrograde during diastole [40]. The amplitude of these movements depends on the level of the arterial pressure, the arteriovenous pressure difference, and the intracranial pressure (Figs. 5.25, 5.26).

4. Besides the rhythmic fluctuations in brain volume (which are very apparent during craniotomies), the pulsations of superficial arteries are transmitted to the ambient CSF. This can be observed in cervical myelography, cisternography, and central ventriculography. Thus, the pulsations of the basilar artery can be transmitted through the thin floor of the third ventricle to the fluid within. Similar local pulsation effects from the tortuous superficial vessels occur in the rest of the basal CSF spaces (circle of Willis, vertebral arteries, basilar artery), in the course of the large branches of the middle cerebral artery (sylvian fissure, insular cisterns), in the the anterior cerebral artery (interhemispheric fissure), in the posterior cerebral arteries (ambient cistern), and in the spinal canal.
5. Respiration affects CSF movements by altering the heart rate and arteriovenous pressure difference.

Thus, the pulsations cited above effect global as well as local, rhythmic modulations in the quantity, direction, and velocity of the CSF flow. Taken together, these forces, which act from various directions, produce laminar, turbulent, oscillatory, and pulsatile flows of varying velocity, which in turn are modulated by the anatomy of the structures they traverse. These *anatomic factors* include:

- The size and shape of the ventricles
- The size and shape of the foramina (Monro, aqueduct, outlet foramina of the fourth ventricle)
- The size of the external CSF spaces (i.e., the extent and localization of cortical atrophy)
- The spatial relation of CSF collections to the large vessels
- The size and shape of the large superficial vessels
- The elasticity of the brain

Velocity of CSF flow: Ventriculographic studies by Du Boulay [30] indicated an oscillatory movement

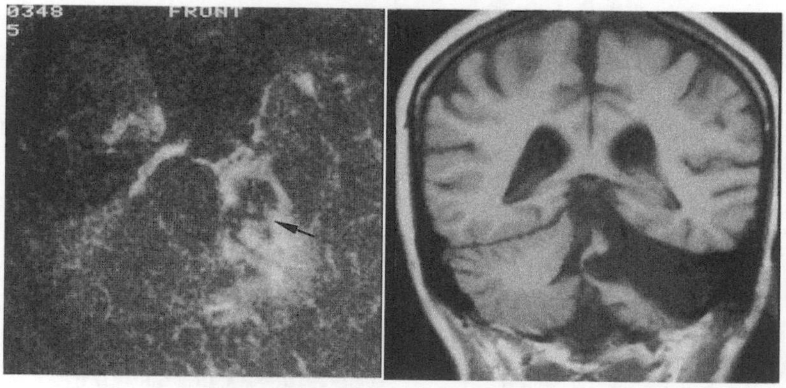

Fig. 5.27 a, b. False-positive finding in the posterior fossa in a 38-year-old woman caused by alteration of the CSF flow pattern after removal of an epidermoid cyst in the right cerebellopontine angle. From the axial MR image (**a**) T2-weighted) tumor recurrence *(arrow)* was suspected. With the coronal scan (**b** SE 0.4 s/17 ms) and contrast-CT cisternography a tumor could be excluded

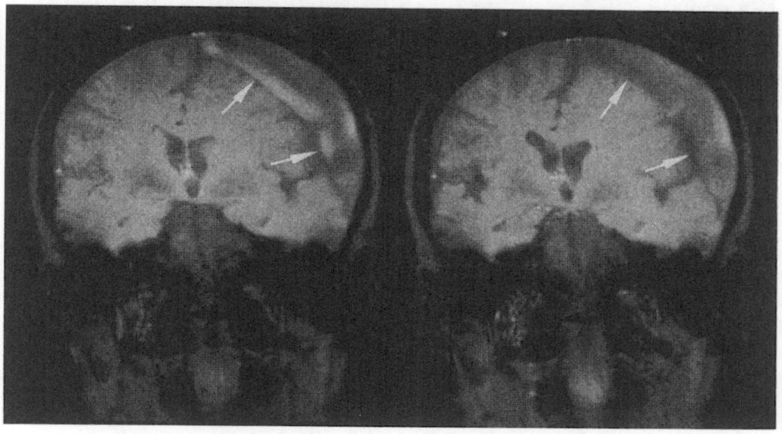

Fig. 5.28 a, b. Chronic subdural hematoma in a 62-year-old man with increasing headache. Coronal scans obtained at different phases of the cardiac cycle: **a** 140 ms and **b** 466 ms after the R wave of the ECG (FLASH 30°/0.79 s/20 ms). The differences of signal intensity within hematoma in **a** *(arrows)* are caused not by differences in the composition of the fluid, but by flow effects. Note also the changing signal pattern within the ventricles

of the CSF in the third ventricle equal to 7-8 mg/min (0.11-0.13 ml/s) at a normal heart rate of 70-80/min [46]. Similarly, the velocity of oscillatory flow in the upper cervical canal is estimated to be 0.8-7.8 cm/s (3-30 mm/pulse according to [38, 47]). The pulsatile movements are greatest in the upper cervical canal and diminish toward the thoracic and lumbar regions.

Higher flow velocities are expected to occur in areas of narrowing within the ventricular system, such as the foramina of Monro, the outlet foramina of the fourth ventricle, and especially the aqueduct of Sylvius (Fig. 5.25). The aqueduct is approximately 12 mm long and varies from 1.85 to 5.1 mm^2 in cross-section [38]. Data on flow velocities in the aqueduct vary greatly and on the whole are inaccurate.

MR Findings

In what way do these flow movements affect the signal intensity of CSF in motion-sensitive sequences?

High flow velocity combined with turbulence leads to signal loss in conventional *SE sequences,* so that the CSF in the aqueduct and possibly in other narrow areas of the ventricular system appears dark. This is also the case on T2-weighted sequences, where stationary CSF yields a high signal. The direction of the flow cannot be ascertained. The jet of CSF flowing from the aqueduct into the fourth ventricle can occasionally be traced as a dark streak on the floor of the rhomboid fossa (Figs. 5.25, 5.26). Sherman et al. [47] saw decreased CSF signal intensity, which they called the CSF flow-void sign (CFVS), in 31 (67%) of 46 normal subjects in the aqueduct, in 15 (32%) in the caudal fourth ventricle, and in 2 (4%) in the third ventricle on T2-weighted images. On T1-weighted scans the sign was apparent in only 13% of patients because of poor contrast with the CSF, which appears dark in these sequences. This signal loss is probably due to a combination of time-of-flight effects, phase shift, and view-to-view variation effects.

"Lagoons," or areas that contain very slow-flowing or stagnant CSF, may form in expansions

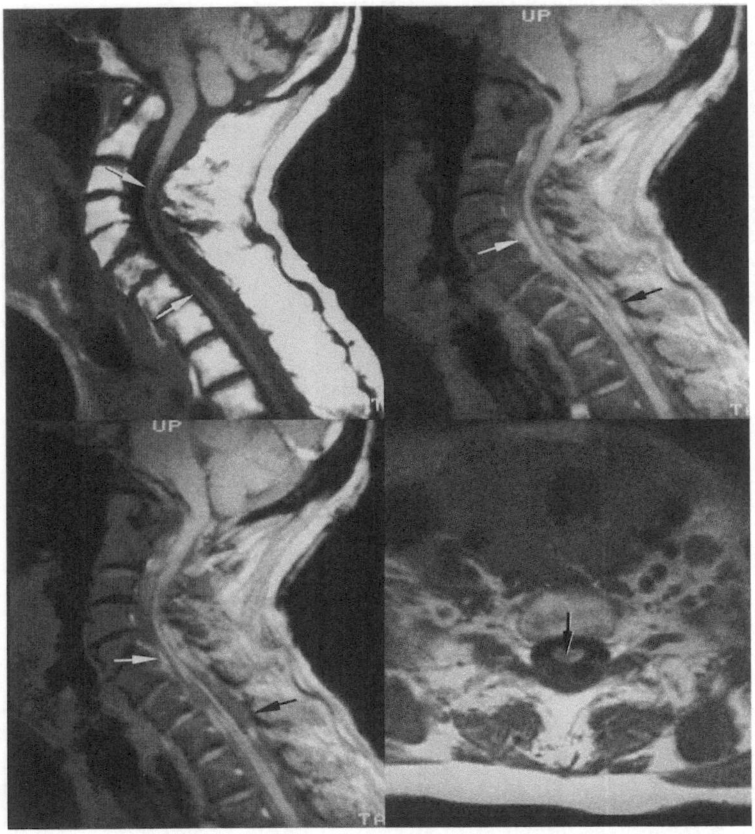

a b c d

Fig. 5.29 a–d. Syringomyelia (*arrows* in **a**) with atrophy of cervical cord in a 71-year-old woman. **a** Midsagittal section, SE 0.6 s/15 ms; **b** pulsatile flow motion of CSF (*arrows* in **b** and **c**) demonstrated by two representative sagittal images 138 ms (**b**) and 369 ms (**c**) after the R wave (ECG), FLASH 40°/0.05 s/10 ms. **d** Flow pattern in an axial section, SE 0.6 s/15 ms (1.5 T)

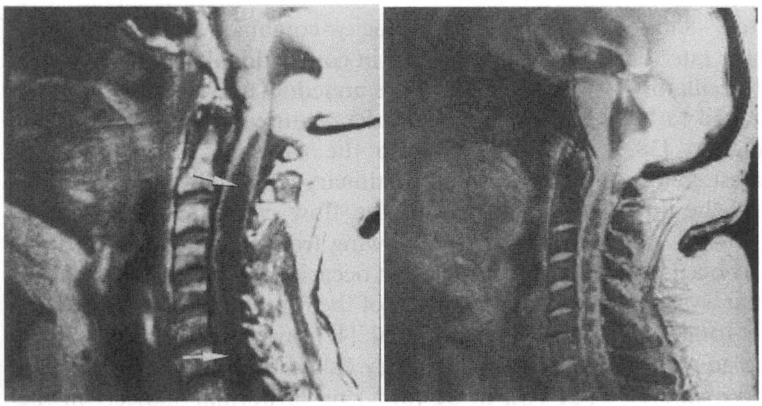

a b

Fig. 5.30 a, b. Syringomyelia (*arrows*) in a 62-year-old woman with spasticity. Midsagittal scans: **a** SE 0.45 s/15 ms; **b** cine study, FLASH 40°/0.03 s/10 ms, 434 ms after the R wave (ECG). The inhomogeneous structure of the cyst in **b** is caused by CSF pulsations

or quiet corners of the ventricles and external CSF spaces (e.g., the internal auditory canal), at nodal points of the complex oscillatory CSF flow in relation to the image plane, or in CSF-filled cavities left by tumor resections (Fig. 5.27). The fluid in these areas gives a higher signal on T2-weighted images than does moving CSF. Hasso et al. [34] explain signal increases seen on T1-weighted images as inflow signal enhancement by to-and-fro movements of unsaturated protons perpendicular to the image plane, and thus as a type of paradoxical enhancement (Fig. 5.28; see also Fig. 5.24).

Fast sequences are particularly sensitive to CSF movements (see Sect. 1.4). ECG-triggered FLASH cine sequences of the cervical spinal canal in the axial projection (flow perpendicular to the image plane) have been able to demonstrate CSF pulsations in temporal resolution. They have shown a diversity of flow directions, with downward flow occurring lateral to the spinal cord and upward flow anterior to the cord. Results of dynamic cine measurements over one ECG cycle have been interpreted as a superposition of oscillatory and directed motion of the CSF [36]. For CSF movements on the image plane, the spins accumulate an additional phase angle which, in the presence of pulsatile flow, causes image artifacts to appear in the phase encode direction [29]. This motion-phase effect has been used, for example, to demonstrate small changes of flow direction in the fast imaging with steady precession (FISP) sequence (Fig. 5.25). The sequence utilizes the steady-state free precession (SSFP) that is established by periodic RF excitation of the spin system. By symmetrical switching of all gradient pulses with respect to the echo center, this SSFP condition is achieved in a dynamic equilibrium of both longitudinal and transverse magnetization. With large pulse angles (90°), a very high signal is obtained from spins whose T2 value is comparable to its T1 value, i.e., for tissues whose T1/T2 ratio is equal to 1. For that reason fluids, especially CSF, appear very bright despite the short repetition time (TR ca. 20 ms). If rephasing of the spins is disturbed, as by movements of the CSF, the signal intensity is greatly decreased (Fig. 5.25). The CSF signal intensity is very sensitive to changes in TE, which provide a selective compensation for the dephasing effect of the fluid motion.

Artifacts of pulsatile flow occurring in the phase encode direction can be significantly reduced by ECG gating. Regardless of the ECG cycle, the additional phases that are generated by uniform and/or accelerated motion can be compensated with *bipolar sequences* for arbitrary values of TR [42, 43].

Flow phenomena carry a danger of *misinterpretation* and false-positive diagnosis. In the spinal canal they can appear as pseudo-mass lesions and pseudodiscs when CSF motion is confined to pockets or limited by arachnoid septa; this can also occur in root cysts. In Fig. 5.27 they mimic a recurrence of tumor in a resection cavity. Flow effects in the internal auditory canal can simulate the presence of a small neuroma [32]. The true nature of these effects can be disclosed by repeating the scan on a different plane, by phase mapping (see above), by rotation of the phase encode gradient, by ECG gating [22], or by cine studies with fast imaging techniques (Fig. 5.29). In basal CSF collections, flow effects need to be distinguished from artifacts that emanate from large vessels (carotid arteries, venous sinuses) in the direction of the phase encode gradient ("ghost images"). Similar effects may be seen above the convexity of the hemispheres if the subarachnoid spaces are large.

CSF flow effects within closed cysts can be of diagnostic assistance when it is necessary to exclude communication of the cyst with the ventricular system. The slower-moving or stationary fluid in these cysts gives a higher signal on T2-weighted images than the surrounding, pulsating CSF. By showing, for example, that the cyst does not communicate with the ventricular CSF, the need for ventriculography can be eliminated. Thus, the higher signal of the cystic fluid does not necessarily indicate a difference in chemical properties (Fig. 5.28). ECG gating can be used to cancel out the motion-related signal difference, producing isointensity between the intracystic and the extracystic fluid. CSF flow effects can also be helpful in distinguishing hydro- or syringomyelia from the weak signal of a pencil glioma (Fig. 5.29–5.30). In intramedullary cysts pulsatile and nonpulsatile fluid can be observed, pulsations being more prominent in larger than in smaller cysts. The presence of pulsations seems to indicate a nonneoplastic cyst. Tumor cysts were found to show no pulsations even when large [31].

Tumor cysts can give a bright signal on T2-weighted mixed images of the SE sequence in cases where a high protein content of the cystic fluid imparts a strong T1 component to the signal.

The goal of future research will be to extract more diagnostic information from CSF movements. A major task will be to characterize the patterns of normal CSF flow and investigate how changes in these patterns correlate with intracranial diseases. With a velocity imaging technique at high resolution (0.4 mm/s) requiring 64 cardiac cycles per image, Feinberg et al. [33] demonstrated and measured vascular-driven movements of the entire brain, which act as the pumping force for CSF circulation. These studies may well provide a noninvasive means for evaluating the intracranial pressure, the CSF dynamics of communicating hydrocephalus, the functional status of shunt systems, and many other questions. In one case of normal pressure hydrocephalus with shunt incompetence, Bradley et al. [23] were able to measure an acceleration of the CSF flow to a velocity 4 times greater than normal. Sherman et al. [47] have published initial observations in 27 patients with obstructions of the ventricular pathways. The presence of the CFVS indicated patency of the ventricular pathways in which it occurred. Its absence may be inconsequential in approximately 18% of normal cases [35], but in pathologic cases it may signify an obstruction of flow. Thus, the CFVS is ambiguous and requires further investigation so that it can be correctly interpreted.

5.4 Effects of Radiotherapy on Brain and Spinal Cord Tumors

I. Baer

The rationale for the radiotherapy of CNS tumors is based on the relatively high radiosensitivity of most neoplasms compared with surrounding healthy brain. In the past it has been difficult to evaluate treatment response even with CT, because late radionecrosis of the treated area (see below) and the associated edema create a mass effect on CT scans that can closely mimic a tumor recurrence. There is hope that the new imaging modality of MR will permit more accurate study and differentiation of the various tissue responses to radiation therapy.

Pathoanatomic Effects of Ionizing Radiation on the CNS and Surrounding Tissues

Connective tissue reacts to ionizing radiation with swelling of its fibrocytes and depolymerization of its macromolecules (polysaccharides).

Blood vessels respond with capillary dilatation, leading to a rise of capillary permeability, swelling of the cell nuclei, and endothelial detachment, so that the basement membrane borders directly on the blood stream. In other cases endothelial proliferation can occur, causing occlusion of the vessel.

Radiation effects on the *cerebrum*, and especially the cerebral cortex, are specific to that tissue and relate to the fact that this area lacks significant pericapillary spaces like those found in other body regions, and the parenchymal cells (astrocytes) have processes that insert directly on the capillary wall [56].

Only the *basement membranes* separate the membranes of the endothelial cells and the adjacent brain cells. The intercellular junctions between the membranes of adjacent cells are only 15-20 nm wide. This structure forms the basis for the phenomenon of the *blood-brain barrier* [56]. The transport of water and most ions in the brain is accomplished through extensions and processes of the glial cells, mainly the astrocytes, and not through the intercellular space.

In the *cerebellar cortex*, too, more than 90% of the blood capillaries lack a perivascular space. This contrasts with the *spinal cord*, in which all of the capillaries possess small perivascular spaces [53].

Certain pathologic conditions in the brain can lead to the formation of pericapillary spaces. This can occur, for example, in the boundary zone of a traumatic cerebrocortical necrosis associated with heavy astrocytic gliosis and fibrosis. In this case there is a splitting of the basement membrane resulting in the creation of pericapillary spaces containing fibroblasts and collagenous fibrils, which may fibrose at a later time.

Unlike the capillaries, the arteries and veins in all regions of the CNS are surrounded by a perivascular space [50, 57].

The cellular effects of ionizing radiation include the arrest of cell division, the inactivation of enzymes, the formation of free radicals and valencies in molecules and atoms, and ultimately the death of the cell through a breakdown of its molecular structure.

An important effect of ionizing radiation in the body is the *radiolysis of water* in tissues, with corresponding secondary effects from OH and H radicals, which may react, for example, with amino acids or with SH groups on the membranes of cells and organelles.

The irradiation of *bone marrow* incites a fatty degeneration process in which hematopoietic tissue is replaced by fat cells. Normal bone marrow is composed approximately 30% of fat and 60% of water, with the fat content increasing with age, especially in females [52].

The clinical classification of radiation injury to the brain and spinal cord is based largely on the time course of the effects. The principal manifestations of radiation injury are as follows [61]:

1. Acute radionecrosis
2. Early changes
3. Transient radiation injury
4. Late injury of early onset
5. Late injury of delayed onset

Radiation always injures both the vessel walls and the parenchyma, with damage to the oligodendroglia and remaining parenchyma predominating in the early stages, and vascular wall changes predominating in the late stages.

The key pathogenic factor is the damage to the reproductive capacity of the cell. CNS cells that are capable of division, such as the endothelial and muscle cells of the vessel walls and the neuroglia, are far more vulnerable than cells having no mitotic activity. This accounts for the high radiosensitivity of the developing pediatric brain, in which the white matter is still maturing [69], and for the vulnerability of the aged brain with its fragile repair mechanisms [71].

Some time is needed before cells exposed to a primarily nonlethal but mutagenic radiation insult undergo sufficient mitotic divisions to produce gross structural tissue change. This factor, plus differences in radiosensitivities, causes the effects on different tissue components to appear at different times. Thus, for example, medullary sheaths may manifest lesions shortly after damage to the oligodendroglial cells, well before overt vascular lesions have had time to develop.

The extent of the radiation injury depends mainly on the irradiated volume, the total dose, the dose rate, and the mode of fractionation. A basic rule is that the latent period preceding the appearance of gross tissue damage lengthens as the radiation dose is decreased.

Acute Radionecrosis

Acute radionecrosis (e.g., from local irradiation with the betatron) affects the gray and white matter equally above a dose of 70 Gy. Doses of 50–70 Gy produce partial necrosis at the center of the irradiated area.

Early Changes

Early changes are manifested between 3 and 6 weeks after exposure, although electron microscopy demonstrates initial changes within a matter of hours [54]. Unless extensive, the changes are reversible.

The acute response involves a disruption of the blood-brain barrier with early development of brain edema. The oligodendroglia is slightly less vulnerable, followed by the astroglia. Neurons are relatively resistant; they show acute swelling, pyknosis, or the features of a severe cellular disease [48]. Perifocal inflammatory reactions occur secondarily. Brain edema is a nonspecific response to a variety of pathogenic influences. Within hours of radiation exposure, intracellular fluid collections are observed in the processes of the glial cells bordering the capillary basement membranes [50, 56, 67]. By 48 h the glial cells themselves appear enlarged [60]. Swollen astrocytic processes may compress the capillaries [70]. An early rise of capillary permeability occurs in the cerebral white matter, and the extracellular spaces become expanded and engorged with fluid [57]. With more severe edema the cell membranes of the glial processes rupture, causing pericapillary fluid collections to appear.

With collateral brain edema in man, the capillary basement membranes enlarge to twice their normal width. Some endothelial cells are enlarged fourfold and contain increased numbers of small vacuoles and fat droplets [68].

Transient Radiation Injury

The spinal cord is more radiosensitive than the cerebrum [65]. This can be attributed to the lower level of bone absorption in the spine and the relatively free penetration of the rays to deeper levels, especially when ultrahard radiation is applied [55]. Added to this is the small diameter and selective radiosensitivity of myelin-containing fibers, which are tightly bundled within the cord, as well as the occurrence of radiation oligodendropathy. The average incidence of radiation myelopathy following a typical therapeutic course of radiation to the spine (55–60 Gy in 5–6 weeks) is between 1% and 5% [61].

The high vulnerability of the oligodendroglia leads to a demyelination that is most pronounced in the dorsal columns and is expressed clinically in Lhermitte's sign.

The transient form is less common than the chronic forms, and its changes are reversible. An average latent period of 4.7 months has been reported.

Late Injury of Early or Delayed Onset

Late effects start to become apparent by 3–6 months after radiotherapy. The average clinical latency is 16.4 months [55].

The acute-onset form of radiation myelopathy develops within days, producing the syndrome of a complete or incomplete transverse cord lesion. Vascular changes are by no means as prominent in this syndrome as are glial injuries with demyelination and necrosis [61].

The progressive form of chronic radiation myelopathy is associated clinically with pronounced sensory disturbances in 54% of cases, motor and sensory disturbances in 21%, and initial paralysis in 22% [55].

Radiation effects on the surrounding brain tissue (including the healthy tissue of the contralateral hemisphere) are characterized histologically by small or larger foci of hemorrhage into the diffusely swollen gray and white matter and by ischemic changes in the neurons.

Changes in the Signal Intensity of Intracranial Tumors During Radiotherapy

It has been our experience [58] that a multiecho SE sequence with a TR of 2.0 s and 16 echoes (TE 30–480 ms) and a T1-weighted SE sequence with a TR of 0.3 s and TE of 30 ms are excellent for evaluating signal changes in brain tumors during and after radiation therapy. The T1 (from two slices) and T2 (from 16 slices) relaxation times are determined from these sequences (Fig. 5.31). The T2 images give a good appreciation of changes during the course of radiotherapy, provided the follow-up scans are made in anatomically identical planes. In patients with various intra-axial and extra-axial tumors (astrocytomas, glioblastomas, metastases, chordoma), we invariably found a significant rise of T2 values at the start of therapy. T1 images are less rewarding, because the proton density of the affected area is only slightly increased, and in many cases the lesion is not delineated (see Fig. 5.31). Contrast agents (e.g., gadolinium chelate; see Fig. 5.32) are helpful in defining the outer tumor boundary. With continuation of the radiotherapy, the T2 values gradually shorten again; the tumor becomes smaller and its borders less distinct (see Fig. 5.33). The surrounding edema shows virtually no change during the therapy, or may regress slightly, as we have observed in patients treated with corticosteroids (see Fig. 5.34). In most cases, follow-up scans taken 1–2 months after the conclusion of radiotherapy will show a marked reduction in the size of the surrounding vasogenic edema.

We have found a tissue discrimination program to be helpful in evaluating therapeutic response. By applying an "adaptable classifier system" and the MR sequences described above, the signal pattern and signal distribution pattern of the individual patient can be "learned" from the appearance of the tumor tissue and adjacent reference tissue (CSF, white matter, edema) (Fig. 5.35). The discrimination program is used in follow-up examinations to identify tumor tissue on the basis of the learned features. Of course, tumor tissue changes during radiotherapy as it undergoes necrotic transformation and is no longer recognized as tumor by the program. Nevertheless, the tissues that were still "recognized" as tumor correlated very well with clinical and CT findings, and so the visible reduction of this tissue area may be taken as a useful index of tumor regression and thus of the success of the radiotherapy.

In patients undergoing whole-brain or partial-brain irradiation, we have found increases in the T2 times of the surrounding healthy white matter. Presumably this represents a mild, acute radiation injury with disruption of the blood-brain barrier (see subsection "Early Changes" above). Curnes et al. [49] found a long T2 in the periventricular white matter of patients who had received combined cranial irradiation and chemotherapy. MR proved superior to CT in its ability to delineate the white matter injury.

Dooms et al. [51] saw radiation lesions in 8 of 55 patients who presented for late MR and CT follow-up after radiotherapy. The lesions appeared as areas of prolonged T1 and T2 in sequences with a long TR (2.0 s) and appeared isointense with the white matter when the TR was short (0.5 s). Tumor recurrence, residual tumor, and tumor necrosis were indistinguishable. Neither was our tissue discrimination program of assistance in this respect. A marked rise of signal intensity can be seen in the bone marrow of vertebral bodies following the radiotherapy of spinal cord tumors [62]. The chemical shift imaging method must be applied to determine whether the change in relaxation times relates to the fat component or to the water component of the tissue [63, 64].

In the *planning* of radiotherapy, the multiplanar facility of MR can contribute valuable information on the size, shape, and location of tumors, thereby reducing the risk of inaccurate localization as the greatest source of error [59, 66]. According to initial observations, low-grade gliomas often appear more extensive on MR images than on CT scans, although the margin between tumor and edema can be difficult to resolve. Degenerated portions of higher-grade tumors can be brought out with intravenous contrast material (e.g., gadolinium chelate).

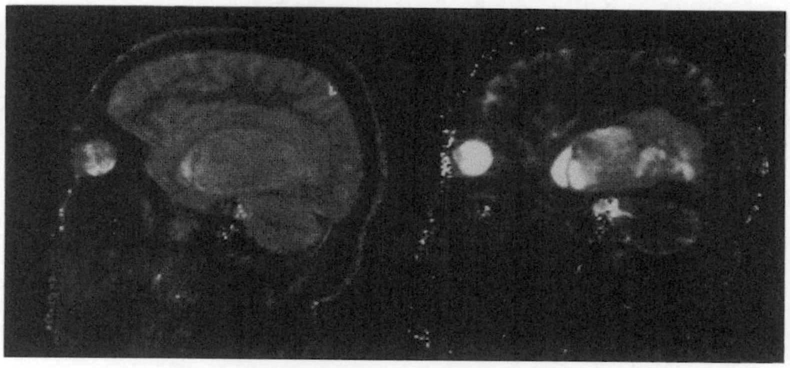

a b

Fig. 5.31. Patient with temporal glioblastoma, before (**a**) and after (**b**) radiotherapy (55 Gy). *Top:* T1 images, calculated from two different images (TR = 300 ms and 2000 ms) at echo time TE = 30 ms; *bottom:* T2 images, calculated from 16 echoes

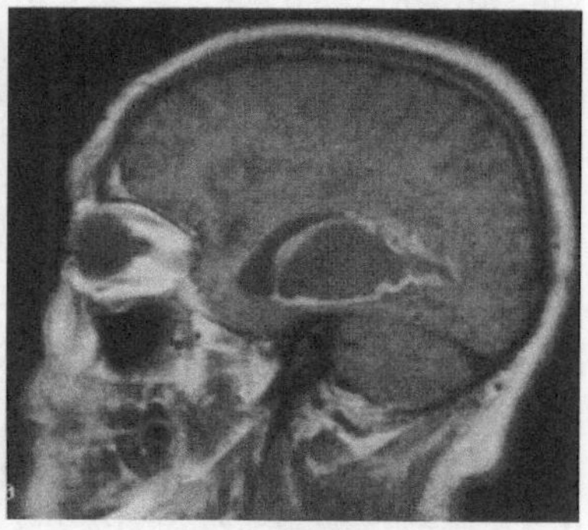

Fig. 5.32. Some patient as in Fig. 5.31 before radiotherapy. Post-contrast picture (gadolinium chelate): TR = 600 ms, TE = 28 ms

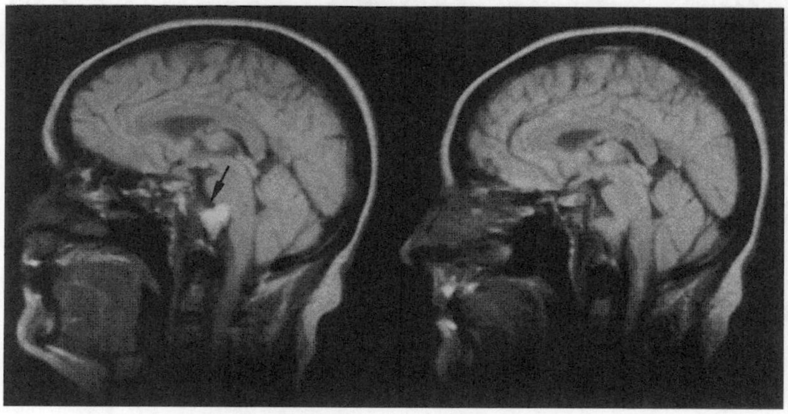

a b

Fig. 5.33. a, b. Chordoma *(arrow)* in a 50-year-old female before (**a**) and after (**b**) radiotherapy (55 Gy). Midsagittal scan, SE 2.0 s/30 ms (1.0 T)

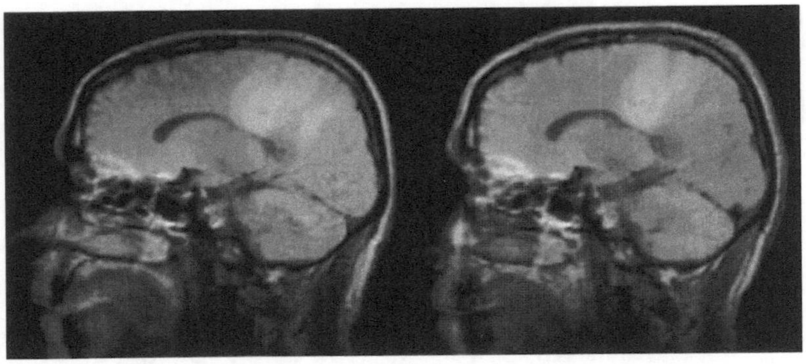
a b

Fig. 5.34 a, b. Metastasis of malignant melanoma with perifocal edema in a 55-year-old male before (**a**) and after (**b**) whole-brain radiotherapy (50 Gy). Sagittal scans, SE 2.0 s/30 ms (1.0 T)

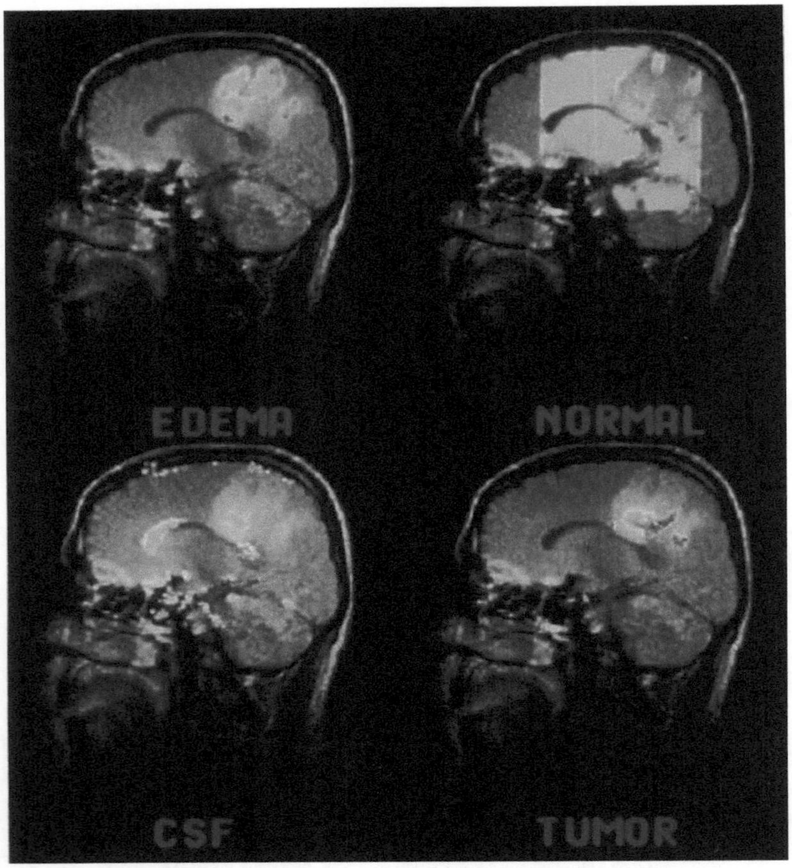

Fig. 5.35. Superimposed color probability images for the four different tissue types learned, calculated only in the region of interest. *Bright yellow* corresponds to high, *dark red* to low probability. Pixels with a probability of less than 0.6 are displayed in their normal gray value

5.5 Effect of Contrast Agent (Gadolinium-DTPA) on the MR Appearance of Normal Tissue

W. J. Huk

The physical and pharmacologic aspects of the mechanism of action of paramagnetic contrast agents for MR imaging have been discussed in Sect. 1.3.3.

The first practical, clinical experience in this area was obtained with the agent gadolinium-DTPA. A *dose* of 0.1 mmol/kg body weight has proved suitable for diagnostically useful contrast enhancement. This dose is well tolerated. Even a dose of 0.2 mmol/kg may be given without concern if this should prove necessary [73].

Intravenous injection of the contrast agent is simple. It is recommended that an i.v. line be established before the patient is moved into the scanner. Extension tubing is used to bring the line out through the opening of the scanner. Following the orientation or noncontrast scan, the contrast agent can then be administered without having to remove the patient from the magnet. So far only few patients were reported to have experienced minor side effects where a connection with the application of the contrast medium has to be discussed. In one patient with no known allergic disposition, who was examined in a private MR-unit in Erlangen, FRG, a severe allergic reaction was seen immediately after the intravenous injection of gadolinium-DTPA. There for it should be standard practice to maintain constant surveillance of patients in the scanner after the agent has been administered.

Concerning potential *limitations* on the use of gadolinium-DTPA, which at this writing was still undergoing phase III clinical trials, we refer the reader to the prescribing information supplied with the marketed product.

Optimum *contrast enhancement* is obtained on T1-weighted image sequences, such as SE sequences with a TR of 0.5 s and a very short TE. In T2-weighted sequences, little if any difference is apparent between contrast and noncontrast scans. Very heavily T1-weighted sequences (e.g., inversion recovery) will also delineate edematous zones. In the absence of perifocal edema, it can be far more difficult to separate a lesion from the surrounding white matter, which also gives a high signal [78].

The *time course* of contrast enhancement corresponds roughly to that of the iodinated contrast media used in CT. Most tumors show enhancement very soon after injection of the contrast agent. In lesions with less perfusion or a less pronounced disruption of the blood-brain barrier, such as MS plaques, enhancement may be delayed. Lesions without a blood-brain barrier, such as pituitary tumors, meningiomas, and metastases, generally show enhancement immediately after the material is injected. Thus, previous experience indicates that "late views" are seldom necessary for tumor detection, although the change in signal distribution on later images may give additional information on the structure of the lesion. In some circumstances the concurrent staining of normal tissues can mask a tumorous growth (e.g., at the skull base or in the paranasal sinuses). But because normal tissues usually release the contrast agent at a faster rate than pathologic tissues [72], the lesion should be conspicuous on later scans (e.g., after 45-60 min).

Time-signal intensity curves can be very useful in differential diagnosis [75, 76] (Fig. 5.36a-c). T1-weighted fast sequences provide serial views only a few seconds after contrast injection, permitting dynamic studies as in CT. The few reports of experience to date are discussed in the relevant clinical chapters.

Gadolinium-DTPA appears to provide greater contrast enhancement than the iodinated media used in CT. Gadolinium-DTPA has also provided substantially longer lasting enhancement of infarcted brain areas than CT [77], although it has not demonstrated a higher specificity.

Effect of Gadolinium-DTPA on the Appearance of Normal Structures

Normal structures that are delineated with contrast material generally show enhancement a few minutes after the i.v. injection of gadolinium-DTPA.

The *brain tissues*, the gray and white matter, do not show a significant increase of signal when the blood-brain barrier is intact.

The *dura*, especially in the region of the falx cerebri and tentorium cerebelli, shows only partial contrast uptake on MR scans. Besides the relatively scant dural blood supply, this may relate to a paucity of free extracellular water, which is necessary for contrast enhancement with gadolinium-DTPA. The iodinated contrast media for CT effect the density increase themselves, which accounts for the prominence of the dura on CT scans.

The signal from *small blood vessels* (arteries and veins) with a low flow velocity is increased, because

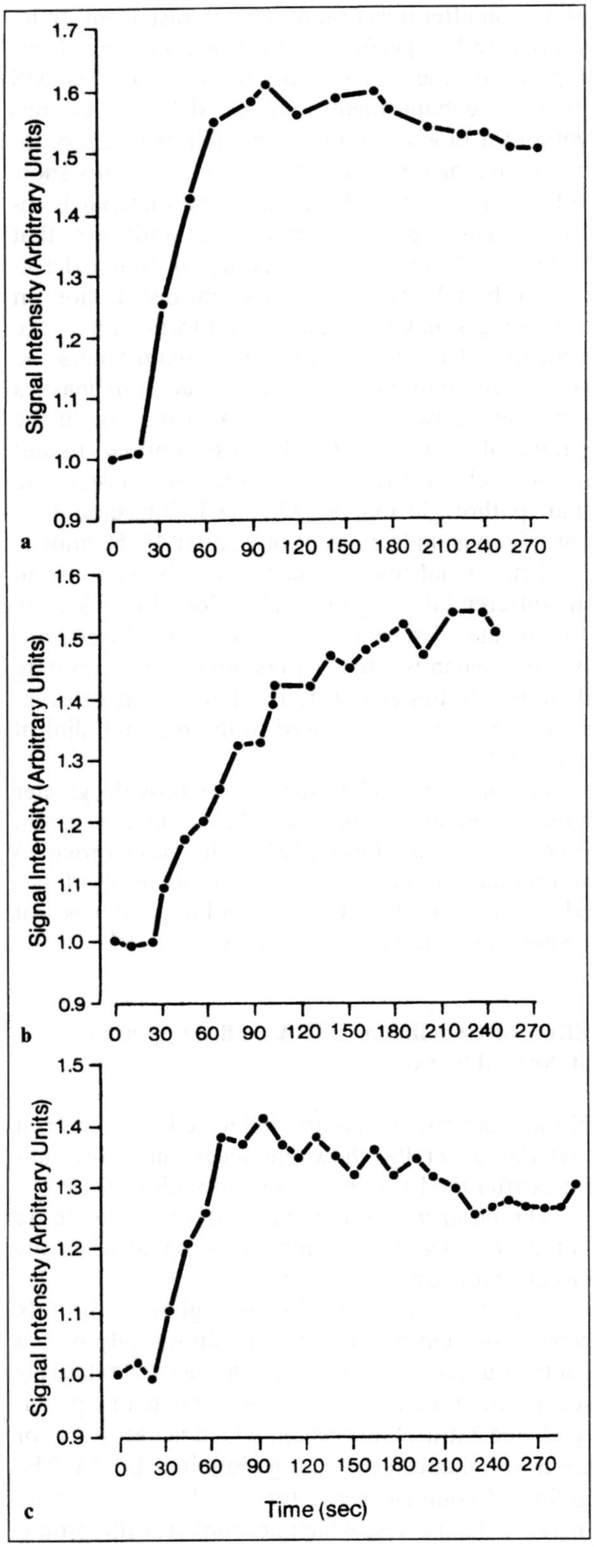

Fig. 5.36 a–c. Time-signal intensity curve of meningioma (**a**), spinal neuroma (**b**), and pituitary adenoma (**c**). (From Laniado et al. 1986)

the contrast agent shortens the T1 relaxation time of the blood. It also raises the cutoff velocity for the same reason (see Sect. 1.4).

The *choroid plexus,* composed of a network of small vessels, appears hyperintense. Vessels with rapidly flowing blood, such as the larger arteries (carotid, basilar) and the venous sinuses, give a low signal.

The heavily vascularized normal *pituitary gland and pituitary stalk,* which do not have a blood-brain barrier, likewise show a marked signal increase when contrast material is used.

In the *sellar region* the *cavernous sinus* shows varying degrees of contrast enhancement, probably depending on the velocity and direction of its blood flow. The dura of the cavernous sinus and the adjacent Meckel's cavity show marked enhancement. Increased signal is also seen in *cranial nerves* III–VI, which traverse the cavernous sinus, in the Gasserian ganglion, and in the second and third divisions of the trigeminal nerve in the skull base region. Enhancement of the proximal, cisternal segment of the trigeminal nerve is not normally seen [74]. The *optic chiasm* likewise remains unchanged.

In the *orbital region* we see no significant enhancement of the external ocular muscles or of the globe. Only the retina may show a signal increase. Small blood vessels and lesions that show contrast uptake may become lost in the retrobulbar fat, which also appears bright on T1-weighted images (see Fig. 10.43).

A strong signal increase is observed in the *mucosae of the paranasal sinuses and nasopharynx.* This is particularly evident on MR scans, because the bone appears dark; contrast is less pronounced on CT scans because of the high density of the bone.

An increase in the density of the blood vessels and dura on CT scans provides the visible evidence that contrast material has been administered. Analogous reference structures on MR scans are the paranasal sinus mucosae, the pituitary, and the choroid plexus.

References

1. Castro ME, Boisvert DP, Treiber ED, Lunt JA, Allen PS (1984) Effect of CSF albumin concentration on NMR relaxation parameters. In: Inaba Y, Klatzo I, Spatz M (eds) Brain edema, Springer, Berlin Heidelberg New York, pp 594–600
2. Fishman RA (1975) Brain edema. N Engl J Med 293: 706–711
3. Fullerton GD, Cameron IL, Ord VA (1984) Frequency dependence of magnetic resonance spin-lattice relaxation of protons in biological materials. Radiology 151: 135–138

4. Reulen HJ, Graham R, Spatz M, Klatzo I (1977) Role of pressure gradients and bulk flow in dynamics of vasogenic brain edema. J Neurosurg 46: 24-35
5. Shaller CA, Jacques DB, Shelden CH (1980) The pathophysiology of stroke: a review with molecular considerations. Surg Neurol 14: 433-443
6. Bradley WG (1987) Pathophysiologic correlates in signal alterations. In: Brant-Zawadzki M, Norman D (eds) Magnetic resonance imaging of the central nervous system. Raven, New York, pp 23-42
7. Bradley WG, Schmidt PG (1985) Effect of methemoglobin formation on the MR appearance of subarachnoid hemorrhage. Radiology 156: 99-103
8. DiChiro G, Brooks RA, Girton ME, Caporale T, Wright DC, Dwyer AJ, Horne MK III (1986) Sequential MR studies of intracerebral hematomas in monkeys. AJNR 7: 193-199
9. Diezel PB (1955) Iron in the brain: a chemical and histochemical examination. In: Biochemistry of the developing nervous system. Academic, New York, pp 145-152
10. Drayer B, Burger P, Darwin R, Riederer S, Herfkens R, Johnson GA (1986) MRI of brain iron. AJR 147: 103-110
11. Edelmann RR, Johnson K, Buxton R, Shoukimas G, Rosen BR, Davis KR, Brady TJ (1986) MRI of hemorrhage: a new approach. AJNR 7: 751-756
12. Gomori JM, Grossman RI, Goldberg HI, Zimmerman RA, Bilaniuk LT (1985) Intracranial hematomas: imaging by high field MR. Radiology 157: 87-93
13. Gomori JM, Grossman RI, Goldberg HI, Zimmerman RA, Bilaniuk LT (1986) Occult cerebrovascular malformations: high field MR imaging. Radiology 158: 707-713
14. Hallgren B, Sourander P (1958) The effect of age on nonhaemin iron in the human brain. J Neurochem 3: 41-51
15. Han JS, Kaufman B, Alfidi RJ, Yeung HN, Benson JE, Haaga JR, El Yousef SJ, Clampitt NE, Boustelle CT, Huss R (1984) Head trauma evaluated by magnetic resonance and computed tomography: a comparison. Radiology 150: 71-77
16. Hill JM, Switzer RC III (1984) The regional distribution and cellular localization of iron in the rat. Neuroscience 11: 595-603
17. Jaffe ER (1964) Metabolic processes involved in the formation and reduction of methemoglobin in human erythrocytes. In: Bishop C, Surgenor D (eds) The red blood cell. Academic, New York, pp 397-403
18. New PF, Ojeman RG, Davis KR, Rosen BR, Heros R, Kjellberg RN, Adams RD, Richardson EP (1986) MR and CT of occult vascular malformations of the brain. AJNR 7: 771-779
19. Rutledge JN, Hilal SK, Silver AJ, Defendini R, Fahn S (1987) Study of movement disorders and brain iron. AJNR 8: 397-411
20. Wintrobe MM, Lee GR, Boggs DR et al. (1981) Clinical hematology. Lea and Febiger, Philadelphia, pp 88-102
21. Zimmerman RD, Snow RB, Heier LA, Lin DPC, Deck MDF (1986) MRI features of acute traumatic and spontaneous intracerebral hemorrhage. Presented at the 24th Annual Meeting of the American Society of Neuroradiology, Jan 18-23, San Diego
22. Bergstrand G, Bergström M, Nordell B, Stahlberg F, Ericsson A, Hemmingsson A, Sperber G, Thuomas KA, Jung B (1985) Cardiac gated MR imaging of cerebrospinal fluid flow. J Comput Assist Tomogr 9(6): 1003-1006
23. Bradley WG, Feinberg D, Openshaw KL, Klein B, Otto R (1986) Comparison of MR cardiac-gated aqueductal flow velocity measurements in healthy individuals and in patients with hydrocephalus. Presented at the RSNA '86, Chicago
24. Bradley WG, Waluch V (1985) Blood flow: magnetic resonance imaging. Radiology 154: 443-450
25. Bradley WG, Waluch V, Lai K, Fernandez E, Spalter C (1984) The appearance of rapidly flowing blood on magnetic resonance images. AJR 143: 1167-1174
26. Brant-Zawadzki N, Norman D, Newton TH, Kelly WM, Kjos B, Mills CM, Dillon W, Sobel B, Crooks LE (1984) Magnetic resonance of the brain: the optimal screening technique. Radiology 152: 71-77
27. Bydder GM, Young IR (1985) Clinical use of the partial saturation and saturation recovery sequences in MR imaging. J Comput Assist Tomogr 9(6): 1020-1032
28. Cutler RW, Page L, Galicich J, Watters GV (1968) Formation and absorption of cerebrospinal fluid in man. Brain 91: 707-719
29. Deimling M, Müller E, Lenz G, Barth K, Fritschy P, Seiderer M, Reinhardt ER (1986) Description of flow phenomena in magnetic resonance imaging. Diagn Imag Clin Med 55: 37-51
30. Du Boulay GH (1966) Pulsatile movements in the CSF pathways. Br J Radiol 39: 255-262
31. Enzmann RD, O'Donohue J, Rubin JB, Shuer L, Cogen P, Silverberg G (1987) CSF pulsations within nonneoplastic spinal cord cysts. AJR 149: 149-157
32. Enzmann DR, Rubin JB, DeLaPaz R, Wright A (1986) Cerebrospinal fluid pulsation: benefits and pitfalls in MR imaging. Radiology 161: 773-778
33. Feinberg DA, Mark AS (1987) Human brain motion and cerebrospinal fluid circulation demonstrated with MR velocity imaging. Radiology 163: 793-799
34. Hasso AN, Kucharczyk W, Colombo N, Norman D, Newton H (1986) "Entry" section phenomena in multisection MR imaging of cerebrospinal fluid. Presented at the RSNA '86, Chicago USA
35. Hoffmann K, Quencer RM, Post MJD, Diaz R, Shapiro R (1986) MR image appearance of cerebrospinal fluid flow. Presented at the RSNA '86, Chicago
36. Klose U, Requardt H, Schroth G, Deimling M (1987) MR-tomographische Darstellung von Liquorpulsationen. RÖFO 147(3): 313-320
37. Kucharczyk W, Kelly WM, Davis DO, Norman D, Newton TH (1986) Intracranial lesions: flow related enhancement on MR images using time-of-flight effects. Radiology 161: 767-772
38. Lane B, Kricheff IT (1974) Cerebrospinal fluid pulsations at myelography: videodensitometric study. Radiology 110: 579-587
39. Lukes SA, Crooks LE, Aminoff MJ, Kaufman L, Panitch HS, Mills CM, Norman D (1983) Nuclear magnetic resonance imaging in multiple sclerosis. Ann Neurol 13: 592-601
40. Mark AS, Feinberg DA (1986) CSF flow: correlation between signal void and CSF velocity measured by gated velocity phase-encoded MR imaging. Presented at the RSNA '86, Chicago
41. Milhorat TH (1975) The third circulation revisited. J Neurosurg 42: 629-645
42. Moran PR (1982) A flow velocity zeugmatography interlace for NMR imaging in humans. Magn Reson Imaging 1: 197-203
43. Nayler GL, Firmin DN, Longmore DB (1986) Blood flow imaging by cine magnetic resonance. J Comput Assist Tomogr 10(5): 715

44. Ortendahl DA, Posin JP, Hylton NM, Mills CM (1986) Optimal visualization of the cerebrospinal fluid in MRI. AJNR 7: 403-407
45. Reuther G (1987) Blutgefäßdarstellung in der Kernspintomographie unter Berücksichtigung der Spin-Echo-Pulssequenz. Thesis, Friedrich-Alexander University, Erlangen
46. Sherman JL, Citrin CM (1986) Magnetic resonance demonstration of normal CSF flow. AJNR 7: 3-6
47. Sherman JL, Citrin CM, Bowen BJ, Gangarosa RE (1986) MR demonstration of altered cerebrospinal fluid flow by obstructive lesions. AJNR 7: 571-579
48. Arnold A, Bailey P (1954) Alterations in the glial cells following irradiation of the brain in primates. Arch Pathol 57: 383
49. Curnes JT, Laster DW, Ball MR, Moody DM, Witkofski RL (1986) MRI of radiation injury to the brain. AJR 147: 119-124
50. David H (1967) Elektronenmikroskopische Organpathologie. VEB, Berlin
51. Dooms GC, Hecht S, Brant-Zawadzki M, Berthiaume Y, Norman D, Newton TH (1986) Brain radiation lesions: MR imaging. Radiology 158: 149-155
52. Dooms GC, Fisher MR, Hricak H, Richardson M, Crooks LE, Genant HK (1985) Bone marrow imaging: magnetic resonance studies related to age and sex. Radiology 155: 429-432
53. Ferszt R, Cervos-Navarro J, Sasaki S (1974) Pericapillary spaces in the human spinal cord. In: Cervos-Navarro (ed.) Pathology of cerebral microcirculation. de Gruyter, Berlin, pp 59-66
54. Franke H, Lierse W (1965) Elektronenmikroskopische Untersuchungen über Hirnveränderungen des Meerschweinchens nach Röntgenbestrahlung. RÖFO 102: 78-87
55. Fröscher W (1976) Die Strahlenschädigung des Rückenmarks. Fortschr Neurol Psychiatr 44: 94-135
56. Hager H (1961) Elektronenmikroskopische Untersuchungen über die Feinstruktur der Blutgefäße und perivaskulären Räume im Säugetiergehirn. Acta neuropathol (Berl) 1: 9-33
57. Hager H (1966) Die frühen Alterationen des Nervengewebes nach Hypoxidose und die fortgeschrittene Nekrose im elektronenmikroskopischen Bild. Proc V Internat Congr Neuropath Zürich 1965, Excerpta Medica Amsterdam, pp 64-78
58. König HA, Graf H-P, Baer I, Laub G, Bachus R, Reinhardt ER (1986) Effects of radiotherapy in patients with cerebral tumors by methods of artificial intelligence for tissue characterization with MRI. Fifth Annual Meeting of the Society of Magnetic Resonance in Medicine, August 19-22, Montreal, Quebec
59. Maruyama Y, Chin HW, Young AB, Wang PC, Tibbs P, Beach JL, Goldstein S (1984) Implantation of brain tumors with Cf-252. Radiology 152: 177-181
60. Pitcock JA (1962) An electron microscopic study of acute radiation injury of the rat brain. Lab Invest 11: 32-44
61. Pfeiffer J (1984) Neuropathologie. In: Remmele W (ed) Pathologie, vol 4. Springer, Berlin Heidelberg New York, pp 149-152
62. Ramsey RG, Zacharias ChE (1985) MR imaging of the spine after radiation therapy: easily recognizable effects. AJNR 6: 247-251
63. Rosen BR, Buxton RB, Wismer GL, Zaner K, Kushner D, Pissinos S, Brady TJ (1986) Quantitative assessment of normal and pathologic bone marrow with chemical shift imaging. Fifth Annual Meeting of the Society of Magnetic Resonance in Medicine, August 19-22, Montreal
64. Sepponen RE, Sipponen JT, Tanttu JI (1984) A method for chemical shift imaging: demonstration of bone marrow involvement with proton chemical shift imaging. J Comput Assist Tomogr 8 (4): 585-587
65. Scholz W, Ducho EG, Breit A (1959) Experimentelle Röntgenschäden am Knochenmark des erwachsenen Kaninchens. Psychiatr Neurol Jap 61: 417-441
66. Shuman WP, Griffin RB, Haynor DR, Johnson JS, Jones DC, Cromwell LD, Moss AA (1985) MR imaging in radiation therapy planning. Radiology 156: 143-147
67. Struck G, Kühn M (1963) Vergleichende licht- und elektronenmikroskopische Untersuchungen an der normalen und ödematös veränderten Hirnrinde des Menschen. Arch Psychiatr Nervenkr 204: 209-221
68. Struck G, Umbach W (1964) Vergleichende elektronenoptische Untersuchungen an der menschlichen Hirnrinde vor und nach Ödemtherapie. Virchows Arch Pathol Anat 337: 317-327
69. Sundaresan N, Gutierrez FA, Laresan MP (1978) Radiation myelopathy in children. Ann Neurol 4: 47-50
70. Wolff J (1964) Ein Beitrag zur Ultrastruktur der Blutkapillaren: das nahtlose Endothel. Z Zellforsch 64: 290-300
71. Zülch KJ (1986) Brain tumors, 3rd edn. Springer, Berlin Heidelberg New York
72. Brant-Zawadzki M, Berry I, Osaki L, Brasch R (1986) Temporal evolution of Gd-DTPA contrast enhancement of intracranial lesions viewed with magnetic resonance imaging. In: Runge VM, Claussen C, Felix R, James AE (eds) Contrast agents in magnetic resonance imaging. Excerpta Medica, Amsterdam, pp 118-120
73. Claussen C, Laniado M, Semmler W, Schörner W, Felix R, Niendorf H-P (1986) Dose dependance of Gd-DTPA enhancement of magnetic resonance images of brain tumors. In: Runge VM, Claussen C, Felix R, James AE (eds) Contrast agents in magnetic resonance imaging. Excerpta Medica, Amsterdam, pp 103-105
74. Kilgore DP, Breger RK, Daniels DL, Pojunas KW, Williams AL, Haughton VM (1986) Cranial tissues: normal MR appearance after intravenous injection of Gd-DTPA. Radiology 160: 757-761
75. Koschorek FG, Terwey B (1986) Gd-DTPA-enhanced dynamic magnetic resonance imaging of brain lesions: preliminary results. In: Runge VM, Claussen C, Felix R, James AE (eds) Contrast agents in magnetic resonance imaging. Excerpta Medica, Amsterdam, pp 129-131
76. Laniado M, Kornmesser W, Treisch J, Felix R (1986) Gd-DTPA-enhanced fast magnetic resonance imaging of brain and spinal tumors: early clinical experience. In: Runge VM, Claussen C, Felix R, James AE (eds) Contrast agents in magnetic resonance imaging. Excerpta Medica, Amsterdam, pp 136-140
77. Mancuso AA, Virapongse C, Quisling RG (1986) Early clinical experience with Gd. DTPA-enhanced magnetic resonance imaging in acute cerebral infarction and chronic ischemic changes. In: Runge VM, Claussen C, Felix R, James AE (eds) Contrast agents in mangetic resonance imaging. Excerpta Medica, Amsterdam, pp 127-128
78. Price AC, Runge VM (1986) Optimization of pulse sequence in Gd-DTPA-enhanced magnetic resonance imaging. In: Runge VM, Claussen C, Felix R, James AE (eds) Contrast agents in magnetic resonance imaging. Excerpta Medica, Amsterdam, pp 99-102

6 Magnetic Resonance Imaging of the Brain in Childhood: Development and Pathology

G. M. Bydder and J. M. Pennock

6.1 Introduction

The success of MR imaging of the brain in adults has provided a strong stimulus for use of the technique in children. The avoidance of ionizing radiation has also been important, and with more experience it has become clear that it is possible to sustain adult-level image quality even in the smallest premature infant by using appropriately sized receiver coils.

Other techniques such as ultrasound and X-ray CT are much better developed in terms of ease of operation, simplicity, and speed, but the image quality available with MR is now fully competitive, and the range of image parameters available provides a variety of options for different clinical problems, the potential of which has yet to be explored in depth. Three general reviews of MR imaging of the brain in children have now been published and provide some indication of what has been achieved thus far, although the overall patient numbers are small [1-3].

There are several important differences of technique in the MR imaging of children, and these will be discussed first, followed by a brief description of normal appearances and a summary of MR appearances in a variety of clinical conditions.

6.2 Technical Aspects

For major illness such as cerebral tumor, *general anesthesia* is acceptable for immobilizing infants and children, but for less severe illness and repeat examinations, it is necessary to apply other methods. In neonates (who may also be brain-damaged), we avoid sedation but begin the examination after a feeding. Neonates usually sleep better on their sides, and this position also serves to lower the risk of inhalation of regurgitated milk or vomit. From about 3 months to 4 years of age, we use oral chloral hydrate. From about 4 years onward we avoid *sedation,* but one of the staff remains in the MR unit with the child. A respiratory monitor is used throughout the procedure (see also Chap. 3.3).

Significant improvement in image quality has been obtained by the use of spherical receiver coils made in six different sizes to fit the range of head sizes from small neonates to large children [4]. The coils are fitted like "space helmets" and are well accepted by the children.

The *neonatal brain* contains a higher proportion of water (92%-95%) than the adult brain (82%-85%), and this is associated with a marked prolongation of T1 and T2 [2]. T1 may increase by up to 300%-400%, and this requires modification of the basic pulse sequences in order to obtain comparable images during the first 2 years of life. Indeed, all of the parameters TR, TI, and TE need to be increased as shown for inversion recovery sequences in Table 6.1.

With satisfactory sedation to keep the child still, improved signal-to-noise (S/N) ratio with better coil design, and age-matched sequences, it has proved possible to increase the spatial resolution from 128 × 128 to 256 × 256 and decrease the slice thickness from 10 mm to 5 or 3 mm while maintaining satisfactory soft tissue contrast. Thus, there has been considerable improvement in image quality since the first low-resolution (128 × 128) pediatric images were published in 1982 [5, 6].

These technical advances sometimes create problems both in the appearance of normal controls (used for reference) and in follow-up examinations where earlier images have become obsolete and are no longer comparable with current images.

Each of the major *pulse sequences* used in practice has undergone significant development.

Table 6.1. Age-related inversion recovery sequences in infants

Age of infant	TR (ms)	TI (ms)	TE (ms)
Premature	3600	1200	44
0-3 months	3000	1000	44
3-6 months	2400	800	44
Over 6 months	1800	600	44

The options available with the *partial saturation* (PS) sequence have been expanded by varying the flip angle *(α)* and also by extending TE to increase the T2 dependence of the sequence [7]. This increases the sensitivity of the PS sequence to susceptibility change, making it of considerable value in the detection of hemorrhage [8]. In addition to this effect, two PS sequences with different TE values can be used to construct a phase map which reproduces changes that can be directly related to susceptibility [9].

The scope of the *inversion recovery* (IR) sequence has been increased by use of the short inversion recovery (TI) variant. This sequence has many features in common with the SE sequence, except that it produces higher gray matter-white matter contrast [10]. It is of value in demonstrating periventricular changes in which the CSF signal can be kept less than that of brain.

Variants of the *SE* sequence have been used with TE values up to 200 ms and TR up to 2400 s. These display increased contrast, but there is considerable difficulty in keeping the signal intensity of CSF less than that of brain. In addition, it is possible to obtain flow-dependent sequences by the use of bipolar gradients [11]. Phase maps produced in this way can be modified to detect flow rates on the order of 1 mm/s, reflecting tissue perfusion.

6.3 Normal Appearance

There are several distinctive features which differ from those in adults. The pediatric brain changes rapidly during the first 2 years of life, and this change continues at a slower rate into the second decade.

As mentioned previously, the neonatal brain is notable for its very long T1 and T2 relaxation times. If adult-type sequences are used, the brain may appear noisy (IR) or featureless (SE). In addition, the periventricular regions containing unmyelinated white matter initially have an increased T1 and T2 exceeding that of gray matter. The unmyelinated subcortical white matter also has a T1 longer than gray matter, so that on IR scans the cortical mantle is highlighted between the long T1 of CSF outside the brain and the unmyelinated white matter inside the brain.

The T1 of unmyelinated white matter decreases and by about 3-6 months of age is equal to that of gray matter. Thus the "edge enhancement" appearance of the cortex is lost, and both tissues appear isointense on IR scans.

The process of normal myelination also begins in the neonatal period, proceeding in a stereotypic manner with sensory tracts myelinating before motor tracts, and the internal capsule preceding the great commissures and the lateral hemispheres [12]. These features are all well demonstrated by MR; they are not seen with other techniques.

Establishing a range of normal appearances has its difficulties. The question of consent for normals is more difficult in children than in adults, and even when scans are performed, they need to be obtained with the same technique that will be used for the patient. As techniques evolve these controls may become "obsolete," and so an active program of recruiting is necessary. Twins of the patient are a useful source of age-matched controls, since they often have a documented medical history, including physical examination, even when they are completely normal (apart from being twins). We still have insufficient information to assemble an atlas (comparable to that for bone age) for normal development of the human brain, but the correspondence with pathologic descriptions of myelination has been very good so far.

6.4 Intracranial Hemorrhage

In general terms the appearance of hemorrhage parallels that seen in adults (Sect. 5.2), with an initial long-T1/short-T2 phase followed by a short-T1/short-T2 phase and a long-T1/long-T2 phase some weeks or months later. There are several important differences, however. The pattern of hemorrhage is different; it is associated with anoxic damage and occurs frequently in the subependymal region. Also, hemorrhage in neonates occurs against a background of long normal T1 and T2 of the brain, so that the T2 of hematoma may appear distinctly shorter than that of the surrounding brain. The intraparenchymal hemorrhages evolve, displaying longer T1 and T2 centers and then frequently developing into porencephalic cysts.

Subdural and extradural hematomas have much in common with their adult counterparts.

Intracranial hemorrhage may have important late sequelae including hydrocephalus (Sect. 6.7) and delays or deficits in myelination (Sect. 6.11).

With T2-weighted PS sequences, hemorrhage produces a loss of signal intensity as a result of decrease in T2 and susceptibility effects (Fig. 6.1). This technique provides a high degree of sensitivity in the detection of subarachnoid, parenchymal, and intraventricular changes.

6.5 Infarction

Infarction in the neonatal period is usually manifested as a region of increased T1 and T2, and there may be difficulty in distinguishing such areas from unmyelinated white matter areas normally present in the brain, although cystic areas are well defined. These appearances are also seen at later stages, but other more subtle features are also apparent. There may be a loss of gray matter-white matter contrast in a focal area, with or without a slight increase in T1. Marginal areas of infarction may also occur symmetrically within the parietal occipital lobes, with essentially the same features. With increasing age, some porencephalic cysts decrease in size while others remain the same size, although the growing size of the brain makes them appear smaller. Associated hydrocephalus with porencephalic cysts communicating with the ventricles may produce an apparent increase in the size of cysts (Fig. 6.2).

6.6 Cysts and Leukomalacias

Periventricular cysts are well displayed at the periventricular margins in patients with a history of anoxic injury (Fig. 6.3). The changes can be quite extreme. Sometimes these cysts appear to coalesce and become continuous with the adjacent ventricles, producing hydrocephalus. The appearance of severe or moderately severe cysts in infancy is frequently associated with a delay or deficit in myelination, and four cases of this type have been documented in detail [13].

Precise correlation with the clinical syndrome of *ischemic anoxic encephalopathy* (IAE) in the neonatal period is difficult. IAE produces an exaggeration of the normal appearances of prolonged T1 and T2 in the periventricular regions, and the differentiation between normal appearances and minor degrees of IAE is very difficult (Fig. 6.4).

6.7 Hydrocephalus

Hydrocephalus can arise in a number of circumstances in children and is recognized on essentially the same basis as in adults. It is possible to recognize periventricular edema with both SE and IR sequences (Fig. 6.5), and we have seen this condition regress following satisfactory ventricular shunting. Likewise, we have observed its presence in cases of shunt malfunction.

The ventricular size is readily assessed, and MR has obvious advantages in establishing a baseline and in the long-term follow-up of children with shunts.

The short-TI IR sequence displays periventricular changes in some cases of hydrocephalus, probably signifying a transependymal spread of fluid. However, similar changes may be seen in other diseases such as periventricular leukomalacia, and the changes are probably not specific.

6.8 Congenital Malformations
(see also Chap. 7)

Obvious anatomic deformities are readily identified, including *anencephalopathy, holoprosencephaly, Dandy Walker syndrome,* and other conditions. Many of these conditions, such as agenesis of the corpus callosum, are recognized most easily on the sagittal plane [14] (see Sect. 7.2).

6.9 White Matter Disease
(see also Chap. 8)

Diffuse abnormalities are seen within the white matter in leukodystrophy (Fig. 6.6). Usually the changes are extensive and not confined to the periventricular region. In other forms of white matter disease, such as Alexander's disease, changes may be confined to the frontal lobes. A variety of other abnormalities have been described in different forms of leukodystrophy. We have also seen periventricular abnormalities associated with intrathecal methotrexate therapy in leukemia (see Sect. 8.2.2).

6.10 Infection (see also Chap. 15)

Cerebral abscess displays an increase in T1 and T2. Edema is well displayed, but the exact margins of the abscess may be difficult to resolve [15] without contrast medium (i.e., gadolinium chelate).

Calcification associated with abscess is poorly demonstrated on MR in comparison with CT.

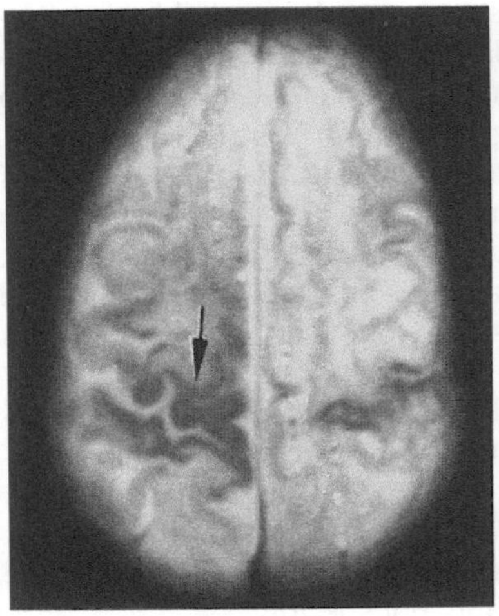

6.1

Fig. 6.1. Parenchymal hemorrhage: PS 500/193 scan. The area of hemorrhage *(arrow)* has a low signal intensity. (A central artifact is noted on this and some subsequent images)

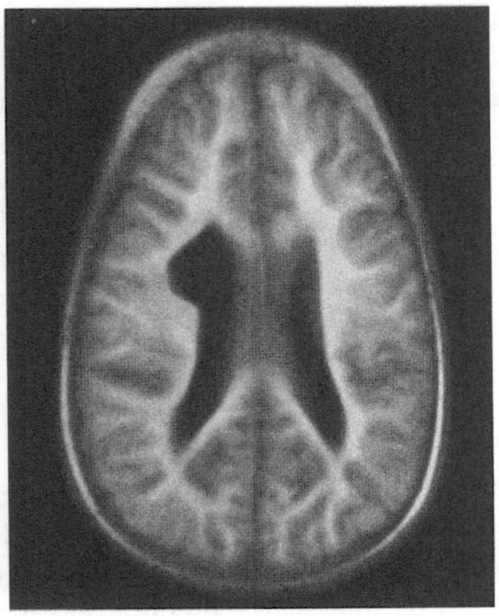

6.2

Fig. 6.2. Porencephalic cyst: IR 1800/600/44 scan. The cyst appears as an extension of the ventricular system

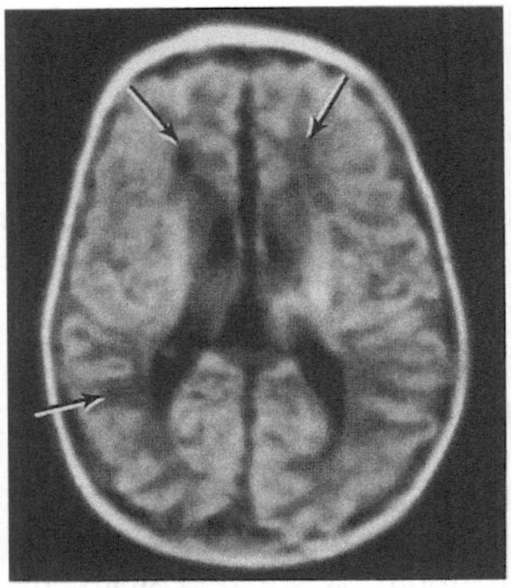

6.3

Fig. 6.3. Cystic leukomalacia: IR 3000/1000/44 scan. Cysts are seen in the periventricular region *(arrows)*

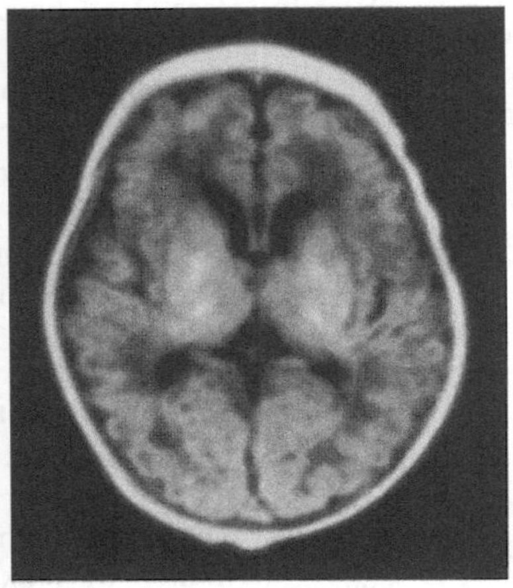

6.4

Fig. 6.4. Ischemic anoxic encephalopathy: IR 3000/1000/44 scan. The periventricular regions appear dark

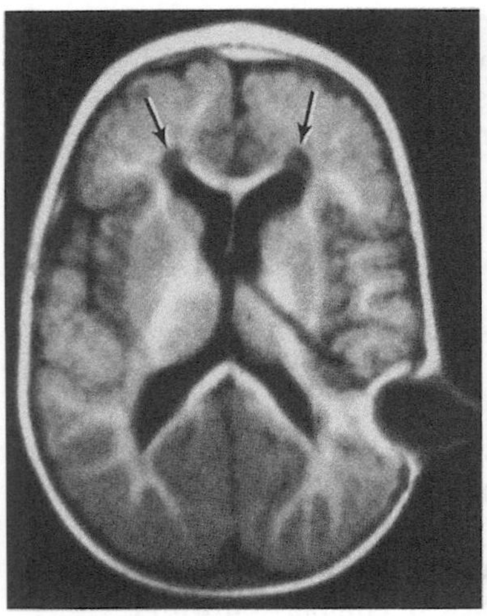

6.5

Fig. 6.5. Periventricular edema: IR 1800/600/44 scan. Areas of periventricular edema are seen *(arrows)* in spite of the shunt

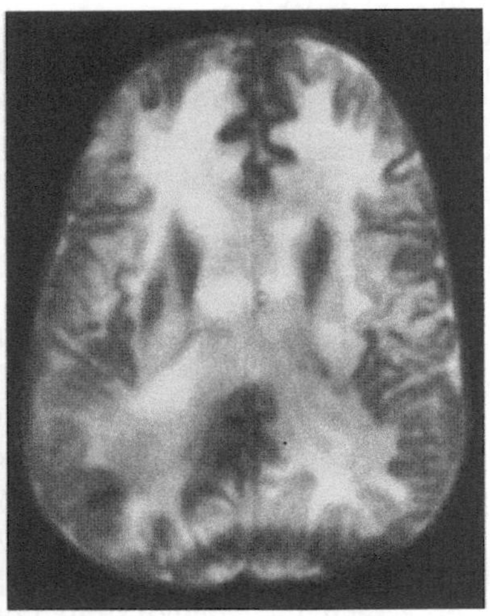

6.6

Fig. 6.6. PS 1660/193 scan. The abnormal white matter is highlighted

In two cases of brainstem *encephalitis,* changes have been seen with very little associated mass effect (Fig. 6.7). This has been the main distinction from tumors on the initial examination, and regression on follow-up provides strong support for the diagnosis, although some caution is necessary as patients are frequently treated with steroids, which may cause some regression of edema associated with a tumor.

6.11 Delays or Deficits in Myelination

Reference to normal controls provides a means of assessing the degree of myelination in children. The most rapid phase of myelination occurs in the first 2 years of life. Delays are difficult to recognize before about 6 months, as relatively little myelin is present. Conversely, after 2 years of age there is time for cases of delayed myelination to "catch up." Delays or deficits are most obvious from 6 to 24 months of age (Fig. 6.8). With only limited information about the normal range, we have preferred to use age-matched controls (twins if possible) and diagnose delays only in the absence of myelination of named tracts or commissures when myelination is present in the control, and both examinations have been performed with the same technique.

Delays or deficits in myelination have been recognized following probable intrauterine rubella infection, in posthemorrhagic hydrocephalus, after IAE, and in cystic leukomalacia.

6.12 Tumors (see also Chaps. 10 and 11)

Generally the features of tumors in children parallel those in adults. However, the incidence of posterior fossa tumors is higher in children, and embryogenic tumors are more frequent [16]. The high incidence of midline tumors lends itself to sagittal imaging, and the clarity with which the posterior fossa is seen is also an advantage.

Most tumors display an increased T1 and T2, providing high contrast with long-TE/long-TR SE sequences, although distinction between tumor and edema may be difficult (Fig. 6.9). Differentiation between a brainstem and cerebellar site is reasonably easy. Craniopharyngiomas and various other lipid-containing tumors may show characteristic features (see Sect. 10.9.3).

Hamartomas may not display a significant change in T1 and T2 and may then need to be recognized by their indirect signs (Fig. 6.10; see Sect. 10.8).

In two cases hypothalamic tumors have been recognized when poorly delineated by CT.

6.13 Other Diseases

Certain other conditions are worth reviewing although they are quite rare.

Delays or deficits in myelination have been recognized in *Hurler's disease,* and these may be reversed following successful bone marrow transplantation [17] (see Sect. 8.2).

Hallervorden-Spatz disease is of particular theoretical interest as a condition in which there is abnormal iron deposition in the brain, and in one case abnormalities have been seen in the basal ganglia [2] (see Sect. 8.3.1).

Wilson's disease is associated with visible abnormalities in the lentiform nucleus and within the thalamus [18] (see Sects. 5.2 and 8.3.1).

In a case of juvenile *Huntington's disease,* the head of the caudate nucleus was found to be atrophic (see p. 216).

6.14 Follow-Up Examination

Follow-up is an essential aspect of pediatric practice. Parameters for which normal appearances and values change include T1 and T2, the presence of periventricular long-T1 areas, the degree of myelination, and the size and shape of the brain. Pathologic changes must be assessed against this changing background.

The lack of known hazards is a strong incentive for pediatric MR imaging. Follow-up examinations are important in conditions where long-term survival is expected and there is a desire to avoid significant cumulative X-ray exposure.

Nevertheless, there are difficulties in obtaining MR scans at the same level and angulation as in the initial studies. There is also a theoretical problem in using age-adjusted sequences, since the machine parameters are different. Genuine advances in techniques also can make comparison difficult.

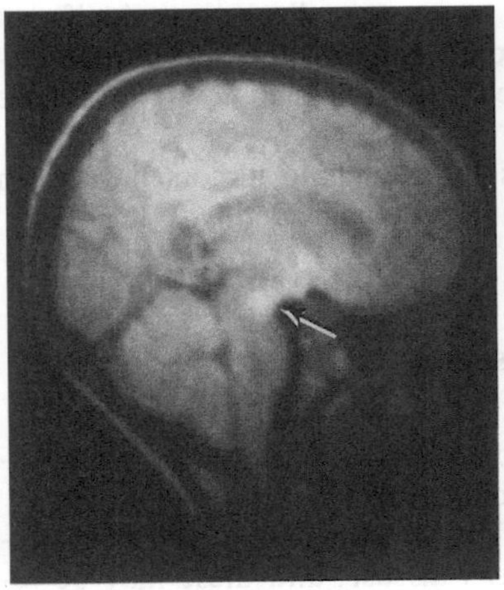

6.7

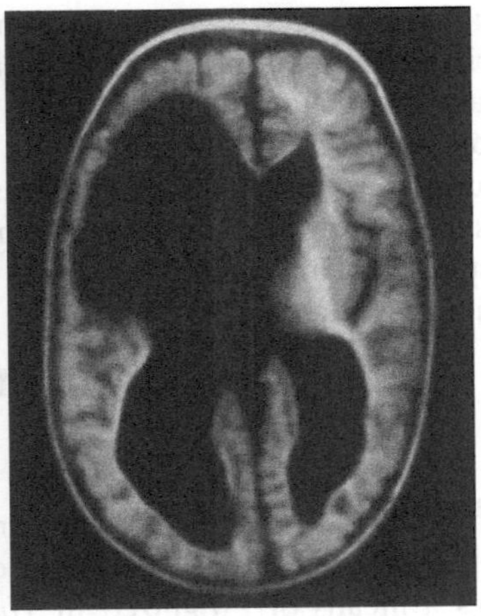

6.8

Fig. 6.7. Brainstem encephalitis: SE 1500/80 scans. There is an abnormal area in the mesencephalon *(arrow)*

Fig. 6.8. Delayed myelination: IR 1800/600/44 scan. There is less white matter anteriorly

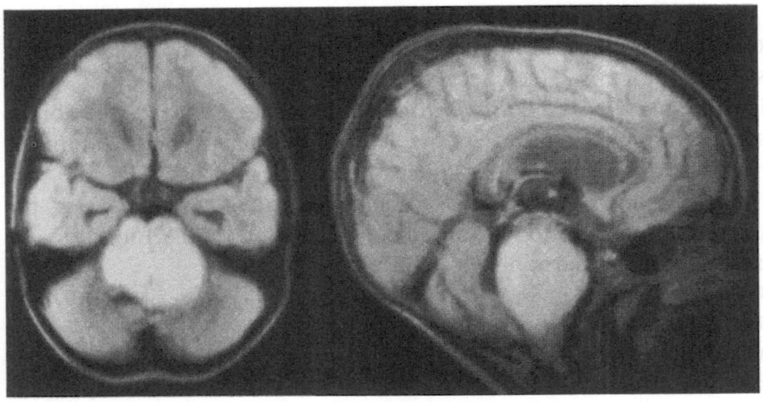

a b

Fig. 6.9 a, b. Brainstem glioma: axial **(a)** and sagittal **(b)** 1500/80 scans. The tumor is well delineated

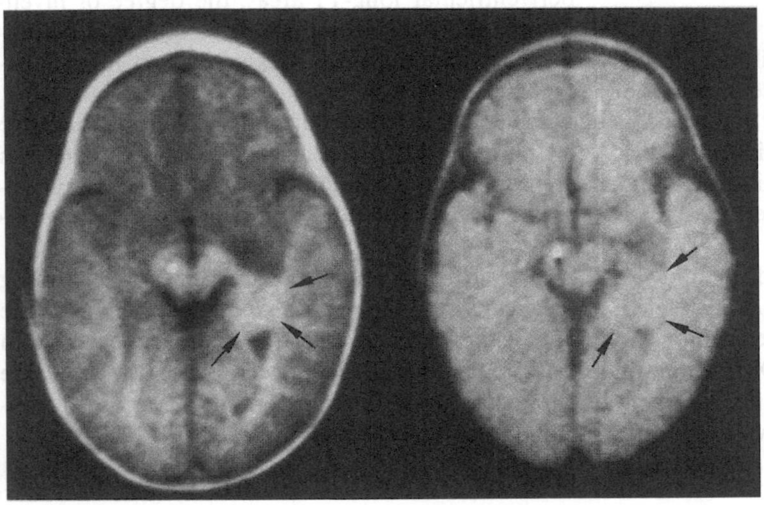

a b

Fig. 6.10 a, b. Hamartoma: IR 1400/400/13 **(a)** and SE 1080/80 **(b)** scans. The tumor is shown in **a** *(arrows)* but is poorly displayed in **b**

6.15 Conclusion

Although developments in pediatric MR imaging lag behind those in adults, the findings in adults can be extrapolated to children to a reasonable degree. There are some problems, however. A population of normal controls is necessary, and with rapid improvements in image quality, these are likely to become obsolete very quickly. Establishing the normal range is even more difficult.

There has been progress in the field of clinical correlation, but the correlation is not precise, and some children may have very large lesions but relatively minor clinical deficits. Large, unsuspected lesions may be found in cases where clinical signs are quite subtle.

The capacity of MR for repeat examination without cumulative radiation exposure has been of value in studying the natural history of a variety of neonatal insults.

Comparability with ultrasound and X-ray CT has been progressing satisfactorily. In general, ultrasound is cheaper, easier to operate, and much more widely available than MR, but its limitations due to closure of the fontanelles are well known. CT has previously been the basic examination for the pediatric brain. In many ways CT is more comparable to MR, and it is a mature technology rather than a developing one.

Several new developments now used in adults have yet to be applied in children. One of these is the intravenous contrast agent gadolinium-DTPA [19], which has been of value in defining benign tumors as well as separating edema from tumor in malignant cases. Chemical shift imaging has not yet been applied in pediatric practice.

The versatility of MR, with its basic image parameters, T1, T2, chemical shift, flow, susceptibility, and diffusion effects, provides for a wide range of approaches to the various problems encountered in clinical practice, and only a small number of these options have yet been utilized.

The overall prospects of MR imaging in pediatrics are excellent. It is difficult to imagine such a versatile, noninvasive, and hazard-free technique failing to have some impact on pediatric neuroradiologic practice in the near future, although the low sensitivity to calcification is a significant drawback.

Acknowledgments. We are grateful to Ian Young of Picker International for his considerable help. We also wish to thank the Department of Health and Social Security and the Medical Research Council for their continued support.

References

1. Smith FW (1983) The value of NMR imaging in pediatric practice: a preliminary report. Pediatr Radiology 13: 141-147
2. Johnson MA, Pennock JM, Bydder GM et al. (1983) Clinical NMR imaging of the brain in children: normal and neurological disease. AJR 141: 1005-1018; AJNR 4: 1013-1026
3. Han JS, Benson JE, Kaufman B et al. (1985) MR imaging of pediatric cerebral abnormalities. J Comput Assist Tomogr 9: 103-114
4. Bydder GM, Butson PR, Harman RR, Gilderdale GJ, Young IR (1985) Use of spherical receiver coils in magnetic resonance imaging of the brain. J Comput Assist Tomogr 9: 413-414
5. Levene MI, Whitelaw A, Dubowitz V et al. (1982) Nuclear magnetic resonance imaging of the brain in children. Br Med J [Clin Res] 285: 774-776
6. Bydder GM, Steiner RE, Young IR (1982) Clinical NMR imaging of the brain: 140 cases. AJR 139: 215-239
7. Bydder GM, Payne JA, Collins AG et al. (1987) Clinical use of rapid T_2 weighted partial saturation sequences. J Comput Assist Tomogr 11 (1): 17-23
8. Edelman RR, Johnson K, Buxton R et al. (1986) MR of hemorrhage: a new approach. AJNR 7: 751-756
9. Young IR, Khenia S, Thomas DGT et al. (1987) Clinical magnetic susceptibility mapping of the brain. J Comput Assist Tomogr 11 (1): 2-6
10. Bydder GM, Young IR (1985) MRI: clinical use of the inversion recovery sequence. J Comput Assist Tomogr 9 (4): 659-675
11. Bryant DJ, Payne JA, Firmin D, Longmore DB (1984) Measurement of flow with NMR imaging using a gradient pulse and phase difference technique. J Comput Assist Tomogr 8 (4): 588-593
12. Yakoulev PI, Lecours AR (1967) The myelogenetic cycles of regional maturation in the brain. In: Minkowski A (ed) Regional development of the brain in early life. Blackwell Scientific, Oxford, pp 3-69
13. Dubowitz LMS, Bydder GM, Mushin J (1985) Developmental sequence of periventricular leukomalacia. Arch Dis Child 60: 349-355
14. Davidson HD, Abraham R, Steiner RE (1985) Magnetic resonance imaging of agenesis of the corpus callosum. Radiology 155: 371-373
15. Davidson HD, Steiner RE (1985) Magnetic resonance imaging of infections of the central nervous system. AJNR 6: 499-504
16. Peterman SB, Bydder GM, Steiner RE (1984) NMR imaging of brain tumors in children and adolescents. AJNR 5 (6): 703-709
17. Johnson MA, Desai S, Hugh-Jones K, Starer F (1984) Magnetic resonance imaging of the brain in Hurler syndrome. AJNR 5: 816-819
18. Lawler GA, Pennock JM, Steiner RE, Jenkins WJ, Sherlock S, Young IR (1983) NMR imaging in Wilson disease. J Comput Assist Tomogr 7 (1): 1-8
19. Carr DH, Brown J, Bydder GM et al. (1984) Gadolinium-DTPA as a contrast agent in MRI: initial clinical experience in 20 patients. AJR 143: 215-224

7 Malformations of the CNS

W. J. Huk

The prenatal development of the CNS can be disturbed by a number of genetic (inherited) and nongenetic (congenital) factors. However, the etiologic classification of the various malformations remains uncertain in many cases, both in terms of the primary cause and the timing of the insult. Adams and Victor [3] suggest classifying malformations according to possible causative factors:

- Malformations caused by the mutation of a single gene
- Malformations in which a hereditary disposition coincides with nongenetic and usually indeterminate factors
- Malformations associated with chromosomal abnormalities
- Malformations due entirely to exogenous factors (virus, other infectious agents, X-irradiation, toxins)
- Malformations of undetermined cause (60% of cases)

7.1 Review of Ontogeny

To understand the malformations of the brain and spinal cord, we must be familiar with the normal development of the CNS. The steps in the various developmental processes and the sequence of involvement of the embryonic structures in neural tube anomalies remain controversial. According to Noetzel [105] and Mori [98], CNS malformations can be assigned to specific developmental stages according to the following scheme:

1. *Blastemic period* (1st-4th weeks of gestation): The initial divisions of the fertilized ovum are followed quickly by the differentiation of ectoderm, entoderm, and mesoderm. In the 2nd week, under the influence of the mesoderm, the neural plate begins to develop from the ectoderm. In the 3rd week the neural folds alongside the central groove become elevated and fuse dorsally to form the neural tube. This process takes place in craniocaudal direction and is complete by 24-26 days gestational age. Meanwhile the forebrain develops from the neural plate and the face from the entoderm. Disturbances at this stage of development lead to *neural tube defects* (dysraphic disorders or midline closure defects, see Table 7.1). Because all three germ layers may be involved, the spectrum of dysraphias range from circumscribed bony defects of the cranial vault (crania lacunosa) and spinal anomalies to partial or extensive malformations of the neural tube. In the 4th week, the prosencephalic, mesencephalic, and rhombencephalic vesicles begin to grow at the anterior portion of the neural tube in anterior-caudal order.

2. *Embryonic period* (2nd-4th lunar months): In the 5th week the telencephalic vesicles develop on both sides of the prosencephalic vesicle. At first they communicate widely with the cavity of the prosencephalic vesicle. Backward growth of the lateral vesicles results in the formation of the two cerebral hemispheres. As this growth progresses, the connections between the lateral vesicles and the primary prosencephalic cavity become narrowed, forming the foramina of Monro. The midline prosencephalic cavity and the diencephalic cavity form the third ventricle.

In the meantime (6th week) the telencephalic wall, which began as the anterior wall of the prosencephalic cavity, changes. From this area, known also as the lamina terminalis, originate the forebrain commissures and related structures. The lamina terminalis extends from the optic chiasm up to the velum transversum. It divides into two parts: the lamina terminalis proper, which eventually becomes the lamina terminalis, an inert, hypocellular structure that borders the third ventricle anteriorly; and the lamina reuniens of His, which is highly cellular and thickened [118]. The dorsal part of the lamina reuniens invaginates between the growing telencephalic vesicles and forms a median groove

Table 7.1. Classification of malformations of the CNS

1. **Midline closure defects (neural tube defects, dysraphic disorders)** [43]
a) Of the brain
- Craniorachischisis
- Anencephaly
- Encephalocele and cranial meningocele
  - Cranium bifidum occultum
  - Occipital encephaloceles
  - Parietal meningoencephaloceles
  - Anterior encephaloceles
b) Of the cerebellum
- Agenesis of the cerebellum
- Hypoplasia of the cerebellum
- Hypoplasia of the vermis
- Dandy-Walker syndrome
- Arnold-Chiari deformity
c) Of the spine
- Spina bifida occulta
- Spina bifida cystica
  - Meningocele
  - Myelomeningocele
- Ventral spinal defects
d) Of the spinal cord
- Hydromyelia and syringomyelia
- Duplication of the spinal cord
  - Dimyelia
  - Diplomyelia
  - Diastematomyelia
- Tethered cord
- Lipoma
- Dermoid, epidermoid, dermal sinus
- Teratomas
	3. **Anomalies of cell migration**
	- Ectopias and heterotopias
	- Agyria, pachygyria, lissencephaly
	- Polymicrogyria, stenogyria
	- Status verrucosus
	- (Ulegyria)
	
	4. **Destructive lesions/abnormalities** [43]
	- Hydranencephaly
	- Porencephaly
	- Schizencephaly
	- Multicystic encephalopathy
	- Hippocampal sclerosis, status marmoratus, status demyelinisatus
	- Ulegyria (see 3)
	- Hemispheric atrophy
	- Putaminal necrosis
	
	5. **Neuroectodermal dysplasias, phakomatosis**
	- Tuberous sclerosis
	- Neurofibromatosis (von Recklinghausen's disease)
	- Encephalofacial angiomatosis (Sturge-Weber syndrome)
	- Von Hippel-Lindau disease
	- Other phakomatosis
	  - Encephaloretinal angiomatosis
	  - Ataxia-teleangiectasia
	  - Neurocutaneous melanosis
	  - Linear nevus sebaceus syndrome
	  - Incontinentia pigmenti

2. **Malformations of the commissures and midline structures**
- Holoprosencephaly
  - Alobar prosencephaly
  - Semilobar prosencephaly
  - Lobar prosencephaly
- Agenesis of the corpus callosum
- Anomalies of the septum pellucidum
- Septo-optic dysplasia
- Cavum septi pellucidi, cavum vergae, cavum veli interpositi
	6. **Miscellaneous abnormalities**
	- Hydrocephalus
	- Microcephaly, micrencephaly
	- Macrencephaly
	- Arachnoid cyst

(called the sulcus medianus telencephali medii). Thus the lamina reuniens consists of two separate parts: a ventral part above the lamina terminalis (the area precommissuralis), which gives rise to the septal nucleus, the rhinencephalon, and the anterior commissure; and a dorsal part (the massa commissuralis), from which the hippocampus and archicortex, the corpus callosum, the hippocampal commissure, and the fornix develop. When the lamina reuniens infolds, a small sac is formed which becomes the cavum septi pellucidi within the sulcus medianus telencephali medii. It is bounded dorsally by the corpus callosum, which develops in the massa commissuralis and grows in a caudal direction with growth of the hemispheres.

Given these relationships, it is clear that a significant early injury to the anterior telencephalic wall will lead to *malformations of the commissures and midline structures* (see Table 7.1). A defect in the entire lamina reuniens will result in agenesis of the corpus callosum, the anterior commissure, and the hippocampal commissure. If the defect involves mostly the dorsal part of the lamina reuniens, development of the anterior commissure (from the area precommissuralis) may be unaffected, while the corpus callosum is totally absent. Focal injury to midline structures later in morphogenesis can cause partial agenesis of the corpus callosum alone. Defects in the more ventrally situated area precommissuralis would interfere with the development of the rhinencephalon and the olfactory bulbs and tracts [88, 23]. Injuries at this stage also lead to facial anomalies such as cyclopia, cebocephaly, and cleft lip and palate.

Between the 4th and 6th weeks the choroid plexus is formed, and the openings at the outlet of the fourth ventricle (foramina of Magendie and Luschka) appear. The secretion, circulation, and absorption of CSF begin. Defects in the development of the membranes involved in the formation of the subarachnoid spaces are responsible for *arachnoidal cysts* and *communicating hydrocephalus*. Because the cerebellar vermis (superior and inferior) forms at this stage from fusion of the cerebellar primordia, the origins of *Dandy-Walker syndrome* also can be traced to this period.

Starting in the 3rd week and paralleling the development of the cerebral vesicles, a cellular germ layer (matrix, germinal layer) begins to form on the inner surface of the vesicles. The initially undifferentiated cells of this primitive ependymal zone proliferate and become neuroblasts. A disturbance of this cell proliferation can result in cerebellar hypoplasia or *Dandy-Walker syndrome*. Excessive proliferation, on the other hand, leads to *neurofibromatosis* in perineural fibroblasts, *tuberous sclerosis* in astrocytes, and *Sturge-Weber syndrome* in endothelial cells [98].

Afterward, especially in the 6th and 7th weeks, neuroblasts gather in a mantle zone (first migration) representing primitive basal ganglia. Primitive white matter is formed by an adjacent, more external marginal zone composed of neuronal processes and containing few cells. The first migration is followed in the 7th week by a second neuroblast migration through the marginal zone to form the cortical plate, a primitive gray matter, at the growing surface of the brain. Disturbances of these processes result in *anomalies of cell migration* (see Table 7.1). Proponents of the congenital etiology of *hydranencephaly* and *schizencephaly* consider this to be the time of possible injury.

Further development of the brain surface continues at a relatively late stage, in the 20th week, as the cortical plate thickens and forms primary sulci. A failure of this differentiation can result in *lissencephaly* (complete absence of the cerebral sulci), *polymicrogyria* (numerous small convolutions), or *pachygyria* (widened gyri).

3. *Fetal period* (5th–9th lunar months): Secondary gyri develop between the 24th and 40th weeks, and tertiary gyri and sulci appear between the 36th and 60th weeks. With disturbances in this stage the affected developmental step remains incomplete, and the resulting defect persists as growth proceeds.

4. *Perinatal period:* Perinatal brain lesions are usually the result of acquired factors such as hypoxia, intoxication, and infection. With increasing maturation of the brain, the effects of these insults resemble those in the mature brain.

Children with malformations and severe perinatal disorders may survive and suffer a variety of deficits (idiocy, paralysis, epilepsy, etc.), which may become manifest only after an apparently normal development (e.g., seizures resulting from heterotopias) or may produce no symptoms until later life (e.g., in hydromyelia) [106].

Lack of certainty in the interpretation of causal and temporal relationships is reflected in the diversity of classifications of congenital anomalies. In areas where uncertainties persist, providing some amount of latitude in classification, we have attempted to tailor our discussion to the practical concerns of diagnostic imaging (see Table 7.1). The more common malformations are treated in somewhat greater detail; less common conditions are described in detail only where informative cases were available.

7.2 MR Imaging of CNS Malformations

The basic role of diagnostic imaging in malformations is to permit a detailed analysis of the anatomic abnormalities that are present. MR imaging has surpassed CT in its ability to perform this role. Direct coronal and sagittal images can be obtained without bone artifact, making it possible to evaluate morphologic defects in these planes without limitation of spatial resolution.

Because certain basic aspects of the MR examination are common to all types of CNS malformation, we shall begin by discussing them in order to avoid unnecessary repetition in cases where the malformation is adequately characterized by the description of its pathoanatomic features. For complex malformations, problems of differential diagnosis, and disorders where there has been considerable experience with MR, the MR and CT findings associated with the condition will be described individually.

Selection of Imaging Sequence

Most malformations are associated with dilatation or shape change in the CSF spaces. Mori [98] has classified these alterations into four groups: (1) hydrocephalus, (2) abnormal CSF cavities off the midline, (3) abnormal CSF cavities on the midline, and (4) dysgeneses of the brain tissue.

Owing to the *good contrast* between the CSF (dark) and the brain tissue (light), *T1-weighted image sequences* (short-TR/TE SE, inversion recovery) are best suited for demonstrating the CSF spaces. T1-weighted sequences, by virtue of their differentiation of CSF, spinal cord, nerve, syrinx, fat and soft tissue, also are useful for analyzing malformations of the spinal canal. Fat in lipomas, dermoids, epidermoids, and in the marrow of cancellous bone spurs yields a high-intensity signal, whereas CSF, dura, and fibrous membranes give low signals. The differentiation of pathologic fatty tissue from normal subcutaneous and epidural fat remains problematic, however.

T2-weighted sequences are necessary for evaluating structural changes in the brain parenchyma (e.g., ectopias and heterotopias, phakomatoses, demyelinating processes, congenital tumors) and for comparing the characteristics of fluids in adjacent cavities (cysts, ventricles). If different signal intensities are noted, it is unlikely that free communication exists between adjacent cystic cavities, although there is a danger of signal distortion from flow effects induced by cardiac and respiratory movements (see Sect. 5.3). It is also necessary to exclude communications between CSF cavities and cysts, which create a mass effect through the deformation and displacement of nearby structures. Local edematous reactions and areas of periventricular interstitial edema signifying an obstruction of CSF drainage with a rise of intraventricular pressure are especially well displayed on T2-weighted and proton-density images.

Calcifications give low signals on T1-weighted and T2-weighted sequences and are virtually indistinguishable from other hypointense structures. Calcium deposits are relatively easy to identify on noncontrast CT scans, although they may be confused with fresh hemorrhage and old (oily) contrast residues.

Selection of Imaging Plane

The imaging plane is selected in accordance with the specific requirements of the malformation in question.

With *malformations of the midline,* such as corpus callosum anomalies, Arnold-Chiari deformity, etc., scans in the sagittal and coronal planes provide the best source of information. The same applies to malformations of the spinal canal and spinal cord. Abnormal curvatures of the spine can create difficulties during the examination and call for ingenuity on the part of the examiner and cooperativeness on the part of the patient. On the technical side, three-dimensional data acquisition can be helpful in this situation. The phase encoding gradient can be modified, fast sequencing and presaturation of prevertebral tissues can be employed to eliminate respiratory and bowel-motion artifacts, which can obscure anatomic details on the sagittal image. Despite all measures, patient cooperation remains an essential ingredient. Barnes et al. [11] recommend careful compression of the abdomen with a strap to reduce respiratory and bowel-motion artifacts in lumbar spine imaging. This technique is said to be especially helpful in children.

Because partial volume effects and CSF flow artifacts are quite likely to occur on sagittal and coronal images of the spinal canal, axial scans can contribute significantly to the diagnosis. The axial plane is also useful for establishing the relationship of intraspinal structures to the spinal cord (i.e., intra- or extramedullary).

Sagittal and coronal sections are preferred for the imaging of *migration disorders,* because they display the abnormal gyral pattern of the brain surface better than axial images. The latter may have adjunctive value, however.

With congenital tumors such as tuberous sclerosis and von Hippel-Landau disease, the use of *contrast agents* (e.g., gadolinium chelate) can assist in the differential diagnosis of the lesion and the determination of its biologic behavior.

There are situations where it is useful to determine the *course of the major intracranial blood vessels.* This is helpful, for instance, in differentiating a severe internal hydrocephalus (anterior cerebral artery and superficial arteries stretched over the hemispheres) from hydranencephaly (a few atretic vessels at the base).

The aforementioned *motion artifacts* in larger fluid-filled cavities can vary in appearance in different sequences and different image planes. The nature of the artifacts can be disclosed by modifying the pulse sequence and scan plane and also by employing ECG and respiratory triggering.

7.3 Midline Closure Defects (Neural Tube Defects, Dysraphic Disorders)

7.3.1 Midline Closure Defects of the Brain

Craniorachischisis

Craniorachischisis is the severest form of dysraphia in which cranioschisis and rachischisis coexist. The entire neural groove (brain and spinal cord) is exposed to the exterior and may be severely damaged. Besides the malformed skull base, the spinal column is shortened because of synostosis and block vertebrae [106].

Anencephaly

Anencephaly results from failure of closure of the neural tube. The cranial vault and its contents may be totally absent (holoanencephaly) or may exhibit major defects (meroanencephaly) [76, 88].

Encephalocele and Cranial Meningocele

Encephalocele and cranial meningocele involve the protrusion of brain tissue and/or meninges through a bony defect in the cranial vault.

Cranium bifidum occultum is the mildest form of this anomaly. Often there is skin involvement in the form of a dermal sinus, which communicates with an intracranial dermoid cyst through a congenital bony defect [78].

Occipital encephalocele: The occipital herniation of brain, with or without involvement of the foramen magnum, is quite common (70% according to Matson [95]). The herniation may occur in association with Meckel's syndrome (microcephaly, microphthalmia, craniofacial clefts, and other visceral and skeletal anomalies) [77]. Differentiation is required from dermoids and epidermoids, small, often cystic cell residues occurring in proximity to midline sutures and in conjunction with a bony defect having intracranial extension [43]. MR is excellent for confirming occipital encephalocele, for it can clearly define the shape, size, and contents of the sac and thus establish its origin, especially when sagittal images are made (Figs. 7.1 and 7.2).

Parietal meningoencephaloceles are relatively uncommon [90, 77]. Accompanying brain malformations include asymmetry of the hemispheres, ventricular wall deformities, agenesis of the corpus callosum, and hydrocephalus. Diebler and Dulac [30] state that the posterior portion of the interhemispheric fissure is always expanded and is associated with brain herniation.

Anterior encephaloceles are most common at the frontoethmoidal junction, from which they may project into the nasal cavity (Fig. 7.3 a, b), the ethmoid or sphenoid sinus [76, 15], the epipharynx, or the orbit [148]. Interfrontal cephaloceles are often located in the pars inferior of the metopic suture, and are frequently quite large. The asymmetric distribution of the herniating brain can cause significant displacement and rotation of the hemispheres [30] (Fig. 7.3 b).

- *Frontal encephaloceles* can occur in conjunction with lipomas of the corpus callosum [70]. In the few cases published to date, the bony defect was located in the pars superior of the metopic suture. Lipomas of the corpus callosum are congenital masses. Because they extend into the upper part of the interhemispheric fissure, they are believed to interfere with normal induction of the membranous roof by the brain [126].
- *Transsphenoidal encephaloceles* are relatively rare. They may coexist with facial anomalies like cleft lip and palate [30] and with midline malformations of the brain [78]. With herniation of only the meninges into the paranasal sinuses, clinical diagnosis can be difficult and may be aided by the presence of spontaneous CSF rhinorrhea. Additional symptoms are hypertelurism, ophthalmologic disorders (coloboma, hypoplasia of the orbit, eye, and optic nerve), and endocrine disorders (hormonal deficits) [30] (Fig. 7.4). In rare cases the opening of the sac may close so that the contents no longer communicate with analogous intracranial structures. This could account for "nasal gliomas" or the neuronal tissue occasionally found within the scalp [82, 22, 64]. *MR scans* may demonstrate structures isointense with brain or CSF within the ethmoid cells or sphenoid sinus. Multiple projections may be necessary to demonstrate the exact shape and localization of these sacs and disclose accompanying malformations of the brain. *CT findings* reported in the literature include herniation of the third ventricle from the suprasellar cistern through the sella turcica into the sphenoid sinus [30].

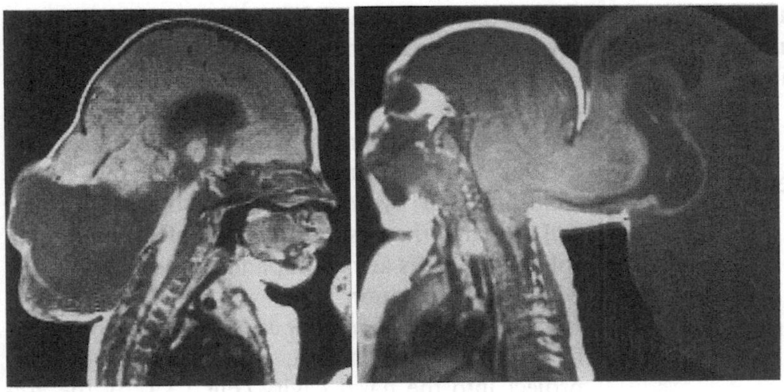

a b

Fig. 7.1. **a** Suboccipital encephalocele in a 18-day-old baby. A large cyst replacing the cerebellum is herniated through a wide defect over the posterior fossa. There is also partial protrusion of the occipital lobes. The ventricles are enlarged. Since the upper cervical vertebrae seem to be involved, also a myelocerebellomeningocele (Arnold-Chiari type III deformity) has to be considered. Mediosagittal (**a**) sections, SE 2.0 s/30 ms (1.0 T). **b** Large suboccipital encephalocele, in a 9-week-old girl, containing brain tissue and large cystic spaces, which probably represent ventricles. There are no ventricles seen intracranially. In the frontotemporal region normal gyri were seen. Sagittal scan, SE 0.45 s/15 ms (1.5 T)

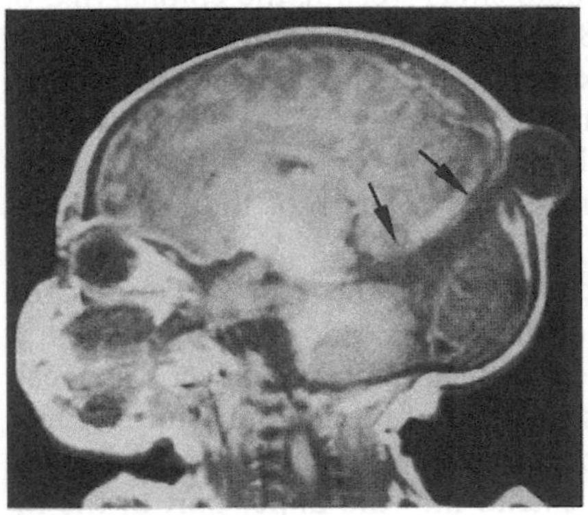

Fig. 7.2. Occipital encephalomeningocele in a 2-day-old baby. The dark band (*arrows*) probably is caused by a CSF-containing tube in the falx which connects the vermian cistern with the cele; at surgery no communication between the cyst and the intracranial CSF space was found. Sagittal scan, SE 0.5 s/15 ms (1.5 T)

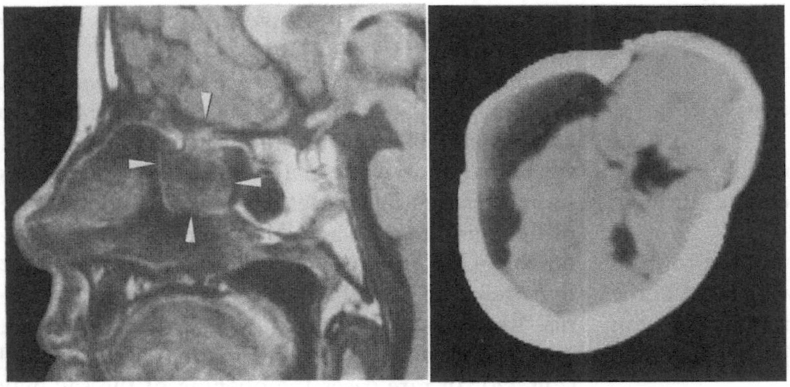

a b

Fig. 7.3. **a** Anterior encephalocele in a 7-year-old girl with nasal liquorrhea and a history of meningitis. A defect is seen in the middle of the left olfactory groove *(arrow)* connecting the intracranial cavity with the cele *(arrowheads)* in the left nasal cavity. Midsagittal scan (**a**) SE 0.5 s/15 ms (1.5 T). **b** Frontal encephalocele in an 11-year-old boy with mental retardation and seizures. Axial CT scans show the large encephalocele and the dislocation and rotation of the brain

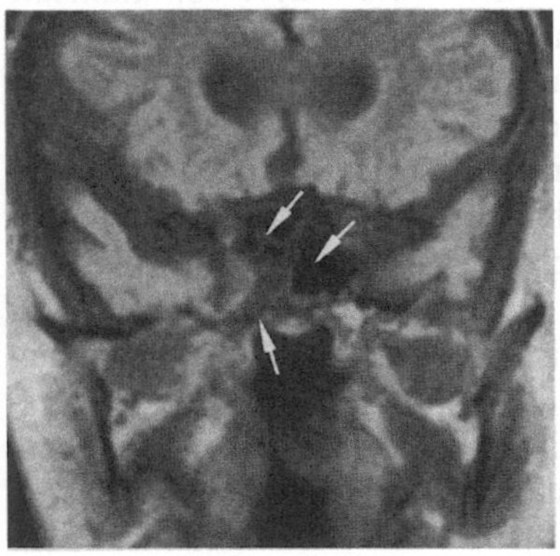

Fig. 7.4. Transsphenoidal encephalocele in a 44-year-old woman with spontaneous rhinoliquorrhea. The coronal section shows bulging of the dura into the right sphenoid sinus *(arrows)* SE 1.6 s/30 ms (0.35 T)

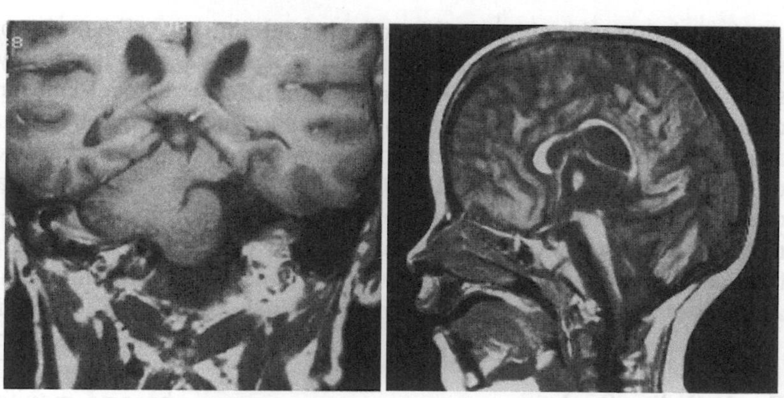

Fig. 7.5. a, b. Aplasia of cerebellum. **a** Aplasia of left cerebellar hemisphere in a 65-year-old woman with slightly unsteady gait. Asymmetric posterior fossa with shifting of the brainstem to the side of the missing cerebellar hemisphere. Coronal scan, SE 0.45 s/15 ms (1.5 T). **b** A 2½-year-old girl with lumbar meningomyelocele, rudimentary cerebellum, hypoplastic and elongated brainstem and midbrain, and hydrocephalus. The tentorium and rectus sinus cannot be identified. Midsagittal scan, SE 0.6 s/15 ms (1.5 T)

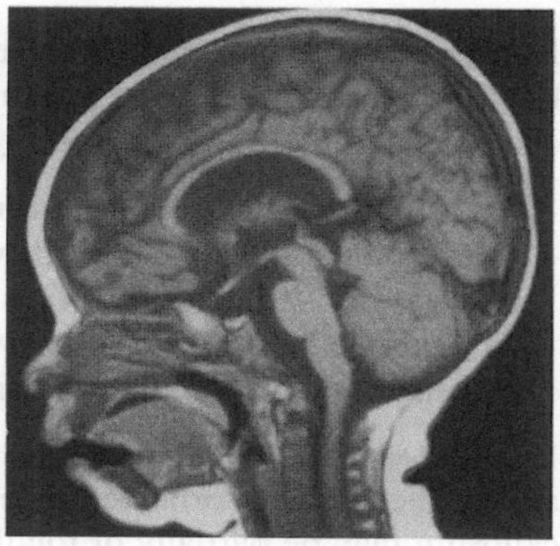

Fig. 7.6. Aplasia of posterior vermis and flocculus in a 6-month-old boy with macrocephaly, psychomotor retardation, and paresis of cranial nerves III and VII. Only a small part of the anterior vermis is present; the flocculus cannot be identified. The cerebellum is of normal size but does not show its characteristic gyration. Further anomalies include ventricular enlargement with thinning out and upward bulging of the corpus callosum, and atrophy of both hemispheres. Sagittal scan, SE 0.4 s/17 ms (1.0 T)

7.3.2 Midline Closure Defects of the Cerebellum

Agenesis of the Cerebellum

Agenesis of the cerebellum is extremely rate. It has been described in the setting of arthrogryposis multiplex congenita. The unilateral absence of a hemisphere is also very unusual. Disturbance in the growth of rhombic lip neurons at different times and stages in the development of the cerebellum can give rise to varying combinations of cerebellar and brainstem anomalies [88]. With total or subtotal absence of the cerebellum, hypoplasia or malformation may also be apparent in related structures like the pontine nuclei, inferior olives, and cerebellar peduncles [76].

Hypoplasia of the Cerebellum

The term "hypoplasia of the cerebellum" encompasses a large and heterogeneous group of anomalies [76]. The small volume of the cerebellum may result from a congenital malformation, a systemic degenerative process, perinatal ischemia, or other destructive factors that are associated with necrosis, demyelination, atrophy, and various combinations of aplasia or hypoplasia of the involved structures (dentate nucleus, brainstem nuclei, cell layers of the cerebellum, etc.) (Fig. 7.5).

MR Findings

Depending on the changes in the architecture and internal structure of the hypoplastic cerebellum, its shape and structure on MR images will deviate to some degree from the normal signal pattern and intensity, although these changes may not be suggestive of a specific disorder.

Hypoplasia of the Vermis

Hypoplasia of the vermis is seen more frequently. It has been described in isolation or as part of a syndrome, such as Dandy-Walker syndrome [76]. With isolated hypoplasia, the inferior vermis is usually hypoplastic or absent. Partial or complete absence of the cerebellar vermis associated with complex deformities of the cerebral hemispheres has been described less frequently [96] (Fig. 7.6).

Association with abnormalities of other midline structures has also been mentioned, such as agenesis or hypoplasia of corpus callosum, septum pellucidum, and fornix, cranioschisis, meningoceles, diastematobulbia [68], and absence of segmentation of the tectum [16]. Joubert et al. [68] describe a syndrome of episodic hyperpnea, abnormal eye movements, ataxia, and retardation in conjunction with familial agenesis of the cerebellar vermis. Isolated agenesis of the vermis may be asymptomatic [68].

Dandy-Walker-Syndrome

Dandy-Walker syndrome [20] refers to a group of hindbrain malformations in patients of all ages. It is characterized by following (see Fig. 7.7):

- Aplasia or hypoplasia of the cerebellar vermis
- Cystic dilatation of the fourth ventricle with anterosuperior displacement of a small cerebellum
- An enlarged posterior fossa with upward displacement of the torcular and sinuses

In addition, there may be dilatation of the aqueduct and of the supratentorial ventricles, and the corpus callosum may be partially or totally absent.

The *etiology* of the Dandy-Walker cyst remains unclear. Genetic, infectious, and chemical factors have been implicated, as well as multifactorial causes. Despite various theories, the *pathogenesis* also remains unexplained [77, 98]. Originally it was felt that development of the cerebellum was retarded by obstruction of the foramina of Luschka and Magendie, leading to cystic dilatation of the fourth ventricle (atresia theory) [98]. However, the finding of patent foramina in many patients [134, 117] seems to make the atresia theory untenable. Raimondi et al. [117] state that a more likely pathogenesis involves a disturbance in the development of the embryonic roof of the fourth ventricle (neuroschisis), thus pointing to the anterior membranaceous area as the responsible factor.

There is growing evidence that the Dandy-Walker syndrome is very frequently accompanied by various other anomalies of the CNS and other systems [55, 63, 98].

Associated anomalies of the CNS include [98]: holoprosencephaly, cerebral gyral abnormalities, malformations of the inferior olives, cerebellar folial anomalies and heterotopias, microcephaly, lipomas, agenesis of the corpus callosum, and occipital encephaloceles [98].

Examples of *coexisting anomalies in other body regions* are polydactyly and syndactyly, cleft palate, Klippel-Feil syndrome, Cornelia de Lange deformity, spinal anomalies, renal cysts, diaphragmatic hernia, and cardiac malformations [98].

Hydrocephalus is often the *initial presenting feature* of Dandy-Walker syndrome in children. The rise of intracranial pressure accounts for other symptoms such as headache and vomiting. If retardation of mental development is also noted, a search should be made for coexisting anomalies of the cerebrum. Occasionally these complaints do not become manifest until adulthood, when they are precipitated by trauma or infection and require differentiation from a posterior fossa tumor.

The so-called *Dandy-Walker variant* (or diverticular variant) involves an expansion of the roof of the fourth ventricle, which communicates with a posteriorly situated cystic cavity of variable size through an enlarged foramen of Magendie. These cysts tend to be smaller than the Dandy-Walker cyst. The inferior vermis (uvula, nodulus, pyramid) is hypoplastic, the cerebellar hemispheres are frequently small, and the torcular and sinus rectus are normally positioned (Fig. 7.8).

Dandy-Walker syndrome has to be distinguished from *other cystic anomalies of the posterior fossa*. In particular, large arachnoid cysts (retrocerebellar arachnoid pouch or Blake's pouch) can closely resemble a Dandy-Walker cysts (Fig. 7.9). In these cases the cerebellar vermis and fourth ventricle are normal, though displaced. The tela choroidea of the fourth ventricle extends far dorsally along the upper and lower surface of the vermis. As development of the brain proceeds, a membrane-like outpouching forms in the roof of the fourth ventricle in the area of the later apertures (foramen of Magendie), which atrophies and creates a communication between the ventricles and the subarachnoid space. If the membrane does not open, the outpouching can persist as Blake's pouch [50]. The cysts may communicate freely or only poorly with the subarachnoid space. Whether a one-way valve effect and/or another mechanism (i.e., arachnoid adhesions) create the mass effect in communicating cysts is not yet clear (Fig. 7.10). Dilated supratentorial ventricles, displacement of the fourth ventricle and adjacent cerebellum, and clinical symptoms indicating intracranial hypertension are indications for decompression of the ventricles and/or shunting of the cyst. A similar pathogenetic mechanism is postulated for the large cisterna magna; it likewise is always smaller than the Dandy-

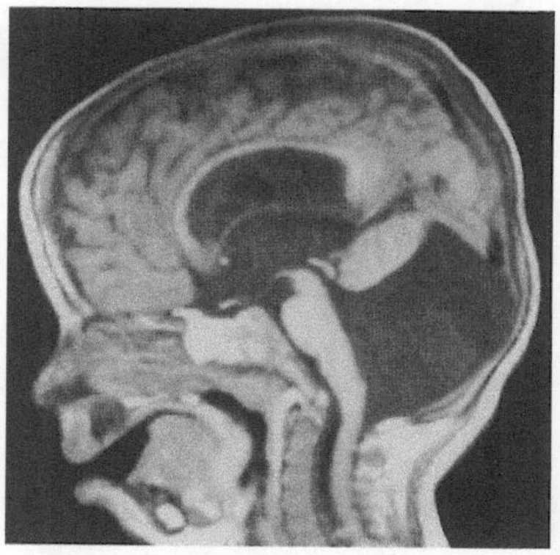

Fig. 7.7. Dandy-Walker syndrome in a 4-month-old boy with large head and hydrocephalus. Enlarged posterior fossa, elongation and hydrocephalic configuration of corpus callosum and fornix, perforated septum pellucidum. Midsagittal section, SE 0.4 s/17 ms (1.0 T)

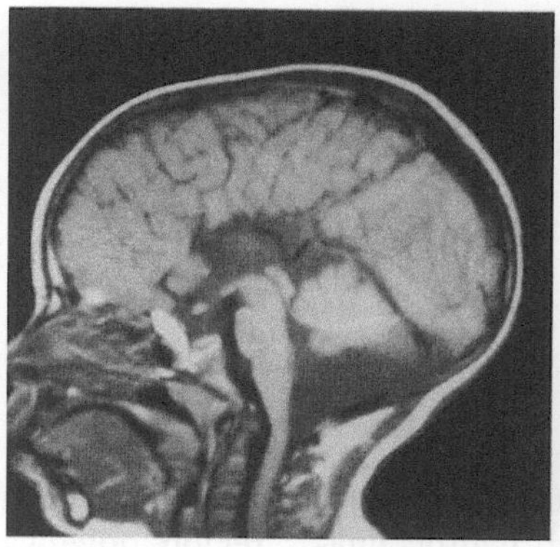

7.8

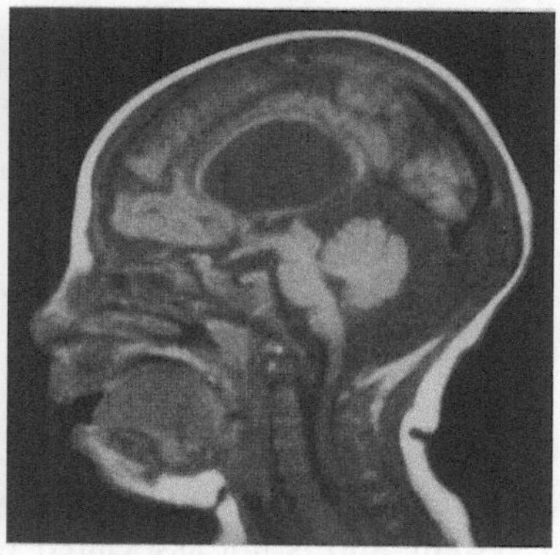

7.9

Fig. 7.8. Dandy-Walker variant in a 3-year-old girl with psychomotor retardation. Hypoplasia of the lower vermis and partial aplasia of the left cerebellar hemisphere. Wide foramen of Magendie. Agenesis of corpus callosum and enlargement of lateral ventricles. Midsagittal section, SE 0.7 s/30 ms (1.0 T)

Fig. 7.9. Retrocerebellar arachnoid pouch (Blake's pouch); enlarged posterior fossa, normal development of vermis and cerebellum, large cystic retro-, supra-, and infracerebellar space, in some cases high insertion of the tentorium and extensions of the cyst dorsal and above the torcular. A 4-month-old boy with similar findings, but additional diverticulum dorsal and above the torcular Herophili and atrophy of both hemispheres. Midsagittal scan, SE 0.7 s/17 ms (1.0 T)

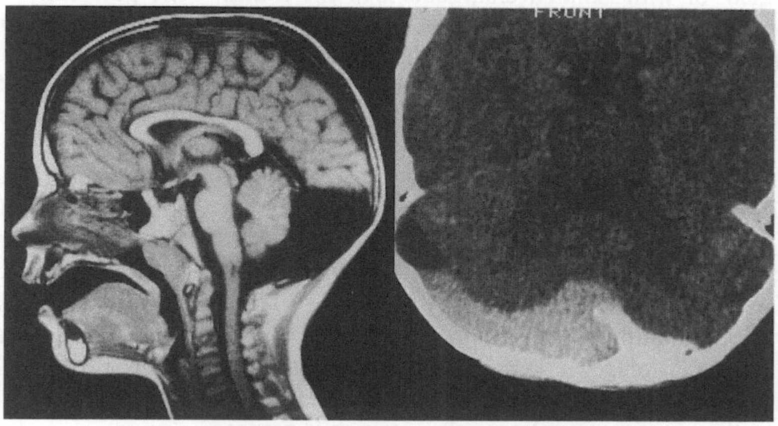

a b

Fig. 7.10 a, b. Retrocerebellar arachnoid pouch without hydrocephalus in a 6-year-old boy with intermittent headache, nausea and slight disturbance of equilibrium, suggesting increased intracranial pressure. **a** Midsagittal MR image, SE 0.4 s/17 ms. **b** After intrathecal application of contrast medium, delayed enhancement of the cyst is seen on CT: note different concentration of contrast medium in the left and right compartments of the cyst in the initial phase (**b**)

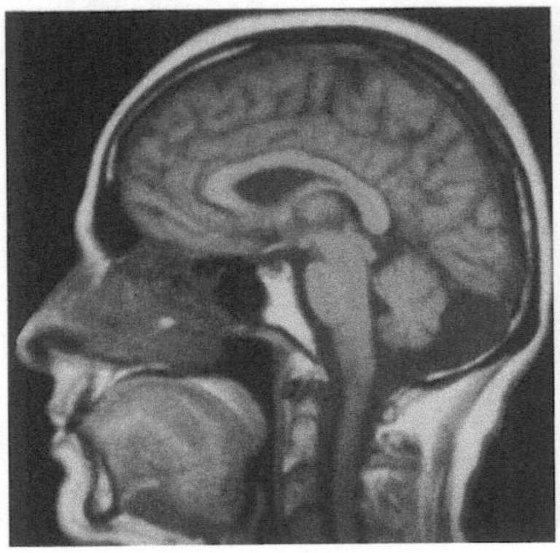

7.11

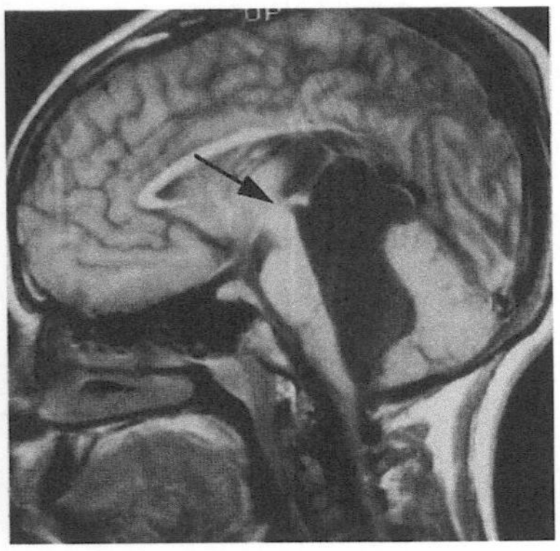

7.12

Fig. 7.11. Enlarged cisterna magna (incidental finding) in a 47-year-old woman. Midsagittal section, SE 0.4 s/17 ms (1.0 T)

Fig. 7.12. Occluded fourth ventricle in an 11-year-old boy with ventriculoatrial shunt because of hydrocephalus and cystic dilatation of fourth ventricle on CT. MR reveals occlusion of aqueduct *(arrow)* and outlet foramina of enlarged fourth ventricle with marked outpouching of anterior velum medullare. Associated malformation of corpus callosum. Midsagittal scans, SE 0.6 s/15 ms (1.5 T)

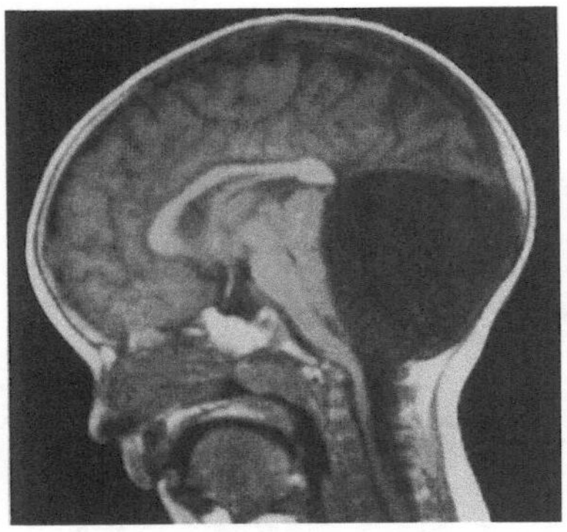

Fig. 7.13. Retrocerebellar arachnoid cyst in a 3-year-old boy with enlargement of the posterior fossa and compression and dislocation of the cerebellum, brainstem and fourth ventricle by a large cyst extending into the vercical canal. No hydrocephalus after shunt operation soon after birth. The axial CT scan could be misinterpreted as Dandy-Walker syndrome. Midsagittal section, SE 0.7 s/30 ms (1.0 T)

Walker cyst, communicates freely with the ventricular system, and is not associated with hydrocephalus (Fig. 7.11).

Secondary occlusion of the outlet foramina of the fourth ventricle is associated with dilatation of that ventricle along with the rest of the ventricular system, or with isolated enlargement of the fourth ventricle if there is concomitant obstruction of the aqueduct (Fig. 7.12). However, the cerebellum is normally developed, and the posterior fossa is not enlarged.

CT and MR Findings

Selection of MR technique and imaging planes is discussed in Sect. 7.2.

Special importance should be attached to the midsagittal image. Like a midline tomogram in pneumoencephalography, this view is able to display the anterior medullary velum, which is continuous above with the posterior wall of the aqueduct and below with the wall of the enlarged fourth ventricle. This scan also can confirm absence of the inferior vermis, displacement of the superior vermis between the tentorial incisure and quadrigeminal region, downward displacement of the midportions of the floor of the fourth ventricle, and high insertion of the tentorium, findings which are pathognomonic for Dandy-Walker syndrome [117].

An important preoperative question concerns the possibility of compression of the aqueduct by the posterior fossa cyst, which would necessitate drainage of the cyst in addition to the lateral ventricles. In doubtful cases intrathecal contrast material may be introduced to see whether the cyst communicates with the remaining CSF cavities. The described technique of MR imaging is also considered the first-line method for differentiating Dandy-Walker cyst from other cystic abnormalities of the posterior fossa. Differentiation among Dandy-Walker cyst, Dandy-Walker variant, and Blake's pouch can be difficult on the basis of axial CT scans alone [56] (Fig. 7.13).

Arnold-Chiari Deformity

Arnold-Chiari deformity (Chiari 1891, 1896; Arnold 1894 cited in [23]) involves a complex malfor-

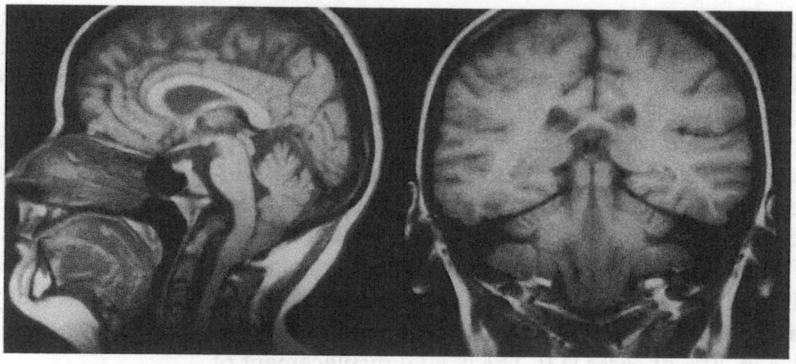

Fig. 7.14 a, b. Arnold-Chiari type I deformity in a 20-year-old woman with hemifacial pain. Small, funnel-shaped posterior fossa with enlarged foramen magnum, mild basilar impression, elongation of the medulla oblongata, and caudal displacement of the cerebellar tonsils, which surround the cord. No hydrocephalus. **a** Midsagittal, **b** coronal scans, SE 0.5 s/30 ms (1.0 T)

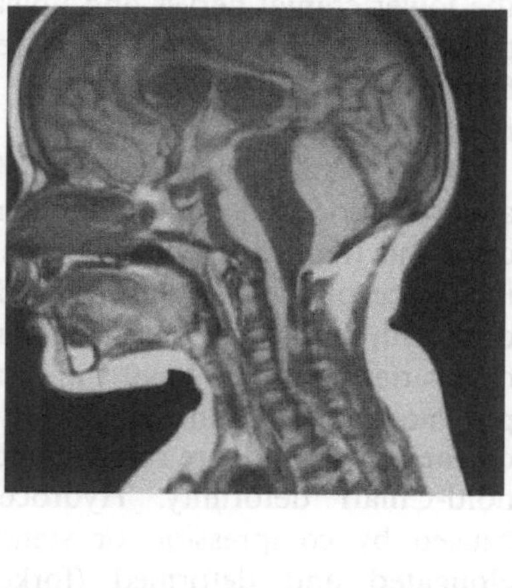

Fig. 7.15. Arnold-Chiari type II deformity in a 4-year-old boy after meningitis and ventriculitis, the infection occurring through an open meningocele. The sagittal section shows the kinking of the cord, a syringo-/hydromyelia, widening of the upper cervical canal, and hypoplasia of the corpus callosum. The enlarged fourth ventricle (secondary to inflammatory adhesions at its foramina) extends far above the tentorium with deformation of the tectum. Sagittal section, SE 0.7 s/30 ms (1.0 T)

mation of the cerebellum and brainstem. The individual components of this anomaly can occur in various combinations and with varying degrees of severity. Chiari [23] described four types of lesion:

Type I: Ectopia of the cerebellar tonsils, which cup the medulla oblongata, and minimal caudal displacement of the slightly elongated brainstem, which does not overlie the spinal cord. Hydrocephalus is possible, but generally very mild [56]. Basilar impression may coexist in up to 50% of cases [56], and hydromyelia or syringomyelia in up to 30% of cases [111] (Fig. 7.14). Meningomyeloceles are rare. Mild cerebellar symptoms usually do not appear until adulthood [76], although the malformation may remain clinically silent [1].

Type II: This type represents the classic Arnold-Chiari deformity. Its hallmark is caudal displacement of the elongated cerebellar vermis and tonsils through the foramen magnum into the cervical canal along with the lower portion of the fourth ventricle and its choroid plexus. The dorsal part of the medulla oblongata is also displaced caudally and overlies the upper cervical cord (Fig. 7.15). In 50%–70% of cases this produces a characteristic Z-shaped "kink" at the junction of the medulla oblongata and cervical cord [38, 101, 76, 88], which usually is found between C2 and C4 but may occur as low as T1. The displaced cerebellar tissue overlies the dorsal medulla and is often tightly bound to it by fibrovascular adhesions of the leptomeninges. The herniated tissue may be firm and gliotic.

Almost complete loss of cerebellar substance has been reported by Yuh et al. [145] in constellation with typical signs of Arnold-Chiari type II deformity in a 7-year-old girl. However, this finding is not considered pathognomonic for Arnold-Chiari type II deformity but rather seems to provide evidence against this diagnosis [145].

The fourth ventricle is visible in 70% of cases. It may appear flattened, occupying a normal or slightly caudal position (15%), or it may show cystic expansion (5%) [102], and there may be ventricular clefts extending deep into the cerebellar white matter [88]. The foramen of Magendie may be absent. The leptomeninges are fibrotic. There is vascular engorgement caused by chronic venous congestion, and in some cases there is vascular proliferation so severe that it resembles a vascular malformation [88].

The posterior fossa is small, widened, and flat with a low attachment of the often rudimentary tentorium cerebelli and correspondingly low-lying venous sinuses. The tentorial incisure is widened as a result of poor development of the leaves [88]. Upward displacement of the cerebellum into the widened tentorial notch produces a "bullet-shaped" configuration on the axial CT scan [103, 101]. The foramen magnum is round and frequently enlarged. Usually the upper cervical canal is also enlarged and shows incomplete closure of the arch of the atlas in 70% of cases [13]. The caudal displacement of the brainstem and medulla results in elongation of the lower cranial nerves and upward angulation of the cervical spinal roots. This feature disappears farther down the cervical spine, and the thoracic roots have a normal course.

The Arnold-Chiari type II deformity is almost always associated with a lumbar myelomeningocele, and frequently with hydrocephalus [101]. The incidence of the Arnold-Chiari deformity in children with thoracolumbar or lumbar myelomeningocele varies from 40% to 90% in different series. Simple meningoceles and sacral myelomeningoceles, on the other hand, are rarely combined with an Arnold-Chiari deformity. Hydrocephalus may be caused by compression or stenosis of the often elongated and deformed (forked) aqueduct or blockage of the foramen of Magendie by glial tissue, or may relate to secondary meningitis or surgical closure of the sac in patients with open spinal defects.

Numerous other anomalies have been seen in association with the Arnold-Chiari deformity: polymicrogyria/stenogyria, partial agenesis of corpus callosum, enlarged massa intermedia, elevated hypothalamus, craniolacunia, hypoplasia of the falx, forking or gliosis of the aqueduct, fusion of the colliculi of the quadrigeminal region, heterotopias within the cerebellar white matter, anomalies of the base of the skull (i.e. basilar impression, anomalies of the atlanto-occipital joints, concave clivus), hydromyelia, myelomeningocele.

The pathogenesis of the Arnold-Chiari type II deformity remains unexplained and is a subject of great controversy. Three main theories have been postulated: (1) the traction theory, (2) the hydrocephalus theory, and (3) the maldevelopment theory [98]. None of these, however, can satisfactorily account for all the variants of the syndrome. All three theories describe an abnormal occipital bone with a disproportion between the flat, undersized posterior fossa and the normally developed cerebellum and brainstem. The malformation arises early, between the 4th and 10th weeks of gestation.

Type III consists of cervical spina bifida with herniation of almost the entire cerebellum through the deficient foramen magnum, forming a suboccipital myelocerebellomeningocele [77]. This very rare type is considered a form of neural tube defect.

Type IV consists of cerebellar hypoplasia alone. Chiari included it in his group of malformations in 1896, but today it is considered to be a separate anomaly.

MR Findings

Selection of MR techniques and imaging planes is discussed in Sect. 7.2.

T1-weighted images are best for demonstrating the pathoanatomic features of the Arnold-Chiari type II deformity described above [26, 97, 54, 1, 83, 131, 138]. Care should be taken to obtain an exact midsagittal scan, which displays most effectively the malformations of the brainstem, aqueduct, fourth ventricle, posterior fossa, and cervical cord. According to Aboulezz et al. [1], Arnold-Chiari deformity may be diagnosed when the cerebellar tonsils extend for more than 5 mm below the foramen magnum. Other criteria are a narrowed fourth ventricle in connection with slightly elongated tonsils, and a sagittal diameter of the foramen magnum greater than 42 mm. More detailed questions concerning the presence of associated anomalies, for example, can be answered by taking additional projections. Venes et al. [138] state that three major types of fourth ventricle anomaly are seen with MR imaging in the Arnold-Chiari type II deformity:

Type A: The fourth ventricle continues caudally as a narrow canal. The peg of the elongated cerebellar vermis produces dorsal cord compression. Dense fibrous adhesions are usually present.

Type B: There is intracranial dilatation of the fourth ventricle and aqueduct with no apparent communication between the third and fourth ventricles. The dilated fourth ventricle may extend into the spinal canal.

Type C: There is intraspinal dilatation of the fourth ventricle without intracranial dilatation. This can occur in two forms: (1) a cystic expansion of the fourth ventricle caudal to the vermian peg and dorsal to the spinal cord, and (2) occlusion of the foramen of Magendie with a saclike prolongation of the fourth ventricle which passes caudally within the

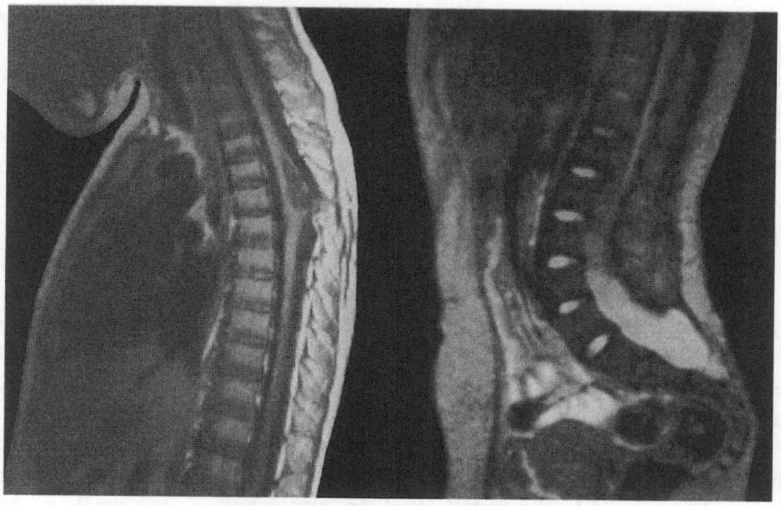

Fig. 7.16. **a** Small meningomyelocele at T5-T6 in a 7-year-old boy with gait disturbances. **a** Sagital scan, SE 0.4 s/17 ms (1.0 T). **b** Lumbosacral meningocele in a 28-year old woman with neurogenic bladder dysfunction. CSF-filled sac herniating into a dorsal defect of the lumbosacral spine, probably associated with tethered cord. Hyperlordosis of the lumbar spine. In (**b**) the signal intensity of CSF reflects the difference of pulsatile motion between the lower and upper parts of the lumbar canal (see also Sect. 5.3). Midsagittal section SE 1.6 s/90 ms (1.0 T)

gray matter of the cord dorsal to the central canal (Fig. 7.15). A cystic prolongation of the fourth ventricle into the cervical cord can mimic hydromyelia on MR scans.

Recognition of the type of anomaly aids in designing a treatment approach specifically for that condition. It is particularly important to identify a trapped fourth ventricle, since deterioration in patients with a type C deformity can be rapid [138]. The frequency of spinal malformations in Arnold-Chiari deformity, including tethering of the cord, lipomatous tissue, and meningomyelocele (see below), should always prompt a concurrent examination of the spinal column in these patients.

7.3.3 Midline Closure Defects of the Spine

Spinal dysraphias involve the outer ectoderm, the mesoderm, and the nervous tissues. They are variable in degree, and they are among the most common malformations in humans [47].

Spina Bifida Occulta (Posterior)

Spina bifida occulta is present in 1%-24% of the general population. This most innocent defect is characterized by incomplete closure of the neural arch, typically at L5 or S1 and usually without dysraphia of the adjacent nervous tissues. In a number of cases, however, fibrous bands fix the spinal cord to the bone, and diastematomyelia is fairly prevalent [61, 66].

Spina bifida occulta may also coexist with a lipoma or dermal sinus. Often these anomalies are manifested by a small vascular malformation in the skin or by hypertrichosis.

Spina Bifida Cystica

Spina bifida cystica is spina bifida in which there is protrusion of a CSF-filled cyst outside the normal spinal canal [43]. Eighty percent of lesions of this type occur in the lumbar region. A meningocele or meningomyelocele may be present, depending on the contents of the sac:

Meningocele: Ten to twenty percent of cases of spina bifida cystica are associated with herniation of the meninges (dura and arachnoid) through the spinal defect in the form of a CSF-filled sac (Fig. 7.16b).

Meningomyelocele: The remaining 80%-90% of cases of spina bifida cystica are associated with the herniation of meninges and spinal cord through the midline vertebral defect. Almost all thoracolumbar and lumbar meningomyeloceles are accompanied by an Arnold-Chiari type II deformity (see above).

The vertebral malformation involves absence of the spinous process, eversion of the lamina, and widening of the interpeduncular distance. In meningocele the conus medullaris is usually at a low level and is fixed in an expanded dural sheath. In meningomyelocele the cord is closed, but usually flattened and deformed, lying close to the posterior surface of the sac. In meningomyelocystocele the central canal is grossly dilated and the thinned-out posterior part of the cord herniates into the sac. The dorsal surface of the sac may be closed and covered with skin (Fig. 7.16a), but in more severe cases it lies exposed like an open and expanded neural tube (area medullovasculosa).

The ventral nerve roots emerge from the area medullovasculosa in their "normal" position, while the dorsal roots emerge from its lateral edges in a less regular fashion. CSF drains from the opened central canal within the area medullovasculosa. From 80% to 90% of meningomyeloceles occur in the lower thoracolumbar region, but the bony defects often extend to the sacral level. In some cases lipomas, often intermixed with the spinal cord, are seen in the area of the sac, classifying the lesion as a *lipomeningomyelocele* (see below).

It is not unusual to find a hydromyelia (29%) or syringomyelia (14%) in spinal cord segments proximal to the myelocele [37]. In the area of the sac itself, an open neural plate is seen in 35% of cases and a total or partial diastematomyelia in 36%. A diastematomyelia is found distal to the sac in 25%, and double or multiple spinal cord canals in 29%. The sac also may contain keratin, dermoid cysts, and hair [88]. Frequently these malformations are combined with hydrocephalus, whose mechanism is not always clear. CSF stasis with a rapidly progressive ventricular dilatation is usually seen following the surgical closure of open meningomyeloceles.

MR Findings. In MR, signal intensity difference can be observed between the contents of meningomyelocystoceles, meningomyeloceles, and normal subarachnoid CSF. Normally there is a concentration gradient of protein from a low level in the ventricles (5–15 mg%) to a high level of 20–50 mg% in the lumbar region. The increased amount of "bound water" (hydration layer) in fluids with a higher amount of protein shortens the relaxation time T1 of the fluid. Increased protein content of the lumbar CSF may be due to an increased permeability of the blood-CSF barrier to proteins in the spinal region compared to the intracranial subarachnoid space. In meningomyelocele and meningomyelocystocele sacs a presumed higher protein content may also be secondary to stagnation of the fluid [41, 136]. With reduced pulsatile flow in the wide sac of the cele compared to the normal canal of the adjacent lumbar spine, the signal intensity of the cele is increased (Fig. 7.16). Nerve roots within meningomyeloceles are very difficult to visualize. The reason for this may be seen mainly in partial volume effects of thick slices and/or motion of the nerve roots with pulsatile flow of CSF, rather than in a lack of tissue contrast.

Ventral Spinal Defects

Ventral defects of the spinal canal include neuroenteric (enterogenic) cysts, anterior sacral meningoceles, and teratomas.

Neurenteric cysts are rare and result from a persistent communication between the embryonic endoderm and the neuroectoderm (notochord). In the 3rd week of embryogenesis, a temporary connection (neurenteric canal) exists between the neuroectoderm and the endoderm. The neuroectoderm may draw a pedicle of endoderm into the forming neural tube, so that complete closure of the neural tube is prevented by the mesoderm. This results in associated vertebral anomalies (butterfly vertebrae or anterior spina bifida) [69]. The cysts generally occur in the cervicothoracic region. They are intraspinal, sometimes intramedullary, and communicate with respiratory or digestive organs through a defect in the vertebral body.

MR findings of an enterogenous cyst were described by Aoki et al. [5] in a 22-year-old female at the level of the upper cervical canal. The cyst was hypointense, its relaxation times being prolonged, similar to those of CSF (T1 = 2.8 s, T2 = 140 ms). The wall of the cyst, which had caused enlargement of the cervical canal with thinning of the vertebral laminae, was thin except for a thick portion which was adherent to the cord. A communication with respiratory or digestive organs was not mentioned.

Anterior sacral meningocele involves a protrusion of dura and leptomeninges through a ventral defect in the sacrum [88].

Teratomatous cysts in the spinal canal were described by [120].

7.3.4 Dysraphic Disorders of the Spinal Cord

Hydromyelia and Syringomyelia

Hydromyelia

Hydromyelia is a congenital dilatation of the central canal of variable extent which chiefly affects

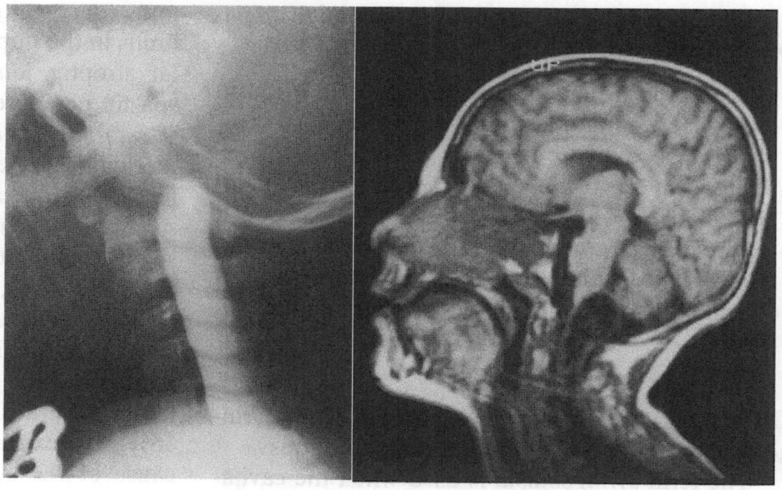

Fig. 7.17 a, b. Hydromyelia/syringomyelia in a 9-year-old girl with extreme scoliosis but no major neurological deficits. **a** Myelography at the age of 3 years with contrast medium in the syrinx which reached from the medulla oblongata to the tethered conus. No communication with the IVth ventricle. **b** MRI at the age of 9 years reveals corresponding finding of the medulla and adjacent cervical cord. SE 0.4 s/17 ms (1.0 T)

the cervical cord [106] (Fig. 7.17). It may be discovered as an incidental finding on sagittal or coronal scans of the spinal cord made in asymptomatic patients. (Often the central canal is still patent at birth.)

The congenital dilatation of the central canal may result from a delayed opening of the outlet foramina of the fourth ventricle; this may cause tonsilar and vermian herniation in the foramen magnum due to obstructive hydrocephalus in the fetus. Besides other abnormalities this mechanism directs the ventricular pulse wave into the central canal, thus increasing the CSF pressure within the central canal.

Several other theories have been proposed to explain the pathogenesis of hydromyelia [10]:
The theory of Ball and Dayan [9] is also based on a foramen magnum lesion, which in their opinion acts as a one-way valve, allowing CSF to enter the spinal subarachnoid space but blocking its return into the cranial cavity. The increased CSF pressure in the spinal canal then forces CSF via the Virchow-Robin spaces into the central canal. According to Aboulker [2] this increased intraspinal pressure secondary to foramen magnum obstruction causes longstanding spinal cord edema, leading eventually to cavitations within the cord tissue.

A differing view of the valvular action of the foramen magnum is taken by Williams [140], who states that it causes a craniospinal pressure gradient which is maintained by the milking or pumping action of the changing volume of epidural veins. This pressure dissociation caused CSF to be "sucked" into the central canal during phases of low venous pressure, thus extending the syrinx at its caudal portion. In phases of high venous pressure, "sloshing" of the syrinx fluid occurs in the upward direction, causing extension of the syrinx in its cranial portion.

This "suck and slosh" effect may also be the underlying mechanism of the extension of traumatic syringomyelia, when a narrowing of the spinal canal develops secondary to a fracture or degenerative changes of the vertebrae [10].

In time the ependymal lining of the hydromyelic cavity may be replaced by a wall of gliosis [88].

A typical finding on myelography is the "collapsing cord sign," or variation of spinal cord width in the recumbent and upright positions. A low position of the cerebellar tonsils combined with expansion of the spinal cord is considered strong evidence for hydromyelia. With concomitant atrophy, however, the cord also may appear thinned out [125].

Hydromyelia may coexist with an Arnold-Chiari deformity in 40% of cases [89], and meningomyelocele is seen in approximately 30% [125].

Syringomyelia

Hydromyelia needs to be differentiated from syringomyelia, which also involves a cavitation of the spinal cord. The distinction is that the cavities of syringomyelia often do not communicate with the central canal. Some cases may be based on a dysraphic disorder, although many are believed to be secondary to trauma or other conditions [106].

Dubois [34] lists the following potential *origins* of syringomyelia:

- Secondary to inadequate drainage of the fourth ventricle (communicating syringomyelia, syringohydromyelia, hydromyelia)
- Late sequela of severe (or occasionally mild) trauma (see below)
- Secondary to arachnoiditis of the spinal canal
- Secondary to tumors of the spinal cord (or, less frequently, extramedullary or intracranial tumors)
- Idiopathic

Differentiation between hydromyelia and syringomyelia can be quite difficult, even at autopsy.

The term *syringobulbia* is used when the cavitation involves the medulla oblongata.

The cavity of syringomyelia is usually largest in the cervical region but is often absent from the first cervical segment. The syrinx extends for a varying distance caudally into the thoracic cord; the lumbosacral region is rarely involved [76]. In cross section the cavity in the cervical cord extends across the cord, involving the anterior horns and passing across the midline behind the central canal. In the thoracic cord the cavity is more often unilateral than bilateral and is most commonly found in the area of the posterior horns. It chiefly involves the gray matter but may also extend into the posterior and lateral columns at the tip of the dorsal horns as far as the pial surface [76] (see Fig. 7.22).

The walls of the cavity vary greatly in character, and this may depend upon the age of the lesion [76]. Where there is recent expansion, the wall is irregular and consists of degenerated neuroglial and neural elements. The myelin around the syrinx shows changes similar to edematous white matter, probably due to tearing of the tissues and transudation of serous fluid into them. Older cavities are surrounded by glial hyperplasia which finally forms a dense concentric wall of neuroglial sclerosis 1-2 mm thick. Strands of collagen or blood vessels with hyalinized walls may traverse the cavity. Where the cavity communicates with the central canal, parts of the cavity wall may be lined with ependymal cells [76]. The syrinx is usually filled with CSF-like fluid, which may have an elevated protein content.

Syringomyelia is manifested clinically in the second or third decade of life by a progressive myelopathy in the form of dissociated sensory disturbances in the shoulder girdle and upper limbs (damage to spinothalamic fibers), autonomic symptoms (damage to cells of the intermediolateral columns in the upper thoracic segments), pain, muscular atrophy, joint neuropathy, kyphoscoliosis, and spastic paraparesis [34]. The symptoms may progress rapidly or remain stationary. The condition is rarely fatal, except with syringobulbia, but generally leads to significant disability.

In *secondary syringomyelia* resulting from adhesive arachnoiditis, hematomyelia, malacia, or trauma (see below), the cavities tend to be smaller, but cavities associated with tumors can be very extensive. A coexisting syringomelia has been found in approximately one-third (31%) of intramedullary tumors. In a smaller proportion of cases (about 16%), a coexisting tumor has been identified as the cause of the syringomyelia [115]. Thus the syringomyelia may be clinically apparent and accessible to diagnosis before the tumor itself is detected. Most are based on tumors of ependymal character or hemangioblastomas. The cavity is produced by transudation from the tumor [76].

CT and MR Findings

Selection of MR techniques and imaging planes is discussed in Sect. 5.3.2. T1-weighted sequences are best for depicting the spinal cord and its cavities. The physiologic curvatures of the vertebral column make sagittal images preferable to coronal images. MR images will often demonstrate much more of the cavity than is displayed on CT scans [36]. However, the extent of the lesion often shows little correlation with the severity of the neurologic deficits, an observation that is relevant to therapeutic decision making [60].

The spinal cord is usually expanded in the presence of intramedullary cavities, but it may also appear normal or even thinned out [114, 71, 83] (Figs. 7.18-7.20). The collapsing cord sign seen on myelograms is not useful in explaining a narrowed spinal cord, because a hydrostatic pressure difference between the cyst and subarachnoid space does not exist as in myelography. A plausible cause appears to be an associated atrophy of the spinal cord and a variable state of cavitary filling, which has been noted in serial MR examinations.

The cysts usually display CSF-like signal intensities. The presence of circumferential gliotic bands can give the syrinx a haustrated or "beaded" appearance [129] (Fig. 7.18). The signal pattern can be altered by a high protein content and also by hemorrhage. Encapsulated cysts may then show T1 and

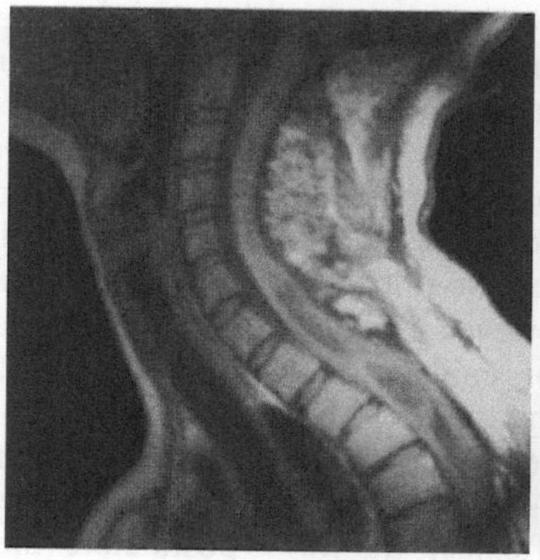

7.18

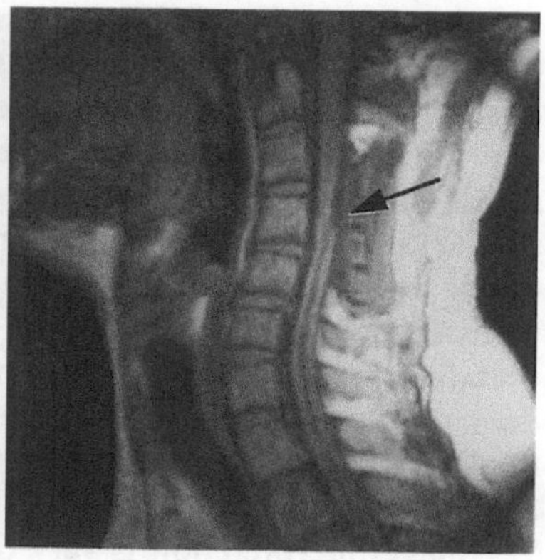

7.19

Fig. 7.18. Syringomyelia in a 34-year-old woman with progressive paraspastic paresis of her legs. Haustrated cervicothoracic syrinx. At surgery, demyelination, gliosis, and hemosiderin deposits were found; no sign of tumor. MR shows slight increase of signal intensity of cord tissue adjacent to the cyst. Midsagittal scan SE 0.7 s/30 ms (1.0 T)

Fig. 7.19. Syringomyelia in a 35-year-old man with spastic tetraparesis and sensory dissociation. Syrinx cavity extending from the medulla oblongata to the conus. After implantation of a cystosubarachnoid shunt *(arrow)*, narrowing of the cyst is seen, predominantly of the cranial portion. Midsagittal scan, SE 0.4 s/17 ms (1.0 T)

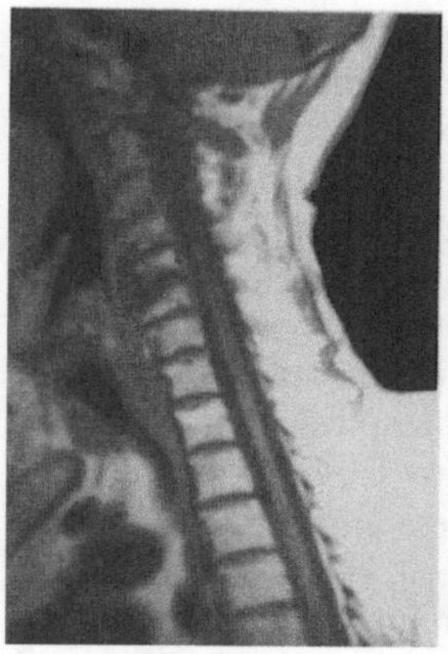

7.20

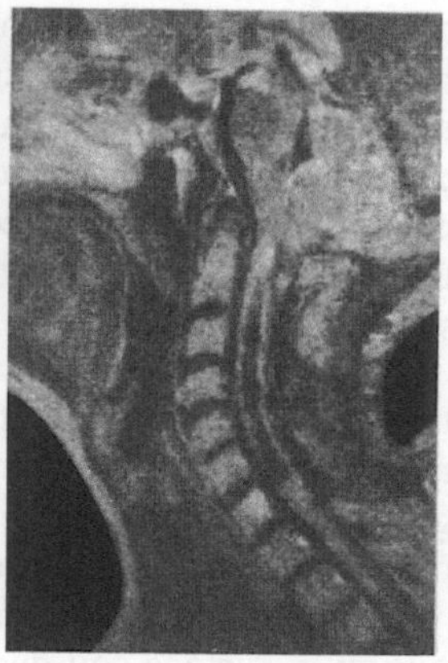

7.21

Fig. 7.20. Syringomyelia with atrophic cord in a 65-year-old man with slowly progressive spastic tetraparesis. Sagittal scan, both SE 0.4 s/17 ms (1.0 T)

Fig. 7.21. Syringomyelia. Pulsatile flow within the syrinx causes flow void sign in the T_2-weighted image. Midsagittal scan, SE 1.6 s/120 ms (0.35 T). (Courtesy of Drs. Kuhn, Steen, and Terwey, Oldenburg, FRG)

T2 relaxation times equal to those of the surrounding cord, while the signal of edematous cord (e.g., in myelomalacia) can resemble that of cystic fluid [114]. However, the pulsatile movements of the syrinx fluid can cause the fluid to give a lower signal than its relaxation times would imply (CSF flow-void sign, Sherman and Citrin [128] (Fig. 7.21), so that the characteristics of the fluid cannot be evaluated on that basis. Flow-sensitive sequences, including cine studies with "fast" gradient echo sequences, can be employed to differentiate pulsatile and nonpulsatile flow within cystic intramedullary fluid spaces. Pulsatile flow usually is more extensive in larger cysts than in smaller fluid collections. Nonpulsatile cysts are described in association with malformations and trauma; tumor cysts also seem to be nonpulsatile in most cases [39, 129]. According to the initial experience of Enzman et al. [39], the absence or reduction of pulsatile flow seems to be an indicator of success after shunt operations of intramedullary cysts.

Partially cystic intramedullary gliomas can lead to similar problems of distinguishing solid and cystic tumor components, with potential for misinterpretation [123]. Cicatricial, gliotic reactions of nervous tissue can likewise alter the relaxation times, and this can pose problems of differentiation from tumorous causes (Fig. 7.18; see also Sect. 17.2.1).

The relaxation times, then, do not seem to provide an adequate criterion for differentiating tumor from cyst. Attention also must be given to morphologic features such as circularity, well-defined margins, and fluid-fluid levels. The ability to detect a cyst and evaluate its size and nature is crucial to proper patient selection for intramedullary tumor surgery and assessment of the prognosis.

The enhancement of tumor tissue on T1-weighted sequences after the intravenous injection of contrast agent (gadolinium chelate) enables more precise differentiation of tumor, cyst, and normal spinal cord. In our opinion, contrast medium should be used in all cases of syringomyelia, since a tumor as the underlying cause cannot be ruled out with certainty in the native scan. However, misinterpretation is still possible if tumor enhancement does not occur, or in cases where the cavity wall is thickened, scarred, and sclerotic. (For examples see Sect. 17.2.1.)

Image interpretation is very difficult in the frequent cases where cavitation of the spinal cord is accompanied by kyphoscoliosis of the spine, because the deformity prevents visualization of a long spinal segment and often leads to troublesome partial volume effects. If doubt exists, axial scans can help to avoid false-negative findings in sagittal images due to partial volume effects and can also demonstrate the eccentric or central position of the cavity within the spinal cord [114, 36, 71, 60], which is of major interest for the explanation of clinical symptoms (Fig. 7.22).

Image quality in the thoracic spine region can be degraded by cardiac and respiratory movements, making it necessary to employ ECG and respiratory gating, fast image sequences, and surface coils to overcome these difficulties.

Further improvements in image quality aided by optimum surface coil designs, zoom technique, and three-dimensional data acquisition will refine the diagnosis of spinal cord cavities, rendering conventional myelography and CT myelography obsolete. To differentiate patent and occluded tubes after shunt operations in syringomyelia by means of MR, thin slices will be necessary in order to avoid volume averaging. Intrathecal contrast medium is still necessary, however, to determine whether the intramedullary cavities communicate with the ventricular system or with the subarachnoid space. Potential artifacts caused by pulsatile CSF flow on MR images of the spinal canal are discussed in Sect. 5.3 (see Figs. 5.30, 5.31).

Duplication of the Spinal Cord

Hori et al. [59] have subdivided duplication of the spinal cord into three groups:

Dimyelia is a complete duplication of the spinal cord in which each cord has a complete set of roots.

In *diplomyelia* an isolated accessory spinal cord lies either ventral or dorsal to the normal cord and lacks nerve roots [88].

Diastematomyelia involves a bifurcation of the spinal cord into two hemicords. They may occupy a common dural sheath, separated from each other by vascular connective tissue, or each may have its own dural sheath, the two sheaths being separated by a bony or fibrous septum [66, 76, 88]. If a septum does not exist, individual pial sheaths are present, but the dural and arachnoid sheaths are shared [88]. Although several reasonable theories have been postulated, the pathogenesis of diastematomyelia remains unclear. There is always an associated spina bifida, usually occult, and scoliosis exists in 50% of cases. If a septum is present, scans generally will show a narrowing of the intervertebral spaces at the affected level, decreased height of the vertebral bodies, and anomalies of the laminae [58].

CT and MR Findings

It is important to distinguish between diplomyelia and diastematomyelia, as the surgical treatment of the former involves excision of the accessory spinal cord, which has no connection with the normal cord, whereas the treatment of diastematomyelia involves removal of the fibrous, bony, or cartilaginous spur [59].

CT studies have shown that diastematomyelia without a septum (split cord) is twice as common as the spur variety [127] (Figs. 7.23, 7.24).

In the absence of a bony spur, the vertebral anomalies are less pronounced. Whereas the split spinal cord may reunite caudal to the spur in the septum variety (Fig. 7.25), each cord has a low tethered conus in the type without a septum. Usually the hemicords are approximately the same size [43].

MR is superior to CT in its ability to display this malformation in its entirety, although CT can demonstrate a bony spur with greater clarity than MR [53]. The radiopacity of compact bone is unmistakable on CT scans, whereas its low signal on MR images can have multiple interpretations.

Statements made in Sect. 7.2 apply with equal validity to examinations of this spinal cord anomaly. Fatty tissues (bone marrow, lipoma) can be identified by their intense, often nonhomogeneous signal when short imaging parameters are used. The signal from cysts (syringomyelia) is homogeneous, but its intensity depends on the nature of the cystic contents (see above). Proton-density and T2-weight-

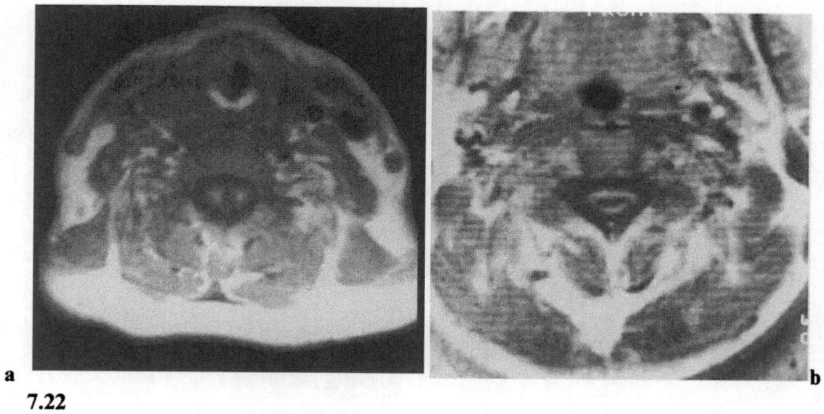

Fig. 7.22 a, b. Syringomyelia with different kinds of transverse extension of the cavity: **a** in the sagittal plane; **b** in the coronal plane. Axial scans: **a** SE 0.5 s/30 ms (1.0 T); **b** SE 0.6 s/30 ms (0.5 T). (Courtesy of Drs. Kuhn, Steen, and Terwey, Oldenburg, FRG)

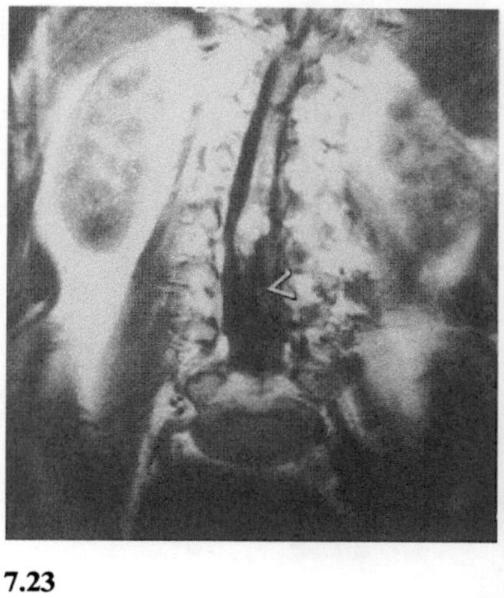

Fig. 7.23. Diastematomyelia in a 50-year-old man with spina bifida, myelocele, and incomplete paraparesis; disturbances of bladder function during childhood. Widening of lumbosacral canal, tethered split cord with bony spur *(arrowhead);* the partly hyperintense signal of the thickened cord indicates lipoma. Coronal section, SE 0.6 s/30 ms (0.5 T). (Courtesy of Drs. Kuhn, Steen, and Terwey, Oldenburg, FRG)

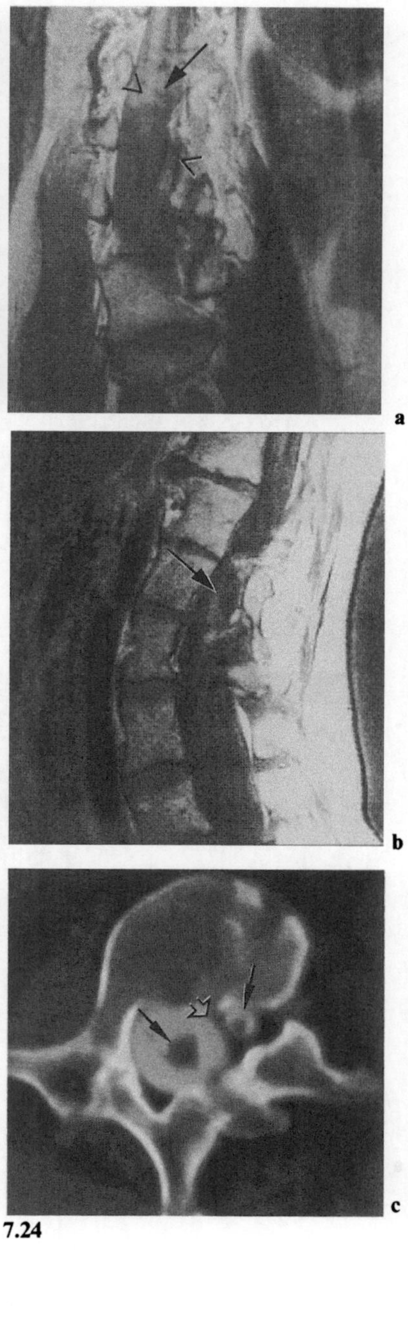

Fig. 7.24 a–c. Diastematomyelia, spur variety, in a 46-year-old woman with spasticity of lower extremities. Marked deformity of lumbar spine and vertebrae with enlarged spinal canal. **a** Split cord *(arrowheads)* on both sides of a spur *(arrow)*. CT myelography shows septum between the two cords (**c** open arrow), separate CSF spaces, and rotation of the two hemicords (arrows). **a** Coronal scan, **b** sagittal scan, SE 0.6 s/24 ms (1.0 T)

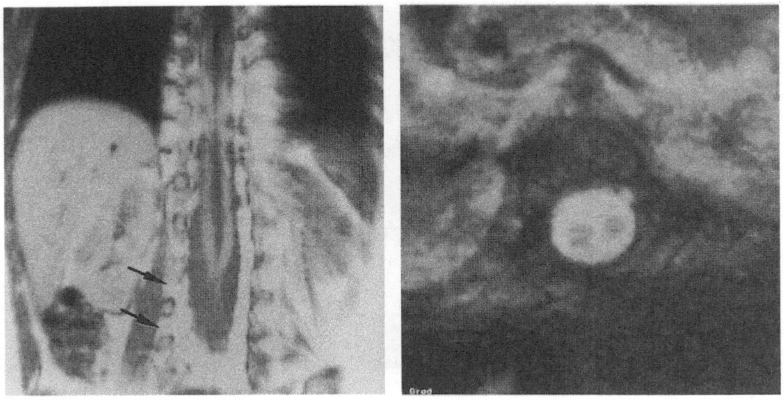

a b

Fig. 7.25 a, b. Diastematomyelia in a 3½-year-old girl with hypotrophy and loss of tendon reflexes of left leg, nevus and doughy swelling in the lumbar region. Spina bifida on CT. MR shows widening of lumbosacral canal and low tethered conus; the split cord reunites at its lower end. In the lower portion of the spinal canal, epidural lipoma is seen with nerve roots *(arrows)* on the right side. Differences of signal intensity of CSF are probably due to flow effects. Coronal scan (**a**) SE 0.4 s/30 ms, axial scan (**b**) FLASH 10°/100 ms/16 ms (1.5 T). (Courtesy of Dr. Schroth, University of Tübingen, FRG)

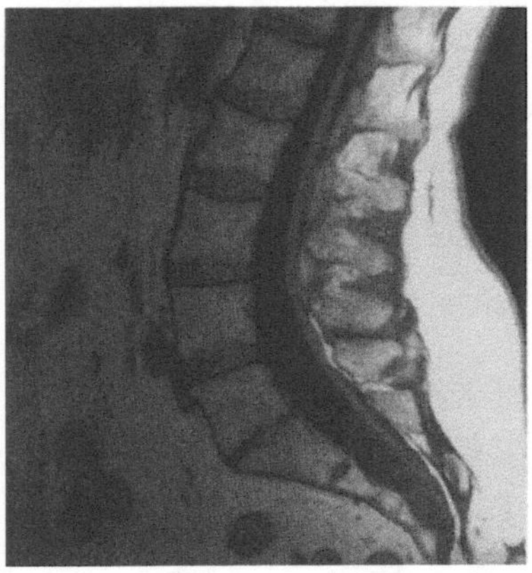

Fig. 7.26. Tethered cord in a 63-year-old woman with progressive disturbance of micturition and bowel movements. Enlargement of sacral canal, thickened filum stretched against the posterior wall of the lumbosacral canal (finding confirmed by surgery). Midsagittal section, SE 0.5 ms/17 ms (1.0 T)

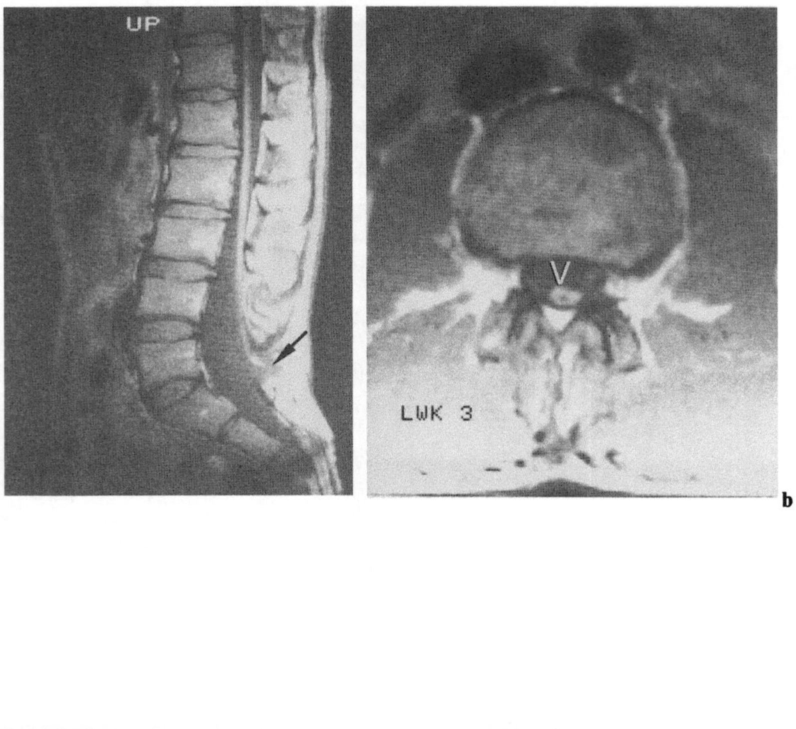

a b

Fig. 7.27 a, b. Tethered cord in a 32-year-old man with back pain, spastic paraparesis, and disturbances of micturition and bowel movement. **a** Wide lumbosacral canal; the low tip of the conus is fixed to a dysraphic defect *(arrow)*. **b** At the level of L3 hydromyelia is visible *(arrowhead)*. **a** Midsagittal scan, **b** axial scan, SE 0.5 s/22 ms (0.5 T). (Courtesy of Drs. Kuhn, Steen, and Terwey, Oldenburg, FRG)

ed sequences can be used to differentiate the various components of a septum (bone, cartilage, fibrous septum) and other extramedullary structures with an accuracy not attainable on T1-weighted scans. A bony spur can be identified by the fat signal of its marrow [53].

Tethered Cord

Tethered cord or conus, known also as tethered filum or filum terminale syndrome, involves an abnormally low position of the conus medullaris, usually accompanied by a thickened filum terminale. The tip of the conus is normally at the level of L2–L3 at the age of 2 years and at the mid-L2 level in 12-year-olds [45]. A conus tip below the L2–L3 interspace is considered to be pathologic.

Normally the filum terminale is lax and occupies a dorsal position in the spinal canal, terminating at the sacral ligament. In the tethered cord, the filum appears tightly stretched against the posterior wall of the lumbar spinal canal (Figs. 7.26, 7.27; see also Fig. 7.16).

The embryology of this malformation is based on inhibition of the normal ascent of the spinal cord.

As longitudinal body growth proceeds a variety of symptoms can appear, such as leg weakness or shortening, abnormal reflexes, foot deformities, scoliosis, back pain, and bladder dysfunction [48, 57, 78]. Cutaneous abnormalities such as hypertrichosis or hemangioma may be noted over the lumbar region and sacrum.

Morphologic findings in tethered cord vary with the severity of the malformation:

Type 1: The conus ends a whole or a half vertebra lower than normal, and the filum terminale is thickened (normal diameter 1.5 mm).

Type 2: Irregularities containing fatty tissue are seen over part or all the length of the abnormal filum terminale (Fig. 7.28).

Type 3: The conus lacks a well-defined tip and gradually tapers to a tube of irregular thickness (5–8 mm in diameter). This tube may represent a filum terminale surrounded by fatty tissue, but often it consists of cord tissue, and a definite filum is not present [44, 78]. In the latter case the long lumbar roots do not pass downward at a sharp angle, but appear shortened and course laterally from the low conus to the corresponding intervertebral foramina.

Lipomas (see below) are commonly seen in association with a tethered cord. Most occur on the dorsal aspect of the spinal cord. With tethered cord the dysraphic changes are less pronounced, and the intraspinal lipoma generally lacks communication with the subcutaneous fat, as is seen in lipomeningomyelocele (Figs. 7.29, 7.30). However, type 3 tethered cord can be difficult to distinguish from lipomeningomyelocele (see above) in cases where the lipoma has infiltrated the spinal cord and has transdural extensions [44, 78].

Besides the patient's neurologic status, Chuang et al. [17] believe that the demonstration of a low position of the conus or a thickened filum is sufficient indication for surgical treatment.

Lipoma

Intraspinal lipomas occur in association with various dysraphic conditions (see above) but can also occur as isolated lesions; these account for less than 1% of spinal tumors [124, 78], and most commonly involve the cervical and thoracic portions of the spine [78]. They generally lie posterior to the spinal cord, often spanning several segments, and may proceed to infiltrate the cord. Isolated lipomas of the cervical and thoracic region are described more frequently in males, and most remain asymptomatic until adulthood (see Fig. 17.22) [4, 43]. Lumbar lipomas are associated with progressive neurologic deficits in 56% of cases where there is a coexisting tethered cord and involvement of the cauda equina roots (e.g., hypertrophy, atrophy, infiltration with fibrous tissue or fat) [113].

With penetration of the dura, the possibility of a lipomeningomyelocele should be considered.

Dermoids, Epidermoids and Dermal Sinuses

Dermoids, epidermoids, and dermal sinuses develop from heterotopic epithelial cell rests that became isolated due to incomplete separation of the cutaneous and neural ectoderm during neural tube closure [7, 43]. Epidermoids contain only superficial skin elements (Fig. 7.31), while dermoids include glandular follicular elements [44, 78]. They are more prevalent in females than males [56, 43]; most are extramedullary and involve the lumbar region. Dermoids and epidermoids comprise 10% of all intraspinal tumors in patients under 15 years of age [51, 43].

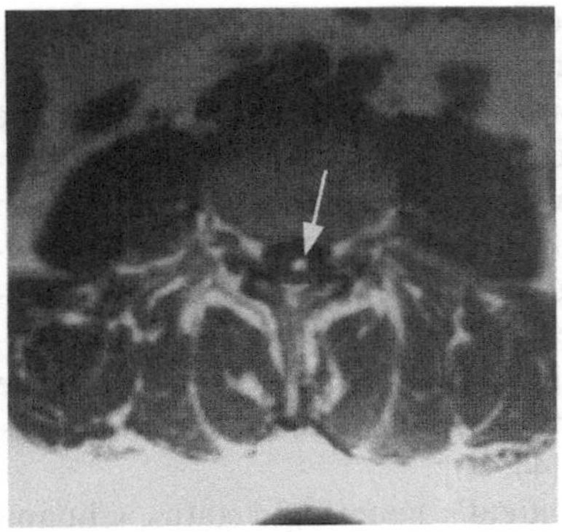

Fig. 7.28. Tethered cord in a 51-year-old man with slight symptoms of bladder dysfunction. The thickened filum or cord contains fatty tissue causing the high signal intensity *(arrow)*. Axial scan at level of L4, both SE 0.7 s/30 ms (1.0 T)

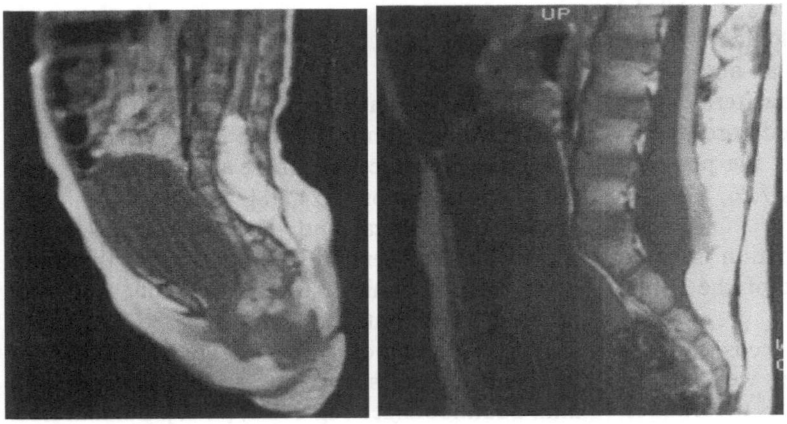

a b

Fig. 7.29 a, b. Tethered cord with lipomeningocele in a 6-month-old girl with bladder dysfunction and weekness of left leg, and dermal sinus of the lumbar region. **a** Large lumbosacral canal and large intraspinal (and intradural) lipoma with extension into the subcutaneous fat. At surgery the lipoma was infiltrating the spinal cord and roots. **b** Control at the age of 2 years. Midsagittal sections: a SE 1.8 s/30 ms (1.0 T); b SE 0.6 s/15 ms (1.5 T)

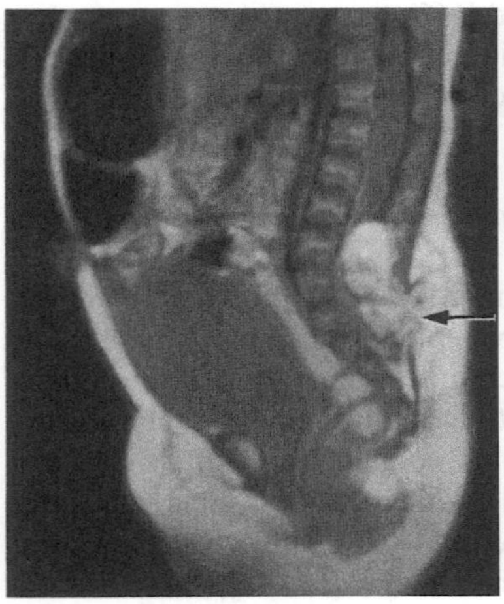

7.30

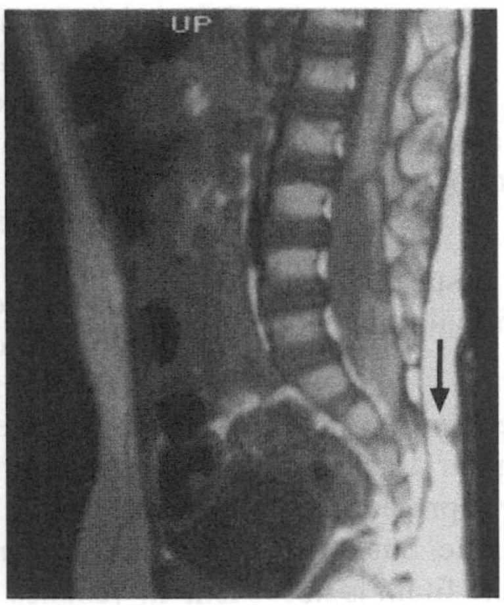

7.31

Fig. 7.30. Lipomyelomeningocele and hydromyelia of tethered cord in a 10-week-old girl with paraparesis and dysfunction of bladder and bowel. Enlarged caudal spinal canal with syringo-/hydromyelia of the tethered cord over a length of at least five segments. Large intraspinal lipoma in the lumbosacral region merging with a subcutaneous lipoma through a major dysraphic defect *(arrow)*. Midsagittal scan, SE 1.6 s/35 ms (1.0 T)

Fig. 7.31. Epidermoid in a 19-month-old girl with dermal sinus and a history of meningitis soon after birth. Dilated lumbar canal filled with a tumor that extends from the conus to the sacrum. In the T1-weighted image an inhomogeneous structure of the tumor is seen. At surgery an epidermoid tumor was found which included fatty contents and also hair. The nerve roots were attached to the tumor sac on both sides. The dermal sinus is indicated by a hypointense band *(arrow)* within the subcutaneous fat. Sagittal scan SE 0.5 s/30 ms (1.0 T)

Teratomas

Teratomas are very rare congenital tumors that contain tissues from all three germ layers. Most are small, spanning only one or two spinal segments. They may be intramedullary and/or extramedullary in location [44] and have both solid and cystic components that may contain fatty tissue and calcifications [130]. If nonsolid elements are identified, the diagnosis can be made without difficulty. Solid tumor elements are indistinguishable from astrocytoma. A cyst with no fatty components can mimic both forms.

MR Findings

The selection of MR techniques and imaging planes is discussed in Sect. 7.2.

Fat in dermoids, epidermoids, lipomas, and in the marrow of cancellous bone spurs appears light on T1-weighted images, while CSF, dura, and fibrous membranes appear dark. It is difficult or impossible to separate pathologic fatty tissue from normal subcutaneous and epidural fat.

One should be alert for partial volume artifacts in the spinal canal, which on sagittal scans can mimic a thickening of the conus medullaris at the junction of the conus and cauda equina. With significant lumbar lordosis or thoracic kyphosis, this can also create the impression of an abnormally low-sited conus, especially when imaging is performed with a long TR and TE [11]. In these cases coronal sections will indicate the position of the conus more accurately.

The value of intraspinal findings is somewhat limited by artifacts produced by CSF pulsations in the spinal canal. It is especially important to eliminate these artifacts when attempting to evaluate small medullary lesions (see also Sect. 5.3).

A dermal sinus is manifested externally by a small skin depression over the center of the lumbosacral spine. Some contain an opening to a fistulous tract that may extend into the spinal canal and communicate with a dermoid cyst. Bacterial infection and even meningitis may develop over the fistulous canal. The majority of dermal sinuses occur without associated tracts, however [56, 43].

7.4 Malformations of the Commissures and Midline Structures

7.4.1 Holoprosencephaly

Holoprosencephaly, the most severe malformation of the anterior telencephalic wall involves a failure of evagination of the telencephalic vesicles, and the prosencephalon remains "whole" (Greek: *holos*). The degree of involvement depends on the timing, location, and severity of the causal insult. Thus, for example, holotelencephaly, arhinencephaly, and olfactory hypoplasia may occur together or as isolated anomalies (see Sect. 7.1).

Demyer and coworkers [28, 29] have classified the holoprosencephalies into three forms:

- In *alobar holoprosencephaly* the telencephalon is not separated into hemispheres or lobes, instead forming a single mass with a single large ventricle. There is fusion of the thalami and corpora striata. The falx and corpus callosum are absent, a circumstance which distinguishes holoprosencephaly from extreme hydrocephalus, where a falx is present and the basal ganglia are separated [78]. The superior and inferior sagittal sinuses, straight sinus, and the internal veins are also absent [142]. Heterotopic gray matter may be demonstrated on the ventricular walls [116].

- In *semilobar holoprosencephaly* the prosencephalon is divided into hemispheres by a narrow, cranial longitudinal sulcus. The lobar structure is rudimentary, the corpus callosum is absent, and the basal ganglia may be fused. A rudimentary third ventricle, a posterior interhemispheric fissure, and a falx can usually be identified.

- In *lobar holoprosencephaly* the hemispheres are largely separated except in their anterior portions. The cortex of the hemispheres remains connected at the base of the longitudinal fissure. The frontal lobes are hypoplastic, and the pituitary is absent. The corpus callosum and rhinencephalon may be absent or incomplete, a communication exists between the bodies of the lateral ventricles, and the thalami and basal ganglia may be fused. The frontal horns may have a square shape and the roof of the ventricles may be flattened as a result of hypoplasia of the corpus callosum (see also septo-optic dysplasia) [78]. A hydrocephalus is present in 80% of cases [92] (Fig. 7.32).

Coexisting anomalies include facial dysplasias, with cyclopia as the most severe form, hypo- and hypertelorism, medial cleft lip and palate, CNS malformations (migration disorders, hydrocephalus, dysraphic anomalies, etc.), and occipital encephalocele.

CT and MR Findings

The pathologic changes of this syndrome can be analyzed best with MR. Selection of MR techniques and imaging planes is discussed in Sect. 7.2.

In the *alobar form,* the single ventricle may present a horseshoe shape on axial CT and MR images because of the central thalami, and this can mimic the development of temporal horns [42].

Differentiation of the semilobar and lobar forms, which relies chiefly on the configuration of the ventricular system, can be difficult with CT [43]. In the *semilobar type* with absence of the anterior interhemispheric fissure, the anterior cerebral artery courses on the outer surface of the prosencephalon; in the *lobar type* the vessel lies deeper between the hemispheres. MR can demonstrate the course of the arteries in relation to the abnormal anatomy of the brain, facilitating the differential diagnosis. The good gray matter-white matter contrast makes it easy to distinguish cerebral cortex below the interhemispheric fissure from a corpus callosum (e.g., in the lobar form) on coronal scans. Similarly, heterotopic gray matter can be identified far more readily with MR than with CT.

7.4.2 Agenesis of the Corpus Callosum

Agenesis of the corpus callosum is an accompanying feature of holoprosencephaly, Dandy-Walker syndrome, Aicardi's syndrome, and other complex malformations, but it may also occur as an isolated anomaly. Absence of the corpus callosum may be either partial or complete, and usually the posterior part is more severely affected when the agenesis is partial. The anterior, posterior, and hippocampal commissures also may be absent. The third ventricle is often dilated posteriorly and may open directly onto the surface of the brain. A thick, longitudinal bundle of myelinated fibers (Probst's bundle), often found on the superior surface of the lateral ventricles, is thought to contain misdirected fibers intended for the corpus callosum (Fig. 7.33).

On coronal sections the ventricles present pointed upper corners ("bat-wing" ventricular shape) [76, 88], whereas holospheric ventricles present a round margin even when they are partially separated. In the axial projection the lateral ventricles are parallel to each other and are spaced abnormally far apart [42]. Frequently the occipital horns are dilated (Fig. 7.40).

In the sagittal projection the supracallosal gyri present a radial arrangement, the cingulate gyrus is absent, and the parieto-occipital and calcarine sulci fail to intersect. The hippocampus is hypoplastic. The leaves of the septum pellucidum, which often is absent, are widely separated and arise from a band of gray and white matter consisting of the central gray nuclei and extending from the paraolfactory cortex up to the bundle of Probst (Fig. 7.33). Agenesis of the corpus callosum is commonly accompanied by a central cyst, whose location between the hemispheres serves to distinguish it from the cyst of holoprosencephaly, which lies above and behind the solitary ventricle (Fig. 7.34).

CT and MR Findings

MR is the method of choice for the direct visualization of agenesis of the corpus callosum [21, 53]. Johnson and Bydder [67] have traced the normal development of the corpus callosum on MR images. The corpus callosum develops in a rostrocaudal direction, dorsal to the lamina terminalis, the splenium being the last part to appear [19]. T1-weighted sagittal and coronal images can clearly demonstrate the absence of the corpus callosum, the abnormal gyral contour, and the upward and backward course of the anterior cerebral artery at the level of the internal veins.

Axial MR images and axial CT scans may fail to demonstrate hypoplasia or partial agenesis of the corpus callosum, especially in children.

Partial agenesis tends to affect the posterior part of the corpus and the splenium most severely (Fig. 7.33). The ratio of corpus callosum to cerebrum, determined by measuring the greatest anteroposterior diameter of both structures, is less than the normal value of 0.45 [21, 19]. Along with the corpus callosum, development of the *limbic system* also is deficient in most cases [6].

Partial or complete agenesis of the corpus callosum may be associated with an interhemispheric cyst or lipoma, encephalocele, and heterotopia of gray matter (see below) (Figs. 7.34, 7.35, 7.39).

Changes in the normal shape of the corpus callosum can have diagnostic significance, as, for example, in Aicardi's syndrome [19]. The splenium may be hypoplastic (the normal diameter being

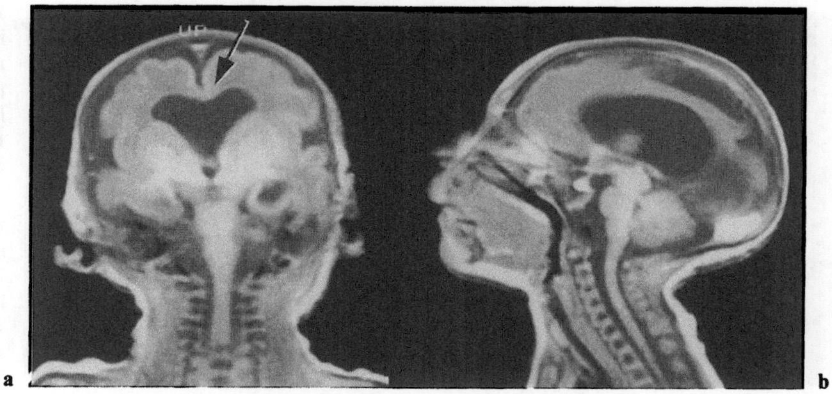

Fig. 7.32 a, b. Lobar holoprosencephaly in an 11-day-old-boy. The hemispheres are connected at the base of the interhemispheric fissure *(arrow)*; the corpus callosum is absent. The pituitary seems to be present. **a** Coronal scan, **b** midsagittal scan, SE 0.7 s/30 ms (1.0 T)

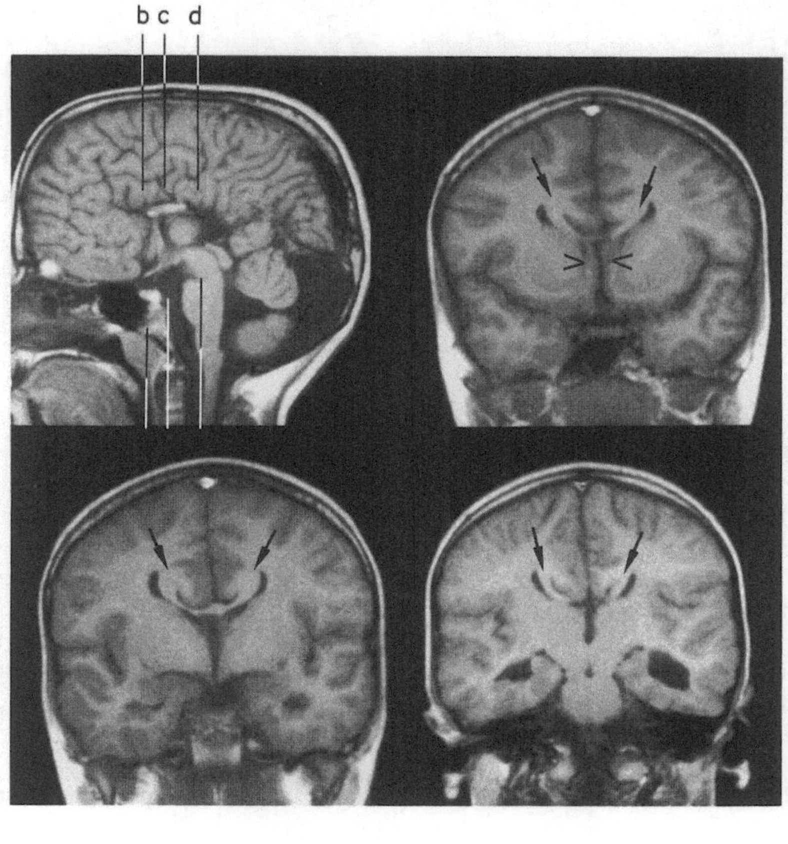

Fig. 7.33 a–d. Subtotal agenesis of corpus callosum in a 12-year-old girl with cerebral seizures. Macrocephaly, stenogyria/polymicrogyria, ectopias, subtotal aplasia of corpus callosum, hypoplastic fornix, separation of leaves of septum pellucidum *(arrowheads)*, Dandy-Walker variant. See also text. Notice the course of Probst's bundle *(arrows)* separating like a "zipper" in anterior-posterior direction. Lines in (**a**) indicate the position of the coronal sections (**b–d**). All images SE 0.4 s/17 ms (1.0 T)

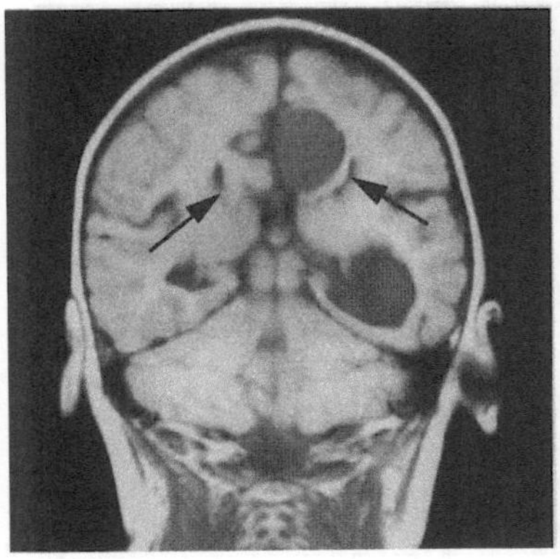

Fig. 7.34

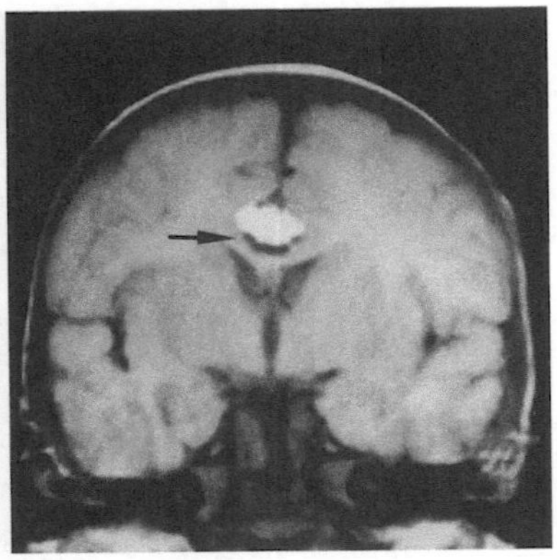

Fig. 7.35

Fig. 7.34. Agenesis of corpus callosum in a 1-year-old girl with psychomotor retardation. Complete absence of corpus callosum, interhemispheric cyst, unilateral hydrocephalus, and polygyria. Probst's bundle *(arrows)*. Coronal Scan, SE 0.5 s/30 ms (1.0 T)

Fig. 7.35. Lipoma of the corpus callosum in a 1½-year-old girl with seizures. Hypoplasia of corpus callosum. Large lipoma overlying the splenium. The low signal of peripheral calcifications *(arrow)* is nonspecific. Coronal scan, SE 2.5 s/35 ms (1.0 T)

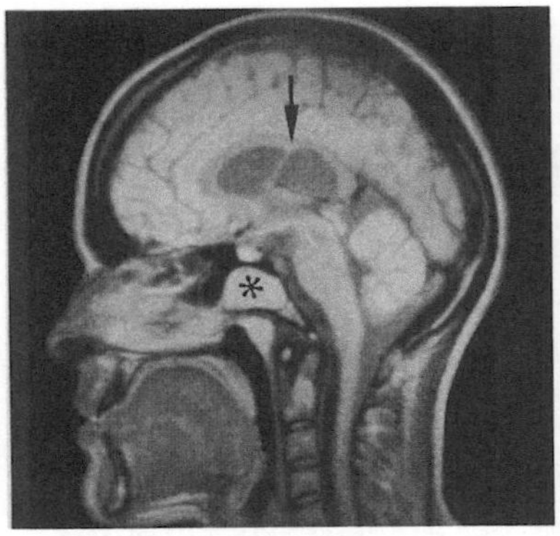

Fig. 7.36

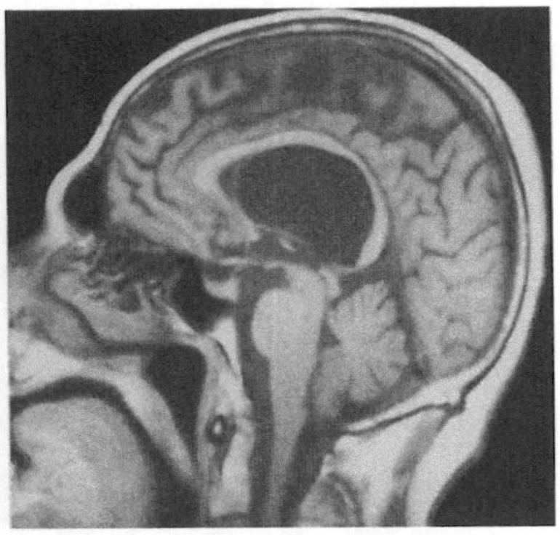

Fig. 7.37

Fig. 7.36. Cavum septi pellucidi and cavum vergae in a 20-year-old woman with headache. The fornix *(arrow)* indicates the borderline between the cysts. No signs of hydrocephalus; the mucocele of the sphenoid sinus *(asterisk)* is probably the cause of the patient's complaints. Midsagittal scan, SE 1.6 s/35 ms (1.0 T)

Fig. 7.37. Cavum vergae cyst in a 54-year-old man with headache and occasional dizziness. Large cyst with upward bulging and elongation of corpus callosum and macrocephaly. No signs of acute obstruction of CSF flow. Midsagittal scan, SE 0.4 s/17 ms (1.0 T)

1.5–2.0 cm according to Ben-Amour and Billewicz [12], leading to absence of the normal clublike thickening and abnormal dilatation of the galenic cistern.

Lipomas of the corpus callosum are conspicuous on T1-weighted images because of their high signal intensity. However, the peripheral calcifications usually present in these tumors are not displayed as well as on CT scans (Fig. 7.35).

7.4.3 Anomalies of the Septum Pellucidum

One or both leaves of the septum pellucidum may be absent in anomalies of this structure. The defect may be the only brain anomaly, or it may be part of a complex malformation (see above). It must, however, be distinguished from cases of secondary destruction of the septum pellucidum due to hydrocephalus. In these cases small remnants of the septum may be seen [88]. Absence of the septum pellucidum may resemble a mild form of lobar holoprosencephaly but is distinguished by the fact that the frontal horns of the lateral ventricles are less square and show an approximately normal configuration. A similar differentiation can be made, according to Probst [116], by identifying the fornices on the floor of the frontal horns of the lateral ventricles in patients with aplasia of the septum pellucidum (see Fig. 7.33).

Septo-optic Dysplasia

Septo-optic dysplasia [27, 42] consists of agenesis of the septum pellucidum and hypoplasia of the optic pathways (optic discs, chiasm, optic nerves and pituitary infundibulum). The frontal horns of the lateral ventricles are usually slightly dilated and present an angular outline that tapers to a point inferiorly. The roofs of the ventricles are flat, and the falx and interhemispheric fissure are normally

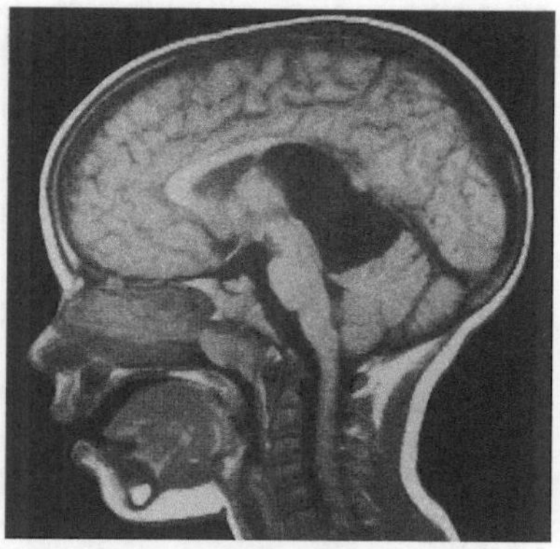

Fig. 7.38. Cyst of cavum veli interpositi in a 5-year-old boy with suspected hydrocephalus. Large cyst in the region of the quadrigeminal cistern with deformation of adjacent anatomical structures (e.g., tectum, corpus callosum, vermis, thalamus). Occlusive hydrocephalus of posterior portions of left lateral ventricle. As the cyst probably does not communicate with the subarachnoid space, an arachnoid cyst has to be included in the differential diagnosis. Midsagittal scan, SE 0.4 s/30 ms (0.5 T). Courtesy of Drs. Kuhn, Steen, and Terwey, Oldenburg, FRG)

developed. The optic recess of the slightly dilated third ventricle is enlarged, the infundibular recess is hypoplastic, and there is concomitant expansion of the chiasmatic cistern [78]. Both optic nerves are small [56].

CT and MR Findings

The pathoanatomic features of septo-optic dysplasia are best appreciated on multiplanar MR images obtained with T1-weighted sequences.

The slight dilatation of the third ventricle and enlargement of the optic recess, which Newton et al. [104] interpret as a persistent expansion of the primitive optic ventricle, are not displayed well on axial CT or MR images. The same can be said of the vertical configuration of the optic chiasm that frequently exists in this anomaly [19].

Cavum Septi Pellucidi, Cavum Vergae, and Cavum Veli Interpositi

With the rostrocaudal development of the corpus callosum, the cavity of the septum pellucidum extends farther dorsally. Sometimes the cavum septi pellucidi has a posterior extension, the cavum vergae, each cavity communicating freely with the other. Very rarely [88] a cavum vergae may be present without a cavum septi pellucidi, but Larroche [76] states that this is never the case.

The *cavum septi pellucidi* is always patent in the fetus and is lined by glial tissue [141]. The cavity persists in up to 82% of newborns [100] and in 12%-20% of adults, at which time it is lined by ependyma [86]. Generally these cavities are asymptomatic when they communicate freely with the ventricular system, but some may exist as large cysts which can block the foramen of Monro and lead to ventricular dilatation with an (often intermittent) rise of pressure (Fig. 7.36).

A *cavum vergae* can be demonstrated in only 30% of newborns [100]. The narrow passage between the cavum septi pellucidi and the cavum vergae is formed by the fornices. The cavum vergae is bounded posteriorly by the splenium of the corpus callosum (Figs. 7.36, 7.37).

The *cavum veli interpositi* is a CSF-filled cistern that lies upon the third ventricle and below the corpus callosum. It tends to communicate with the quadrigeminal cistern rather than with the ventricular system and occurs in association with a cavum septi pellucidi and cavum vergae [78] (Fig. 7.38).

MR Findings

Selection of MR techniques and imaging planes is discussed in Sect. 7.2.

These anomalies of the central ventricles of the brain are displayed most effectively on sagittal and coronal T1-weighted images.

7.5 Anomalies of Cell Migration

The excellent gray matter-white matter contrast of proton-density SE images, T2-weighted images, and especially IR images, together with the ability to demonstrate anatomy on all spatial planes, provides a unique opportunity to study these structural anomalies of the brain parenchyma, which are not displayed well with CT.

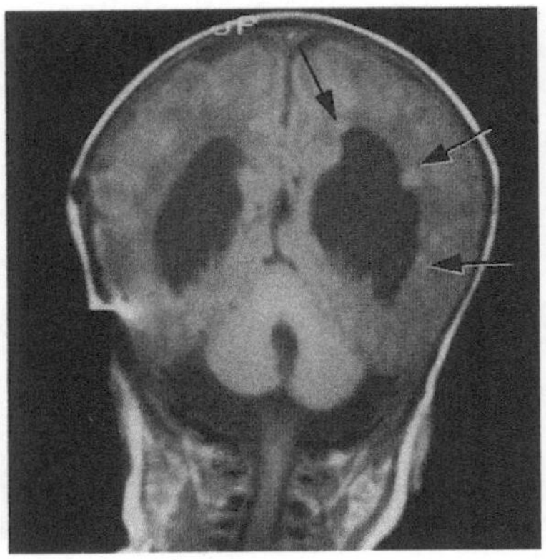

7.39

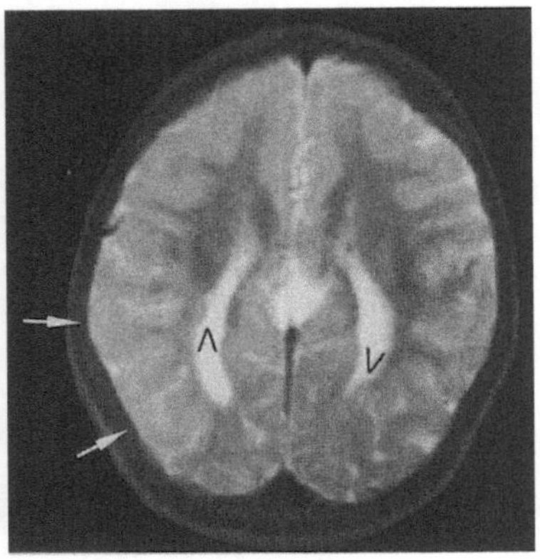

7.40

Fig. 7.39. Complex malformation in a 6-week-old boy: hydrocephalus associated with agenesis of corpus callosum, hypoplasia of cerebellum, and multiple ectopic foci of gray matter *(arrows)* on the wall of the ventricles. Coronal scan, SE 0.6 s/15 ms (1.5 T)

Fig. 7.40. Heterotopia in a 6-year-old boy with microcephaly and retardation of growth. Small nodules of ectopic gray matter at the lateral wall of the lateral ventricles *(arrowheads)* and regional anomalies of gyral architecture *(arrows)*, associated with partial agenesis of corpus callosum. Axial scan, SE 2.7 s/120 ms (1.0 T)

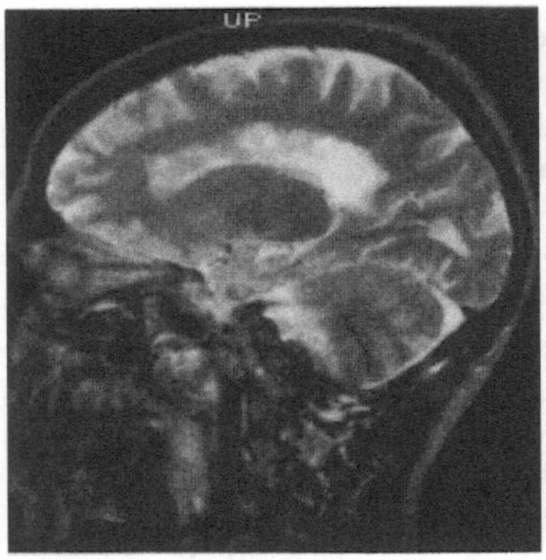

7.41

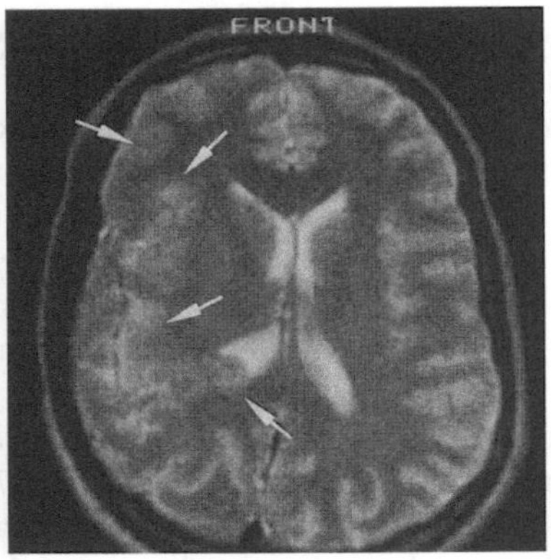

7.42

Fig. 7.41. Heterotopias in a 66-year-old woman with grand mal seizures. Pseudogyri are visible along the lateral walls of both lateral ventricules. Parasagittal scan, SE 3.0 s/120 ms (1.0 T)

Fig. 7.42. Heterotopias in a 24-year-old woman with epilepsy. Extensive area of ectopic gray matter *(arrows)* of the right hemisphere simulating glioma. Axial scan: SE 2.0 s/120 ms (1.0 T). (Courtesy of Dr. Dangel, Stuttgart, FRG)

7.5.1 Ectopias and Heterotopias

The ontogenic aspects of ectopias and heterotopias are discussed in Sect. 7.1.

These malformations consist of masses of nerve cells that become displaced during their migration from the periventricular germinal layer to their final cortical destination within the white matter. These ectopic neurons form irregularly shaped, nodular structures within the parenchyma located at varying distances from the ventricle, concentric stripes in the white matter, or radially arranged columns that recapitulate a normal neuronal migration [76]. These masses of ectopic gray matter vary in size from microscopically small foci (Fig. 7.39) to conglomerates up to 3 cm in diameter [135]. When they occur as small nodules on the walls of the lateral ventricles, the absence of associated calcification or gliosis distinguishes them from the subependymal nodules of tuberous sclerosis [24, 88].

Heterotopias and ectopic neurons occur most commonly in the cerebellum. They may be found in conjunction with polymicrogyria, pachygyria, agyria, microcephaly, or other complex malformations [76, 88] such as congenital aqueductal stenosis, agenesis of the corpus callosum, and dysgenesis of the cerebellum (see below) [135] (Fig. 7.40).

Patients with pronounced heterotopias may present with cerebral seizures and may manifest impairment of psychomotor development [8, 35, 79].

CT and MR Findings

These displaced foci of gray matter are easily missed on CT scans, or may be misidentified as tumorous masses [35]. On MR images the ectopic gray matter appears isointense with the cerebral cortex in all sequences [8, 24], a finding that may be regarded as pathognomonic.

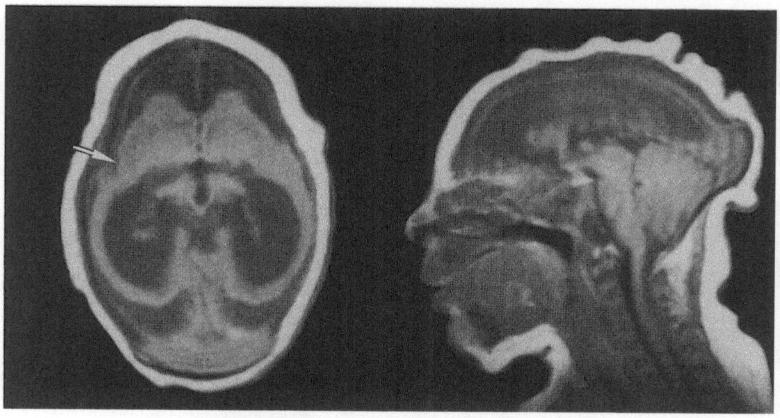

a b

Fig. 7.43 a, b. Lissencephaly in a 3-week-old boy. Microcephaly, smooth cortex with a shallow groove indicating the Sylvian fissure *(arrow)*, similar to fetal brain. The corpus callosum is absent. The small basal ganglia are not fused, the choroid plexus is present. Additionally the posterior fossa, cerebellum, and brainstem show Arnold-Chiari deformity. **a** axial scan, **b** sagittal scan, both SE 0.6 s/15 ms (1.5 T)

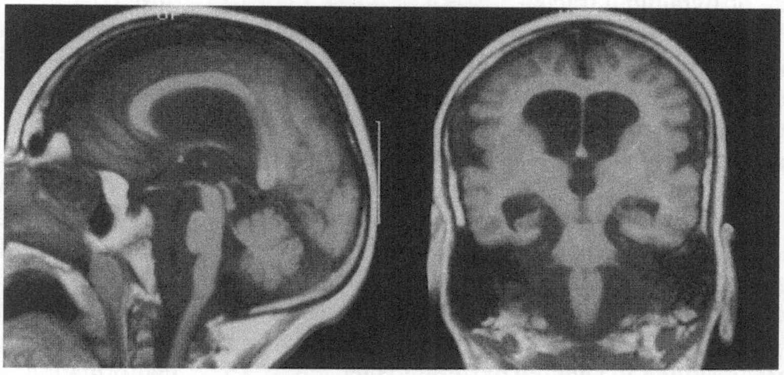

a b

Fig. 7.44 a, b. Pachygyria and lissencephaly in a 7-year-old boy with severe mental deficits, seizures, and microcephalus. Small brain with reduced number of broad gyri, diminution of white matter, hypotrophic brainstem, exposed operculum, hypoplastic claustrum, elongated corpus callosum, short falx. Diagnosis confirmed by biopsy. **a** Sagittal, **b** coronal scans, SE 0.4 s/17 ms (1.0 T)

Figure 7.41 shows parasagittal images from a 66-year-old woman exhibiting small, radially arranged gyri on the lateral ventricular wall that are isointense with the regular cerebral cortex. Correct identification of the heterotopic foci of gray matter is of clinical importance mainly when they occur as solitary nodules requiring differentiation from other focal masses. MR is superior to all other modalities in accomplishing this task (Fig. 7.42).

7.5.2 Agyria, Pachygyria, Lissencephaly; Polymicrogyria, Stenogyria; Status Verrucosus

Anomalies in the formation of cerebral fissures, gyri, and sulci are the combined result of failures of several developmental steps: migration of neuroepithelial cells from the periventricular germinal layer to the cortical mantle; further maturation of these cells once they have reached the cortical mantle; and, in many cases, adequate cell proliferation, as many of these brains are small. The latter failure also may be explained in terms of increased cell death [88].

Agyria, pachygyria, lissencephaly are the most severe forms of these neuronal migration defects. They are characterized by the presence of a few broad gyri separated by only the primary fissures and sulci. These changes may be focal or generalized (Figs. 7.43, 7.44). The *gray matter* is abnormally thick and may extend almost to the ventricular wall. The cortex consists microscopically of four layers: a molecular layer, a thick gray zone of densely packed nerve cells, a layer of white matter, and a layer of periventricular gray matter [76]. The fourth layer is often the thickest and is thought to contain neurons arrested in their migration [88]. In many cases, however, the four-layered structure is not found; instead, there is a single, thick, relatively homogeneous layer of cells in which it is difficult to

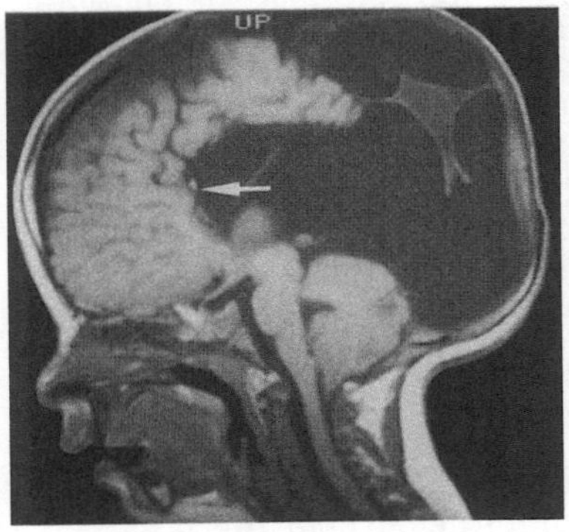

Fig. 7.45. Complex malformation in a 2-year-old boy with severe mental retardation. Macrocephaly, agenesis of corpus callosum (anterior commissure is present: *arrow*), polymicrogyria/stenogyria, large monoventricle with wide opening to the interhemispheric fissure, porencephalic defects, probably atresia of aqueduct, Arnold-Chiari type I deformity. The pituitary is not seen. Sagittal scan, SE 0.6 s/15 ms (1.0 T)

recognize individual laminae [88]. A marked reduction of white matter is related to the diminution in size of pyramidal tracts.

The falx is either short or absent, the ventricles may be enlarged (colpocephaly), and nodules of heterotopic gray matter bulge beneath the ependyma [76]. The claustrum, which shares its origin with the insular cortex, often is missing bilaterally [31].

Polymicrogyria is more common than pachygyria [18]. It consists of an increased number of small, closely packed gyri that resemble the surface of a cauliflower or create an appearance that has been described as "cobblestones" or "moroccan leather" [76, 88]. The molecular layers of several gyri may fuse, resulting in shallow or absent sulci.

The microgyria may occur in irregular patches or diffusely and may be confined to a single vascular distribution, usually that of the middle cerebral artery. The cortical pattern varies from area to area [88]. A four-layered cortical structure similar to that in pachygyria is occasionally seen in polymicrogyria and is important for the diagnosis of this anomaly. In other cases the cells of the cortex may show a chaotic arrangement [76].

Regarding the pathogenesis and time of occurrence of polymicrogyria, authors have postulated both a malformative cause and a postdestructive cause occurring at a somewhat later stage in development [106].

Microgyria has also been described in association with other syndromes, such as incontinentia pigmenti. Polymicrogyria must be distinguished from ulegyria, which is described in Sect. 7.6.

The term *"stenogyria"* was introduced by Muller [99] to describe a condition where an increased number of small, closely packed gyri is seen (Fig. 7.45). In contrast to polymicrogyria, the architecture of the cellular layers of the cortex is undisturbed in stenogyria. This anomaly has been described in association with malformations of the corpus callosum and in the Arnold-Chiari syndrome.

Status verrucosus, also known as nodular cortical dysplasia (Friede 1975), is very rare. It consists of superficial round cortical nodules composed of nerve and glial cells that are irregularly oriented and gliotic ("brain warts") [18]. In these nodules the second and third cellular layers prolapse through the molecular layer, which is frequently thinned or absent. Sometimes the nodule contains a blood vessel at its center. The "warts" may be found on an otherwise normal brain but often are associated with polymicrogyria (see above) [18, 76] or another malformation.

MR Findings

MR is the modality of choice for the diagnosis of these anomalies (see also Sect. 7.2).

Sequences providing good gray matter-white matter contrast demonstrate the altered "interdigitation" of the white and gray matter, heterotopias, and ectopias; enlarged ventricles are seen in many cases. These changes are well displayed on axial and coronal scans. The altered cortical pattern is best appreciated on T1-weighted sagittal and coronal images.

In lissencephaly there is a lack of development of the frontal and temporal opercula, creating the appearance of a deep or only shallow cleft in the region of the sylvian fissure [78], with widening of the subarachnoid spaces (Fig. 7.43). In a case published by Krawinkel et al. [72] the ratio of gray to white matter was altered, the claustrum was absent, and only the frontal part of the external capsule was visible.

The IR sequence is best for evaluating the abnormal four-cell-layer cortex, because it gives the best gray matter–white matter contrast. At present the spatial resolution of MR is inadequate to define the lamination of the cortex, but use of the zoom technique may enable the cortical architecture to be studied in greater detail.

7.6 Destructive Anomalies

Destructive lesions may involve most of the white matter, with extensive cavitation, or may be limited to the territory of one or more cerebral arteries. The divisions between hydranencephaly, porencephaly, and multicystic encephalopathy are ill defined, as the development of these lesions depends on the timing and extent of the damage and on survival time [76].

7.6.1 Hydranencephaly

Hydranencephaly, the most severe of the destructive anomalies, is characterized by an almost complete absence of the cerebral hemispheres except for the basal portions and the occipital and temporal lobes (Fig. 7.46). A large membranous sac whose wall consists of pia-arachnoid and a gliotic layer occupies the cranial cavity. Usually the basal ganglia are normal, but they may be hypertrophied and deformed [143, 144]. The head size in patients with hydranencephaly may be normal or increased.

MR Findings

Selection of MR techniques and imaging planes is discussed in Sect. 7.2.

MR shows remnants of cerebral tissue and can demonstrate anatomic details that are helpful in making a differential diagnosis: If very little brain tissue is present, the condition can resemble an extreme hydrocephalus. But whereas the cerebral arteries in hydrocephalus are found to be tightly stretched over the hemispheres, only a few atretic vessels are seen at the base of the brain in hydranencephaly.

Occasionally it is necessary to consider alobar holoprosencephaly (see Sect. 7.4) in the differential diagnosis. This condition is characterized by the presence of an unpaired anterior cerebral artery, which apposes to the far anterior part of the cranial vault due to the absence of hemispheric separation [78]. These diagnostically important cerebral arteries can be delineated with MR. Usually the falx cerebri is well developed in patients with hydranencephaly [42].

7.6.2 Porencephaly

Yakovlev et al. [142, 144] originally subdivided the porencephalies into encephaloclastic defects (due to destructive or vascular insults) and developmental defects [119]. Ludwin and Norman [88] believe that almost all such lesions are due to necrosis of the brain tissue from various causes, and that a migrational disorder results when the damage occurs during cell migration. For example, a vascular insult occurring during or after the 24th week can lead to polymicrogyria, evidence of a local failure of migration or a disorganized, incomplete repair of the defect. In porencephaly, funnel-shaped or trough-shaped defects tend to develop in the distribution of the middle cerebral artery, internal veins, or terminal veins (at the lateral border of the lateral ventricle). The cavities often communicate freely with the ventricular system and, unlike vascular parenchymal defects in adults, have smooth walls [106].

MR Findings

Selection of MR techniques and imaging planes is discussed in Sect. 7.2.

Besides T1-weighted sequences to demonstrate the pathoanatomic changes in all three projections, T2-weighted images are indicated when there is suspicion of ischemic injury (white matter damage, edema) or heterotopias.

7.6.3 Schizencephaly

The term "schizencephaly" was introduced by Yakovlev et al. [142, 144] to describe what they believed to be a malformative defect (anomalous development of one segment of the germinal matrix or a defect of neuronal migration) in the zones of cleavage of the primary cerebral mantle [77]. Today the pathogenesis is believed to relate more to ischemia during brain development in the critical period of cell migration [107, 77, 88]. Two different forms of schizencephaly are described:

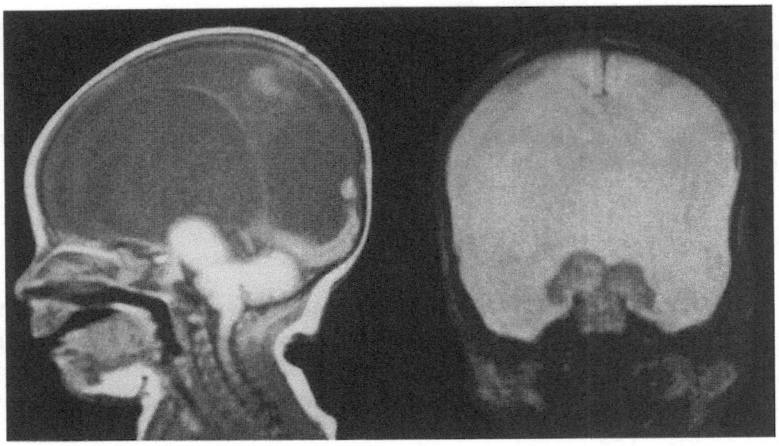

a b

Fig. 7.46 a, b. Hydranencephaly in a newborn baby. Normal size head. Only small basal portions of the occipital lobes are seen, the falx is present; the basal ganglia seem to be separated (**b**). The anterior cerebral artery cannot be seen in this case, probably due to the small size of the vessels, partial volume effect and CSF motion. Midsagittal scan (**a**) SE 0.7 s/30 ms; coronal scan (**b**) SE 2.5 s/120 ms (1.0 T)

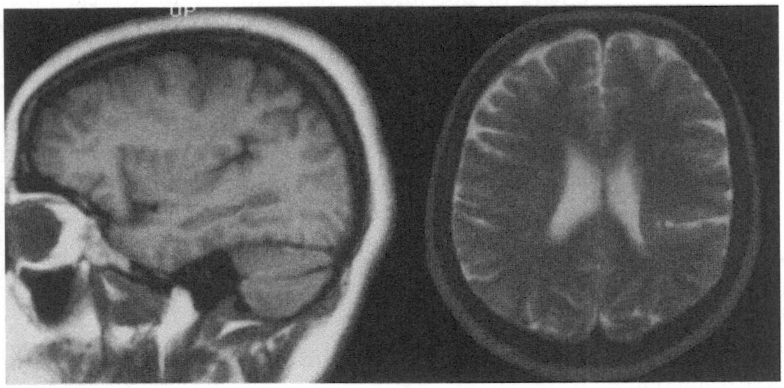

a b

Fig. 7.47 a, b. Schizencephaly (with lips fused) in a 30-year-old woman with epilepsy. Deep cleft in the right parietal region. **a** axial scan, SE 3.0 s/120 ms; **b** parasagittal scan, SE 0.6 s/30 ms (1.0 T)

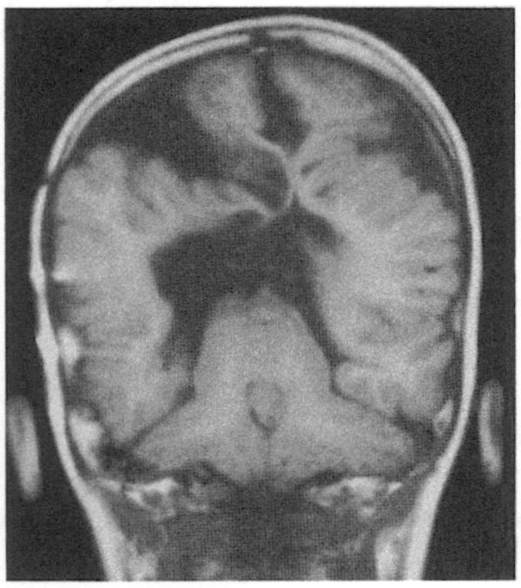

Fig. 7.48. Complex malformation in a 6-year-old boy with severe mental retardation (after bilateral shunt operation for hydrocephalus). Incomplete agenesis of corpus callosum, bizarre ventricular space, probably atresia of aqueduct, schizencephaly with separated lips, large areas of polymicrogyria/stenogyria, shallow posterior fossa with enlarged incisura tentorii. Coronal section, SE 0.4 s/17 ms (1.0 T)

- Schizencephaly with *fused lips:* In this form there are superficial bilateral clefts at the center of the hemispheres near the sylvian fissure and the central or medial orbital fissures. As the name implies, the borders of the clefts are fused together (Fig. 7.47). The cleft involves the entire thickness of the cerebral wall. No communication exists between the subarachnoid space and the ventricular system, and there is no hydrocephalus. The lumen of the porus represents a true expansion of the ventricular cavity and thus contains no vascular remnant [119]. Pia and ependyma closely approach the edges of the furrows, forming "pial-ependymal seams" [143, 144]. Schizencephalic brains show no gliosis. Based on experience with pneumoencephalography and CT studies after the intrathecal injection of contrast material, Fitz [43] believes that a communication indeed exists between the porencephalic defects and the ventricular system. Figure 7.47 shows a unilateral cerebral cleft with fused lips. Friede [47] points out, however, that unilateral schizencephaly is very rare, and that a less pronounced anomaly can usually be discovered in the contralateral hemisphere.

- Schizencephaly with *separated lips:* This second form is characterized by hydrocephalus and by a cleft whose lips are separated by a porus. Usually the clefts are bilateral and symmetrical. This form may be associated with other malformations, such as agenesis of the corpus callosum and absence of the septum pellucidum. The defects may be bordered by microgyria and heterotopic foci [147] (Fig. 7.48).

MR Findings

Selection of MR techniques and imaging planes is discussed in Sect. 7.2. T1-weighted sequences are best suited to demonstrate the distorted anatomy.

7.6.4 Multicystic Encephalopathy

Multicystic encephalopathy is the end result of an injury occurring late in gestation. It is characterized by the presence of cystic cavities situated mostly in the subcortical portion of the white matter [50], sparing the periventricular zone [119]. The lesions have been described in children following severe birth trauma, venous stasis, and cerebral ischemia. The herpes simplex virus also has been implicated as a cause of the disease in children. The multicystic cavities are separated from one another by gliotic tissue [47].

7.6.5 Ammon's Horn Sclerosis, Status Marmoratus, Status Demyelinisatus

Ammon's horn sclerosis (hippocampal sclerosis) secondary to birth asphyxia can be a cause of epileptic seizures. It consists of neuronal loss and gliosis, sometimes associated with ulegyria and status marmoratus and demyelinisatus [106] (see Chap. 9).

In *status marmoratus,* areas of parenchymal necrosis prior to or during myelin formation in the putamen and caudate nucleus caused by an oxygen deficit are replaced by scars of myelinated glial fibers [106, 73].

Status demyelinisatus has a similar ischemic etiology and affects mainly the pallidum. There is a diffuse gliosis with partial demyelination [106], which presumably would affect the MR signal.

MR Findings

Selection of MR techniques and imaging planes is discussed in Sect. 7.2.

MR can demonstrate the white matter lesions as areas with prolonged relaxation times (cystic fluid, edema). Because the damage occurs in the perinatal period and affects a relatively mature brain, adjacent brain tissues would be expected to show glial scarring with a consequent lengthening of relaxation times. MR appears to be the first modality capable of displaying the cicatricial changes that are the morphologic substrate of temporal lobe epilepsy (see Chap. 9).

7.6.6 Ulegyria

Ulegyria is the result of perinatal hypoxic-ischemic damage to normally formed cerebral convolutions [106]. Scarring of the gyri occurs chiefly in the distribution of the internal or middle cerebral artery or in the "watershed areas" of the three major arteries (and veins), and is associated with atrophy of the vascular territories and expansion of the adjacent portions of the ventricles. The normal cortical lamination is disturbed. The characteristic *plaques fibromyeliniques* are formed by myelinated glial fibers radiating into the altered cortex [106].

MR Findings

The morphologic features of ulegyria resemble those of polymicrogyria (see Sect. 7.5.2). T1-weighted sequences in the sagittal and coronal projections are probably best able to display the scarred, shrunken convolutions in the affected vascular area. T2-weighted sequences can also bring out gliotic changes in the brain tissue and foci of demyelination.

7.6.7 Hemispheric Atrophy

Hemispheric atrophy is more often unilateral than bilateral and may be caused by perinatal insult, traumatic mass lesions (hematomas), or infection in early childhood. The late stage is characterized by shrunken, ulegyric convolutions (see above) denuded of ganglion cells with sclerosis and cavitation of the white matter (Fig. 7.49). Atrophy of the pons, medulla oblongata, and cerebellum can occur secondarily [106].

MR Findings

Selection of MR techniques and imaging planes is discussed in Sect. 7.2.

The sclerosis and demyelination of the damaged white matter prolongs the relaxation times, and this can be demonstrated with proton-density and T2-weighted sequences (Fig. 7.49). The altered surface contours of the affected hemisphere are best seen on coronal and sagittal T1-weighted scans.

7.6.8 Putaminal Necrosis

A variety of toxic, metabolic, and chronic degenerative disorders cause lesions of the striatum in the form of well-circumscribed areas of loss of substance confined to the putamen and neighboring structures (Fig. 7.50).

CT and MR Findings

The CT features have been described by Kretzschmar et al. [73] for a variety of etiologies and together with MR findings by Druschky [33] for a case of hereditary putaminal necrosis: elongated lesions of the putamen and caudate nucleus that appear hypodense on CT scans give a low signal on T1-weighted MR images and a high signal on T2-weighted scans because of the prolonged relaxation times. The case described by Druschky [33] additionally showed bilateral involvement of the area subcallosa (Fig. 7.51). The explanation for these lesions is still a matter of controversy. Differentiation is required from Wilson's disease, Hallervorden-Spatz disease (see above), and Leigh's syndrome (including brainstem and cerebellar atrophy).

7.7 Neuroectodermal Dysplasias

In this section we describe a class of disorders that show features of proliferation, neoplasia, and malformation. They are considered to represent fundamental disturbances at an embryonic and often a genetic level. The skin and nervous system are equally involved (see Sect. 7.1) [49, 88].

7.7.1 Tuberous Sclerosis

Tuberous sclerosis (Bourneville's disease, Bourneville-Pringle disease) is a familial disease with an autosomal dominant mode of inheritance that produces characteristic lesions of the skin (adenoma sebaceum) and viscera. The brain is the organ most frequently involved and may be micrencephalic, macrencephalic, or of normal weight. Clinical signs include mental deficiency and seizures [139]. Formes frustes occur with some frequency and should always be suspected in cases of macrencephaly or mental retardation with seizures [62].

The disease shows three characteristic features (Figs. 7.52, 7.53):

1. Multiple tubers scattered over the cortical surface. These may occur at the crests of the gyri or in the depths of sulci. They obscure the gray matter-white matter junction and expand the normal gyrus [112]. The tubers consist of aggregations of cells that distort the normal architecture of the cortex. Cortical calcifications may occur in these tubers or in heterotopias [49].
2. Subependymal nodules on the walls of the lateral ventricles, in the third and fourth ventricles, and even in the aqueduct. They frequently occur about the foramen of Monro, which may become obstructed leading to hydrocephalus. The nodules are firm, and many contain calcifications.

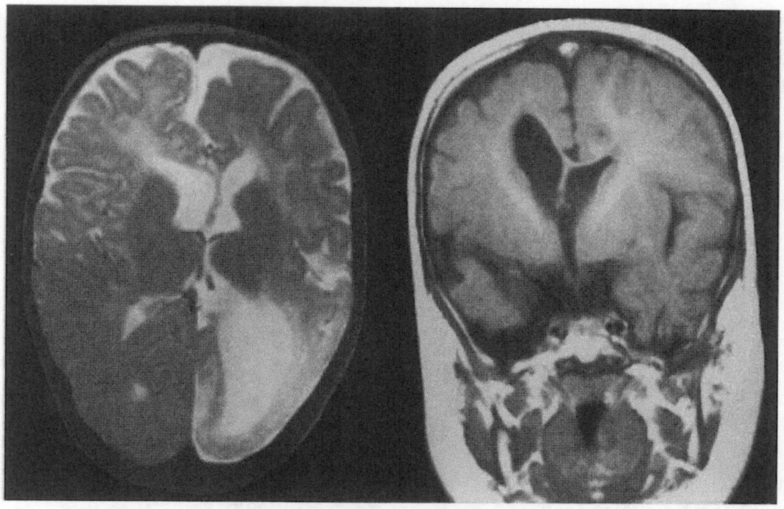

a b

Fig. 7.49 a, b. Hemispheric atrophy in a 1-year-old boy with hemispasticity and seizures. Atrophy of right hemisphere, dilatation of lateral ventricle, demyelination, glial scar, and disturbed gyral pattern of temporo-occipito-parietal region. **a** Axial scan, SE 3.0 s/90 ms; **b** coronal scan, SE 0.6 s/15 ms (1.5 T)

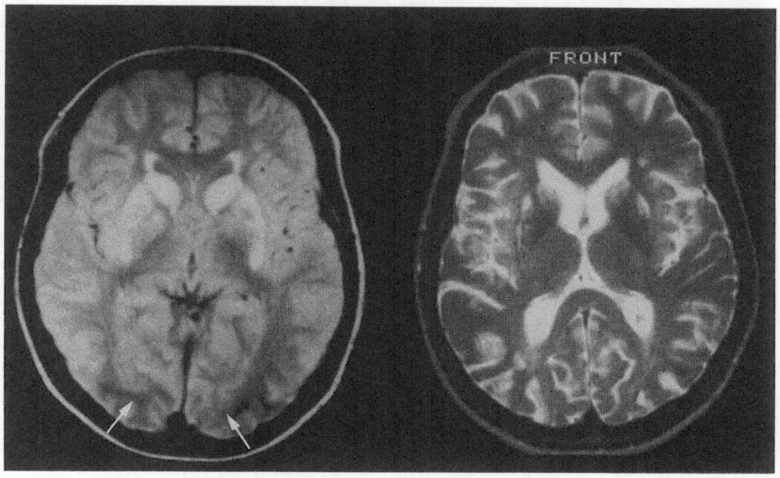

a b

Fig. 7.50 a, b. Bilateral lesions of the basal ganglia due to severe hypoxia in a 29-year-old female 6 weeks after cardiac and respiratory arrest secondary to asthmatic state with tetraparesis and cortical blindness. **a** The hypointense areas in both occipital lobes *(arrows)* may be caused by hemosiderin deposits secondary to hemorrhagic infarction. Axial scan: 3 s/40 ms (1.0 T). **b** Control scan about 4 months later after incomplete recovery of the patient (only slight spasticity and tremor of both hands, normal vision) shows a reduction in the size and signal intensity of the lesions. The hypointense occipital areas are not seen in this section. Axial scan, SE 3.5 s/90 ms (1.5 T)

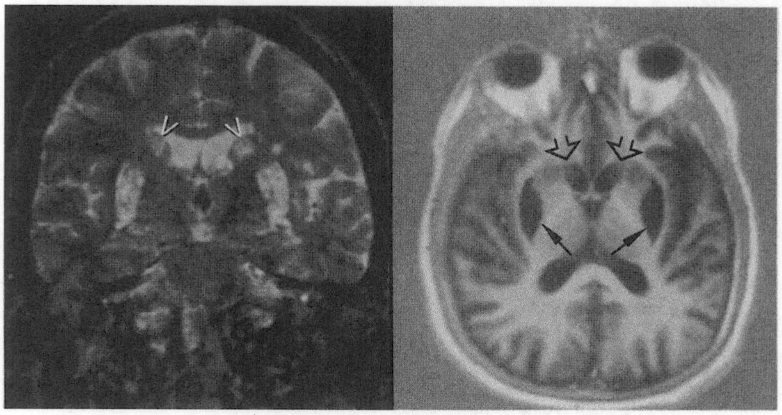

a b

Fig. 7.51 a, b. Putaminal necrosis in a 64-year-old man with dysarthria, atactic disturbances in writing with athetoid movements of the right hand, and slight dysphagia. Well-delineated bilateral lesions of putamen *(arrows)*, caudate nucleus *(arrowheads)*, and area subcallosa *(open arrows)*. Coronal scan (**a**) SE 2.5 s/120 ms; axial scan (**b**) IR 1.5 s/400 ms/30 ms (1.0 T)

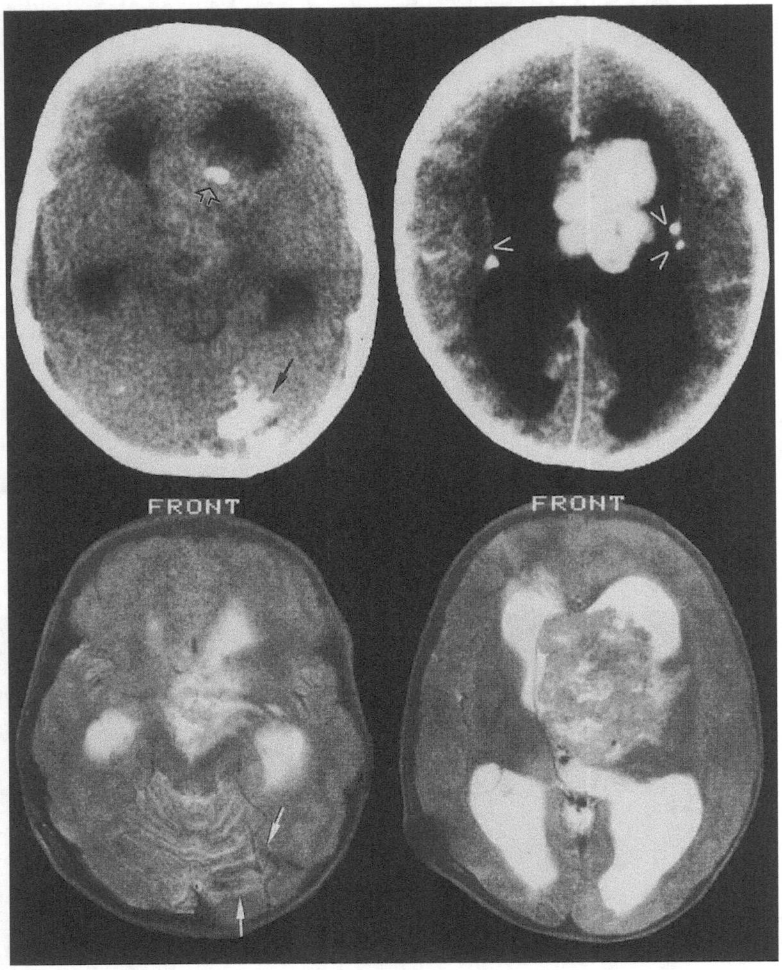

Fig. 7.52 a–d. Tuberous sclerosis in an 1-year-old boy with epilepsy, symptoms of intracranial hypertension, and gait disturbances. **a, b** CT reveals occlusive hydrocephalus secondary to obstruction of the foramina of Monro by a larger tumor (giant cell astrocytoma) which shows distinct contrast enhancement. Calcifications are seen in subependymal nodules *(arrowheads)*, in the astrocytoma *(open arrow)*, and in an area of disruption of the cortical architecture of the cerebellum *(arrow)*. **c, d** MR depicts the large intraventricular tumor with inhomogeneous structure; the mural nodules and the cerebellar calcifications *(arrows)* are poorly visualized. **c, d** Axial scans, SE 3.0 s/90 ms (1.5 T)

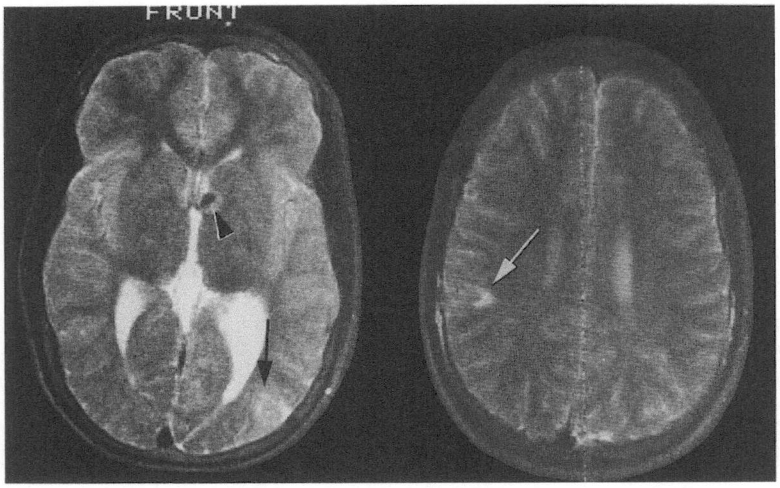

Fig. 7.53 a, b. Tuberous sclerosis in a 17-year-old boy with cerebral seizures. Small, partly calcified tumor *(arrowheads)* near the left foramen of Monro and hyperintense areas in the left temporo-occipital and right parietal cortex *(arrows)*, probably indicating cortical tubers. Axial sections: **a, b** SE 3.0 s/140 ms (0.5 T). (Courtesy of Drs. Kuhn, Steen, and Terwey, Oldenburg, FRG)

3. The subependymal nodules may become "giant cell astrocytomas," which do not always contain calcifications. These lesions consist of numerous multinucleated cells (giant cells) whose origin (spongioblasts, astrocytes?) is still unexplained.

CT and MR Findings

An important diagnostic criterion for this disorder is the presence of calcifications in the subependymal (or other) tumors. CT is superior in this regard, because the calcifications are not easily distinguished from other low-signal areas on MR scans. This may be because the subependymal nodules do not represent gross, isolated calcifications, but rather gliotic areas that contain only microscopic calcified foci [46]. The nodules usually are isointense on T1-weighted images, whereas the T2 relaxation time may be slightly prolonged [91].

The giant cell astrocytoma may contain no calcifications. It appears relatively isodense or slightly hyperdense on plain CT scans and shows enhancement after intravenous administration of contrast material. Subependymal lesions appearing hypodense on CT scans are extremely rare, and diagnosis can be very difficult when these lesions occur in isolation [49]. But contrast material will pass through the abnormal blood-brain barrier of the neoplasm, thereby distinguishing it from the nonenhancing subependymal nodule [81, 49, 78]. Similar considerations apply to MR imaging with use of contrast agents (e.g., gadolinium chelate).

Low-density lesions of the cortex on CT scans usually represent the cortical tubers, which do not show contrast enhancement [49]. On MR they possess prolonged relaxation times. T2-weighted MR sequences can demonstrate tubers as high-signal areas that are not visible with CT [32, 137]. This observation underscores the importance of MR in cases where there is suspicion of tuberous sclerosis but CT fails to show the characteristic subependymal calcifications. MR can also demonstrate the expansion of the gyri by the tubers. Calcifications of the cortical tubers or of areas of cortical architecture disruption appear hypointense (Fig. 7.53); they have also been described in the cerebellar cortex [49].

Frequently, enlargement of the ventricles is seen. This may be induced by obstruction of the foramen of Monro by tumor growth, or secondary to dysplasia [91].

Differentiation is required from multiple subependymal calcifications of other etiology, such as hypoparathyroidism, Fahr's disease, toxoplasmosis, or cytomegalic inclusion disease. The inflammatory processes generally produce other cerebral abnormalities, e.g., micrencephaly and hydrocephalus [78]. If cutaneous manifestations and subependymal calcifications are absent, one should also consider heterotopias (see above, Sect. 7.5), cortical dysplasia, and astrocytoma.

7.7.2 Neurofibromatosis

Neurofibromatosis (von Recklinghausen's disease) is a relatively common disease that is transmitted as an autosomal dominant trait. Males are predominantly affected. The cutaneous manifestations consist of cafe-au-lait spots and multiple neurofibromas. The variations in the clinical manifestation of the disease seem to justify a classification into central, peripheral, and transitional types. Neurofibromatosis is thaught to be secondary to differences in the production of a nerve growth factor cross-reacting protein and the response of the tissues affected [40, 146]. CNS lesions include tumors of the peripheral and autonomic nerves, cranial nerves, and spinal roots (neurilemmomas and neurofibromas), which often are multiple [88] (Figs. 7.54-7.56). Malignant transformation of these tumors has been reported. Other CNS tumors commonly seen in this disease are (multiple) meningiomas, optic nerve gliomas (mostly slow-growing pilocytic astrocytomas, especially in children), pilocytic astrocytomas of the third ventricle, and diffuse cerebral gliomas. Acoustic neuromas tend to develop earlier in patients with neurofibromatosis, and many are bilateral [49].

Neurofibromatosis may also be associated with disturbed ossification of the sphenoid bone, leading to dysplastic defects and asymmetries of the orbits, paranasal sinuses, skull base, posterior fossa, and skull (Fig. 7.57) [146]. Other associated conditions are macrencephaly, pachygyria, polymicrogyria, heterotopias, meningoceles, syringomyelia, seizures, and mental retardation [49, 88, 98].

CT and MR Findings

The CT and MR features of intracranial neoplastic changes in neurofibromatosis are described in Sect. 11.2.

Because of the frequent bilateral occurrence of acoustic neuromas, the porus acusticus internus should always be carefully examined on both sides

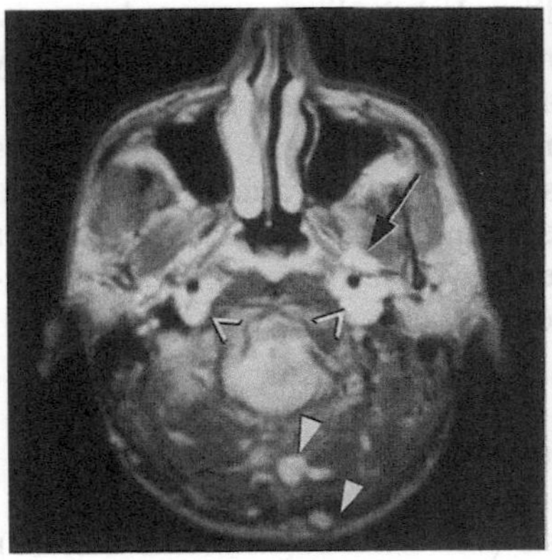

7.54

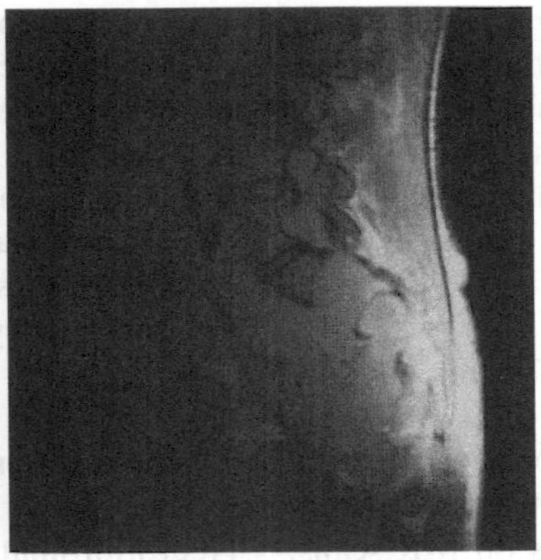

7.55

Fig. 7.54. Known von Recklinghausen's disease in a 14-year-old boy with facial pain. Multiple neurinomas of subcutaneous nerves *(filled arrowheads)*, autonomous carotid body nerves *(open arrowheads)*, and trigeminal nerves *(arrow)*. Axial scan (**a**) SE 3.0 s/45 ms, (1.0 T)

Fig. 7.55. Known von Recklinghausen's disease in a 20-year-old man: slowly progressive flaccid paraparesis of both legs, same symptoms beginning in both arms. Huge tumor masses with prolonged relaxation times in the lower spinal canal extending through enlarged intervertebral foramina into the abdomen and pelvis. Sagittal scan, SE 2.0 s/30 ms (1.0 T)

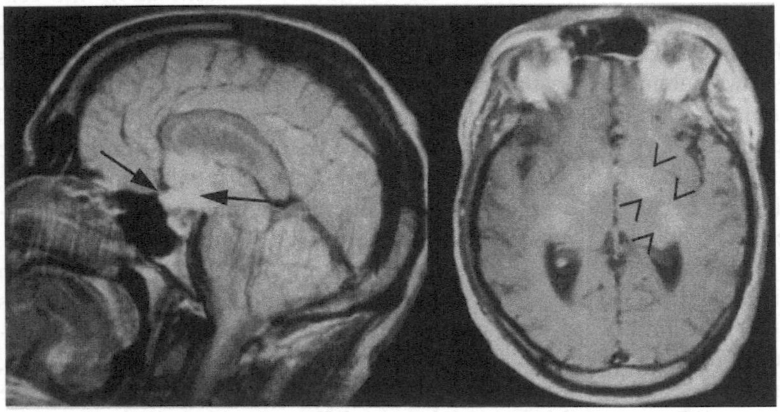

a b

Fig. 7.56 a, b. Known von Recklinghausen's disease in a 22-year-old man with bitemporal visual field defects. Increased signal intensity of the enlarged chiasm *(arrows)* extending along the optic tracts to the thalami on both sides *(arrowheads)*, probably indicating low-grade glioma. Discrete enhancement after i.v. injection of gadolinium-DTPA. (**a**) Sagittal scan, SE 2.5 s/35 ms, (**b**) axial scan, SE 0.7 s/30 ms (1.0 T)

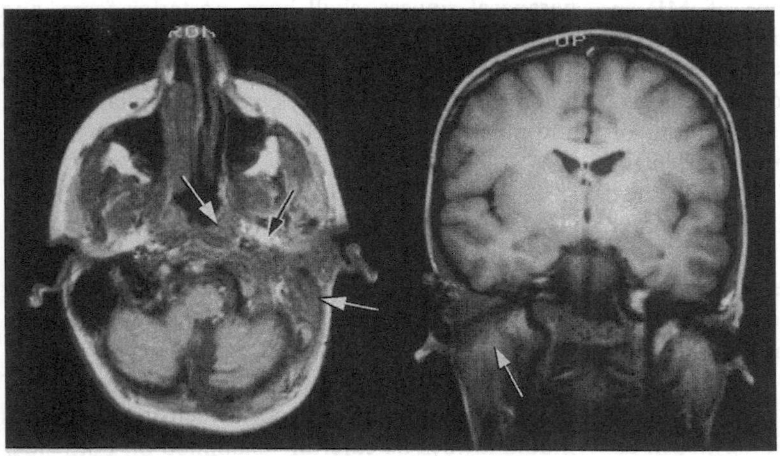

a b

Fig. 7.57 a, b. Disturbed ossification of right sphenoid bone *(arrows)* in von Recklinghausen's disease: 10-year-old girl with cafe-au-lait spots presenting with transient facial palsy on the left. Axial (**a**) and coronal (**b**) scans, SE 0.6 s/15 ms (1.5 T)

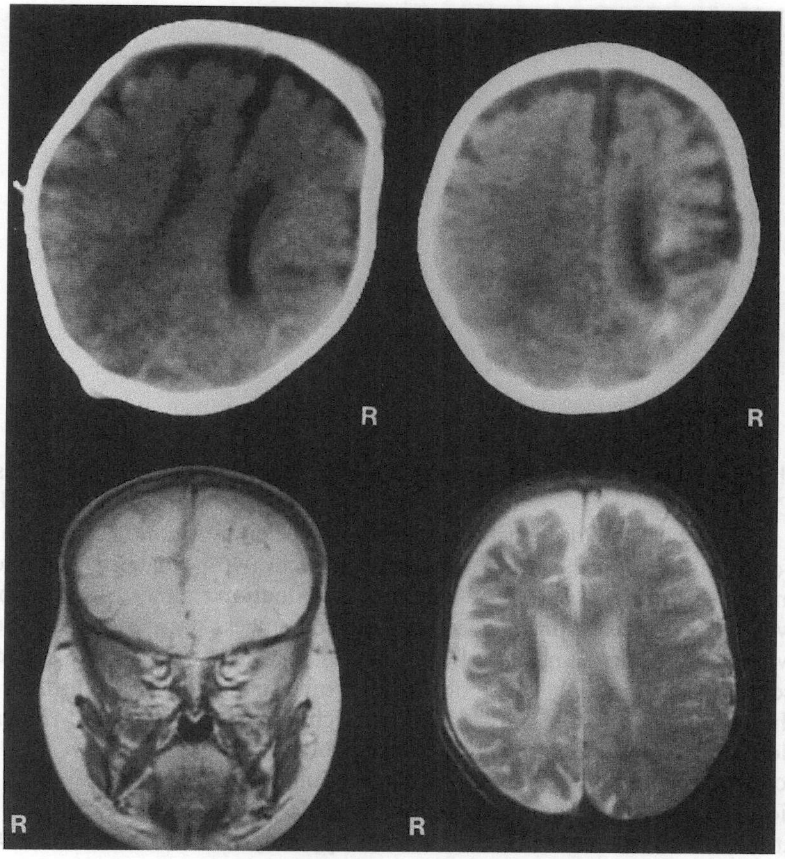

Fig. 7.58 a–d. Sturge-Weber syndrome in a 3-year-old boy with grand mal seizures. **a, b** CT reveals progressive atrophy of right hemisphere from the age of 4 months (**a**) to 12 months (**b**), and gyriform calcifications. **c, d** MR at the age of 18 months confirms the atrophy. The calcifications cannot be identified; however, increased signal intensity of frontal and parietal white matter indicates demyelination and gliosis. In the left frontal lobe the angioma seems to extend into the brain (**c**). **c** Coronal scan, SE 2.5 s/35 ms; **d** axial scan, SE 3.0 s/120 ms (1.0 T)

to enable the prompt detection of an intracanalicular growth. Intravenous contrast medium (i.e. gadolinium chelate) may be necessary in doubtful cases. The smaller the tumor at the time of surgical treatment, the better the chance of preserving the hearing.

7.7.3 Encephalofacial Angiomatosis

Encephalofacial (encephalotrigeminal) angiomatosis (Sturge-Weber syndrome) is a rare, nonfamilial disease characterized by hemangiomatosis of the face and leptomeninges. The angioma is thought to form at 4–8 weeks of gestation [52]. The typical intracranial changes are as follows (Fig. 7.58):

1. Leptomeningeal angiomatosis, usually involving the area of the parieto-occipital cortex and occasionally spreading into the brain
2. Cerebral calcifications
3. Cerebral atrophy

The calcifications can vary in size from small, amorphous, perivascular nodules to large mulberry-shaped masses. Typically they are gyriform or serpentine, tend to affect the more posterior brain areas, and are bilateral in about 15% of cases [14, 49]. Cerebral anoxia caused by vascular changes leads to neuronal loss, atrophy, and gliosis. In some cases angiomatosis does not cause calcification but only hampers development of the hemispheres, producing a hemiatrophy or lobar atrophy, sometimes associated with asymmetry of the cranial vault and pneumatized spaces [49, 88].

Clinical symptoms include convulsions in early childhood, ipsilateral glaucoma, homonymous hemianopsia, hemiplegia, and mental retardation [98].

CT and MR Findings

The focal or hemispheric atrophy is well displayed on MR images, while the gyriform calcifications

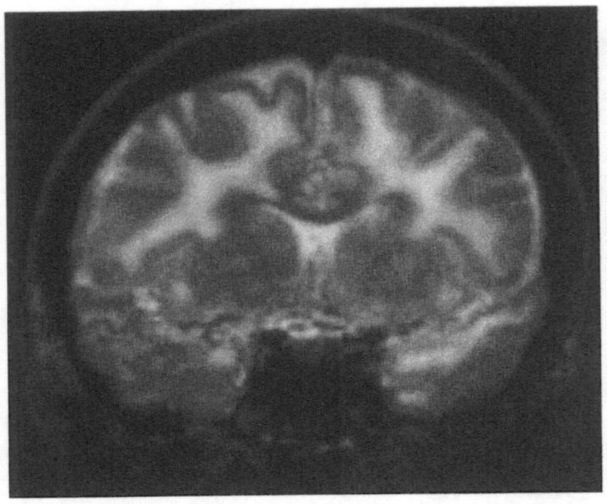

Fig. 7.59. Incontinentia pigmenti (Bloch-Sulzberger syndrome) in a 26-year-old woman with cutaneous lesions, dental anomalies, and cerebral seizures (clinical diagnosis). Prolonged relaxation times of white matter, no enlargement of ventricles. Coronal scan SE 2.0 s/100 ms (0.5 T)

show relatively little contrast and are best seen on CT scans.

Jacoby et al. [65] describe a pattern of accelerated myelination in the abnormal hemisphere in two infants with this disease. The extent of myelination was most apparent on T1-weighted IR sequences, while T2-weighted images reflect changes in water content. The probable cause of this phenomenon is thought to be ischemia of the brain parenchyma underlying the leptomeningeal angioma, which leads to hypermyelination once the process of myelination has started. A similar ischemic-hypoxic insult at birth is considered to be the cause of hypermyelination in status marmoratus [65].

Enlargement of the choroid plexus on the same side as the facial and intracranial lesions, as described by Stimac et al. [33], was not seen in our cases.

7.7.4 Von Hippel-Lindau Disease

Von Hippel-Lindau disease is a dominantly inherited disease affecting the CNS as well as the kidneys, retina, pancreas, and skin. Hemangioblastomas most commonly occur in the cerebellum but are also found in the medulla, area postrema, spinal cord, and retina. The tumors may occur as small mural nodes within a large cyst, as solid tumors, or as solid tumors with multiple associated cysts. The cysts contain a xanthochromic fluid (see also Sect. 11.2).

CT and MR Findings

Contrast CT scans show marked enhancement of the solid tumor nodule alongside the cystic components. The cysts appear light (like CSF) on T2-weighted MR images. Cysts with a high protein content give an intense signal even when shorter imaging parameters are used. Solid tumor parts may show enhancement on T1-weighted scans, analogous to their appearance on CT. Small mural nodes situated close to the bone may be obscured by bone artifact on CT scans but are displayed well on serial MR scans covering the entire region of interest.

7.7.5 Other Neuroectodermal Dysplasias

The typical changes occurring in other neuroectodermal dysplasias [49] are outlined below. At present, few descriptions of MR findings are available for these conditions.

- *Encephaloretinal angiomatosis* involves a combined occurrence of vascular nevi in the face and angiomas extending from the retina to the brainstem [80].

- *Ataxia-teleangiectasia* (Louis-Bar syndrome or Border-Sedgwick syndrome): The hallmark of this disease is cerebellar atrophy due to degeneration of the Purkinje cells, with enlargement of the fourth ventricle and cisterna magna. This is accompanied by teleangiectasias of the skin (face) and mucosae (conjunctiva) which begin in childhood and are progressive. The small vessels of the pia and white matter of the brain show an expansion and thinning of the vessel wall [98]. Clinical manifestations include cerebellar symptoms, impaired ocular motility, and motor disturbances [87, 98].

- *Neurocutaneous melanosis* is characterized by a proliferation of melanin-containing cells in the skin, the meninges, the leptomeninges, and the brain pa-

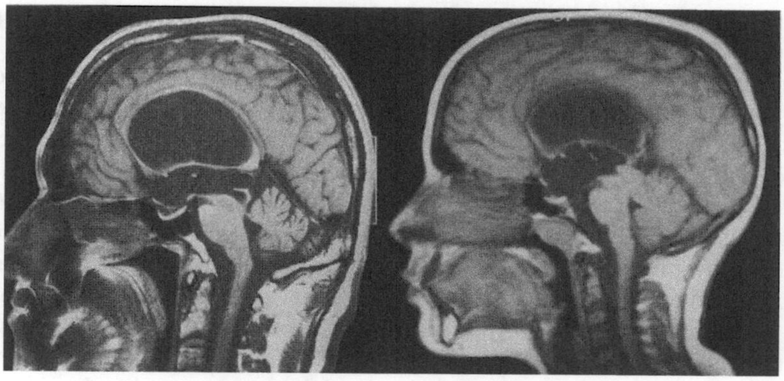

a b

Fig. 7.60 a, b. Stenosis/occlusion of the aqueduct with arrested hydrocephalus: **a** 48-year-old male with repeated dizzy spells; **b** 11-year-old girl with known hydrocephalus and occasional headache. Elongation and thinning of the corpus callosum, bulging of the floor of the third ventricle into the enlarged sella, gaping of the orifice of the aqueduct (**a** and **b**, see also Fig. 7.12); in **b**, atypical shape of the quadrigeminal plate. **a, b** Midsagittal scans, SE 0.4 s/17 ms (1.0 T)

renchyma. Secondary hydrocephalus has been described with CT [49].

- *Linear naevus sebaceus syndrome* involves a combination of porencephaly, cranial asymmetry, hemiatrophy of the brain, and hamartomas [84].

- *Incontinentia pigmenti* (Bloch-Sulzberger syndrome): The clinical picture of this sex-linked (X-chromosomal) hereditary disorder is dominated by skin lesions and malformations of various organs, which become apparent in the first weeks of life. CNS involvement occurs in 35%-40% of cases and is manifested by seizures, spastic paralysis, and mental retardation [109]. Associated anomalies have been described and consist of microgyria [110] and ventricular dilatation secondary to deficient development of the white matter [109].

CT and MR Findings

CT may demonstrate micrencephaly, hydrocephalus, or porencephalic cysts [49]. In one of our own cases, MR imaging showed prolonged T1 and T2 relaxation times throughout the cerebral white matter with no significant ventricular dilatation (Fig. 7.59).

7.8 Miscellaneous Abnormalities

7.8.1 Congenital Hydrocephalus

Congenital hydrocephalus may occur in the setting of complex syndromes (e.g., Dandy-Walker syndrome, Arnold-Chiari deformity) or in isolation. Often the condition is based on an obstructive anomaly of the cerebral aqueduct such as stenosis, forking, or atresia. The aqueduct develops beneath the tectal plate from the lumen of the neural tube. Because of the wide variation in the normal lumen of the aqueduct (4-12 mm^2), it is difficult to define the point at which the aqueduct becomes obstructive to CSF flow. Obstruction by membrane formation also has been described. Gliosis around the aqueduct, usually due to inflammatory causes, likewise can restrict or completely obstruct the lumen (Fig. 7.60). The ependyma of the dilated ventricular walls is replaced by a layer of gliotic tissue.

The cause of these stenosing lesions remains a subject of controversy. Because inflammatory processes in the fetal brain can heal, leaving no residual evidence of inflammation, there is very little basis for distinguishing between postinflammatory and maldevelopmental causes.

A hydrocephalus ex vacuo can result from severe hypoxic-ischemic prenatal brain damage. In premature infants with leukomalacia progressing to sclerosis or spongiform changes in the white matter, asymmetric involvement can lead to unilateral ventricular enlargement. Other cases of congenital hydrocephalus have an obscure etiology. Unclassified, bizarre, and complex malformations of the brain, fluid-filled cysts over the hemispheres, cerebellar agenesis, and abnormal meninges and vessels [107] have been found, but none of these anomalies bears a definite relationship to the hydrocephalus [77].

MR Findings

Selection of MR techniques and imaging planes is discussed in Sect. 7.2.

T1-weighted sequences in various planes can demonstrate the large ventricular cavities, an expanded infundibulum reduced to a thin membrane, a fenestrated or absent septum pellucidum, an atrophic corpus callosum, and an accentuation of ventricular dilatation in the occipital and temporal horns. The cortex is well preserved, while the white matter is markedly reduced. Diffusion of CSF into the periventricular white matter creates interstitial edema, which appears on T2-weighted and proton-density images as a periventricular zone of high signal intensity. When a shunt procedure is undertaken at the proper time, reexpansion of the cerebral mantle may be observed on scans.

The finding of a flow-induced signal loss in the cerebral aqueduct on midsagittal and/or paraxial coronal scans made parallel to the axis of the aqueduct signifies patency, although it does not necessarily confirm the functional soundness of this CSF pathway. Conversely, the absence of signal loss in the aqueduct may be interpreted as evidence of ventricular disease [85, 94].

The technique of visualizing flow movements appears to hold great promise for the evaluation of pulsatile CSF flow dynamics and is of potential value in the study of questions relating to normal pressure hydrocephalus, insufficiency of ventricular drainage systems, syringomyelia, and spinal block (see also Sect. 5.3).

7.8.2 Microcephaly, Micrencephaly

The normal weight of the brain varies widely, but a mature brain that weighs less than 900 g is generally regarded as abnormal.

Microcephaly and micrencephaly are not pathologic entities. They can have diverse etiologies and may be associated with degenerative, destructive, or malformative conditions. They may follow congenital infections such as rubella, toxoplasmosis, cytomegaly, meningitis, toxins, irradiations, phenylketonuria, or Tay-Sachs disease [108, 88]. Microcephaly can occur in association with congenital malformations such as migration disorders, holoprosencephaly, and agenesis of the corpus callosum.

In most cases all parts of the brain are small, although the frontal and temporal lobes may be affected more than the others. The gyral pattern can vary considerably. Generally the basal ganglia are unaffected and may appear disproportionately large [88].

Familial cases of microcephaly are associated with pronounced cerebral anomalies [121], a simplified gyral pattern, atrophy of gyri, calcifications similar to those in Fahr's disease, and large ventricles.

7.8.3 Macrencephaly

The definition of macrencephaly is as imprecise as that of microcephaly. Brain weights in excess of 1700 g have been described. Macrencephaly has occasionally been found in individuals with superior intelligence, but is more commonly associated with mental retardation.

Dekaban and Sakuragawa [25] classify macrencephaly into three groups:

Primary macrencephaly may occur as an isolated finding or in association with achondroplasia and endocrine disorders.

Secondary macrencephaly accompanies genetic disorders such as Tay-Sachs disease, Hunter-Hurler syndrome, Alexander's disease, metachromatic leukodystrophy, and migration disorders. The cerebral mantle (cortex and white matter) is usually thickened, but the corpus callosum may be poorly developed.

Unilateral macrencephaly: In this form the neuronal and glial cells may appear cytologically abnormal and bizarre [93]. Friede [47] attributes the condition to an overproduction of neurons during brain development secondary to a failure of normal bionecrosis. Additional disturbance of migration of neurons and cortical architecture must be assumed.

Patients with unilateral macrencephaly often show an associated overgrowth of the face, limbs, or the entire body half. In cases with abnormal neurons and glia, the possibility of a forme fruste of tuberous sclerosis or von Recklinghausen's disease should be ruled out [88].

CT and MR Findings

Selection of MR techniques and imaging planes is discussed in Sect. 7.2.

The pathoanatomic details outlined above are best appreciated on T1-weighted MR sequences. Both CT and MR show an enlarged brain with proportional expansion of the ventricles. The brain tissue itself appears normal. In unilateral macrencephaly enlargement of one hemisphere with dilated ventricle, ill-defined thick and disordered cortex with abnormal gyration, and heterotopic neurons in subcortical white matter can be found; as in Fig. 7.61 the high signal of the white matter may indicate early myelination compared to the hypointense white matter of the normal hemisphere.

The specific CT and MR features of the various syndromes and diseases that are associated with ab-

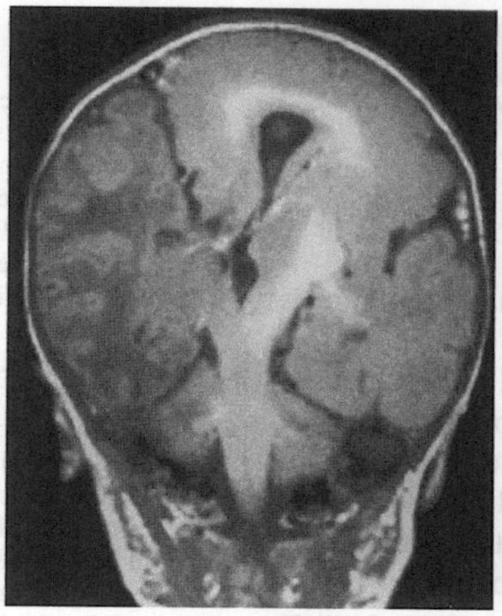

7.61

Fig. 7.61. Unilateral macrencephaly in a newborn girl. Enlargement of left hemisphere with abnormal gyration, disordered thick cortex, and enlarged ventricle, cerebral peduncle, and medulla oblongata. The white matter seems to be myelinated compared to the hypointense white matter of the normal right hemisphere. Coronal scan, SE 0.6 s/19 ms (1.5 T)

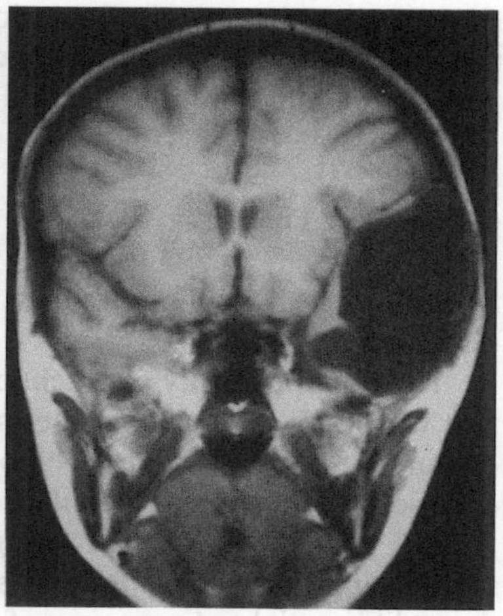

7.62

Fig. 7.62. Arachnoid cyst in a 9-year-old girl with headache. Large cyst of the right temporal region with deformity of temporal bone, enlargement of middle cranial fossa; no midline shift. Signal intensity consistent with CSF. Coronal section, SE 0.5 s/30 ms (1.0 T)

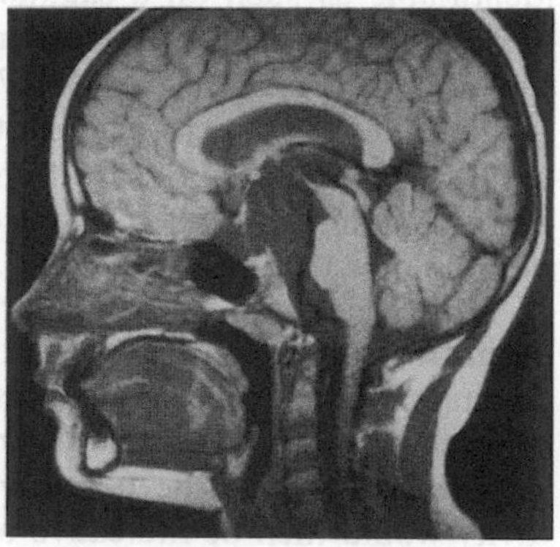

Fig. 7.63. Suprasellar arachnoid cyst in an 8-year-old girl complaining of headache. Large cyst of suprasellar cistern with distinct mass effect on the adjacent structures. Midsagittal section, SE 0.7 s/30 ms (1.0 T)

normalities of brain size are described under the appropriate headings.

7.8.4 Arachnoid Cyst

The origin of arachnoid cysts is believed to relate to a maldevelopment of the meninges [132]. The cyst results from a splitting of the arachnoid, which is thickened by a layer of collagenous tissue [77]. The mature cyst usually has no connection with the ventricles, although a free communication with the subarachnoid space has been suggested.

The most common sites of occurrence of the cysts are the sylvian fissure, the cerebellopontine angle, the supracollicular area, the vermis, the interhemispheric fissure, the cerebral convexity, the clivus, and the interpeduncular area.

It is common for arachnoid cysts to cause deformation of the adjacent cranial bone, such as enlargement of the middle fossa with deformation of the sphenoid wing, or thinning and bulging of the cranial vault (Fig. 7.62). Temporal lobe agenesis also is associated with bulging of the temporal squama and elevation of the lesser sphenoid wing [122].

Arachnoid cysts contain a clear, colorless fluid that resembles CSF. Occasionally the protein content of the fluid may be elevated due to hemorrhage [75].

Arachnoid cysts have to be distinguished from ependymal cysts (see Fig. 10.59), whose walls contain glia ("glial ependymal" cysts), from an expanded cavum veli interpositi (see above), and from other subdural or subarachnoid processes that result in a localized collection of fluid.

Occasionally it may be difficult to differentiate unilateral or bilateral temporal lobe agenesis from an arachnoid cyst. A defect of brain tissue seems to be present when the large size of the fluid collection does not correspond to its small mass effect. A straight posterior margin for lesions originating in the middle cerebral fossa has been described as a pathognomonic sign of arachnoid cysts [74].

CT and MR Findings

Selection of MR techniques and imaging planes is discussed in Sect. 5.3.2.

The signal intensity of arachnoid cysts is consistent with CSF. Relaxation times shorter than those of pure CSF may be due to blood elements or increased protein contents, similar to tumor cysts.

MR images, especially T1-weighted scans in the sagittal and coronal planes, are superior to CT in the differential diagnosis of cystic cavities (Fig. 7.62). Thus, while a suprasellar cyst is clearly identifiable as such on a sagittal MR image, it is difficult to distinguish from an enlarged third ventricle on an axial CT scan (Fig. 7.63). The same is true of other cysts occurring near the ventricles. It is unlikely to be possible to differentiate arachnoid and ependymal cysts, because of their similar gross morphologic features.

It is common to find an enlarged cisterna magna in the posterior fossa without evidence of concomitant displacement or compression of the fourth ventricle. An asymmetrically enlarged posterior fossa with thinning of the bone over the fluid-filled cavity would then be indicative of a noncommunicating cyst. In doubtful cases, CT contrast cisternography may be necessary to establish the degree of communication with the subarachnoid cistern.

Hypodense low-grade gliomas may be confused with arachnoid cysts on CT scans, as the two lesions have similar absorption coefficients. But while the cyst is sharply marginated in all projections, the tumor usually shows some degree of irregularity [78]. On MR, a greater difference of signal intensity can be measured in these cases. In doubtful cases a careful search to exclude a mural tumor nodule is necessary before the lesion can be assumed to be a benign cyst.

The relaxation times of gliomas on MR images are somewhat shorter than those of the free cystic fluid. Also, MR is more sensitive than CT in its ability to depict structural inhomogeneities, making differentiation easier.

In arachnoid cysts, no abnormal signal of the displaced brain tissue adjacent to the cyst can be observed. This feature helps to differentiate arachnoid cysts from cavities of encephalomalacia and tumor cysts.

References

1. Aboulezz AD, Sartor K, Geyer CA, Gado MH (1985) Position of cerebellar tonsils in the normal population and in patients with Chiari malformation: a quantitative approach with MR imaging. J Comput Assist Tomogr 9 (6): 1033-1036
2. Aboulker J (1979) La syringomyelie et les liquides intra rachidiens. Neurochirurgie 25 [Suppl 1]: 1-44
3. Adams RD, Victor M (1985) Principles of neurology, 3rd edn. McGraw-Hill, New York
4. Ammerman BJ, Henry JM, De Girolami U, Major MC, Earle KM (1976) Intradural lipomas of the spinal cord. J Neurosurg 44: 331-336
5. Aoki S, Machida T, Sasaki Y, Yoshikawa K, Iio M, Sasaki T, Takakura K (1987) Enterogenous cyst of cervical spine: clinical and radiological aspects (including CT and MRI). Neuroradiology 29: 291-293
6. Atlas SW, Zimmerman RA, Bilaniuk LT, Rorke L, Hackney DB, Goldberg HI, Grossman RI (1986) Corpus callosum and limbic system: Neuroanatomic MR evaluation of development anomalies. Radiology 160: 355-362
7. Bailey IC (1970) Dermoid tumours of the spinal cord. J Neurosurg 33: 676-681
8. Bairamian D, Di Chiro G, Theodore WH, Holmes MD, Dorwart RH, Larson SM (1985) MR imaging and positron emission tomography of cortical heterotopia. J Comput Assist Tomogr 9 (6): 1137-1139
9. Ball MJ, Dayan AD (1972) Pathogenesis of syringomyelia. Lancet II: 799-801
10. Barkovich AJ, Sherman JL, Citrin CM, Wippold FJ II (1987) MR of postoperative syringomyelia. AJNR 8: 319-327
11. Barnes PD, Lester P, Yamanashi WS, Prince JR (1986) MRI in infants and children with spinal dysraphism. AJR 147: 339-346
12. Ben-Amour M, Billewicz O (1970) The posterior cerebral vein. Neuroradiology 1: 179-182
13. Blaauw G (1971) Defect in posterior arch of atlas in myelomeningocele. Dev Med Child Neurol [Suppl] 25: 113-115
14. Boltshauser E, Wilson J, Hoare RD (1976) Sturge-Weber syndrome with bilateral intracranial calcification. J Neurol Neurosurg Psychiatry 39: 429-43
15. Buchfelder M, Thierauf P, Huk W, Fahlbusch R (1986) Rhinoliquorrhoe bei transsphenoidaler Encephalocele. Presented at the 37th Annual Meeting of the German Society of Neurosurgery, May 4-7, 1986
16. Calogero Ja (1977) Vermian agenesis and unsegmented midbrain tectum. Case report. J Neurosurg 47: 605-608
17. Chuang S, Hochhauser L, Harwood-Nash DC, Fritz CR, Armstrong D, Savoic J (1986) The tethered cord syndrome revisited. Presented at the XIII Symposium Neuroradiologicum, June 23-28, Stockholm
18. Crome L (1952) Microgyrie. J Pathol Bacteriol 64: 479-495
19. Curnes JT, Laster WD, Koubek TD, Moody DM, Ball MR, Witcofski RL (1986) MRI of callosal syndromes. AJNR 7: 617-622
20. Dandy WE (1921) The diagnosis and treatment of hydrocephalus due to occlusion of the foramina of Magendie and Luschka. Surg Gynecol Obstet 32: 112-124
21. Davidson HD, Abraham R, Steiner RE (1985) Agenesis of corpus callosum: magnetic resonance imaging. Radiology 155: 371-373

22. Davis DH Jr, Alexander E Jr (1959) Congenital nasofrontal encephalomingoceles and teratomas. J Neurosurg 16: 365-377
23. Davis RL, Robertson DM (1985) Textbook of neuropathology. Williams and Wilkins, Baltimore
24. Deeb ZL, Rothfus WE, Maroon JC (1985) MR imaging of heterotopic gray matter. J Comput Assist Tomogr 9 (6): 1140-1141
25. Dekaban AS, Sakuragawa N (1977) Megalencephaly. In: Vinken PJ, Bruyn GW (eds) Handbook of clinical neurology, vol 30. North-Holland, Amsterdam, pp 647-660
26. De La Paz RL, Brady TJ, Buonanno FS, New PFJ, Kistler JP, McGinnis BD, Pykett IL, Taveras JM (1983) Case report. Nuclear magnetic resonance (NMR) imaging of Arnold-Chiari Type I malformation with hydromyelia. J Comput Assist Tomogr 7: 126-129
27. De Morsier G (1956) Etudes sur les dysraphies cranio-encephaliques, agenesie du septum lucidum avec malformation du tractus optique. La dysraphie septo-optique. Schweiz Arch Neurol Psychiat 77: 267-292
28. De Myer W, Zeman W (1963) Alobar holoprosencephaly (arhinencephaly) with median cleft lips and palate: clinical, electroencephalographic and nosologic considerations. Confin Neurol 23: 1-36
29. De Myer W, Zeman W, Palmer CG (1964) The face predicts the brain: diagnostic significance of median facial anomalies for holoprosencephaly (arhinencephaly). Pediatrics 35: 256-263
30. Diebler C, Dulac O (1983) Cephaloceles: clinical and neuroradiological appearance. Associated cerebral malformation. Neuroradiology 25: 199-216
31. Dignan PSJ, Warkany J (1978) Congenital malformations: lissencephaly, agyria, pachygyria. Ment Ret Dev Disabil 10: 77-91
32. Dörnemann H, Petsch R, Braitinger S, Neulinger P, Heller H (1986) Vergleichende Darstellung der tuberösen Hirnsklerose im Computertomogramm und Kernspintomogramm. RÖFO 144 (5): 614-616
33. Druschky KF (1986) Hereditary putaminal necrosis (Paterson). In: Vinken PJ, Bruyn GW, Klawans HL (eds) Handbook of clinical neurology, vol 5 (49): Extrapyramidal Disorders. Elsevier Science Publishers B.v., pp 493-498
34. Dubois PJ (1984) Syringomyelia. In: Rosenberg RN, Heinz ER (eds) The clinical neurosciences, sect IV. Neuroradiology. Livingstone, New York, pp 931-942
35. Dunn V, Mock T, Bell WE, Smith W (1986) Detection of heterotopic gray matter in children by magnetic resonance imaging. Magn Reson Imaging 4: 33-39
36. Von Einsiedel H, Stepan R (1985) Magnetic resonance imaging of spinal cord syndromes. Eur J Radiol 5: 127-132
37. Emery JL, Lendon RG (1973) The local cord lesion in neurospinal dysraphism (meningomyelocele). J Pathol 110: 83-96
38. Emery JL, Mac Kenzie N (1973) Medullo-cervical dislocation deformity (Chiari II deformity) related to neurospinal dysraphism (meningomyelocele). Brain 96: 155-162
39. Enzman DR, O'Donohue JO, Rubin JB, Shuer L, Cogen P, Silverberg G (1987) CSF pulsations within nonneoplastic spinal cord cysts. AJR 149: 149-157
40. Fabricant RN, Todaro GJ, Eldridge R (1979) Increased levels of a nerve-growth-factor cross-reacting protein in central neurofibromatosis. Lancer 2: 4-7
41. Fishman RA (1980) Composition of cerebrospinal fluid. In: Fishman RA (ed) Cerebrospinal fluid in diseases of the nervous system. Saunders, Philadelphia, pp 168-252
42. Fitz CR (1983) Holoprosencephaly and related entities. Neuroradiology 25: 225-238
43. Fitz CR (1984) Developmental abnormalities of the brain. In: Rosenberg RN, Heinz ER (eds) The clinical neurosciences. Neuroradiology. Churchill Livingstone, New York, pp 215-246
44. Fitz CR (1985) Congenital anomalies of the spine and spinal cord. In: Latchaw RE (ed) Computed tomography of the head, neck, and spine. Year Book, Chicago, pp 715-736
45. Fitz CR, Harwood-Nash DC (1975) The tethered conus. Am J Roentgenol Radium Ther Nucl Med 125: 515-523
46. Franek A, Werner S (1984) Hirnsonographischer Befund bei tuberöser Hirnsklerose - ein Vergleich mit röntgenologischen Darstellungsmethoden und dem pathologisch-anatomischen Befund. Monatsschr Kinderheilkd 132: 543
47. Friede RL (1975) Developmental neuropathology. Springer, Berlin Heidelberg New York
48. Garceau GJ (1953) The filum terminale syndrome. J Bone Joint Surg 35: 711-716
49. Gardeur D, Palmieri A, Mashaly R (1983) Cranial computed tomography in the phakomatoses. Neuroradiology 25: 293-304
50. Gilles FH (1985) Perinatal neuropathology. In: Davis RL, Robertson DM (eds) Textbook of neuropathology. Williams and Wilkins, Baltimore, pp 243-283
51. Guidetti B, Gagliardi FM (1977) Epidemoid and dermoid cysts. J Neurosurg 47: 12-18
52. Haberland C (1977) Encephalofacial angiomatosis (Sturge-Weber-Dimitri syndrome). In: Vinken PJ, Bruyn GW (eds) Handbook of clinical neurology, vol 31. North-Holland, Amsterdam, pp 18-24
53. Han JS, Benson JE, Kaufman B, Rekate HL, Alfidi RJ, Bohlman HH, Kaufman B (1985) Demonstration of diastematomyelia and associated abnormalities with MR imaging. AJNR 6: 215-219
54. Han JS, Benson JE, Kaufman B, Rekate HL, Alfidi RJ, Huss RG, Sacco D, Yoon YS, Morrison SC (1985) MR imaging in pediatric cerebral abnormalities. J Comput Assit Tomogr 9 (1): 103-114
55. Hart MN, Malamud N, Ellis WG (1972) The Dandy-Walker syndrome. A clinicopathological study based on 28 cases. Neurology 22: 771-780
56. Harwood-Nash DC, Fitz CR (1976) Neuroradiology in infants and children. Mosby, St Louis
57. Hendrick EB, Hoffmann JH, Humphreys RP (1977) Tethered cord syndrome. In: Mc Laurin R (ed) Myelomeningocele. Grune and Statton, New York
58. Hilal SK, Marton D, Pollach E (1974) Diastematomyelia in children. Radiology 112: 609-621
59. Hori A, Fischer G, Dietrich-Schott B, Ikeda K (1982) Dimyelia, diplomyelia and diastematomyelia. Clin Neuropathol 1: 23-30
60. Hülser PJ, Schroth G, Petersen D (1986) Gegenüberstellung von klinischem Befund und Kernspintomogramm bei Syringomyelie und intramedullären Tumoren. Fortschr Neurol Psychiatr 54 (2): 54-58
61. Hughes JT (1966) Developmental disorders. In: Pathology of the spinal cord. Lloyd-Luke, London
62. Huk WJ, Rott H-D (1980) Computertomographische Befunde bei der tuberösen Sklerose Bourneville-Pringle.

In: Spranger J, Tolksdorf M (eds) Klinische Genetik in der Pädiatrie. Thieme, Stuttgart, pp 154-158
63. Huong TT, Goldbatt E, Simpson DA (1975) Dandy-Walker syndrome associated with congenital heart disease. Report of three cases. Dev Med Child Neurol 35 [Suppl]: pp 35-42
64. Jackson FE, Moore BS (1969) Ectopic glial tissue in the occipital scalp. Arch Dis Child 44: 428-430
65. Jacoby CG, Yuh WTC, Afifi AK, Bell WE, Schelper RL, Sato Y (1987) Accelerated myelination in early Sturge-Weber syndrome demonstrated by MR imaging. J Comput Assist Tomogr 11 (2): 226-231
66. James CCM, Lassman LP (1972) Spinal dysraphism: spina bifida occulta. Butterworth, London
67. Johnson MA, Bydder GM (1984) NMR imaging of the brain in children. Br Med Bull 40: 175-178
68. Joubert M, Eisenring JJ, Robb JP, Andermann F (1969) Familial agenesis of the cerebellar vermis. Neurology 19: 813-825
69. Kantrowitz LR, Pais MJ, Burnett K, Choi B, Pritz MB (1986) Intraspinal neurenteric cyst containing gastric mucosa: CT and MR findings. Pediatr Radiol 16: 324-32
70. Kazner E, Stochdorph D, Wendl S, Grumme T (1980) Intracranial lipoma. J Neurosurg 52: 234-245
71. Köhler D, Treisch J, Hertel G, Schörner W, Fiegler W (1985) Die magnetische Resonanztomographie der Syringomyelie. RÖFO 143 (6): 617-622
72. Krawinkel M, Steen-H-J, Terwey B (1987) Magnetic resonance imaging in lissencaphaly. Eur J Pediatr 146: 205-208
73. Kretzschmar K, Ludwig B, Krämer G, Collmann H, Kazner E (1986) Bilateral lesions of the putamina. Neuroradiology 28: 87-91
74. Lang C, Lehrl S, Huk WJ (1981) A case of bilateral temporal lobe agenesis. J Neurol Neurosurg Psychiatry 44: 626-630
75. Lang C, Ott G, Reichwein J, Huk WJ (1986) Zur klinischen Bedeutung von Arachnoidalzysten. Nervenarzt 57: 619-623
76. Larroche JC (1984) Malformation of the nervous system. In: Adam JH, Corsellis JAN, Duchen LW (eds) Greenfield's neuropathology. Wiley, New York, pp 385-450
77. Larroche JC (1984) Perinatal brain damage. In: Adam JH, Corsellis JAN, Duchen LW (eds) Greenfield's neuropathology. Wiley, New York, pp 451-489
78. Latchaw RE (1985) Congenital anomalies of the brain. In: Latchaw RE (ed) Computed tomography of the head, neck and spine. Year Book Chicago, pp 439-488
79. Layton DD (1962) Heterotopic cerebral grey matter as an epileptogenic focus. J Neuropathol Exp Neurol 1 (21): 244-249
80. Lecuire J, Dechaume JP, Bret P (1972) Bonnet-Dechaume-Blanc syndrome. In: Vinken PJ, Bruyn GW (eds) North Holland, Amsterdam, pp 260-266 (Handbook of clinical neurology, vol 14)
81. Lee BC, Gawler J (1978) Tuberous sclerosis comparison of CT and conventional neuroradiology. Radiology 127: 403-407
82. Lee CM Jr, Laurin RL (1955) Heterotopic brain tissue as an isolated embryonic rest. J Neurosurg 12: 190-192
83. Lee BCP, Zimmerman RD, Manning JJ, Deck MDF (1985) MR imaging of syringomyelia and hydromyelia. AJNR 6: 221-228
84. Leonidas JC, Wolpert SM, Feingold M, Mc Cauley RGK (1979) Radiographic features of the linear nervus sebaceous syndrome. AJR 132: 277-279
85. Levy LM, Di Chiro G, Brooks RA, Dwyer AJ, Dietz MJ (1986) Changes in cerebral ventricular dimensions related to the cardiac cycle as seen with gated magnetic resonance imaging. Presented at the XIII. Symposium Neuroradiologicum, June 23-28, Stockholm
86. Liss L, Mervis L (1964) The ependymal lining of the cavum septi pellucidi. A histological and histochemical study. J Neuropathol Exp Neurol 23: 355-367
87. Louis-Bar D (1941) Sur un syndrome progressif comprenant des teleangiectasies capillaires cutanees et conjunctivales symmetriques, a disposition naevoide et des troubles cerebelleux. Confin Neurol 4: 32-42
88. Ludwin SK, Norman MG (1985) Congenital malformation of the nervous system. In: Davis RL, Robertson DM (eds) Textbook of neuropathology. Williams and Wilkins, Baltimore, pp 176-242
89. Mackenzie NG, Emery JL (1971) Deformities of the cervical cord in children with neurospinal dysraphism. Dev Med Child Neurol 13 [Suppl 23] 58-61
90. McLaurin RL (1964) Parietal cephalocele. Neurology 14: 764-774
91. McMurdo SK JR, Moore SG, Brant-Zawadzki M, Berg BO, Koch T, Newton TH, Edwards MSB (1987) MR imaging of intracranial tuberous sclerosis. AJNR 8: 77-82
92. Manelfe C, Rochiccioli P (1979) CT of septo-optic dysplasia. AJR 133: 1157-1160
93. Manz JH, Phillips TM, Rowden G, McCullough DC (1979) Unilateral megalencephaly, cerebral cortical dysplasia, neuronal hypertrophy, and heterotopia: cytomorphometric, fluorometric, cytochemical, and biochemical analyses. Acta Neuropathol (Berl) 45: 97-103
94. Mark AS, Feinberg DA, Brant-Zawadzki MN (1986) CSF motion and changes in ventricular size during the cardiac cycle evaluated by gated MR. Presented at the XIII. Symposium Neuroradiologicum, June 23-28, Stockholm
95. Matson DD (1969) Neurosurgery of infancy and childhood, 2nd edn. Charles C Thomas, Springfield
96. Michaud J, Mizrahi EM, Urich H (1982) Agenesis of the vermis with fusion of the cerebellar hemispheres, septo-optic dysplasia and associated anomalies. Report of a case. Acta Neuropathol (Berl) 56: 161-166
97. Modic MT, Weinstein MA, Pavlicek W, Boumphrey F, Starnes D, Duchesneau PM (1983) Magnetic resonance imaging of the cervical spine: technical and clinical observations. AJR 141: 1129-1136
98. Mori K (1985) Anomalies of the central nervous system. In: Nadjmi M, Piepgras U, Vogelsang H (eds) Neuroradiological atlases. Thieme, Stuttgart, and Stratton, New York
99. Muller J (1983) Congenital malformations of the brain. In: Rosenberg RN (ed) The clinical neurosciences, vol 3. Churchill, New York, pp 1-33
100. Nakano S, Hojo H, Kataoka K, Yamasaki S (1981) Age related incidence of cavum septi pellucidi and cavum vergae on CT scans of pediatric patients. J Comput Assist Tomogr 5: 348-349
101. Naidich TP, McLone DG, Fulling KH (1983) The Chiari II malformation, part IV: the hindbrain deformity. Neuroradiology 25: 179-197

102. Naidich TP, Pudlowski RM, Naidich JB (1980a) Computed tomographic signs of the Chiari II malformation, II. Midbrain and cerebellum. Radiology 134: 391-398
103. Naidich TP, Pudlowski RM, Naidich JB (1980b) Computed tomographic signs of the Chiari II malformation. III. Ventricle and cistern. Radiology 134: 657-663
104. Newton TH, Hoyt WF, Glaser JS (1978) Abnormal third ventricle. In: Newton TH, Potts DG (eds) Radiology of the skull and brain, vol 4. Ventricles and cisterns. Mosby, St Louis, pp 3481-3482
105. Noetzel H (1983) Entwicklungsstörungen und Schäden des reifenden Gehirns. In: Berlet H, Noetzel H, Quadbeck G et al (eds) Spezielle pathologische Anatomie, vol 2/II. Pathologie des Nervensystems II. Springer, Berlin Heidelberg New York
106. Noetzel H, Gulotta F (1986) Nervensystem. In: Grundmann E (ed) Spezielle Pathologie. Urban und Schwarzenberg, München, pp 394-439
107. Norman MG (1980) Bilateral encephaloclastic lesions in a 26 week gestation fetus: effect on neuroblast migration. J Can Sci Neurol 7: 191-194
108. Norman RM (1963) Malformations of the nervous system. In: Greenfield JG (ed) Neuropathology, 2nd edn. Edward Arnold, London
109. O'Doherty N (1972) Bloch-Sulzberger syndrome. Incontinentia pigmenti. In: Vinken PJ, Bruyn GW (eds) The phakomatoses, vol 14. North Holland, Amsterdam, pp 213-222 (Handbook of clinical neurology)
110. O'Doherty NJ, Norman RM (1968) Incontinentia pigmenti (Bloch-Sulzberger syndrome) with cerebral malformation. Dev Med Child Neurol 10 (2): 168-174
111. Paul KS, Lye RH, Strang FA, Dutton J (1983) Arnold-Chiari malformation. Review of 71 cases. J Neurosurg 58: 183-187
112. Peters G (1970) Klinische Neuropathologie. Thieme, Stuttgart, pp 314-316
113. Pierre-Kahn A, Lacombe J, Pichon J, Giudicelli Y, Renier D, Sainte-Rose C, Perrigot M, Hirsch JF (1986) Intraspinal lipomas with spina bifida. J Neurosurg 65: 756-761
114. Pojunas K, Williams AL, Daniels DL, Haughton VM (1984) Syringomyelia and hydromyelia: magnetic resonance evaluation. Radiology 153: 679-683
115. Poser CM (1956) The relationship between syringomyelia and neoplasm. Thomas, Springfield
116. Probst FP (1979) The prosencephalies; morphology, neuroradiological appearance and differential diagnosis. Springer, Berlin Heidelberg New York
117. Raimondi AJ, Sato K, Shimoji T (1984) The Dandy-Walker-syndrome. Karger, Basel
118. Rakic P, Yakovlev PI (1968) Development of the corpus callosum and cavum septi in man. J Comp Neurol 132: 45-72
119. Rayboud C (1983) Destructive lesions of the brain. Neuroradiology 25: 265-291
120. Rewcastle NB, Francover J (1962) Teratomous cysts in the spinal canal. Arch Neurol 11: 91-100
121. Robain O, Lyon G (1972) Les microencephalies familiales par malformation cerebrales. Acta Neuropathol (Berl) 20: 96-109
122. Robinson RG (1977) Agenesis and anomalies of other brain structures. In: Vinken PJ, Bruyn GW (eds) Congenital malformations of the brain and skull, vol 30, part I. North Holland, Amsterdam (Handbook of clinical neurology)
123. Rubin JB, Enzmann DR (1986) New concepts in magnetic resonance spine imaging: exploiting CSF pulsation flow phenomenon. Presented at the XIII. Symposium Neuroradiologicum, June 23-28, Stockholm
124. Rubinstein LJ (1972) Tumors of the central nervous system. Armed Forces Institute of Pathology, Washington (Atlas of tumor pathology, Series 2, fasc 6)
125. Samuelsson L, Wallensten R, Aparisi T, Bergström K, Thuomas KA, Hemmingsson A (1986) Magnetic resonance imaging of syringohydromyelia and Chiari malformations in myelomeningocele patients with scoliosis. Presented at the XIII. Symposium Neuroradiologicum, June 23-28, Stockholm
126. Schowing J (1968) Influence inductrice de l'encephale embryonnaire sur le developpment du crane chez le poulet. J Embryol Exp Morphol 19: 1-32
127. Scotti G, Musgrave MA, Harwood-Nash DC, Fitz CR, Chuang SH (1980) Diastematomyelia in children: metrizamide and CT metrizamide myelography. AJNR 1: 403-410
128. Sherman JL, Citrin CM (1986) Magnetic resonance demonstration of normal CSF flow. AJNR 7: 3-6
129. Sherman JL, Barkovich AJ, Citrin CM (1987) The MR appearance of syringomyelia: new observations. AJR 148: 381-391
130. Smoker WRK, Biller J, Moore SA, Beck DW, Hart MN (1986) Intradural spinal teratoma: case report and review of the literature. AJNR 7: 905-910
131. Spinos E, Laster DW, Moody DM, Balt MR, Witcofski RL, Kelly DL Jr (1985) MR evaluation of Chiari malformation at 0.15 T. AJNR 6: 203-208
132. Starkman SP, Brown TC, Linell EA (1958) Cerebral arachnoid cysts. J Neuropathol Exp Neurol 17: 484-500
133. Stimac GK, Solomon MA, Newton TH (1986) CT and MR of angiomatous malformations of the choroid plexus in patients with Sturge-Weber disease. AJNR 7: 623-627
134. Strandgaard L (1970) The Dandy-Walker syndrome - a case with patent foramen of the fourth ventricle demonstrated by encephalography. Br J Radiol 43: 734-738
135. Taylor DC, Falconer MA, Bruton CJ, Corsellis JA (1971) Focal dysplasia of the cerebral cortex in epilepsy. J Neurol Neurosurg Psychiatry 34: 369-387
136. Vade A, Kennard D (1987) Lipomeningomyelocystocele. AJNR 8: 375-377
137. Vaghi M, Visciani A, Testa D, Binelli S, Passerini A (1987) Cerebral MR findings in tuberous sclerosis. J Comput Assist Tomogr 11 (3): 403-406
138. Venes JL, Black KL, Latack JT (1986) Preoperative evaluation and surgical management of the Arnold-Chiari II malformation. J Neurosurg 64: 363-370
139. Vogt H (1908) Zur Diagnostik der tuberösen Sklerose. Z Erforsch Behandl Jugendl Schwachsinns 2: 1-16
140. Williams B (1980) On the pathogenesis of syringomyelia: a review. J R Soc Med 73: 798-806
141. Wolf A, Bamford TE (1935) Cavum septi pellucidi and cavum vergae. Bull Neurol Inst NY 4: 294-309
142. Wolpert SM (1974) Vascular studies of congenital anomalies. In: Newton TH, Potts DC (eds) Radiology of the skull and brain, chapt 87. Mosby, St Louis
143. Yakovlev PI, Wadsworth RC (1964a) Schizencephalies: a study of the congenital clefts in the cerebral mantle. I. Clefts with fused lips. J Neuropathol Exp Neurol 5: 116-130

144. Yakovlev PI, Wadsworth RC (1964b) Schizencephalies: a study of the contenital clefts in the cerebral mantle. II. Clefts with hydrocephalus and lips separated. J Neuropathol Exp Neurol 5: 169-205
145. Yuh WTC, Segall HD, Senac MO, Schultz D (1987) MR imaging of Chiari II malformation associated with dysgenesis of cerebellum and brain stem. J Comput Assist Tomogr 11 (1): 188-191
146. Zanella FE, Mödder U, Benz-Bohm G, Thun F (1984) Die Neurofibromatose im Kindesalter - Computertomographische Befunde im Schädel-Halsbereich. RÖFO 141: 498-504
147. Zimmerman RA, Bilaniuk LT, Grossman RI (1983) Computed tomography in migratory disorders of human brain development. Neuroradiology 25: 257-263
148. Ziter F, Bramwit D (1970) Nasal encephalocele and glioma. Br J Radiol 43: 136

8 Degenerative Disorders of the Brain and White Matter Diseases

W. J. Huk, G. M. Bydder, and W. L. Curati

In this chapter we shall look at diseases of various etiologies that exhibit similar CNS changes on CT and MR images. The etiologies may be congenital (e.g., congenital metabolic diseases) or acquired (e.g., metabolic, inflammatory, toxic insults) and result in diffuse or (multi)focal degenerative changes in central nervous tissues.

In describing the CT and MR appearances of these disorders, it is helpful to classify them less by their metabolic, enzymatic, or pathogenic features than by topographic criteria. Boltshauser [12] has proposed classifying the diseases as follows:

1. Primary neuronal (gray matter) involvement.
2. Primary myelin (white matter) involvement: here we distinguish between *dys*myelinating processes (those that disturb the formation and maintenance of normal myelin, such as congenital enzyme defects) and *de*myelinating processes (those causing secondary destruction of normal myelin, such as multiple sclerosis). Problems relating to the differentiation of pathologic changes from physiologic immaturity of the white matter in small children are discussed more fully in Chap. 6.
3. Primary involvement of the basal ganglia and brainstem.
4. No apparent sites of predilection.

Table 8.1. Classification of degenerative disorders

1. Primary neuronal (gray matter) involvement
   - a) Congenital causes
     - Lipidoses
     - Gangliosidoses
     - Neuronal ceroid lipofuscidosis
     - Mucolipidosis
   - b) Acquired and unexplained causes
     - Creutzfeldt-Jakob syndrome and kuru
     - Alzheimer's disease
     - Pick's disease
2. Primary myelin (white matter) involvement
   - a) Congenital causes
     - Metachromatic leukodystrophy
     - Globoid cell leukodystrophy
     - Orthochromatic (sudanophilic) leukodystrophy
       - Adrenoleukodystrophy
       - Pelizaeus-Merzbacher disease
     - Spongy degeneration
     - Alexander's disease
     - Defects of protein metabolism
       - Maple syrup disease
       - Phenylketonuria
   - b) Acquired and unexplained causes
     - Multiple sclerosis
     - Concentric sclerosis
     - Hypertensive cerebrovascular diseases
       - Binswanger's disease
       - Multi-infarct dementia
     - Progressive multifocal leukoencephalopathy
     - Postinfectious encephalomyelitis
     - Methotrexate-associated disease
     - Radiation damage
3. Primary involvement of the basal ganglia and brainstem
   - a) Congenital causes
     - Wilson's disease
     - Fahr's disease
     - Hallervorden-Spatz syndrome
     - Fabry's disease
     - Glycogen storage disease
     - Huntington's chorea
     - Subacute necrotizing encephalopathy
     - Spinocerebellar degeneration
       - Olivopontocerebellar degeneration
       - Cerebellar heredoataxia
   - b) Acquired and unexplained causes
     - Wernicke's encephalopathy
     - Central pontine myelinolysis
4. Primary involvement with no sites of predilection
   - a) Congenital causes
     - Mucopolysaccharidoses
     - Cerebrotendinous xanthomatosis
     - Farber's disease
     - MELAS, MERRF, and KSS
     - Other, uncommon metabolic diseases
   - b) Acquired and unexplained causes
     - Systemic lupus erythematosus

8.1 Primary Neuronal (Gray Matter) Involvement

8.1.1 Congenital Causes

The nervous system is involved in congenital metabolic disorders with greater frequency than any other system. Depending on the disease, pathologic alterations may or may not be apparent and, when present, may be manifested at an early or late stage. The clinical manifestations of a metabolic disease vary in accordance with the nature of the biochemical defect, the degree of maturation of the nervous system, dietary intake, drug use, and the occurrence of infections [7]. Clinical signs may be caused by a deficiency of a particular enzyme due to degeneration (as in leukodystrophy), by a surplus of protein products that cannot be utilized (as in storage diseases), or by toxic metabolic products (as in diabetes mellitus, uremia, etc.).

These disorders are diagnosed mainly from clinical and laboratory findings, but in some cases imaging procedures can provide information helpful in assessing the degree of severity of the disorder and its response to medical treatment. Below we shall look at the major morphologic, and metabolic characteristics of these disorders which can influence their MR appearance. Where necessary, we have drawn on the literature to supplement our own case data on these rare disorders. In cases where the literature is unrewarding, we must rely on a knowledge of pathologic features for the interpretation of findings. Details on clinical presentation, neuropathology, and etiology would exceed the scope of this text but may be found in the specialized literature.

Lipidosis [7]

Niemann-Pick disease (sphingomyelin lipidosis) involves storage of sphingomyelin in cerebral gray matter:

Type a: Acute neuronopathic form. Brain slightly atrophic, cerebellum severely atrophic. White matter normal. Astrogliosis and histiocytosis throughout the gray matter.
Type b: Non-neuronopathic form.
Type c: Chronic neuronopathic form (biochemical defect remains unknown). Brain atrophy with demyelination.
Type d: Nova Scotia variant.
Type e: Adult non-neuronopathic form.

Gangliosidoses [7]

GM_1 gangliosidosis (low activity of enzyme GM_1-beta-galactosidase-A leading to accumulation of GM_1 ganglioside, neural glycolipids, glycosaminoglycans, oligosaccharides):

Generalized form: Brain atrophy with narrow gyri and dilated ventricles. Surviving neurons swollen.
Juvenile form: Brain severely atrophic, cortex and basal ganglia small, lateral ventricles markedly dilated. Cerebellum only mildly atrophic.

GM_2 gangliosidosis (deficiency of the isoenzyme hexosaminidase A and B, causing several disease states in which GM_2 ganglioside is stored):

Tay-Sachs disease (variant B = deficiency of hexosaminidase A, seen only in Ashkenazic Jews): Macrencephaly in some cases due to neuronal storage and astrogliosis, or brain atrophy due to neuronal loss and demyelination. Cortical ribbon narrowed, centrum semiovale severely demyelinated.

Sandhoff's disease (variant 0 = deficiency of hexosaminidase A and B): Brain normal or slightly enlarged, cerebellum small.
Variant AB (hexosaminidase A and B normal, absence of activator substance): Brain normal or slightly atrophic.

Neuronal Ceroid Lipofuscidosis (Battens's disease)

Neuronal ceroid lipofuscidosis [4, 71] involves accumulation of ceroid and lipofuscin):

Infantile form (Haltia-Santavuori disease): Micrencephaly, axonal loss and demyelination including the subcortical U-fibres, prominent astrogliosis, demyelination of optic nerve.

Late infantile form (Bielschowsky-Jansky-disease): Brain, especially cerebellum, atrophic due to loss of neurons and gliosis in cerebellum and optic nerve. Only slight loss of myelin in the white matter. Preserved neurons in cerebral cortex, basal ganglia, and brainstem.

Late juvenile form (Batten-Spielmeyer-Vogt disease): Mild brain atrophy, cerebellar granule cells sometimes severely reduced. Only little evidence of mylin loss. Optic nerve well preserved, but neurons contain ceroid lipofuscin.

Adult form (Kuf's disease): Moderate atrophy of the brain.

Mucolipidosis

In mucolipidosis oligosaccharidosis both glycosaminoglycans and lipids accumulate in lysosomes as a result of a single enzyme defect. Usually the brain is grossly normal.

MR Findings

Reports on the MR features of these rare diseases are not available at this writing. Dilatation of the internal and external CSF spaces is well displayed on T1-weighted sequences.

Atrophic changes in the cortex and/or white matter are best appreciated on heavily T1-weighted images (inversion recovery; SE with short TR and short TE < = 17 ms).

Demyelination and gliosis prolong the relaxation times of the white matter. Edema, which can occur in response to storage substances, has a similar effect.

8.1.2 Acquired and Unexplained Causes

Creutzfeldt-Jakob Disease and Kuru

Creutzfeldt-Jakob disease (CJD) and kuru are classified among the presenile spongiform encephalopathies, which are believed to be caused by a virus-like agent (slow virus).

The *morphologic features* of these diseases are as follows [38, 44]:

- Widespread loss of neurons in the cerebral cortex, central gray matter, cerebellum, and brainstem.
- Extensive vacuolization of the gray matter in the affected regions. These spongiform lesions are considered to indicate active disease, and their visualization very strongly suggests the presence of the disease.
- Heavy proliferation of astrocytes.
- Small, stellate, occasionally amyloid-containing deposits in the ganglion cell layer of the cerebellum and in some cases the cerebrum (kuru plaques).

If the disease takes a protracted course, involvement of the white matter may become evident.

The *clinical course* often begins with personality change and visual impairment and progresses to profound dementia. It is also characterized by deficits or hypersensitivity of the extrapyramidal system (see Sect. 2.3.5). Death occurs within a few years (usually 1 year) of onset.

CT and MR Findings

The CT and MR appearances of CJD are nonspecific.

The extent of CT findings depends on the stage of the disease. Scans may show progressive atrophic changes with enlargement of the cerebral sulci and ventricles.

Kovanen et al. [37] describe the CT and MR findings (0.17 T; IR and SE sequences with T1- and T2-weighted images) in three patients with CJD, which was histologically confirmed in one case. Both imaging modalities showed cortical atrophy and mild ventricular enlargement, which appeared less pronounced with MR than with CT. The atrophy was predominantly occipital in one case and temporal in another. The parenchymal signal was apparently unchanged.

Involvement of the cerebral white matter is considered an unusual finding, expect for secondary Wallerian degeneration [37]. White matter abnormalities were found no earlier than 3 months before the death of a CJD patient; in this terminal stage the changes apparently resulted from diffuse myelin loss and from microvacuolization resembling spongiform changes [37]. Marked prolongations of T1 and T2 would be expected to occur in association with these white matter changes.

In its early stage, then, CJD can be difficult to distinguish from Alzheimer's disease. Dementia due to vascular causes (multi-infarct type, lacunar state type, Binswanger's disease) shows marked focal signal abnormalities in the white matter which are not found in CJD.

Alzheimer's Disease

Today we distinguish two forms of Alzheimer's disease according to the age of onset: a *presenile* form occurring between 50 and 60 years of age, occasionally earlier, and a *senile* form occurring after 60 years of age.

The gross morphologic changes of Alzheimer's disease consist of cortical atrophy, which is greatest in the region of the frontal lobes, and ventricular enlargement.

Histologic examination shows shrinkage and lipofuscin storage in the ganglion cells, neurofibril-

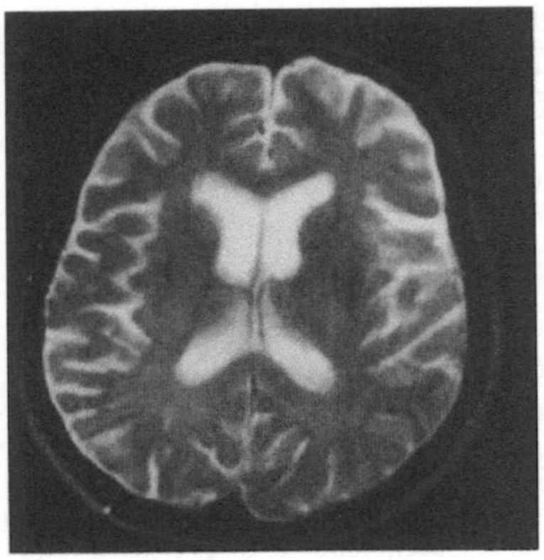

Fig. 8.1. Alzheimer's disease in a 57-year-old woman with dementia (Hachinski score 1). MR shows enlarged ventricles, slight cortical atrophy, and discreet increase of signal intensity of temporoparietal white matter; well-delineated, bilateral, patchy, hyperintense lesions of the subcortical white matter of the island of Reil probably are secondary to vascular disease. Axial scan, SE 3.0 s/120 ms (1.0 T). SPECT 15 min p.i. showed characteristic bilateral temporoparietal reduction of activity

lary tangles in the neurons ("Alzheimer's fibrils"), and senile plaques in the cerebral and cerebellar cortex [44]. These neuropathologic changes are marked in the region of the angular gyrus and the inferior and middle temporal gyri, in the amygdala, and in the hippocampus and parahippocampal gyrus [34].

CT and MR Findings

The cortical atrophy and ventricular enlargement of Alzheimer's disease can be appreciated on CT scans. However, the severity of the atrophy does not necessarily correlate with the degree of cognitive impairment. Also, quantitative measurements of the CT absorption coefficients of the parenchyma are not helpful in distinguishing Alzheimer's disease from atrophic changes of other etiology.

In a review of CT findings in dementing disorders, LeMay [38] describes striking atrophy of the anterior and medial portions of the temporal lobes, leading to a widening of the adjacent CSF spaces as well as the temporal horns of the lateral ventricles. Most patients also showed increased widening of the anterior portion of the sylvian fissure. A similar widening of the superficial gyri can be seen in nondemented elderly individuals, however. Enlargement of the third ventricle relative to the bodies of the lateral ventricles is much more pronounced in Alzheimer's disease patients than in age-matched controls [38].

MR images in various projections permit a detailed evaluation of the atrophic changes of Alzheimer's disease. This is best accomplished with T1-weighted sequences owing to the good contrast between CSF and brain tissue. So far no data are available on characteristic T1 and T2 values. Besson et al. [9] found a significantly higher proton density of the white matter in three Alzheimer's disease patients than in normal controls, leading them to conclude that proton-density measurements of the white matter can be of value in differentiating Alzheimer-type senile dementia from other diffuse atrophic process. This observation is supported by Naeser et al. [43], who found lower CT density values in demented patients than in normal controls. George et al. [23] report that the signal increases on T2-weighted sequences commonly seen in elderly individuals as a sign of leukoencephalopathy are more extensive in patients with Alzheimer's disease (Fig. 8.1).

Pick's Disease

Pick's disease, unlike the diffuse atrophies, is characterized by a selective, frontal cortical atrophy in an otherwise normal brain. The atrophy is often asymmetric and affects the left hemisphere preferentially. Involvement of the temporal and parietal lobes is less frequent and also less pronounced. There is a concomitant loss of white matter in the frontal brain, causing the frontal horns of the lateral ventricles to become enlarged. Marked atrophy of the striatum and thalamus may also occur.

The lesions are based on a loss of ganglion cells and a pigmentary atrophy of the surviving cells. The senile plaques and fibrils of Alzheimer's disease are absent.

Clinical manifestations include personality changes and mental deterioration, especially speech disturbance and a progressive decline in memory. Females are predominantly affected. The disease usually presents between 40 and 50 years of age, and the time from onset to death is 2–15 years [44].

CT and MR Findings

Both CT and MR show a circumscribed cortical atrophy that involves the frontal to frontotemporal regions and often is more pronounced on one side than the other, supporting the clinical suspicion of Pick's disease. The atrophy may involve the basal ganglia. In contrast to Alzheimer's disease, the changes spare the posterior two-thirds of the superior temporal gyrus [38].

8.2 Primary Myelin (White Matter) Involvement

Magnetic resonance has proved to be a very sensitive method in the detection and diagnosis of white matter diseases. The white matter of the brain contains less water than the gray matter (71.6% vs 81.9%) and thus contains relatively few mobile protons with long T1 and T2 relaxation times. The white matter is rich in lipid compounds (16% vs 6.3% in the gray matter), which shorten somewhat the relaxation times of adjacent spins. The gray matter-white matter contrast is determined chiefly by the difference in the population of free water protons. Because the water content of the immature neonatal brain is quite high, at 92%-95% (it subsequently decreases, rapidly at first and then gradually more slowly), the interpretation of MR findings can be difficult in this very young age group. This problem is discussed more fully in Chap. 6.

Diseases of *diverse etiologies* can cause a loss of hydrophobic myelin with an increase in interstitial water and a disruption of the blood-brain barrier. This results in a relatively *nonspecific prolongation of the T1 and T2 relaxation times,* causing the involved areas to give a high signal on proton-density and T2-weighted images and a low signal on T1-weighted images. Such lesions can have similar appearances even though associated with different underlying conditions, e.g., demyelinating diseases and hydrocephalus. Differentiation can be made on the basis of clinical features and also by evaluating the morphology and sites of occurrence of the lesions. In *hydrocephalus* they are plump, irregular, and do not extent to the gray matter-white matter junction. With *diffuse demyelination* the irregular contours of the lesions are sharper, and the lesions extend to the gray matter-white matter junction and form insular areas in the white matter. When diffuse medullary damage of vascular etiology and hydrocephalus coexist in older patients, the conditions can be impossible to separate. Thus, while MR is more sensitive than CT, ultimately it is just as nonspecific.

Approximately 90% of normal patients may show a narrow periventricular border of high MR signal intensity, which usually is enhanced around the frontal horns of the lateral ventricles. This feature cannot be construed as evidence of demyelinating disease. It has been attributed to anatomic peculiarities and physiologic mechanisms [62]:

- A loose arrangement of axons with a low myelin content
- "Ependymitis granularis," i.e., small ependymal defects with astrocytic gliosis
- Bulk flow interstitial water in this region, which becomes confluent in the posterolateral angle of the frontal horns.

8.2.1 Congenital Causes

Metachromatic Leukodystrophy

Metachromatic leukodystrophy, inherited as an autosomal recessive trait, is based on a cerebroside sulfatase disturbance due to a lack of the enzyme arylsulfatase A. It leads to an accumulation of sulfatides in the CNS, peripheral nerves, and kidneys. Three forms are recognized - late infantile, juvenile, and adult - according to the age of symptom onset. *Clinical manifestations* include deterioration of mental faculties, progressive spasticity, and seizures.

The brain shows a diffuse demyelination without involvement of the arcuate fibres. The white matter appears glassy gray, sclerotic, and may show spongy cavitation. The gray matter is spared. Hydrocephalus e vacuo is commonly seen as a result of the white matter damage.

Histologic examination shows a proliferation of glial fibers in the sclerotic white matter and an accumulation of scavenger cells with a weakly positive ("metachromatic") lipid stain that is most pronounced in the marginal zones of lesions [12, 44].

CT and MR Findings

The leukodystrophic changes appear on CT scans as extensive, diffuse, symmetrical, poorly marginated areas of decreased density in the central white matter accompanied by mild ventricular dilatation

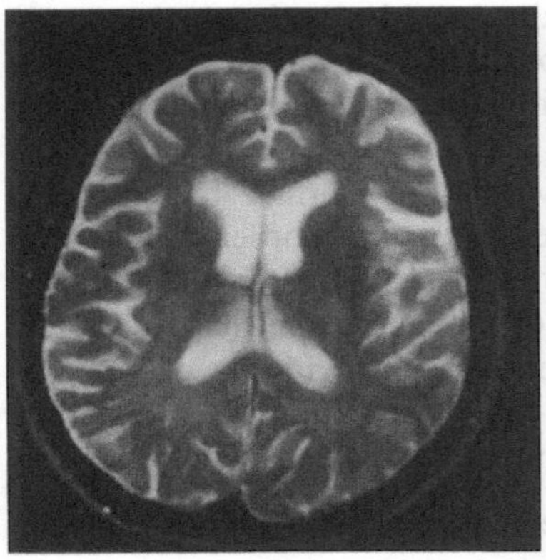

8.2

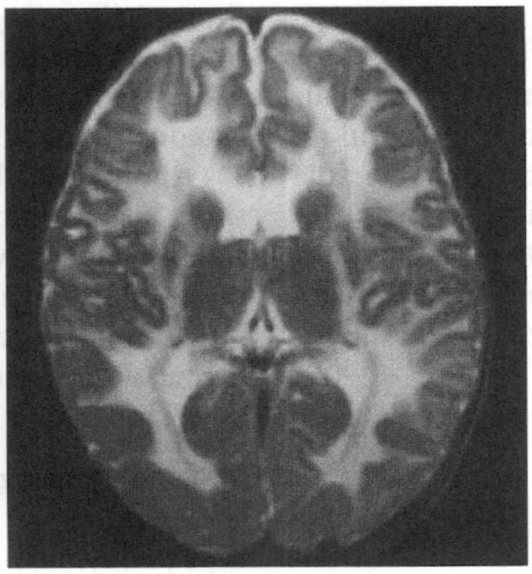

8.3

Fig. 8.2. Metachromatic leukodystrophy, juvenile form, in a 16-year-old girl with tetraparesis, ataxia, and dementia. Prolonged relaxation times of white matter secondary to diffuse demyelination. Axial scan, SE 1.6 s/90 ms (1.0 T)

Fig. 8.3. Orthochromatic leukodystrophy (autopsy finding) in a 6-month-old girl with grand mal seizures and progressive apathy, mental deterioration, and hypotonia. Generalized loss of myelin. Axial scan, SE 3.0 s/110 ms (1.5 T)

(Fig. 8.2). Contrast enhancement is not described [13, 68]. Changes in the white matter appear with even greater clarity as hyperintense areas on proton-density and T2-weighted MR images (Fig. 8.2).

Globoid Cell Leukodystrophy

Globoid cell leukodystrophy (Krabbe's disease), a familial form of leukodystrophy, produces symptoms within the first 1-2 years of life, occasionally later, and takes a rapidly fatal course. It is caused by a deficiency of beta-cerebrosidase, leading to an increased storage of cerebrosides in distended macrophages ("globoid cells") arranged predominantly around vessels in the white matter. The brain is small with a diffuse loss of myelin [68], the subcortical arcuate fibres usually being preserved.

The disease is manifested clinically by spastic paresis, rigor, pseudobulbar symptoms, ataxia, progressive dementia, and decerebrate rigidity. Initial symptoms include increased irritability and extreme sensitivity to light and noise, which elicit myoclonic jerks.

Microscopic examination may show myelin sheath destruction and atrophy of the white matter in the cerebrum (with hydrocephalus e vacuo), cerebellum, and brainstem [12, 44].

CT and MR Findings

Reports on CT findings in globoid cell leukodystrophy are exceedingly rare. Authors have described normal white matter in the questionable low-density areas together with mild ventricular dilatation and widening of the cortical sulci [6, 68].

The CT and MR findings change with progression of the disease. Initially the white and gray matter may still appear normal, or CT may show hypodense areas in the periventricular white matter and centrum semiovale with increased T1 and T2 values on MR scans. These foci may result from edema and active phagocytosis caused by the accumulation of cytotoxic derivatives (galactosylsphingosines). As the disease progresses, CT shows symmetric zones of high density in the thalamus, the posterior limb of the internal capsule, the quadrigeminal region, and the cerebellum [5]. These lesions produce a slightly increased signal on T1-weighted images and a low signal on T2-weighted images, suggesting that a paramagnetic effect (as in hemorrhages) may be involved. Meanwhile the ventricles and external CSF spaces begin to enlarge, later creating the appearance of a diffuse cerebral atrophy [5].

Further observational data are needed before we can assess the specificity of the above findings and their sites of occurrence.

Orthochromatic Leukodystrophy

Orthochromatic (sudanophilic) leukodystrophy is a collective term applied to various subforms of leukodystrophy with a normal breakdown of neutral fats. These disorders are diverse in their age of onset, clinical presentation, and neuropathologic features. The pathogenesis is unexplained but appears to vary from one disorder to the next. A reduction of phospholipids and galactose in the white matter has been demonstrated [44].

The white matter of the hemisphere is vacuolated and shows grayish-yellow discoloration. Ventricular dilatation e vacuo eventually develops.

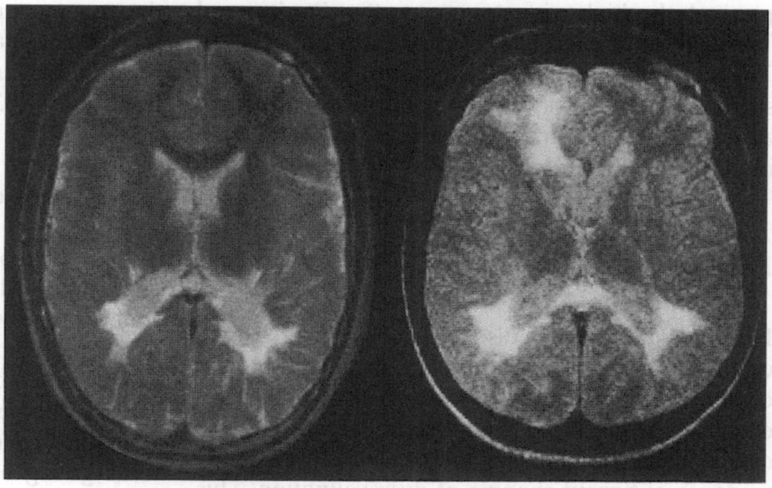

a b

Fig. 8.4 a, b. Adrenoleukodystrophy, juvenile form. **a** In an 18-year-old male with adrenocortical insufficiency and one grand mal seizure. Symmetrical areas of prolonged relaxation times in the parietal white matter and slight ventricular dilatation indicating demyelination with atrophy. Axial scan (**a**) SE 1.6 s/140 ms, (0.5 T). (Courtesy of Drs. Kuhn, Steen, and Terwey, Oldenburg, FRG). **b** Adrenoleukodystrophy, juvenile form, in a 24-year-old man with personality changes, intellectual deterioration, spasticity, and adrenocortical insufficieny. Demyelination is predominantly seen in the temporoparieto-occipital white matter. Axial scan (**b**) SE 1.6 s/70 ms; (1.0 T)

MR Findings

In the advanced stage of orthochromatic leukodystrophy increased signal intensity of the entire white matter secondary to generalized loss of myelin can be seen (Fig. 8.3).

Special forms include adrenoleukodystrophy and Pelizaeus-Merzbacher disease.

Adrenoleukodystrophy

Adrenoleukodystrophy (diffuse cerebral sclerosis and adrenal atrophy; [12]) is associated with a primary adrenal cortical atrophy that usually develops between 4 and 12 years of age. Death typically occurs within a few years of symptom onset. Symptoms include personality change, mental deterioration, visual failure, spasticity, and ataxia. The disease is based on a defect in the breakdown of long-chain saturated fatty acids. The following forms are recognized [12]: the congenital form, the juvenile (classic) form, adrenomyeloneuropathy, and Addison's disease (isolated).

Areas of demyelination, usually symmetrical, occur mainly in the occipital, parietal, and temporal white matter. The subcortical arcuate fibres may be partially involved. The optic nerve and tract, fornix, hippocampal commissure, posterior cingulum, and corpus callosum commonly are severely affected. Changes in the frontal regions are rare, they usually are mild (Fig. 8.4) [4]. Histologic examination shows myelin destruction, sparing of axons, signs of inflammation, and lipophage response, as well as a dense gliosis with loss of oligodendrocytes, myelin, and axons. The result is cerebral atrophy with ventricular dilatation.

CT and MR Findings

The CT and MR findings in adrenoleukodystrophy are localized to the areas of white matter destruction. Three histopathologic zones can be identified from the edge to the center of the lesions [68]:

- An outer zone with destruction of myelin, rarefaction of the axons, and no inflammatory response
- An intermediate zone of increased demyelination with loss of axons, numerous lipid-containing macrophages, and perivascular accumulation of mononuclear cells, signifying a marked inflammatory response
- A central zone with inactive gliosis

CT shows contrast enhancement at the border between the outer zone and the intermediate zone as evidence of disruption of the blood-brain barrier (*type 1*). DiChiro et al. [20] have described a type 2 adrenoleukodystrophy, characterized by enhancement of various white matter tracts (internal capsule, corona radiata, forceps minor, cerebral peduncle). This pattern is believed to be specific for a variant form or an evolving stage of the disease. Calcifications, unilateral parietal manifestation, and atrophy of the pons and cerebellum have also been described [68].

The loss of hydrophobic myelin and the edema-related increase in interstitial water causes a prolongation of T1 and T2 on MR scans. The lesions give particularly high signals on proton-density and T2-weighted images [10, 17]; they appear dark on T_1-weighted sequences. The resolution of MR is insufficient at present to delimit the histopathologic zones, whose margins are irregular and frequently ill-defined.

Pelizaeus-Merzbacher Disease

Pelizaeus-Merzbacher disease is characterized by a chronic, progressive sclerosis of the cerebral and cerebellar white matter, thought to be caused by a defect in the glycerine phosphate metabolism of the myelin sheaths. The diagnosis can only be made evidence of tigroid changes of dysmyelination. This disease is not a single histologic entity [12], and three main subforms are recognized:

- A classical type (Merzbacher) with symptoms appearing in early childhood predominantly in the male sex. The life span is 25 years or less. Clinical symptoms include microcephaly, progressive intellectual deterioration, disturbances of speech and coordination, and tetraparesis secondary to an extensive loss of white matter.
- A connatal type [56] revealed in the postnatal period by a lack of psychomotor development. While axons may be well preserved, the myelin may be missing completely. This form is also found predominantly in males.
- An adult type (Löwenberg-Hill) with onset of symptoms around the age of 42 years and a remaining life expectancy of about 10 years. Clinical symptoms include seizures, disturbances of speech, psychomotor deficits, and dementia in the late stage of the disease. This form is inherited preferentially by females in a dominant mode. Patchy lesions of demyelination are accompanied by an extensive destruction of axons.

CT and MR Findings

The CT findings in the few cases of Pelizaeus-Merzbacher disease published to date comprise cortical atrophy, diffuse or patchy (periventricular) areas of decreased density in the cerebral and cerebellar white matter, and atrophy of the cerebellum.

On MR, marked prolongation of T1 and T2 relaxation times due to lack of myelin is seen throughout the white matter of both the cerebral and cerebellar hemispheres, causing inversion of the gray matter-white matter contrast. These atrophic changes may be associated with more or less severe enlargement of the ventricles and subarachnoid spaces [33, 47] (Fig. 8.5).

Spongy Degeneration

Spongy degeneration (Canavan's disease, van Bogaert-Bertrand disease) is transmitted as an autosomal recessive trait, but its pathogenesis remains unclear. Symptoms usually appear within a few months after birth, and death generally occurs before the 5th year of life.

Clinical symptoms include macrocephaly, hypotonia giving way to spasticity, optic nerve atrophy with blindness, and convulsive seizures. Pathologic findings include spongiform lesions of the subcortical white matter mainly of the centrum semiovale with involvement of the arcuate fibres, giant mitochondria in astrocytes, and intramyelin vacuolation [12]. The basal ganglia and cerebellum may also be affected.

Spongy degeneration is also seen in some inborn errors of amino acid metabolism (see below) and thus may be considered a nonspecific response of the brain to various abnormal metabolites [68].

CT and MR Findings

Diffuse, symmetrical areas of decreased density in the white matter have been reported with CT [68]. These changes would produce increased relaxation times in MR images and would appear more extensive than on CT scans owing to the greater sensitivity of MR (Fig. 8.6).

Alexander's Disease

Alexander's disease, a very rare form of infantile leukodystrophy, likewise has an autosomal recessive mode of inheritance, and its pathogenesis is unexplained. Symptoms appear within 6 months after birth with developmental retardation, macrocephaly, spasticity, and seizure. The average life expectancy is 28 months [53].

Differential diagnosis must rely on biopsy to demonstrate the presence of subpial, subependymal, and perivascular Rosenthal fibers [12, 44]. The profusion, distribution, and radial orientation of the Rosenthal fibers are pathognomonic for this condi-

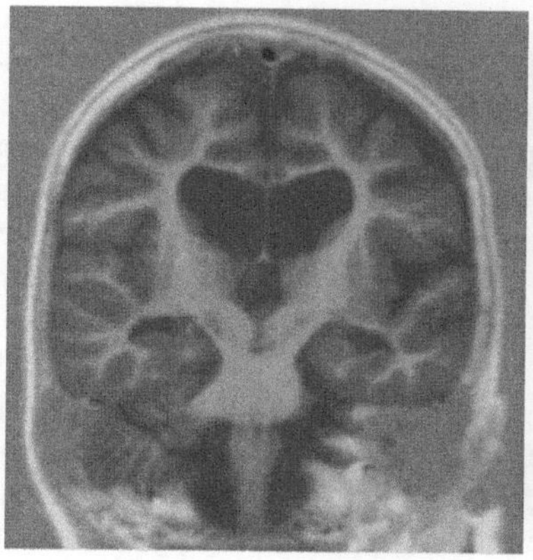

8.5

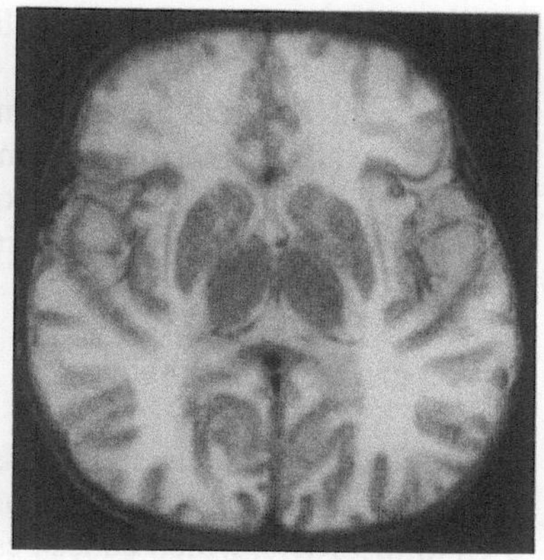

8.6

Fig. 8.5. Extensive loss of white matter with large ventricles, normal cortex, and slightly enlarged sulci in a 5-year-old boy with severe stato-and psychomotor retardation, flaccid trunc and hypertonic musculature of the extremities, divergent strabismus without fixation. Probable diagnosis Pelizaeus-Merzbacher disease! Coronal scan, IR 1,5 s/400 ms/30 ms 1,0 T).

Fig. 8.6. Spongy degeneration in a 9-month-old boy with large head and marked statomotor retardation. The high signal of the entire white matter relates to spongy change and demyelination which also involves the arcuate fibres. Axial scan, SE 2,0 s/105 ms (0,5 T) (Courtesy of Dr. Dangel, Stuttgart, FRG)

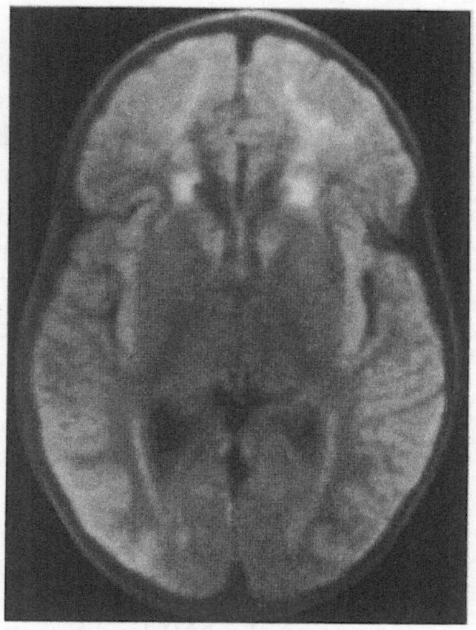

Fig. 8.7. Alexander's disease. Increased signal is seen in both frontal lobes, particularly on the left. Axial scan, SE 1.5 s/80 ms (0.15 T)

tion. Rosenthal fibers themselves are a nonspecific finding, as they have been described in association with multiple sclerosis, slowly growing astrocytic gliomas, and other diseases [27]. They are believed to represent inert metabolic products from the degeneration of astrocytes [68].

CT and MR Findings

Trommer et al. [63] reviewed the literature and followed the course of one patient from birth until death at 13 months. They point out several CT features which in their opinion enable Alexander's disease to be distinguished from other atypical forms of leukodystrophy:

- Marked peripheral extension of the frontal lobe white matter lucency to involve the subarcuate U fibers
- Involvement of the external and extreme capsules with relative sparing of the internal capsule
- Increased density of the optic chiasm and optic radiation, the columns of the fornices, the basal ganglia, the subependymal rim, and the medial portion of forceps minor
- Marked enhancement of areas that appear relatively dense on noncontrast CT

Trommer et al. (1983) believe that contrast enhancement is seen only in the acute stage of the infantile form, and that later the zones of increased density become less distinct and no longer show contrast enhancement. At this stage the low-density areas in the white matter appear more sharply defined, and differentiation from other degenerative diseases of the white matter is more difficult.

The same authors state that the earliest white matter change on CT scans is hyperdensity, and that hypodensity is observed only after a period of 9-33 weeks. They attribute this to a hyperemic stage (vascular congestion) prior to vacuolation of the white matter, which is followed later by loss of myelin, axons, and cavitation with a corresponding decrease in density.

The involved areas of white matter exhibit prolonged relaxation times on MR images (Fig. 8.7). As with CT, enhancement can be expected when MR contrast material is administered in the acute phase.

Defects of Protein Metabolism

Most defects of protein metabolism have an autosomal recessive mode of inheritance, and a few lead to CNS disorders, which consist essentially of spongiform degeneration of the brain.

Maple syrup disease is based on an enzymatic defect in the oxidative decarboxylation of the keto amino acids, leading to an abnormal buildup of valine, leukin, and isoleukin in the blood [44]. The result is a myelination defect with spongy degeneration in the cerebrum, brainstem, and cerebellum.

Phenylketonuria is based on an enzymatic defect in the amino acid breakdown of phenylalanine to tyrosine, resulting in toxic concentrations of phenols, indoles, and phenylpyruvic acid. This leads to spongiform changes in the white matter and damage to ganglion cells [44].

MR Findings

No reports on the MR findings in defects of protein metabolism were available to us at the time of writing. Spongy degeneration is associated with prolongation of relaxation times T1 and T2, so that hyperintense areas in the affected region can be expected in proton-density and T2-weighted sequences.

8.2.2 Acquired and Unexplained Causes

Multiple Sclerosis

Multiple sclerosis (MS) is presently regarded as an autoimmune disease (significant elevation of IgG) that may have a viral or genetic etiology. It is the most common organic disease of the CNS, showing a maximal incidence between 20 and 35 years of age. It often takes a long, progressive course marked by periods of relapse and remission.

The *clinical picture* of MS is protean and features a variety of sensorimotor disturbances and psychic chances whose severity fluctuates with the phases of remission and progression.

Multiple foci of demyelination are found in the white matter as well as in the cortex. Usually this is most pronounced around the ventricles and especially in the angle between the caudate nucleus and corpus callosum, although areas of demyelination may be scattered throughout the parenchyma without regard for structural boundaries or vascular territories (Fig. 8.8). In long-standing cases atrophy becomes apparent with dilatation of the internal and external CSF spaces. Spinal involvement gives rise to similar atrophic changes in the spinal cord.

The lesions of MS show myelin sheath destruction with sparing of glial cells and axis cylinders. Histologically, the acute phase is further characterized by a perivascular infiltration of lymphocytes and mononuclear cells. Older lesions appear as sharply demarcated areas of destroyed myelin sheaths bordered peripherally by a glial wall. Fiber-forming astrocytes gradually replace the parenchymal defect [44].

CT and MR Findings

The CT and MR features of MS are nonspecific and cannot establish the presence of the disease. The major role of MR imaging in MS lies in providing access to clinically silent lesions. The discrepancy between clinical manifestations and the extent of the underlying lesions is important in early diagnosis, when clinical signs may be subtle even though the disease is well established. The absence of changes does not exclude MS, because plaques in the region of the optic nerve cannot yet be demonstrated, and plaques in the spinal cord region are difficult to visualize (see below).

CT displays the lesions of MS as solitary or multiple foci of irregular shape, usually small, that become confluent in the later stages of the disease. They tend to occur around the ventricles, especially the frontal and occipital horns of the lateral ventricles, and in the centrum semiovale. The lesions appear more or less hypodense.

Old lesions show no changes on follow-up and are not enhanced by contrast material.

Fresh lesions or acutely exacerbating older lesions may show enhancement in high-dose delayed-contrast CT, signifying disruption of the blood-brain barrier in the setting of an acute demyelinating process. Follow-up scans may show changes in the shape and size of these foci or the appearance of new lesions (see Fig. 8.9). Lesions large enough to cause a mass effect may show nodular or ringlike

Fig. 8.8 a–d. Variety of lesions in multiple sclerosis: **a** 25-year-old, SE 3.0 s/45 ms; **b–d** 17-year-old (**b, c** SE 3.0 s/40 ms, **d** SE 3.0 s/120 ms): (1.0 T)

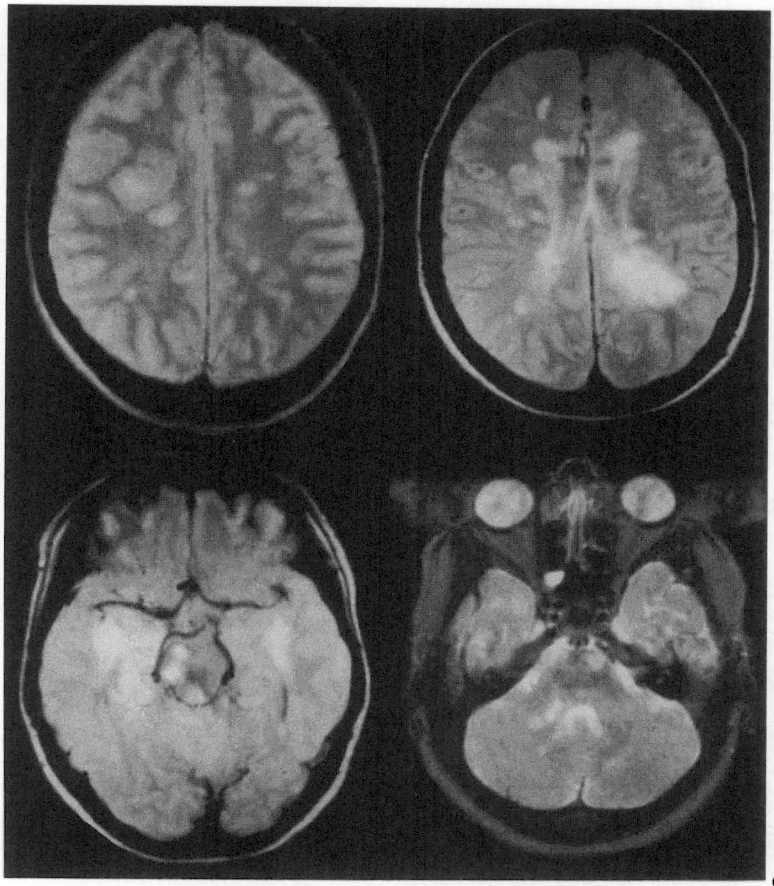

a b c d

Fig. 8.9 a, b. Multiple sclerosis. **a** Multiple hyperintense lesions near the ventricles and scattered throughout the white matter. **b** Control scan 20 months later: marked increase of size and number of lesions. Axial scans, SE 1.5 s/80 ms (0.15 T)

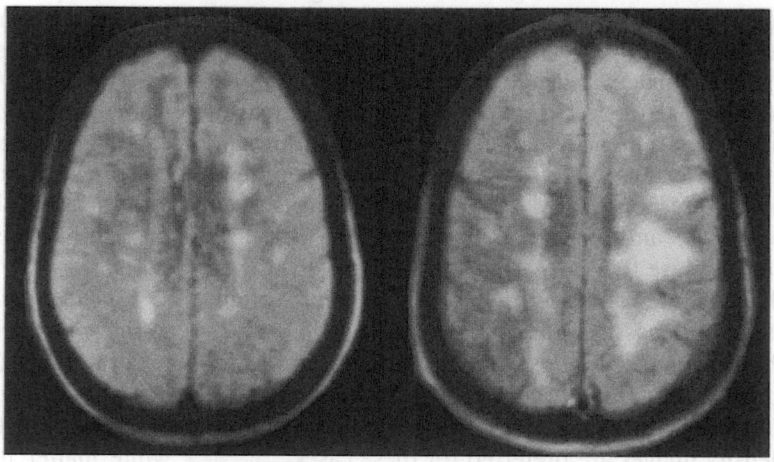

a b

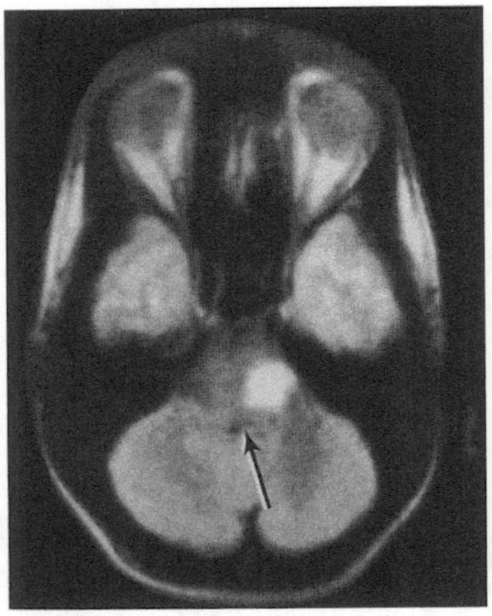

8.10

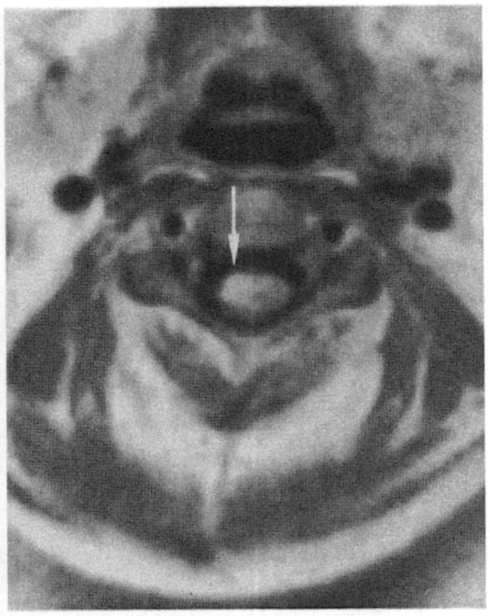

8.11

Fig. 8.10. Multiple sclerosis lesion associated with mass effect. The fourth ventricle *(arrow)* is displaced by the lesion in the pons. Axial scan, SE 1.58 s/80 ms (0.15 T)

Fig. 8.11. Multiple sclerosis of the cervical cord at the level of C2. Axial scan: SE 1.6 s/35 ms, (0.5 T). (Courtesy of Drs. Kuhn, Steen, and Terwey, Oldenburg, FRG)

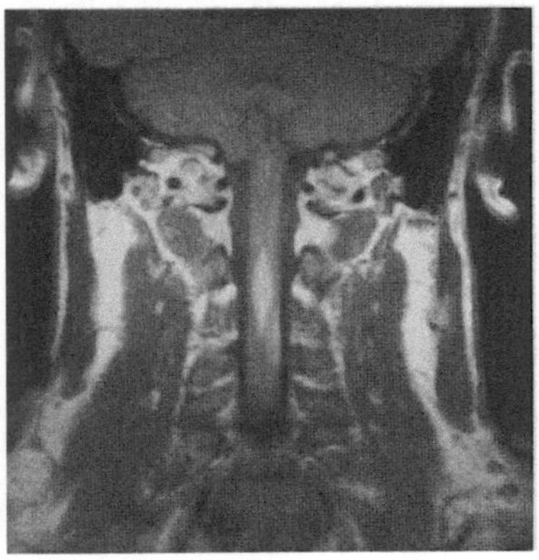

Fig. 8.12. Spinal plaques of multiple sclerosis in a 19-year-old man with bilateral dysesthesia, predominantly on the right, and CSF findings corresponding to MS. The native T1 weighted scan showed only slight thickening of the cord at C3. After i.v. gd-DTPA, enhancement is seen at the level of C3 and C4. Coronal, scan, SE 0.6 s/15 ms (1.5 T)

enhancement simulating a metastasis or glioblastoma. This can be suppressed by treatment with steroids.

MR imaging using proton-density and T2-weighted sequences displays MS lesions as areas of high signal intensity, indicating demyelination and also the edema that accompanies the acute inflammatory response (Fig. 8.9). Because of its greater sensitivity and absence of bone artifact, MR also can disclose foci not visible with CT and can even demonstrate lesions in the corpus callosum, brainstem, and possibly the spinal cord (Figs. 8.8–8.12). Periventricular lesions can be difficult to distinguish from partial volume effects between the CSF and brain on T2-weighted images, and so proton-density images are preferred for these cases.

Another technique that may be of value in detecting MS lesions is the short-TI inversion-recovery sequence, which has the advantage that T1 and T2 contrast is additive following the 180° pulse. These sequences show a high level of tissue contrast, and by shortening TR and TE the CSF signal can be made less than that of brain [14] (Fig. 8.13).

The *age of the lesions* cannot be ascertained from a single MR examination, but follow-up scans can identify the presence of new lesions and the enlargement of known lesions, thereby confirming an acute process (Fig. 8.9). Marked atrophy of the corpus callosum is frequently noted in long-standing cases.

Spinal plaques have signal characteristics similar to those in the brain, with prolonged T1 and T2 relaxation times (Fig. 8.11). They tend to occur in the dorsal and lateral segments and do not respect the boundaries of the tract systems or the gray matter-white matter junction. The detection of spinal lesions places high demands on the resolving power of the equipment (surface coils!) and is made difficult by CSF flow artifacts and by artifacts arising from the heart and major vessels, especially in the

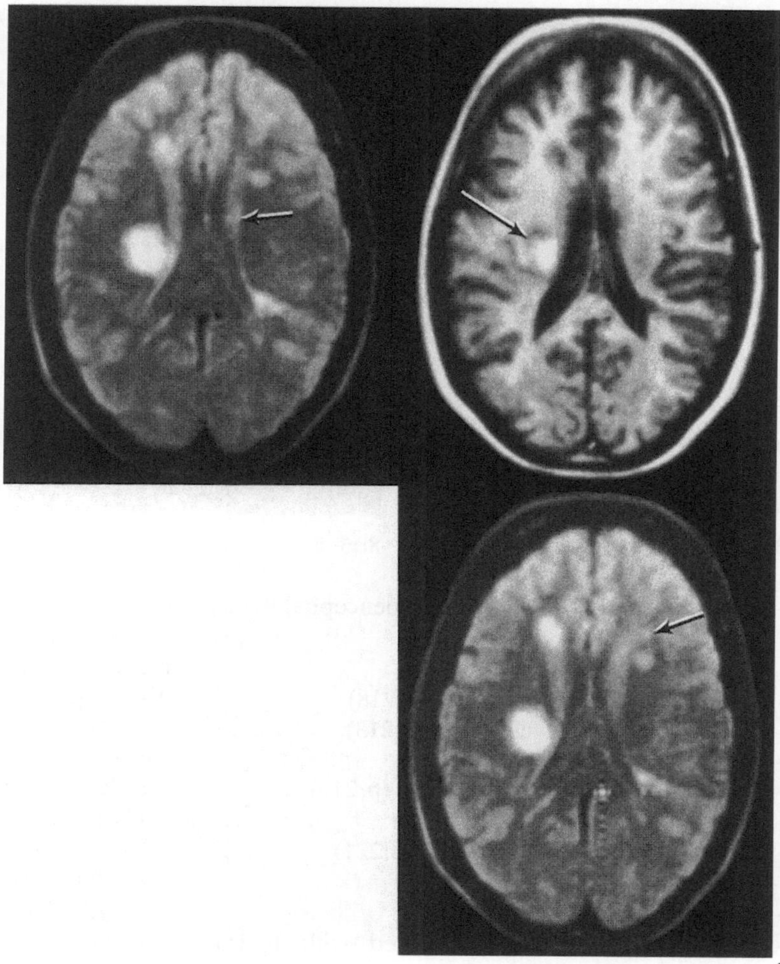

Fig. 8.13 a–c. Multiple sclerosis before (**a**) and after (**c**) i.v. gd-DTPA. The left paraventricular lesion *(arrow)* displays enhancement in **b** but not in **c**. An additional lesion is seen in **c** *(short arrow)*. Axial scans: **b** IR 1.5 s/500 ms/44 ms, **a, c** SE 1.5 s/80 ms (0.15 T)

thoracic region. Suspicious findings should always be confirmed on a second plane.

As with CT, a correlation usually cannot be established between the clinical symptoms and the sites of the lesions on MR scans, so it is prudent to assume the existence of symptomatic lesions that are not detected with MR.

MR has proved far superior to CT in its ability to detect chronically progressive lesions [30]. Contrast MR (e.g., with 0.2 ml/kg gadolinium-DTPA) likewise can demonstrate enhancement of fresh lesions in the stage where there is disruption of the blood-brain barrier (Figs. 8.12, 8.13). Observations by Grossmann et al. [25] indicate that MR is more sensitive than high-dose delayed-contrast CT, and in most of the acute cases examined, the authors were able to find at least one lesion that correlated with neurologic symptoms.

Differential Diagnosis

The nonspecific MR findings in MS must be differentiated from normal paraventricular signal changes seen around the frontal and occipital horns of the lateral ventricles (see p. 201) and from anatomic structures that can resemble focal lesions. The latter include the tail of the caudate nucleus, the superior aspect of the thalamus in midventricular sections, and the body of the caudate nucleus, which is represented by a band of increased T2 within the centrum semiovale just lateral to the lateral ventricles and extending into the frontal lobes. The following white matter diseases in particular can mimic the features of MS:

- Leukodystrophy (p. 201)
- Adrenoleukodystrophy (p. 203)
- Alexander's disease (p. 204)
- Binswanger's disease (p. 210)

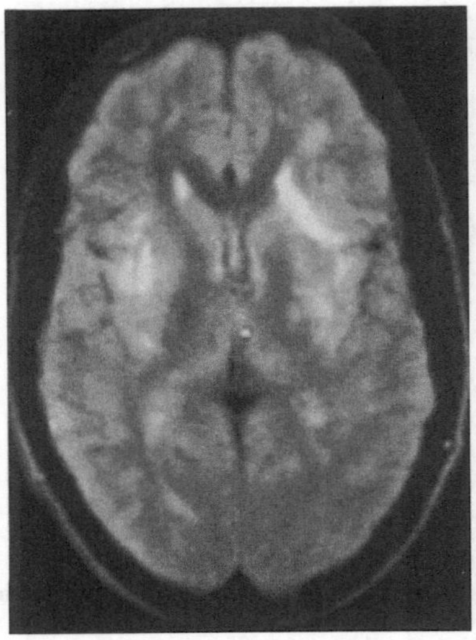

8.14

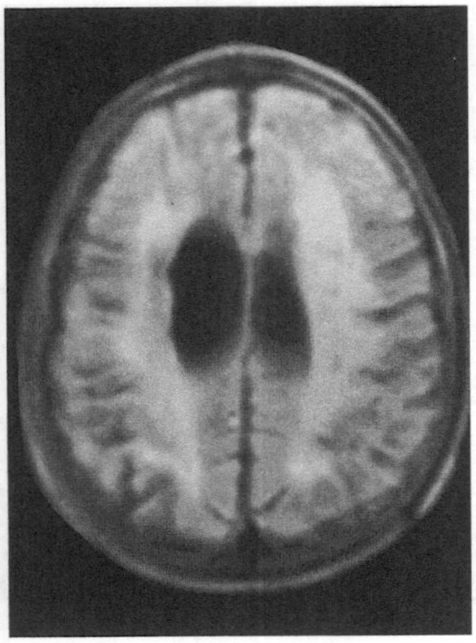

8.15

Fig. 8.14. Vascular disease. Lesions largely within the gray matter. Axial scan: SE 1.5 s/80 ms (0.15 T)

Fig. 8.15. Binswangers's disease. Extensive changes within the centrum semiovale of both hemispheres. Axial scan, SE 1.5 s/80 ms (0.15 T)

- Progressive multifocal leukoencephalopathy (p. 212)
- Fabry's disease (p. 216)
- Central pontine myelinolysis (p. 218)
- Postinfectious demyelination (p. 213)
- Radiation damage (p. 213)
- Methotrexate-associated disease (p. 213)
- Delays or deficits in myelination
- Systemic lupus erythematosus (p. 221)
- Sarcoidosis (p. 357)
- Infectious disease
- Periventricular edema associated with hydrocephalus (p. 115)
- Multiple metastases

Concentric Sclerosis

Concentric sclerosis (Baló's disease) is a rare condition of undetermined etiology that is related to MS. Usually there is only one focus in the white matter of the hemispheres, with the areas of demyelination arranged concentrically around a blood vessel [44].

At the time of writing we have no information on the MR appearance of this special form of MS.

Hypertensive Cerebrovascular Diseases

See also the discussion of peripheral angiopathies in Sect. 13.1.2.

From about 50 years of age on, zones of heightened MR signal intensity may be seen in the periventricular white matter. These zones are significantly more common in individuals with an increased vascular risk (e.g., hypertension, diabetes mellitus) or with overt symptoms of cerebrovascular disease [24].

Like diabetes mellitus and advanced age, a chronic elevation of the blood pressure accelerates the development of cerebral arteriosclerosis, especially in the smaller arteries of the brain (arteriolosclerosis). Arteriolosclerosis can cause small cerebral infarcts (lacunae) and small parenchymal hemorrhages. The generalized changes of hypertensive encephalopathy may be superimposed on these multifocal lesions. Examination of the parenchyma in this situation may show microinfarcts, petechiae, and a status lacunaris in the region of the basal ganglia [22] (Fig. 8.14).

Hypertensive patients also have been found to have an increased water content in the cerebral white matter as well as histologic changes indicative of acute or prior edema.

Additionally, microaneurysms are found in 46% of hypertensive patients, compared with only 7% of normotensives [22]. Sites of predilection for these aneurysms and for concomitant lipohyalinosis of the vessels ("fibrinoid necrosis") are the putamen, thalamus, pons, cerebellum, and cerebral cortex. This accounts for the prevalence of hypertensive hemorrhages and lacunar infarcts in these regions.

Binswanger's Disease

Binswanger's disease is a condition of vascular etiology. Arteriosclerotic changes chiefly involve

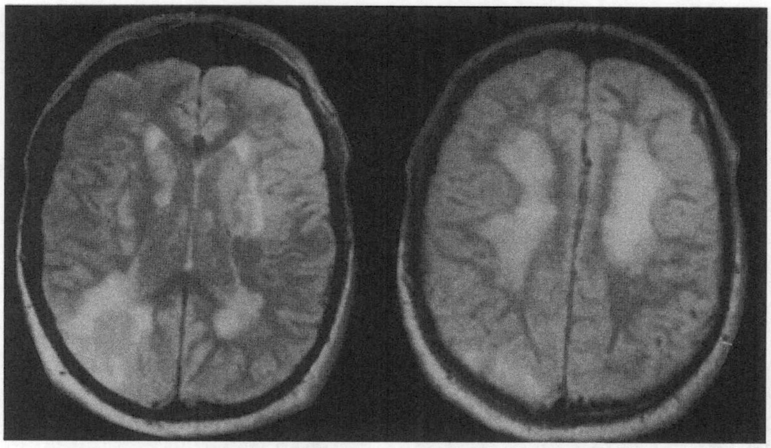

Fig. 8.16 a, b. Multi-infarct dementia in a 73-year-old woman. Multiple patchy areas of increased signal intensity in the basal ganglia, cortex and white matter. Axial scans: **a, b** SE 3.0 s/28 ms, (1.0 T)

the small blood vessels to the white matter about the ventricles and to the basal ganglia. The pathogenesis of the disease is poorly understood. Janota [31] postulates an increased threshold of autoregulation in hypertensive patients, so that periods of hypotension occurring spontaneously or during antihypertensive therapy are tolerated less well than in normotensive persons and can eventually lead to parenchymal damage through diminution of perfusion [60, 31]. Because the white matter is in the peripheral zones of the arterial supply ("watershed areas"), it is jeopardized by the reduction of arterial flow with age and is subject to more frequent ischemic insult from hypertensive crises and microembolisms. The result is a diffuse or circumscribed, patchy demyelination of the white matter, which becomes shrunken and permeated by small cavities. Histologic examination may show diffuse demyelination and axonal loss in the white matter with gliosis and macrophage infiltration, or there may by well-defined foci of white matter damage. These changes may be seen in hypertensive as well as normotensive individuals, however [40].

Clinical manifestations include a gradually progressive mental deterioration, parkinsonoid symptoms, and pseudobulbar paralysis.

CT and MR Findings

CT shows low-density areas in the white matter that may be patchy, confluent, or diffuse with ill-defined borders [51]. There is concomitant widening of the sulci and mild dilatation of the ventricular system. Lacunar infarcts may appear as small, patchy areas of low density having more sharply defined borders. The relative sparing of the cerebral cortex compared with the marked changes in the other regions is noteworthy.

With MR, the low-density areas on CT scans give a somewhat low signal on T1-weighted images and a high signal on T2-weighted images. Thus, MR is considerably more sensitive in its ability to demonstrate these white matter changes and more precise in its characterization of them. The prolonged relaxation times signify a loss of hydrophobic myelin with a concomitant rise in the volume of interstitial water (Fig. 8.15).

Multi-Infarct Dementia

The boundary between multi-infarct dementia and Binswanger's disease is not always clearly defined. The multiple infarcts of varying size and age are a result of arteriosclerotic changes in the large blood vessels supplying the brain. Often hypertension and diabetes mellitus are present as underlying conditions.

CT and MR Findings

The multiple infarcts appear on CT scans as patchy, well-defined, low-density areas of varying size in the region of the basal ganglia, cortex, and white matter. MR is able to demonstrate even small lacunar infarcts as patchy areas of increased T1 and T2 in all three spatial planes, making it possible to localize the lesions with precision. This has particular value in the region of the central nuclei, where even small lesions can produce marked clinical

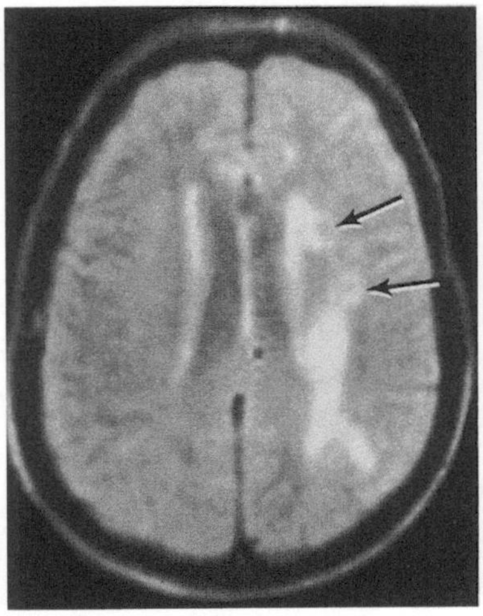

8.17

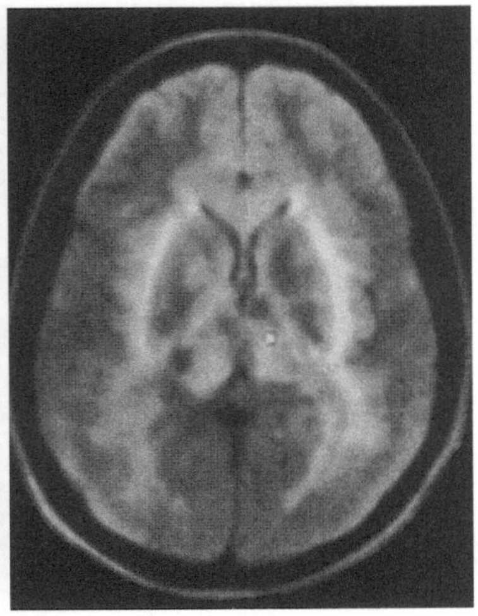

8.18

Fig. 8.17. Progressive multifocal leukoencephalopathy in a 68-year-old woman with carcinoma of the breast accompanied by progressive neurologic deficit without intracranial metastases. Two of the lesions display rings *(arrows)*; a larger lesion is seen posteriorly. Axial scan, SE 1.5 s/40 ms (0.15 T)

Fig. 8.18. Postinfective demyelination in a 43-year-old man with influenza-like illness followed by a catastrophic neurologic illness producing dementia, bilateral long tract motor-sensory signs. The abnormalities are particularly obvious in the external capsule. Axial scans: SE 1.5 s/80 ms (0.15 T)

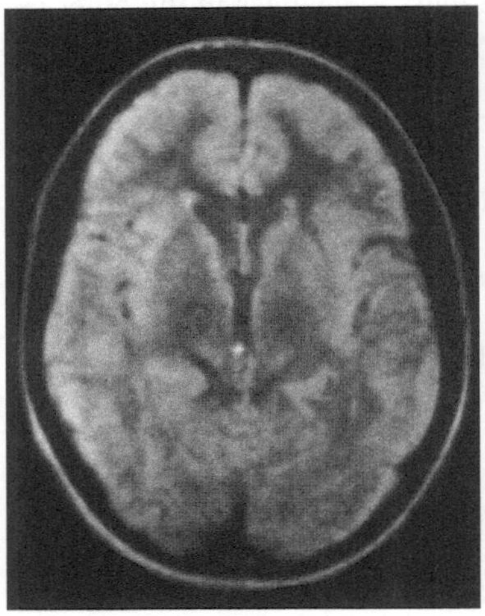

8.19

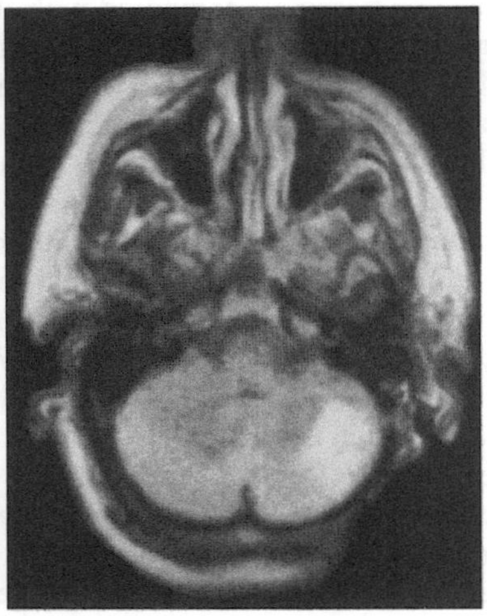

8.20

Fig. 8.19. Methotrexate-associated disease in an 8-year-old child treated with prophylactic intrathecal methotrexate for acute lymphatic leukemia. A margin of increased signal intensity is seen at the medial aspect of the head of the right caudate nucleus and third ventricle. Axial scan, SE 1.5 s/80 ms (0.15 T)

Fig. 8.20. Radiation damage. Increased T2 signal intensity is seen in the cerebellum in the radiation field of the overlying carcinoma of the mastoid. Axial scan, SE 1.5 s/80 ms (0.15 T)

signs (Fig. 8.16). Thus, for example, localized damage to the subthalamic nucleus due to a small hemorrhage, ischemia, or lacunar infarct is considered to be the most frequent cause of hemiballismus [11].

Progressive Multifocal Leukoencephalopathy

Progressive multifocal leukoencephalopathy, which is counted among the paraneoplastic syndromes of the CNS, can occur in the setting of leukoses and reticuloses (leukemia, lymphosarcoma, Hodgkin's disease, Boeck's disease, carcinomatosis, AIDS). It has a viral etiology, being caused by infection with the simian virus 40 and the papovavirus Ic. Scattered, often confluent areas of demyelination of varying size are found mostly in the subcortical white matter of the cerebral hemispheres and occasionally in the spinal cord. Histologically there is a marked proliferation of neoplastoid astrocytes and enlarged oligodendroglial cells that may contain inclusions composed of viral colonies [44].

MR Findings

MR shows multiple ill-defined, focal, ringlike, or confluent foci with prolonged T1 and T2 times in the subcortical white matter that are most pronounced in the parietal and occipital regions (Fig. 8.17).

Postinfectious Encephalomyelitis

Involvement of the CNS can follow a number of viral infections such as measels, chickenpox, rubella, and occasionally influenza, mumps, scarlet fever, and pertussis. The general clinical symptoms - headache, nausea, fever, and stupor - are accompanied by a variety of neurologic symptoms such as nuchal rigidity, strabismus, loss of reflexes, and incontinence. The disease ends fatally in about 15%-20% of cases.

Histologically there is edematous swelling and marked perivascular demyelination, the foci of which may coalesce. Lipid-containing microglial cells form a wall-like border around the lesions, which are scattered throughout the white matter and along the ventricular walls. Involvement of the gray matter is unknown.

The pathogenesis of postinfectious encephalomyelitis may relate to direct injury from an autoimmune response or to an overspill of locally produced immunologic factors hostile to the CNS myelin [50].

MR Findings

The lesions of postinfectious encephalomyelitis appear as nonspecific areas of prolonged T1 and T2 that give a high signal on proton-density and T2-weighted images. They may resemble the lesions of multiple sclerosis (Fig. 8.18).

Methotrexate-Associated Disease

Methotrexate, a folic acid antagonist, is the antineoplastic drug most likely to cause neurologic complications following prolonged, high-dosage systemic and/or intrathecal use (often in conjunction with radiotherapy). The white matter changes have been described as "disseminated necrotizing leukoencephalopathy" [52] and as "subacute encephalopathy" [48]. The lesions consist of discrete foci or larger, confluent foci scattered throughout the white matter and sometimes containing petechial hemorrhages. Histologically these foci show coagulation necrosis, demyelination, vacuolation, and gliosis [54].

MR Findings

The affected white matter regions appear as zones of increased signal intensity on proton-density and T2-weighted images due to their prolonged T1 and T2 relaxation times (Fig. 8.19).

Radiation Damage (see Sect. 5.4)

Not infrequently, radiation therapy of the brain causes damage to the white matter in the form of focal necrosis, vascular proliferation, and atypical astrogliosis. The white matter is especially sensitive to high-energy radiation, whose initial effect is demyelination, followed later by necrosis and axonal degeneration [45].

MR Findings

The radiation-induced changes in the white matter prolong its relaxation times, the location of the changes corresponding essentially to the target areas of the radiotherapy (Fig. 8.20). As fenestrated vessels are found in areas of radionecrosis [28], it can be difficult to distinguish the necrosis from a recurrent tumor, even after administration of contrast material.

8.3 Primary Involvement of the Basal Ganglia and Brainstem

8.3.1 Congenital Causes

Wilson's Disease

Wilson's disease (hepatolenticular degeneration) [69] is a disturbance in copper metabolism that is inherited as an autosomal recessive trait. It is associated with abnormal deposition of copper in various tissues, most notably the liver and brain.

Clinical manifestations include psychic changes, a wide range of tremors, and speech difficulties.

Wilson's disease is associated with cavitation of the lenticular nuclei and neuronal loss in the putamen and caudate, which are shrunken. Later, similar changes are encountered in the pallidum and substantia nigra. There is less severe involvement of the thalamus, brainstem, cerebrum, and cerebellum. In the cortex there may be focal spongy demyelination and also widespread loss of myelin. Noetzel et al. [44] state that the pathologic changes are not specific for hepatolenticular degeneration and may be seen in hepatic cirrhoses of other etiology.

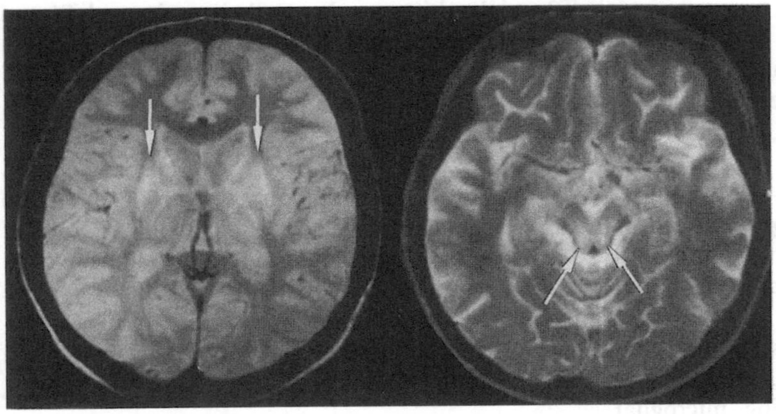

Fig. 8.21 a, b. Wilson's disease in a 30-year-old woman with flapping tremor and speech disturbances. Symmetrical lesions *(arrows)* are seen in the basal ganglia and in the midbrain. Axial scans: **a** SE 3.0 s/45 ms, **b** SE 3.0 s/120 ms (1.0 T)

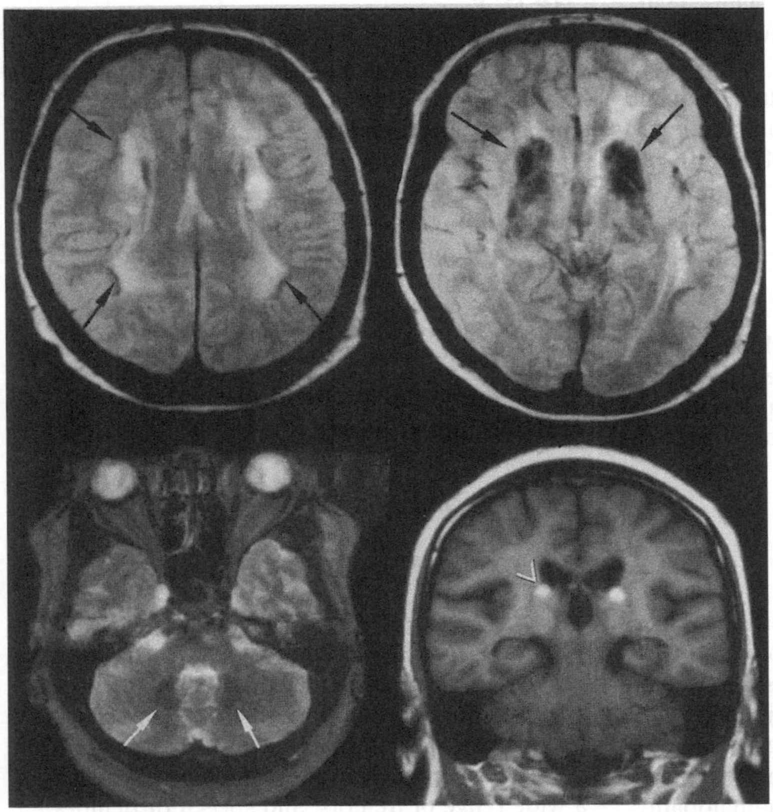

Fig. 8.22 a–d. Hypoparathyroidism in a 48-year-old woman with slight disorder of extrapyramidal movements. Calcium and mineral deposits in the basal ganglia, the subcortical rim *(arrows)*, and the nucleus dentatus associated with white matter changes similar to those seen in Fahr's disease. The hyperdense areas *(arrowhead)* probably indicate mucopolysaccharidosis. Axial scans: **a, b** SE 2.5 s/40 ms, **c** SE 2.5 s/120 ms; coronal scan (**d**) SE 0.4 s/17 ms (1.0 T)

CT and MR Findings

In the florid stage of Wilson's disease the affected areas of the basal ganglia appear hypodense on CT scans. Corresponding areas of high signal are seen on proton-density and T2-weighted MR scans, resembling edematous swelling or demyelination. Edema would appear to be a likely cause of the swelling, for regression can be seen on follow-up CT scans during treatment with penicillamine [41]. The lesions are usually symmetric, although asymmetric distributions may be seen [3]. In the few cases described thus far, MR was more sensitive than CT in its ability to demonstrate the brain lesions of Wilson's disease (Fig. 8.21) [26, 64].

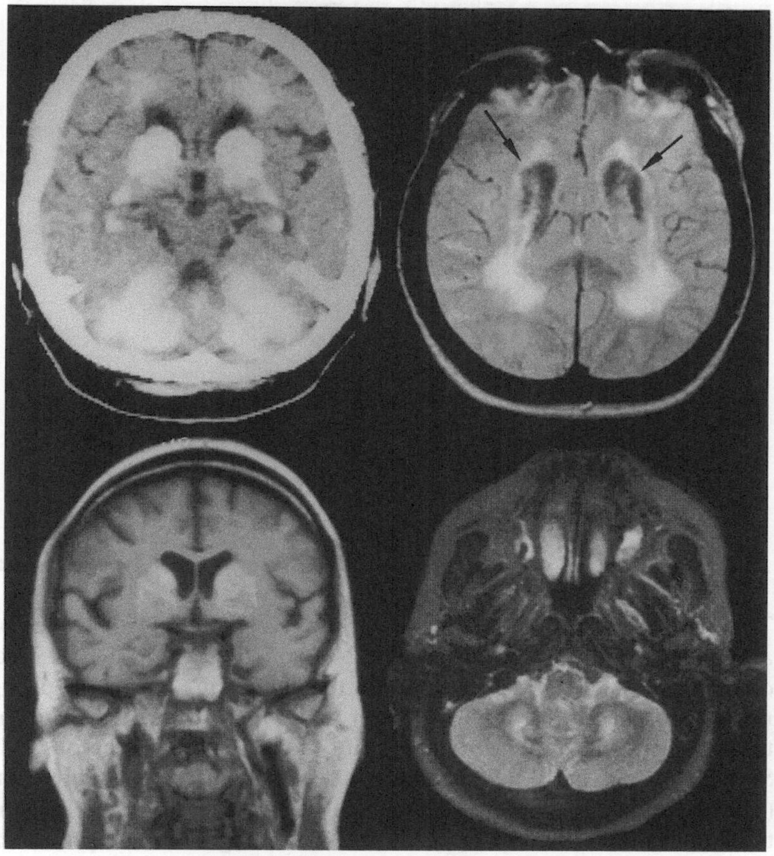

Fig. 8.23 a–d. Fahr's disease: incidental finding in a 62-year-old woman. **a** CT scan: extensive mineral deposits in the basal ganglia, white matter, and cerebellum. **b–c** MR scans: low signal of deposits in basal ganglia (*arrows in* **b**), increased signal (**c**), large hyperintensive areas of white matter (**b**). The deposits within the cerebellar white matter are hyperintense in **d**, but were not seen in the T1-weighted image. **b** Axial scan, SE 3.0 s/45 ms; **c** coronal scan, SE 0.7 s/17 ms; **d** axial scan, SE 3.0 s/120 ms (1.0 T)

Fahr's Disease

In Fahr's disease, whose cause remains unknown, there is an extraordinary degree of mineralization (deposits of calcium, iron, and other metals embedded in a PAS-positive mucopolysaccharide matrix) of the pallidum, the striatum, the dentate nucleus, the hippocampus and the sulcal depths of the cerebral cortex, and the white matter. The mineralization, which is a common incidental finding in asymptomatic persons, is localized to small and medium-size blood vessels. Often there is no parenchymal reaction [45]. Similar, less pronounced calcifications occur in hypoparathyroidism (Fig. 8.22).

CT and MR Findings

The lesions appear on CT scans as uniform areas of high density. With MR, Scotti et al. [55] describe three patterns (also seen in the case in Fig. 8.23):

1. The high signal of the white matter lesions, which cannot be explained by the low proton density of the calcifications and is probably caused by protein and/or mucopolysaccharides binding the mineral ions.
2. The low signal in the basal ganglia, which is most likely due to the low proton density of the calcium and other minerals without a mucopolysaccharide matrix.
3. Nonvisibility of the deposits in the cerebellum which may indicate an intermediate stage of the disease process.

Hallervorden-Spatz Syndrome

Hallervorden-Spatz syndrome is characterized by abnormal iron storage within the cells of the globus pallidus, the reticular zone of the substantia nigra, and the red nucleus. Diffuse disordered myelination is seen and is most marked in tracts between the striatum and the pallidum [39].

Clinical symptoms in clude progressive rigidity of the legs, choreic or athetoid movements, also torsion dystonia, dementia, and seizures.

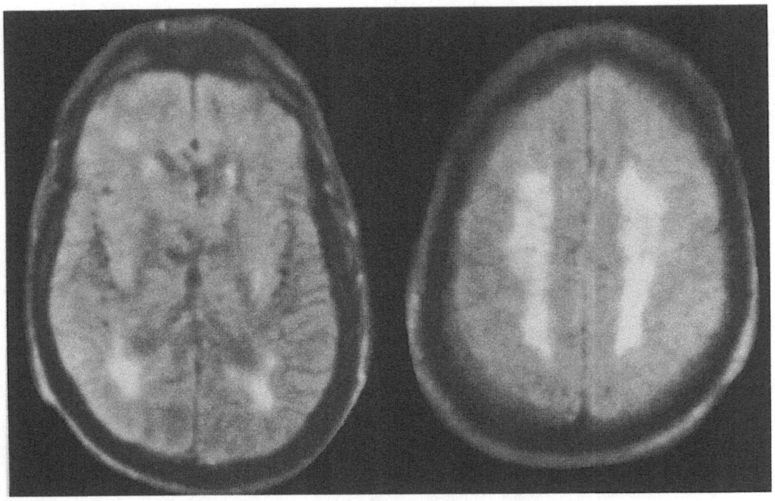
a b

Fig. 8.24 a, b. Fabry's disease. Confluent changes in the centrum semiovale of both hemispheres. The pattern in **a** resembles that in multiple sclerosis, but that in **b** resembles Binswanger's disease. Axial scans, SE 1.5 s/80 ms (0.15 T)

MR Findings

The presence of iron shortens the T1 and T2 relaxation times of the affected areas. T2-weighted sequences show hypointense areas in the lentiform nuclei and perilentiform white matter and hyperintense foci in the periependymal white matter (see Sect. 5.2). Vogl et al. [66] examined two patients (mother and son) with typical clinical manifestations of Hallervorden-Spatz syndrome. The foregoing changes were noted in the region of the putamen in the son, but CT and MR findings in the mother were unremarkable.

Fabry's Disease

Fabry's disease involves a deposition of glycolipids in blood vessels, leading to cerebrovascular abnormalities such as aneurysms, thrombosis, and embolic and hemorrhagic episodes. Glycolipids also accumulate in the nervous system, especially in the basal ganglia and in the nuclei of the midbrain, brainstem, and spinal cord.

MR Findings

Scans may show multifocal areas with long T1 and T2 coalescing in the region of the centrum semiovale and possibly resembling the changes of Binswanger's disease or multiple sclerosis (Fig. 8.24). The effects of vascular involvement, such as hemorrhage or infarction, also can be demonstrated and are nonspecific.

Glycogen Storage Disease

Deficiencies of enzymes involved in glycogen synthesis and breakdown produce a wide clinical spectrum in glycogen storage diseases, with disorders primarily of the liver, heart, musculoskeletal system, or nervous system.

In the infantile form the brain may be grossly normal. Histologically, PAS-positive deposits are most prominent in motor nuclei of the brainstem, the dorsal root ganglia, and the anterior horn cells of the spinal cord, with neuronal loss and astrogliosis occurring in areas of severe damage [7].

Huntington's Chorea

Huntington's chorea is a systemic atrophic disease inherited as an autosomal dominant trait and generally having its onset after 30 years of age. Its pathogenesis is poorly understood. Death occurs after an average illness of 13 years [44]. It has recently been reported that the disease may be linked to a DNA fragment of chromosome 4 [38].

The clinical course is marked by behavioral disturbances, dementia, choreiform movements, seizures, cerebellar symptoms, and rigor.

Pathologic findings include atrophy of the striatum, pallidum, caudate nucleus, subthalamic nucleus, substantia nigra, and dentate nucleus. Atrophy of the caudate nucleus is particularly marked, obliterating the "waist" of the basal ganglia and causing the internal capsule to appear widened. The atrophy is based mainly on a loss of small ganglion cells. The glial cells are increased in number, and there is proliferation of glial fibers [44].

CT and MR Findings

The CT findings are nonspecific and mainly include atrophy of the caudate nucleus [12] with progressive widening of the intercaudate region of the lateral ventricles. The extent of the caudate atrophy does not necessarily parallel the clinical status [38], and so the stage of the disease cannot be established from CT findings.

Besides the caudate atrophy, MR has not demonstrated any unusual signal patterns in the cortex or the basal ganglia [41, 57]. A normal configuration of the caudate nucleus does not exclude the illness.

Subacute Necrotizing Encephalopathy

Subacute necrotizing encephalopathy (Leigh's disease) is transmitted as an autosomal recessive trait and probably affects the pyruvate metabolism. Symptoms appear in infancy or early childhood, occasionally later in adulthood, and death always ensues after a period of illness that is highly variable (from hours to 15 years; [12]).

The clinical symptoms include nonspecific disease manifestations such as nausea and vomiting and variable neurologic disturbances, resembling the pattern of Wernicke's encephalopathy (see p. 218).

Pathologically there is vacuolation secondary to necrosis of gray matter, mainly affecting the putamen, thalamus, hypothalamus, optic chiasm, cerebellum, dentate nucleus, and medulla oblongata, with proliferation of capillaries and macroglia [44].

CT and MR Findings

In the few cases of subacute necrotizing encephalopathy published to date, CT has shown focal, symmetric, hypodense, nonenhancing areas in the striatum, especially in the putamen, but also in other areas of the brain [12, 18].

MR has demonstrated bilateral, symmetric areas of increased signal intensity in the lentiform nucleus as well as lesions in the white matter, brainstem, and cortex [29]. T2-weighted images are best suited to demonstrate the preference for involvement of the gray nuclei of the brainstem.

The CT and MR findings of this disease are nonspecific and may resemble those caused by CO poisoning, hypoxia (see Fig. 8.27 b), acute childhood hemiplegia, and encephalitis [18]. The definite diagnosis can only be established by biopsy. So far we have not personally observed the MR features of this condition.

Spinocerebellar Degeneration

The rare spinocerebellar degenerations are associated with an irreplaceable loss of groups or systems of neurons. Their clinical picture varies with the sites of the atrophic lesions in the brainstem, cerebellum, and spinal cord.

Olivopontocerebellar Degeneration

Olivopontocerebellar degeneration, inherited as an autosomal dominant trait, may begin in early childhood or not until much later and runs a course of 10–20 years. The outstanding clinical features are unsteady gait, motor disturbances, dysarthria and dysphagia, spasticity, cranial nerve deficits, and muscular atrophy.

Histologic examination shows a loss of neurons in the pons, medulla, olive, and cerebellar white matter and atrophy of the lateral portions of the cerebellar hemispheres (due to loss of Purkinje cells) (Fig. 8.25).

Cerebellar Heredoataxia

Cerebellar heredoataxia (Nonne-Pierre Marie disease) also with an autosomal dominant mode of inheritance, usually has its onset between 20 and 40 years of age but may begin later; rare cases appear in early youth. Severe atrophy affects the Purkinje cells and the granule layer of the cerebellar cortex, especially the superior vermis [21] (Fig. 8.26).

CT and MR Findings

CT and MR show more or less pronounced atrophy of the above-named anatomic structures of the posterior fossa. The changes are seen best on sagittal and coronal MR images. Measurements of the sagittal diameter of the brainstem have shown the following average values in adults [36].

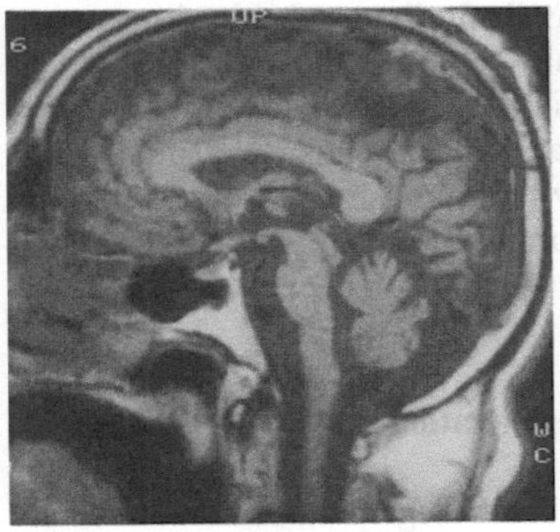

8.25

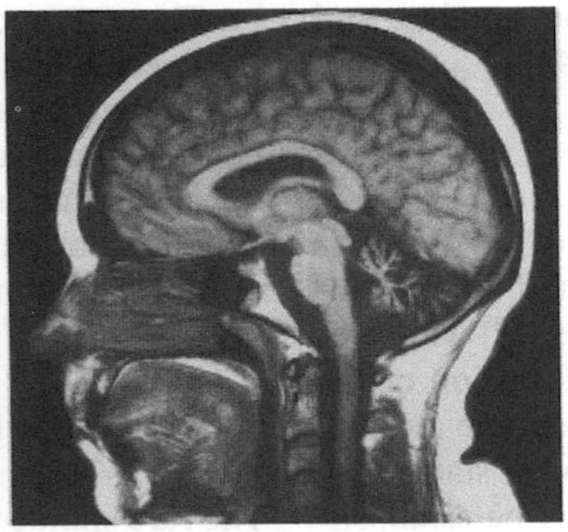

8.26

Fig. 8.25. Olivopontocerebellar atrophy in a 59-year-old man with spinal ataxia. Marked atrophy of the brain stem. Midsagittal scan, SE 0.6 s/30 ms (1.0 T)

Fig. 8.26. Cerebellar heredoataxia (Nonne-Pierre Marie disease) in a 33-year-old woman with ataxia, amaurosis, and dysarthria. Midsagittal scan, SE 0.5 s/30 ms (0.5 T). (Courtesy of Drs. Kuhn, Steen, and Terwey, Oldenburg, FRG)

Distance between

- Interpeduncular fissure and aqueduct 13.2 mm
- Anterior surface of cerebral peduncle and aqueduct 18.1 mm
- Anterior surface of middle of pons and floor of fourth ventricle 26.6 mm
- Anteroposterior diameter of the medulla at the pontomedullary junction 15.3 mm

There is no apparent hypodensity on CT scans or signal change on MR scans relative to normal findings.

The disease must be quite severe before the findings can be related to clinical symptoms. In milder cases differentiation from toxic cerebellar degeneration (alcohol, phenytoin, nonmetastatic effect of cancer) is required.

8.3.2 Acquired and Unexplained Causes

Wernicke's Encephalopathy

Wernicke's encephalopathy (superior hemorrhagic polioencephalitis) occurs as a result of thiamine deficiency in patients with liver damage (e.g., chronic alcohol abuse) or abnormalities of gastrointestinal function (chronic gastrointestinal diseases, hyperemesis gravidarum, heavy metal poisoning, children of mothers with beriberi) [44].

In the acute form there is pericapillary diapedesis in the mamillary bodies, around the third ventricle, in the thalamus, around the aqueduct, the fourth ventricle, and the quadrigeminal region. In the subacute form there is vacuolation of these regions with gliosis and capillary proliferation, combined with atrophy and sclerosis. Iron pigment deposits can be seen following hemorrhages.

Clinically there is a triad of encephalopathy, ataxia, and ophthalmoplegia.

MR Findings

In acute cases the neuropathologic changes would be expected to prolong the relaxation times in the affected areas, which would shows signs of recent and older hemorrhage (see Sect. 5.2).

Chronic cases would presumably show long relaxation times in the vacuolated tissues and/or atrophic changes with dilatation of the third ventricle, the aqueduct and fourth ventricle. Charness et al. [16] reported finding a marked decrease in the volume of the mamillary bodies on MR scans.

Central Pontine Myelinolysis

Central pontine myelinolysis is viewed as a complication of alcoholic as well as nonalcoholic hepatic cirrhosis and may also occur in association with diabetes, chronic debilitating illnesses, and electrolyte abnormalities [1, 19, 44]. The pathogenesis is unknown but may relate to electrolyte disorders.

Pathological findings are characterized by loss of myelin and oligodendroglia spreading centrifugally from the median raphe of the pons, with relative sparing of nerve cells and axis cylinders. There is perivenular inflammatory reaction in early lesions, and proliferation of macroglia and fibrillary gliosis in chronic and inactive lesions.

Besides the typical pontine location, symmetrical lesions of similar histologic type have also been found in other parts of the brain [70] (Fig. 8.27).

CT and MR Findings

CT shows low-density lesions occupying the base of the pons and extending from the lower mesencephalon to the pontomedullary junction. They pro-

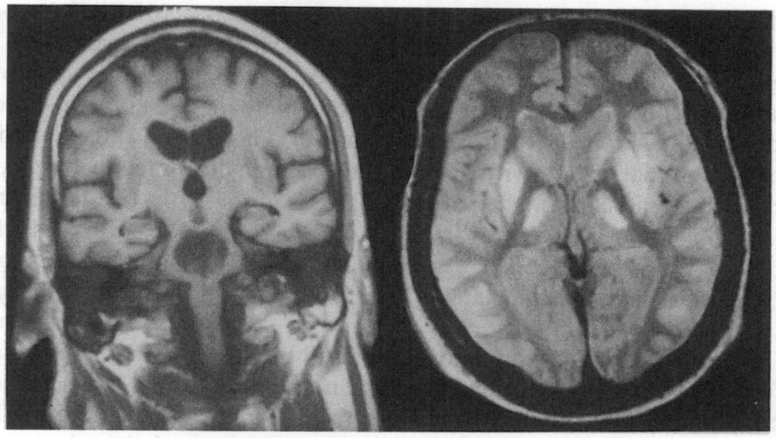

Fig. 8.27 a, b. Central pontine myelinolysis in a 48-year-old man with history of alcoholism, presenting with state of confusion, spastic paraparesis, and electrolyte disturbances. In addition to the typical pontine location, lesions are seen within the basal ganglia; these may also be secondary to a hypoxic state during a short cardiac arrest in the acute phase. Coronal scan (**a**), SE 0.4 s/17 ms; axial scan (**b**) SE 3.0 s/120 ms (1.0 T)

duce no mass effect and are nonenhancing after administration of contrast medium.

MR in the early stage of the disease shows symmetric lesions with prolonged T1 and T2 relaxation times, the latter possibly due to edema. Consequently the lesions appear dark on T1-weighted scans (Fig. 27 a) and bright on T2-weighted scans. As the disease progresses, the T1 and T2 values gradually return to normal.

Central pontine myelinolysis is most accurately diagnosed from the location and symmetry of the lesions and the absence of major mass effect (Fig. 27 a). The signal changes are not specific and can occur in association with tumors or infarcts [19].

8.4 Primary Involvement with No Sites of Predilection

8.4.1 Congenital Causes

Mucopolysaccharidoses

The various types of mucopolysaccharidosis (MPS) are caused by a defect in the metabolism of the mucopolysaccharides (glycosaminoglycans) leading to mucopolysaccharide storage in certain tissues. The mucopolysaccharidoses vary widely in severity. All patients manifest "gargoylism," dysostosis multiplex (except for Morquio's syndrome) and multiple organ involvement. Arteriosclerosis develops with deposits of mucopolysaccharides in arterial smooth muscles. Besides mucopolysaccharides, lipids also accumulate in the brain.

MPS I (Hurler's syndrome): Patients with this type of MPS have a progressively hyperostotic scaphocephalic skull, shallow orbits, poorly developed sinuses, and a large sella turcica. The brain shows cortical atrophy, thickened meninges, large ventricles, dilated perivascular spaces with increased collagen, and clusters of histiocytes.

MPS I-S (Scheie's syndrome): Normal neurologic development.
MPS II (Hunter's syndrome): Inclusion material in meningeal cells and neurons. Diagnosis by direct assay of enzymes in serum and cells.
MPS III (Sanfilippo's syndrome): Atrophy of cerebrum, normal cerebellum, leptomeninges slightly thickened.
MPS IV (Morquio's syndrome): Affection of cortex and basal ganglia. The tendency toward ligamentous laxity leads to atlantoaxial subluxations and consequent cervical myelopathy. The odontoid process is hypoplastic.
MPS VI (Maroteaux-Lamy syndrome): Hydrocephalus secondary to thickening of the leptomeninges.

CT and MR Findings in MPS I

Various nonspecific CT findings have been described, including a symmetric low attenuation of white matter, hydrocephalus, and enlargement of the cortical sulci and interhemispheric fissures [35, 67].

MR findings noted by Johnson et al. [32] include reduced gray matter-white matter contrast, ventricular and cortical sulcal enlargement, and prolonged periventricular T2 in one case. In a second case these were accompanied by delayed or deficient myelination.

The reduced gray matter-white matter contrast with prolongation of T1 and T2 may relate to (a) the deposition of glucolipids and mucopolysaccharides in the lysosomes of neurons and astrocytes of gray and white matter [42, 49]; (b) cavitations around blood vessels with accumulations of foam cells in the Virchow-Robin spaces; and (c) dilated periadventitial spaces with viscous fluid, "gargoyle cells," and mesenchymal elements [32].

Cerebrotendinous Xanthomatosis

Cerebrotendinous xanthomatosis is caused by a defect of hydroxylase with overproduction and accumulation of cholestanol. It is characterized by mild atrophy of the frontal lobes and cerebellar folia, with areas of demyelination in the optic nerves, brainstem, and cerebellum.

CT and MR Findings

In the few cases of cerebrotendinous xanthomatosis that have been published, CT has shown hyperdense nodules in the cerebellum, diffuse hypodensity of the white matter, or focal cerebellar hypodensities [8, 15].

In a case published by Swanson et al.[61] MR showed findings suggesting demyelination in the cerebral white matter and moderate to severe atrophy. The latter could be explained by microscopic findings, including restricted areas of demyelination and collections of foam cells seen in postmortem examinations of patients dying with the disease. The areas of possible demyelination were more extensive on MR scans than on comparable CT scans.

Farber's Disease

Farber's disease is a lipogranulomatosis based on a deficiency of acid aramidase in different tissues. CNS involvement includes the cerebellum, brainstem, anterior horn of the spinal cord, retina, dorsal root, and autonomous ganglia. Most patients die before 2 years of age.

No MR findings were available at the time of writing.

MELAS, MERRF, and KSS

MELAS (mitochondrial myopathy, encephalopathy, lactic acidosis, and strokelike syndrome), MERRF (myoclonus epilepsy and ragged red fibers, and KSS (Kearns-Sayre syndrome) are three distinct syndromes that presumably are caused by an inherited biochemical defect in mitochondria. In all three disorders ragged red fibers are evident on muscle biopsy, and in most cases elevated blood lactate levels are found [46].

Early development is normal. Clinical symptoms include growth failure, cerebral seizures, episodes of hemiparesis, dementia, episodic vomiting, cortical blindness, hearing loss, and aphasia. In MELAS the fluctuation of neurological symptoms is a characteristic sign, in MERRF myoclonism and ataxia are predominant findings, and in KSS ophthalmoplegia, atypical pigmentary degeneration of the retina, and heart block are seen in most cases. Involvement of the spinal cord has only been observed in MERRF [46, 59].

As neuropathological findings, spongy degeneration of the brain, focal encephalomalacia, and basal ganglia calcification have been described in MELAS. In MERRF the spongy state and glial proliferation have been found to involve also the subcortical white matter of the cerebellum and the dentate nuclei and superior cerebellar peduncles, and degeneration has been seen in the spinal cord. Spongy state of the brain has also been encountered in KSS. Since the endothelium of the cerebral capillaries is rich in mitochondria it can be speculated that the mitochondrial defect affects the microvasculature, leading to multifocal ischemia and infarctions [46].

CT and MR Findings

In CT focal lucencies due to cerebral infarctions are described [46]. In MR multilocular lesions of varying size can be revealed involving the cortex, subcortical white matter, and the cerebellum. They may be due to ischemic/hypoxic edema (Fig. 8.28). The lesions may be transient without leaving tissue defects.

Other, Uncommon Metabolic Diseases

Other less common metabolic diseases that are combined with disorders of the CNS include encephalopathies associated with disorders of amino acid metabolism [58] (hyperglycinemia, homocystinuria, Hartnup disease), with hyperammonemia, with metabolic acidosis (organic aciduria, glutaraciduria (Fig. 8.29), congenital lactic acidosis, Lowe's syn-

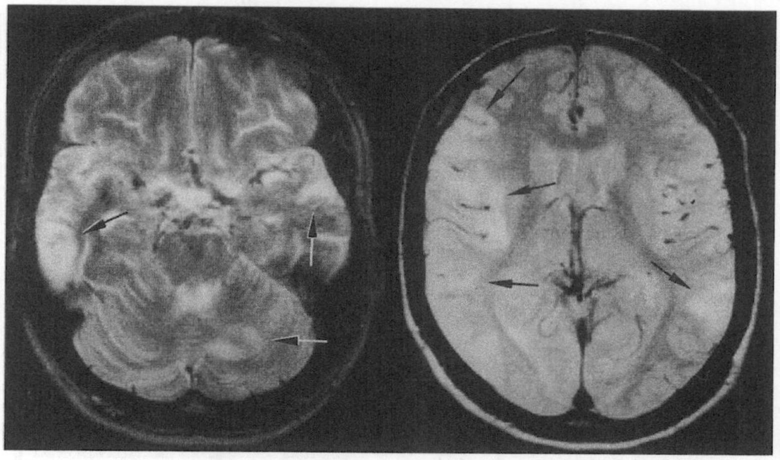

Fig. 8.28 a, b. MELAS in a 28-year-old man with short stature and recurrent, fluctuating symptoms including paresis of left extremities, nausea, aphasia, focal seizures of left side of face, ptosis, and sudden hearing loss. **a, b** Multiple focal hyperintense lesions *(arrows)* in cortex, subcortical white matter, and cerebellum. Axial scans: **a** SE 3.0 s/120 ms, **b** SE 3.0 s/45 ms. Control scan 2 weeks later showed decreasing size of left frontal lesions (1.0 T)

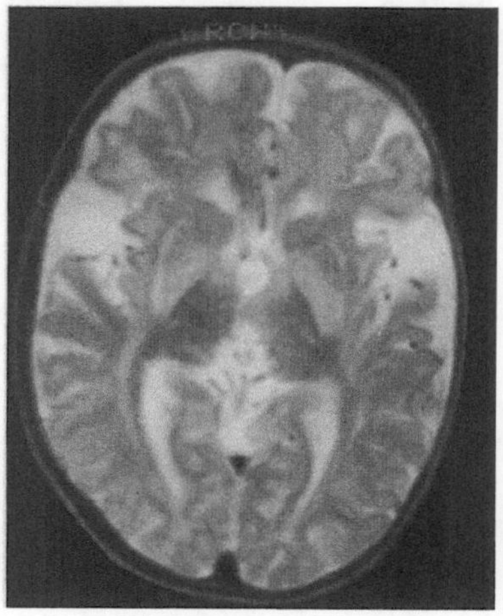

Fig. 8.29. Glutaraciduria type 1 (disturbance of lysine metabolism), in a 3-year-old boy presenting with spasticity, clouding of consciousness, and acidosis. Marked atrophy and prolonged relaxation times in putamen, pallidum, capsula externa, and white matter. Axial scan, SE 2.5 s/120 ms; (1.0 T)

drome), with hypoglycemia (galactosemia), and disorders of copper metabolism (Menke's syndrome, Lesch-Nyhan syndrome).

The CNS lesions in these diseases consist of spongy vacuolation with or without demyelination, ischemic necrosis (in homocystinuria), astrogliosis, neuronal loss, calcifications, subependymal cysts, and hemorrhagic lesions.

8.4.2 Acquired and Unexplained Causes

Systemic Lupus Erythematosus

The prevalence of CNS involvement in systemic lupus erythematosus (SLE) is approximately 75%. SLE is a multisystem autoimmune disorder which in the CNS leads to reactive and proliferative changes in arterioles and capillaries [21]. These changes in turn give rise to multiple microinfarcts and larger infarcts in the cortex and brainstem, hemorrhages (parenchymatous, subarachnoid, subdural), and infections (promoted by steroid therapy).

The lesions are manifested clinically by headache, seizures, disturbances of mental function, and cranial neuropathies, especially in the late stage of the disease.

CT and MR Findings

The SLE finding most widely described with CT is cerebral atrophy, which, however, may also occur after steroid therapy. Patchy hypodensities of variable size have been seen in the cortex and especially in the white matter (Fig. 8.30).

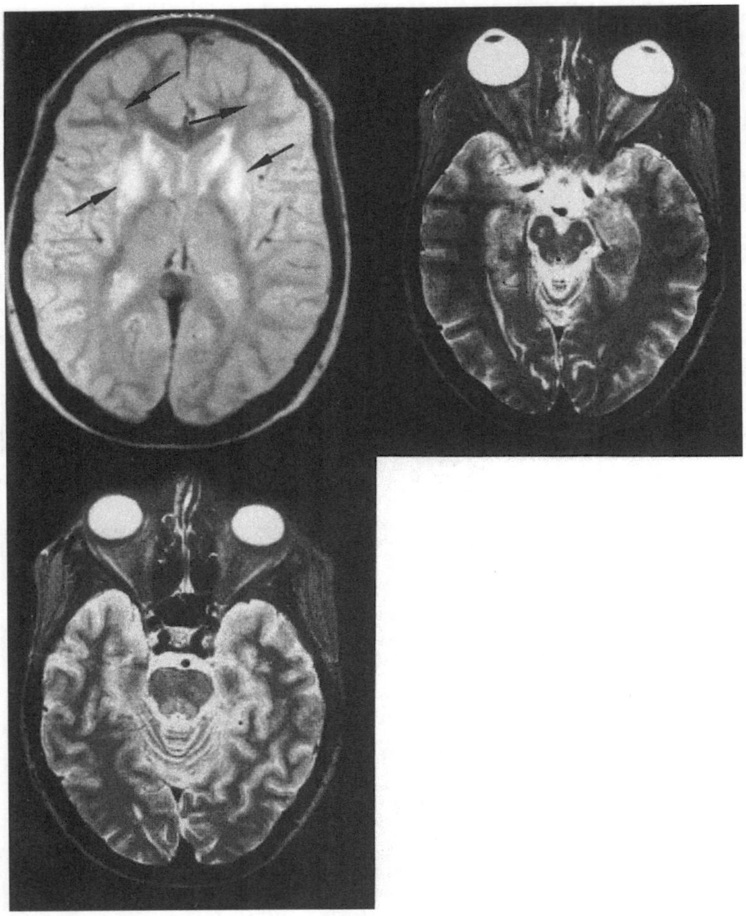

a b c

Fig. 8.30 a–c. Systemic lupus erythematosus in an 18-year-old woman with headache, slight disturbances of mental functions, and partial seizures. Multiple lesions of different size with prolonged T1 and T2 *(arrows)* scattered in the white matter, striatum, and brainstem. Axial scans: **a** SE 3.0 s/45 ms, (1.0 T), **b, c** SE 3.0 s/90 ms (1.5 T)

MR is able to demonstrate lesions that cannot be visualized with CT, and these are displayed with great clarity on proton-density and T2-weighted images. They are probably caused by ischemic edema. It is noteworthy that some CT and MR changes were found to regress with clinical improvement, but these changes could not be used to evaluate the course of the disease [65, 2].

References

1. Adams RD, Victor M, Mancall EL (1959) Central pontine myelinolysis; a hitherto undescribed disease occurring in alcoholic and malnourished patients. Arch Neurol Psychiatry 81: 145-172
2. Aisen AM, Gabrielsen TO, McCune WJ (1985) MR imaging of systemic lupus erythematodes involving the brain. AJNR 6: 197-201
3. Aisen AM, Martel W, Gabrielsen TO, Glazer GM, Brewer G, Young AB, Hill G (1985) Wilson disease of the brain; MR imaging. Radiology 157: 137-141
4. Allen IV (1984) Demyelinating diseases. In: Adams JH, Corsellis JAN, Duchen LW (eds) Greenfield's neuropathology. 4th ed. J. Wiley and sons, New York, pp 338-384
5. Baram TZ, Goldman AM, Perca AK (1986) Krabbe disease: specific MRI and CT findings. Neurology 36: 111-115
6. Barnes DM, Enzman DR (1981) The evolution of white matter diseases as seen on computed tomography. Radiology 138: 379-383
7. Becker LE, Yates A (1985) Inherited metabolic disease. In: Davis RL, Robertson DM (eds) Textbook of neuropathology. Williams and Wilkins, Baltimore, pp 284-371
8. Berginer VM, Berginer J, Salen G, Sheter S, Zimmerman RS (1981) Computed tomography in cerebrotendinous xanthomatosis. Neurology 31: 1463-1465
9. Besson JAO, Corrigan FM, Foreman EI, Ashcroft GW, Eastwood LM, Smith FW (1983) Differentiating senile dementia of Alzheimer type and multi-infarct dementia by proton NMR imaging. Lancet II: 789
10. Bewermeyer H, Bamborschke S, Ebhardt G, Hünermann B, Heiss WD (1985) MR Imaging in adrenoleucomyeloneuropathy. J Comput Assist Tomogr 9(4): 793-796
11. Biller J, Graff-Radford NR, Smoker WRK, Adams HP Jr, Johnston P (1986) MR imaging in "lacunar" hemiballismus. J Comput Assist Tomogr 10(5): 793-797

12. Boltshauser E (1983) Degenerative Erkrankungen des Zentralnervensystems im Kindesalter. Huber, Bern
13. Buonanno FS, Ball MR, Laster W et al. (1978) Computed tomography in late-infantile metachromatic leucodystrophy. Ann Neurol 4: 43-46
14. Bydder GM, Young IR (1985) MRI: clinical use of the inversion-recovery sequence. J Comput Assist Tomogr 9: 659-675
15. Canelas HM, Quintao ECR, Scaff M, Vasconcelos KS, Brotto MWI (1983) Cerebrotendinous xanthomatosis: clinical and laboratory study of 2 cases. Acta Neurol Scand 67: 305-311
16. Charness ME, DeLaPaz RL, Diamond I, Norman D (1986) Diagnostic significance of mamillary body atrophy on MR images in chronic Wernicke disease. Radiology 161 (P): 35 (abstr 68)
17. Cherryman GR, Smith FW (1985) Nuclear magnetic resonance in adrenoleucodystrophy: report of a case. Clin Radiol 36: 539-540
18. Davis PC, Hoffman JC Jr, Braun IF, Ahmann P, Krawiecki N (1987) MR of Leigh's disease (subacute necrotizing encephalomyelopathy). AJNR 8: 71-75
19. DeWitt LD, Buonanno FS, Kistler JP, Zeffiro T, De LaPaz RL, Brady TJ, Rosen BR, Pykett IL (1984) Central pontine myelinosis: demonstration by nuclear magnetic resonance. Neurology 34: 570-576
20. DiChiro G, Eiben EM, Manz HJ et al. (1908) A new CT pattern of adrenoleucodystrophy. Radiology 137: 687-692
21. Erbslöh F (1974) Atrophisierende Prozesse. In: Bodechtel G (ed) Differentialdiagnose neurologischer Krankheitsbilder, Thieme, Stuttgart, pp 607-716
22. Garcia JH (1985) Circulatory disorders and their effects on the brain. In: Davis RL, Robertson DM (eds) Textbook of neuropathology. Williams and Wilkins, Baltimore, pp 548-631
23. George AE, de Leon MJ, Kalnin A, Rosner L, Goodgold A, Chase N (1986) Leucencephalopathy in normal and pathologic aging; 2. MRI of brain lucencies. AJNR 7: 567-570
24. Gerard G, Weisberg LA (1986) MRI periventricular lesions in adults. Neurology 36: 998-1001
25. Grossman RI, Gonzales Sarano F, Atlas SW, Galetta S, Silberberg DH (1986) Multiple sclerosis: gadolinium enhancement in MR imaging. Radiology 161: 721-725
26. Harik SI, Post MJD (1981) Computed tomography in Wilson's disease. Neurology 31: 107-110
27. Herndon RM, Rubinstein LJ, Freeman JM, Mathieson G (1970) Light and electron microscopic observations on Rosenthal fibers in Alexander's disease and in multiple sclerosis. J Neuropathol Exp Neurol 29: 524-551
28. Hirano A (1983) Praktischer Leitfaden der Neuropathologie. Springer, Berlin Heidelberg New York
29. Holland BA (1986) Diseases of white matter. In: Brant-Zawadzki M, Norman D (eds) Magnetic resonance imaging of the central nervous system. Raven, New York, pp 259-277
30. Jackson JA, Leake DR, Schneider NJ, Rolak LA, Kelley GR, Ford JJ, Appel SH, Bryan RN (1985) Magnetic resonance imaging in multiple sclerosis: result in 32 cases. AJNR 6: 171-176
31. Janota I (1981) Dementia, deep white matter damage and hypertensive Binswanger's disease. Psychol Med 11: 39-48
32. Johnson MA, Deai S, Hugh-Jones K, Starer F (1984) Magnetic resonance imaging of the brain in Hurler syndrome. AJNR 5: 816-819
33. Journel H, Roussey M, Gandon Y, Allaire C, Carsin M, le Marec B (1987) Magnetic resonance imaging in Pelizaeus-Merzbacher disease. Neuroradiology 29: 403-405
34. Kemper TL (1984) Neuroanatomical and neuropathological changes in normal aging and in dementia. In: Albert M (ed) Clinical neurology of aging. Oxford University Press, New York, pp 9-52
35. Kendall BE (1979) Symmetrical white matter low attenuation in children. In: Extract no 7. Excerpta Medica, Amsterdam, pp 3-14
36. Koehler PR, Haughton VM, Daniels DL, Williams AL, Yetkin Z, Charles HC, Shutts D (1985) MR measurements of normal and pathologic brainstem diameters. AJNR 6: 425-427
37. Kovanen J, Erkinjuntti T, Iivanainen M, Ketonen L, Haltia M, Sulkava R, Sipponen JT (1985) Cerebral MR and CT imaging in Creutzfeldt-Jakob disease. J Comput Assist Tomogr 9(1): 125-128
38. LeMay M (1986) CT changes in dementing diseases: a review. AJNR 7: 841-853
39. Littrup PJ, Gebarski SS (1985) MR imaging of Hallervorden-Spatz disease. J Comput Assist Tomogr 9(3): 491-493
40. Liozou LA, Jefferson JM, Smith WT (1982) Subcortical arteriosclerotic encephalopathy (Binswanger's type) and cortical infarctions in a young normotensive patient. J Neurol Neuro Surg Psychiatry 45: 409-417
41. Lukes SA, Aminoff HJ, Crooks L, Kaufman L, Mills C, Newton TH (1983) Nuclear magnetic resonance imaging in movement disorders. Ann Neurol 13(6): 690-691
42. Mc Kusick VA, Neufeld EF, Kelly TE (1973) The mucopolysaccharide storage diseases. In: Stanburg JB, Wyngaarden JB, Frederickson DS (eds) The metabolic basis of inherited diseases, 4th edn. Mc Graw-Hill, New York, pp 1282-1288
43. Naeser MA, Gebhardt C, Levine HL (1980) Decreased computerized tomography numbers in patients with presenile dementia: detection in patients with otherwise normal scans. Arch Neurol 37: 401-409
44. Noetzel H, Gulotta F (1986) Nervensystem. In: Grundmann E (ed) Spezielle Pathologie. Urban und Schwarzenberg, München, pp 394-439
45. Norenberg MD, Gregorios JB (1985) Central nervous system manifestations of systemic disease. In: Davis RL, Robertson DM (eds) Textbook of neuropathology. Williams and Wilkins, Baltimore, pp 403-467
46. Pavlakis SG, Phillips PC, DiMauro S, De Vivo DC, Rowland LP (1984) Mitochondrial myopathy, encephalopathy, lactic acidosis, and strokelike episodes: a distinct clinical syndrome. Ann Neurol 16: 481-488
47. Penner MW, Li KC, Gebarski SS, Allen RJ (1987) MR imaging of Pelizaeus-Merzbacher disease. J Comput Assist Tomogr 11(4): 591-593
48. Price RA, Jamieson PA (1975) The central nervous system in childhood leukemia. II. Subacute leukoencephalopathy. Cancer 35: 306-318
49. Purpura DP, Guzuki K (1976) Distortion of neuronal geometry and formation of aberrant synapses in neuronal storage disease. Brain Res 116: 1-21
50. Raine CS (1985) Demyelinating disease. In: Davis RL, Robertson DM (eds) Textbook of neuropathology. Williams and Wilkins, Baltimore, pp 468-547
51. Rosenberg GA, Kornfeld M, Stovring J, Bicknell JM (1979) Subcortical arteriosclerotic encephalopathy (Binswanger): computed tomography. Neurology 29: 1102-1106

52. Rubinstein LJ, Herman MM, Long TF, Wibur JR (1975) Disseminated necrotizing leukoencephalopathy: a complication of treated central nervous system leukemia and lymphoma. Cancer 35: 291-305
53. Russo LS Jr, Aron A, Anderson PJ (1976) Alexander's disease: a report and reappraisal. Neurology 26: 607-614
54. Schochet SS (1985) Exogenous toxic-metabolic disease including vitamin deficiency. In: Davis RL, Robertson DM (eds) Textbook of neuropathology. Williams and Wilkins, Baltimore, pp 372-402
55. Scotti G, Scialfa G, Tampieri D, Landoni L (1985) MR imaging in Fahr disease. J Comput Assist Tomogr 9(4): 790-792
56. Seitelberger F (1970) Pelizaeus-Merzbacher disease. In: Vinken PJ, Bruyn GW (eds) Handbook of clinical neurology, vol 10. North Holland, Amsterdam, pp 150-202
57. Simmons JT, Pastakia B, Chase TN, Shults CW (1986) Magnetic resonance imaging in Huntington Disease. AJNR 7: 25-28
58. Stanbury JB, Wyngaarden JB, Frederickson DS et al. (eds) (1983) The metabolic basis of inherited disease, part 3: disorders of amino acid metabolism, 5th edn. Mc Graw-Hill, New York, p 231
59. Stefan H (1987) MELAS-MERRF-KSS. Dtsch Ärztebl 84(15): 708-711
60. Strandgaards S (1978) Autoregulation of cerebral circulation in hypertension. Acta Neurologica Scand 57 [Suppl 66]: 1-82
61. Swanson PD, Cromwell LD (1986) Magnetic resonance imaging in cerebrotendinous xanthomatosis. Neurology 36: 124-126
62. Sze G, De Armond SJ, Brant-Zawadzki M, Davis RL, Norman D, Newton TH (1986) Foci of MRI signal (pseudo lesions) anterior to the frontal horns: histologic correlations of normal findings. AJR 147: 331-337
63. Trommer BL, Naidich TP, Dal Canto MC, McLone DG, Larsen MB (1983) Noninvasive CT diagnosis of infantile Alexander disease: pathologic correlation. J Comput Assist Tomogr 7(3): 509-516
64. Uhlenbrock D, Straube A, Beyer HK, Leopold HC (1985) Kernspintomographie und Computertomographie des Gehirns zum Nachweis des Morbus Wilson. Digitale Bilddiagn 5: 120-122
65. Vermess M, Bernstein RM, Bydder GM, Steiner RE, Young IR, Hughes GRV (1983) Nuclear magnetic resonance (NMR) imaging of the brain in systemic lupus erythematodes. J Comput Assist Tomogr 7(3): 461-467
66. Vogl TH, Bauer M, Seiderer M, Rath M (1984) Kernspintomographie bei Hallervorden-Spatz Syndrom. Digitale Bilddiagn 4: 66-68
67. Watts RWE, Spellacy E, Kendall BE, du Boulay G, Gibbs DA (1981) Computed tomographic studies on patients with mucopolysaccharidosis. Neuroradiology 21: 9-23
68. Weinstein MA, Modic MT, Keyser CK (1985) Diseases of the white matter. In: Latchaw RE (ed) Computed tomography of the head, neck and spine. Year Book, Chicago
69. Wilson SAK (1912) Progressive lenticular degeneration: a familial nervous disease associated with cirrhosis of the liver. Brain 34: 259-309
70. Wright DG, Laureno R, Victor M (1979) Pontine and extrapontine myelinolysis. Brain 102: 361-385
71. Zeman W, Donahue S, Dyken P (1970) The neuronal ceroid-lipofuscinoses (Batten-Vogt syndrome). In: Vinken PJ, Bruyn GW (eds) Handbook of clinical neurology, vol 10. North-Holland, Amsterdam, pp 588-679

9 Temporal Lobe Epilepsy

W. J. Huk

Temporal lobe epilepsy (TLE) is a problematic condition in which MR imaging has shown significant diagnostic value. In many cases the focal cerebral seizures of TLE cannot be explained in terms of a CT-definable lesion or other organic or neurologic disease. The possible causes of the seizures and the corresponding ages of onset are shown in Table 9.1.

Epileptic seizures occur in approximately 0.5%-1.0% of the population. They are broadly classified into two groups.

1. Primary generalized seizures, in which no epileptogenic activity arising from a local anatomic region can be identified.
2. Partial seizures, in which an epileptic focus and often focal brain disease can be found. These are subdivided into simple partial seizures, where consciousness is not impaired, and complex partial seizures with impairment of consciousness.

Complex partial seizures are the most common type of epilepsy in adults. They usually originate in the temporal lobe, and half of the cases are difficult to control or are refractory to treatment.

The leading causes of these seizures in early childhood are defects acquired during the course of development, hypoxic (ischemic-hypotensive) insult, perinatal infections, metabolic diseases, and tuberous sclerosis. Cerebral seizures are late results of these diseases and insults, which often are of quite long standing. By the time seizures occur, the only demonstrable pathologic substrate may be neuronal loss and glial scarring in the anterior hippocampus of the temporal lobe ("mesial temporal sclerosis"), which can be difficult to interpret.

Besides these sclerotic changes, approximately 30%-50% of patients undergoing surgery because of seizures refractory to medical treatment have been found at operation to have low-grade gliomas. Smaller percentages have shown posttraumatic scarring, glial hamartomas, vascular malformations, and residua of previous infarcts [4].

Because surgical removal of these epileptogenic foci eliminates or markedly reduces seizures in a high percentage of cases, the goal of diagnosis must be the detection and localization of the seizure foci. This may be done by means of EEG (electroencephalography), CT, MR imaging, or PET (positron emission tomography). In view of the therapeutic objective, pathologic diagnosis is of only secondary importance in candidates for operation.

The accurate localization of seizure foci with EEG requires invasive measures involving, for example, the surgical implantation of subdural or intracerebral depth electrodes. This technique carries corresponding risks and is subject to technical er-

Table 9.1. Causes of recurrent seizures in different age groups

Age of onset	Probable cause
Neonatal	Congenital maldevelopment, birth injury, anoxia, metabolic disorders (hypocalcemia, hypoglycemia, vitamin B_6 deficiency, phenylketonuria, and others)
Infancy (1-6 months)	As above Infantile spasms
Early childhood (6 months-3 years)	Infantile spasms, febrile convulsions, birth injury and anoxia, infections, trauma
Childhood (3-10 years)	Perinatal anoxia, injury at birth or later, infections, thrombosis of cerebral arteries or veins, or indeterminate cause ("idiopathic" epilepsy)
Adolescence (10-18 years)	Idiopathic epilepsy, including genetically transmitted types, trauma
Early adulthood (18-25 years)	Idiopathic epilepsy, trauma, neoplasm, withdrawal from alcohol or other sedative-hypnotic drugs
Middle age (35-60 years)	Trauma, neoplasm, vascular disease, alcohol or other drug withdrawal
Late life (over 60 years)	Vascular disease, tumor, degenerative disease, trauma

Note: Meningitis and its complications may be a cause of seizures at any age. In tropical and subtropical countries, parasitic infection of the CNS is a common cause
From Adams and Victor (1985)

rors. PET requires complex equipment, is costly, and is not always available. CT and MR, on the other hand, are noninvasive and are readily accessible in most centers.

Comparisons of the value of these two modalities in the diagnostic evaluation of complex partial seizures have shown MR to be superior for three reasons:

- High sensitivity (high soft tissue contrast and high CSF/brain tissue contrast
- Direct coronal and sagittal plane imaging with high spatial resolution
- Absence of bone artifact

The diagnostic value of MR can be further enhanced by the use of intravenous contrast material such as gadolinium chelate.

9.1 MR Findings

There are basically two changes associated with TLE that are accessible to evaluation by MR imaging:

1. Atrophy of the temporal lobe
2. Areas of increased signal intensity in T2-weighted sequences

Atrophy of the temporal lobe: McLachlan et al. [3] found an asymmetry of the temporal lobes in 12 of 16 patients with complex partial seizures. In 10 cases the smaller, atrophic temporal lobe contained the seizure focus. The local asymmetry of the mesial temporal structures and of the temporal horns had less localizing value than the overall decrease in the volume of the temporal lobe, for, as Latack et al. [2] point out, a discrepancy often exists between focal cerebral substance loss and EEG foci (Fig. 9.1).

The size and shape of the two temporal lobes are most accurately compared on coronal scans that are exactly perpendicular to the sagittal plane. Sagittal and axial scans can provide a more complete spatial picture if required. T1-weighted sequences provide the high contrast between CSF and brain that is necessary for defining anatomic details. Normally the two temporal lobes are equal in size [3].

Focal lesions displaying high signal intensity on T2-weighted SE sequences are described by various authors as a nonspecific sign of the foregoing pathologic changes in the temporal lobe (Figs. 9.2–9.4).

Latack et al. [2] (1986), (using 0.35 T; SE TR 2.0/TE 56) saw abnormal MR signal increases in 10 patients with negative CT studies. Four patients had lesions in the mid- and posterior hippocampus with cerebral substance loss as evidence of scarring, and six had an abnormal signal in the anterior hippocampus, which was attributed to mesial temporal sclerosis. The latter finding is in contradiction to the results of Sperling et al. [5] (see below).

Ormson et al. [4] (using a 0.15-T resistive magnet; SE TR 2.0/TE 60, 120) found, in 12 of 25 operated patients, nine low-grade gliomas in the resected temporal lobe, one posttraumatic scar, one case of temporal lobe atrophy, and one thrombosed arteriovenous malformation (AVM). Figures 9.3 and 9.4 show two examples of cryptic AVMs as causes of complex partial seizures. Eight of the nine histologically diverse gliomas showed a nonspecific signal increase on MR scans, while one small glioma 1.2 cm in diameter was undetected by CT and MR. The posttraumatic scar was better demonstrated by MR imaging, while the thrombosed AVM was detected by CT but not by MR, possibly due to the limited spatial resolution of the low-field scanner used. Thirteen cases of mesial temporal gliosis produced no signal abnormalities on MR scans.

Sperling et al. [5] (using 0.35 T and 0.3 T; SE TR 2.0/TE 56 and TR 2.0/TE 112) found, in 7 of 35 patients, focal high-signal lesions that were shown to be caused by tuberous sclerosis, low-grade gliomas, and a glial hamartoma. In 18 patients with mesial temporal sclerosis (29%–95% cell loss in the anterior hippocampus), MR findings were normal.

Interestingly, none of the patients with MR signal abnormalities had abnormal PET findings in the form of a hypometabolic area in the temporal lobe. Conversely, PET was abnormal in 56% of the 18 patients with normal MR scans. Stefan et al. [6] obtained different results in their study of 10 patients with complex partial seizures. CT demonstrated focal abnormalities in 30%, MR in 80%, and PET in all cases. SPECT (single photon emission computed tomography) was positive in 50% unequivocally and in another 40% questionably, with the same lateralization as indicated by PET.

All the authors agree that MR signal abnormalities are best appreciated on heavily T2-weighted-sequences. A TE of 90 ms and preferably 120 ms should be used, and a long TR can improve the signal-to-noise ratio. The close proximity to the carot-

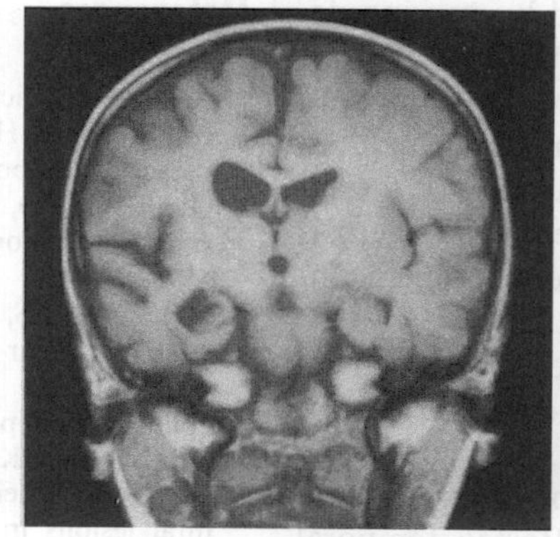

9.1

Fig. 9.1. Astrogliosis of the temporal lobe in a 6-year-old girl with frequent complex partial and partial seizures, probably related to subacute, unspecific, perivascular inflammation (pathologic finding). Atrophy of right hemisphere, including the temporal lobe, without changes of signal intensity. Coronal scan, SE 0.6 s/15 ms (1.0 T)

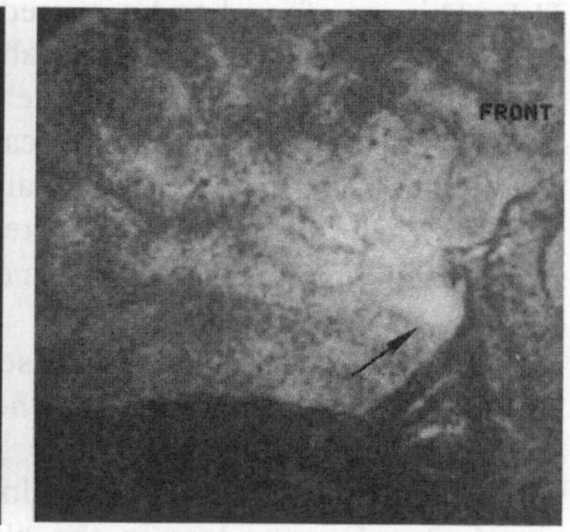

9.2

Fig. 9.2. Gliotic scar of pole of temporal lobe in a 30-year-old man with frequent complex partial seizures refractory to treatment. A hyperintense lesion *(arrow)* is seen at the pole of the right temporal lobe. Intraoperative EEG confirmed the epileptogenic focus in this region, and pathology verified a gliotic scar. Parasagittal scan, SE 1.6 s/140 ms (0.5 T). (Courtesy of Drs. Kuhn, Steen, and Terwey, Oldenburg, FRG)

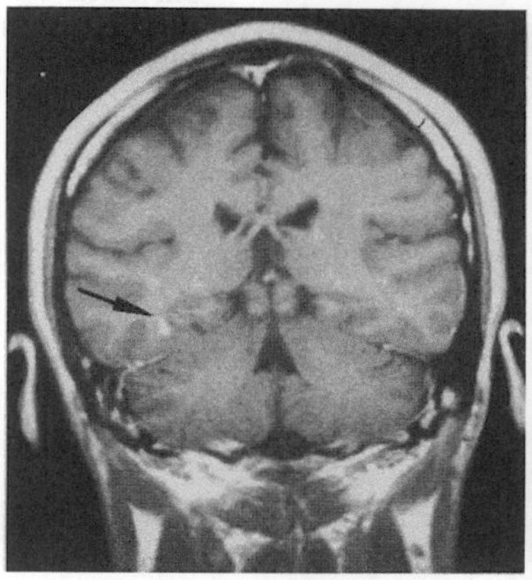

9.3

Fig. 9.3. Occult vascular malformation *(arrows)* of the temporal lobe (confirmed by surgery) in a 26-year-old man with frequent complex parietal seizures. No further seizures occurred after operation. Coronal scan, SE 0.4 s/17 ms, with i.v. gadolinium-DTPA (1.0 T)

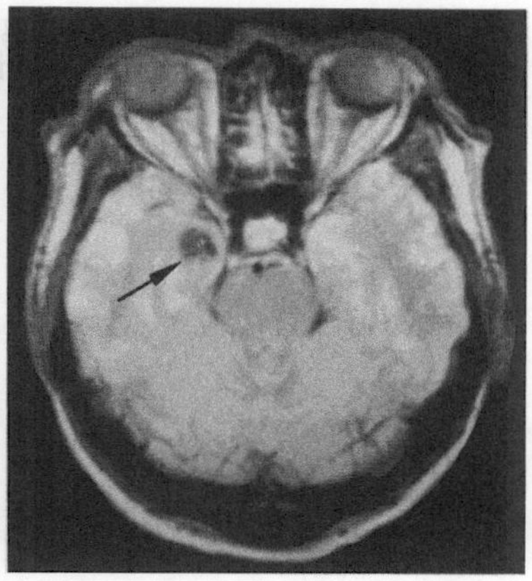

9.4

Fig. 9.4. Occult vascular malformation in a 47-year-old man with uncinate fits. Small round lesion in the uncus indicates a cryptic AVM (see Sect. 14.2) Axial scan SE 3.0 s/40 ms SE 0.5 s/30 ms (1.0 T)

id siphon can lead to superimposed flow artifacts, which are especially troublesome with these imaging parameters. This applies equally to coronal and axial projections. Axial scans also may show artifacts caused by eye movements, requiring that the patient be cautioned to keep his eyes as still as possible. Sagittal scans, which are largely free of these difficulties, can demonstrate the temporal pole with very high clarity, but it does not allow for direct comparison of the temporal lobes. Problem cases may require the use of ECG triggering, changes in the direction of the phase encode gradient, or rephasing sequences to reduce or eliminate flow artifacts. This can also be accomplished by using nonstandard, paraxial sections.

In summary, it may be said that MR imaging is a very sensitive method for the detection of seizure foci in TLE. The involved side can be identified by demonstrating atrophy or substance loss of the affected temporal lobe and a focal signal increase on T2-weighted scans. The high-signal areas are nonspecific, and their exact nature cannot be established (low-grade glioma, posttraumatic scar, hamartoma), with the exception of AVMs, which are characterized by their effects of flow and paramagnetic substances (i.e., methemoglobin) on signal intensity (see Sect. 5.3). Mesial temporal sclerosis, the leading cause of TLE, did not produce MR signal abnormalities in the majority of cases described, whereas PET demonstrated a hypometabolic area in the affected lobe in approximately half of these patients. In the series of McLachlan et al. [3], the temporal lobe atrophy observed with MR was confirmed at lobectomy in seven of eight patients with

TLE. This was found to be caused by varying degrees of gliosis, neuron loss, and abnormal neurons in the hippocampus and neocortex. There was no evidence of tumors or other focal abnormalities. This suggests that asymmetry or atrophy of a temporal lobe can result from mesial temporal sclerosis and therefore can be the seat of an epileptogenic focus.

Thus, if a focal signal increase is not seen on T2-weighted sequences in TLE where EEG has indicated a unilateral seizure focus, scans should be taken that enable the temporal lobes to be compared. A substance loss in the affected temporal lobe correlating with the EEG focus can then provide the sole evidence of a mesial temporal sclerosis as the cause of the seizures. Confirmatory evidence may be sought in these cases in the form of a hypometabolic area on PET scans.

Further studies are necessary, however, to establish the role of the various imaging procedures in TLE and further differentiate their findings.

References

1. Adams RD, Victor M (1985) Principles in neurology, 3rd edn. McGraw-Hill, New York
2. Latack JT, Abou-Khalil BW, Siegel GJ, Sackellares JC, Gabrielsen TO, Aisen AM (1986) Patients with partial seizures: evaluation by MR, CT, and PET imaging. Radiology 159: 159-163
3. McLachlan RS, Nicholson RL, Black S, Carr T, Blume WT (1985) Nuclear magnetic resonance imaging, a new approach to the investigation of refractory temporal lobe epilepsy. Epilepsia 26 (6): 555-562
4. Ormson MJ, Kispert DB, Sharbrough FW, Houser OW, Earnest F, Scheithauer BW, Laws ER (1986) Cryptic structural lesions in refractory partial epilepsy: MR imaging and CT studies. Radiology 160: 215-219
5. Sperling MR, Wilson G, Engel J Jr, Babb TL, Phelp M, Bradley W (1986) Magnetic resonance imaging in intractable partial epilepsy: correlative studies. Ann Neurol 20: 57-62
6. Stefan H, Pawlik G, Böcher-Schwarz H, Biersack HJ; Burr W, Penin H, Heiss WD (1987) Functional and morphological abnormalities in temporal lobe epilepsy: a comparison of interictal and ictal EEG, CT, MRI, SPECT, and PET. J Neurol 234: 377-384

10 Intracranial Tumors

W. J. Huk and W. Heindel

Since Virchow [58] (1847), neuropathologists have attempted to classify the many types of intracranial tumors by morphologic criteria and differentiate them according to their biologic behaviors. The classification of brain tumors has been greatly advanced by the work of Bailey and Cushing [5, 6] (1926, 1930), Kernohan and Sayre [29], Russel and Rubinstein [50] (1977), and Zülch [64-66]. The scheme of Kernohan et al. [28] combines a histologic classification by cell type with a biologic grading of malignancy and recognizes four stages. In 1979 a tumor classification and grading system was developed under the auspices of the World Health Organization [65], and that system will form the basis for the description of MR findings in this text.

We base our description of the MR appearance of intracranial tumors on reports from the literature and our own experience. In the case of rare tumors for which MR findings were not available when the book went to press, we shall follow our usual practice of describing histopathologic features. Rare lesions exhibiting architectures and regressive changes resembling those seen in more familiar tumor types may be expected to present similar signal patterns on MR images.

Table 10.1. WHO classification of intracranial tumors

Tumors of neuroepithelial tissue
1. Astrocytic tumors
   a) Astrocytomas
   b) Pilocytic astrocytomas
   c) Subependymal giant cell astrocytomas (ventricular tumors of tuberous sclerosis)
   d) Astroblastomas
   e) Anaplastic (malignant) astrocytomas
2. Oligodendroglial tumors
   a) Oligodendrogliomas
   b) Mixed oligoastrocytomas
   c) Anaplastic (malignant) oligodendrogliomas
3. Poorly differentiated and embryonal tumors
   a) Glioblastomas
   b) Medulloblastomas
   c) Medulloepitheliomas
   d) Primitive polar spongioblastomas
   e) Gliomatosis cerebri
4. Ependymal and choroid plexus tumors
   a) Ependymomas
   b) Anaplastic ependymomas
   c) Choroid plexus papillomas
   d) Anaplastic choroid plexus papillomas
5. Pineal cell tumors
   a) Pineocytomas
   b) Pineoblastomas
   c) Pinealomas, germinomas
   d) Embryonal carcinomas
6. Neuronal tumors
   a) Gangliocytomas
   b) Gangliogliomas
   c) Ganglioneuroblastomas
   d) Anaplastic (malignant) gangliocytomas/gangliogliomas
   e) Neuroblastomas
   f) Primitive neuroectodermal tumors

Tumors of the nerve sheath cells
1. Neurilemmomas
2. Anaplastic (malignant) neurilemmomas
3. Neurofibromas
4. Anaplastic (malignant) neurofibromas

Tumors of meningeal and related tissues
1. Meningiomas
2. Meningeal sarcomas
3. Primary melanotic tumors (melanomas and meningeal melanomatosis)

Primary malignant lymphomas
1. Primary tumors of the lymphoreticular system

Tumors of blood vessel origin
1. Hemangioblastomas
2. Monstrocellular sarcomas

Germ cell tumors
1. Germinomas
2. Embryonal carcinomas
3. Teratomas

Other malformative tumors and tumor-like lesions
1. Craniopharyngiomas
2. Rathke's cleft cysts
3. Epidermoid and dermoid cysts
4. Colloid cysts
5. Enterogenous cysts
6. Ependymal cysts
7. Lipomas
8. Hypothalamic neuronal hamartomas
9. Nasal glial heterotopias

Tumors of the pituitary
1. Tumors of the anterior pituitary
   a) Pituitary adenomas
   b) Pituitary adenocarcinomas
2. Lesions of the posterior lobe

Local extensions from regional tumors
1. Glomus jugulare tumors
2. Chordomas
3. Chondromas
4. Chondrosarcomas
5. Olfactory neuroblastomas
6. Adenoid cystic carcinomas

Metastatic tumors

Pseudotumor cerebri

From Zülch [66]

The order in which the various tumor types are presented in the text deviates somewhat from this outline where considered appropriate for reasons of common diagnostic criteria.

The *goals of imaging procedures* in intracranial tumors are:

- Detection of the tumor
- Localization of the tumor
- Differential diagnosis of the tumor (identification of tumor type)

10.1 General Aspects of the Detection of Intracranial Tumors with MR

Experience to date indicates that MR imaging is more sensitive than CT in the detection of intracranial and especially cerebral tumors. Tumors, especially of the glioma type, generally show a greater extent on MR than on CT. MR can also detect tumors earlier than CT, although the early stage of tumor growth is still inaccessible to both modalities (Fig. 10.1). The tumor becomes visible with MR, and later with CT, only when the volume of free intracellular or extracellular water has increased sufficiently. This means that the extent of signal changes on MR scans is not always equivalent to the extent of tumor growth. These observations are supported by the results of stereotaxic serial biopsies performed by Kelly et al. [27] showing that in some cases tumor cell infiltration may extend even beyond the limits defined by T2-weighted MR images. In the planning of radiation therapy, MR images are more reliable for the identification of potential tumor-bearing tissue.

The direct visualization of coronal and sagittal sections and the absence of bone artifact enable a better and more accurate description of the shape and characteristics of a tumor and of its position relative to adjacent, normal anatomic structures. This information is important for assessing the operability of a tumor and selecting the surgical approach; it can also contribute to the differential diagnosis.

Other *criteria for the differential diagnosis* of intracranial tumors are:

1. Signal contrast with normal brain
2. Tumor structure
3. Tumor margins
4. Presence, absence, and extent of perifocal edema
5. Indirect tumor signs
6. Relation of tumor to blood vessels, richness of tumor blood supply
7. Degree of contrast enhancement

1. The *signal contrast* is based on differences in proton density and differences in the T1 and T2 relaxation times. Shortening of relaxation times is rarely seen in neoplasms and can occur only in lesions with a high content of fat (lipomas) or lipid-containing substances (e.g., craniopharyngiomatous cysts). These tumors give a bright signal on T1-weighted sequences.

The majority of tumors have prolonged relaxation times. The prolongation may be small, as in meningiomas, or substantial, as in gliomas. It results from an increase of intracellular and/or extracellular free water and produces a high signal intensity on T2-weighted images. If the tumor signal is isointense with brain, as in some meningiomas, the presence of the tumor may still be indicated by perifocal edema (see point 4 below). In the absence of this edema, detection must rely on indirect tumor signs (see point 5 below). Contrast material may be used in doubtful cases.

2. The *tumor structure,* as assessed by the signal pattern within the lesion, may be homogeneous or nonhomogeneous. The homogeneous structure in turn may be hypointense (giving a low signal), isointense (giving a signal equal to that of surrounding tissue), or hyperintense (giving a high signal). The imaging parameters must always be known so that the relaxation times can be correctly interpreted. A homogeneous signal pattern is suggestive of benignity (e.g., meningiomas, many low-grade gliomas, cysts), whereas the majority of malignant, blastomatous lesions present a relatively chaotic, non-

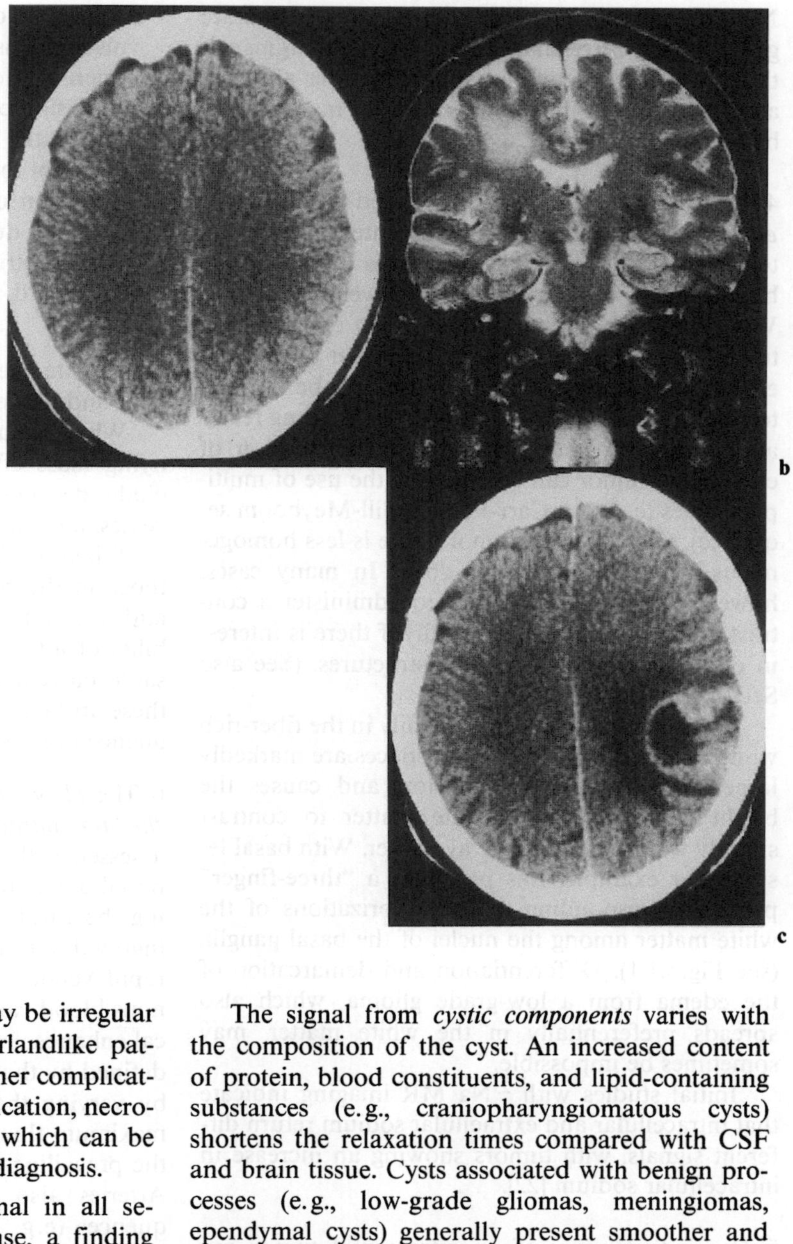

Fig. 10.1 a–c. Early MR findings in glioblastoma multiforme in a 59-year-old woman examined after one focal seizure: **a** Negative CT with IV contrast medium. **b** MR on the same day as CT reveals unspecific hyperintense area in the right parietal white matter. Coronal scan, SE 3.0 s/120 ms (1.0 T). **c** Ten weeks later CT shows the ring-shaped glioblastoma confirmed by surgery

homogeneous structure. The latter may be irregular and patchy, although ringlike or garlandlike patterns are also seen. The picture is further complicated by regressive changes such a calcification, necrosis, hemorrhage, and cyst formation, which can be very helpful in making a differential diagnosis.

Calcifications produce a low signal in all sequences. They are always hypointense, a finding that is nonspecific compared with CT imaging [45]. Calcifications are most commonly associated with slow-growing, benign tumors, although they do not afford proof of benignity. Discrete calcium inclusions in the tissue generally cannot be visualized with MR.

Hemorrhages, which usually are seen in their subacute or chronic stage, appear bright initially on T1-weighted images and later on T2-weighted scans. Acute hemorrhages and sites of *iron deposition* (hemosiderin) appear dark on T2-weighted sequences (see Sect. 5.2, p. 116).

The signal from *cystic components* varies with the composition of the cyst. An increased content of protein, blood constituents, and lipid-containing substances (e.g., craniopharyngiomatous cysts) shortens the relaxation times compared with CSF and brain tissue. Cysts associated with benign processes (e.g., low-grade gliomas, meningiomas, ependymal cysts) generally present smoother and more regular margins than the liquefied necrotic cavities of malignant growths (e.g., glioblastoma); epidermoids are exceptions to this rule. Sometimes fluid levels can be seen (e.g., in pituitary adenomas), signifying corpuscular elements of older hemorrhages.

3. The *tumor margins* can show all gradations from smooth and regular to irregular, indistinct, or ill-defined. Homogeneous signal changes may be sharp and regular, they may present lobulated borders, (e.g., meningiomas), or they may present indistinct margins suggesting infiltration, (e.g., gliomas).

Nonhomogeneous tumors with a patchy structure generally have irregular and ill-defined margins, although their borders may appear sharper after the administration of intravenous contrast material (see below).

4. Most brain tumors are surrounded by vasogenic *edema,* which, owing to its high content of free water, displays long relaxation times and appears bright on proton-density and T2-weighted scans. With the water, plasma proteins also enter the extravascular space. The margin between tumor and edema may be clearly defined or it may be difficult to resolve, especially in tumors that have long relaxation times. In some cases the differentiation of edema and tumor can be aided by the use of multiple echoes (e.g., the Carr-Purcell-Gill-Meyboom sequence). Generally the tumor tissue is less homogeneous than the edematous zone. In many cases, however, it will be necessary to administer a contrast agent (see below), especially if there is interest in delineating small anatomic structures. (See also Sect. 5.1, p. 115.)

The edema spreads most readily in the fiber-rich white matter, whose interstitial spaces are markedly larger than those of the cortex, and causes the bright contours of the white matter to contrast sharply with those of the gray matter. With basal lesions, for example, this produces a "three-finger" pattern corresponding to the arborizations of the white matter among the nuclei of the basal ganglia (see Fig. 5.1.1). Differentiation and demarcation of the edema from a low-grade glioma, which also spreads preferentially in the white matter, may sometimes be impossible.

Initial studies with ^{23}Na MR imaging indicate that intracellular and extraellular sodium return different signals, with tumors showing an increase in intracellular sodium [22].

5. The *indirect signs* of an intracranial tumor are produced by the deformation and displacement of normal adjacent structures. The examiner should be alert for the following changes, often quite subtle, in cases where the tumor itself is not clearly visualized:

- Compression and deformation of adjacent portions of the ventricles, including the displacement of entire lateral ventricles and midline structures
- Compression of adjacent sulci
- Compression of the basal CSF spaces, or filling of these spaces by tumor tissue
- Expansion of the lateral ventricle of the uninvolved hemisphere through constriction of the foramen of Monro or the third ventricle
- Expansion of the prepontine and peripontine cisterns on the involved side by displacement of the brainstem toward the opposite side
- Expansion of the supratentorial portions of the ventricles due to plugging of the aqueduct or fourth ventricle
- Downward displacement of the cerebellar tonsils

Evaluation of these signs requires the use of T1-weighted sequences with good contrast between CSF and tissue.

When signal changes are seen with no accompanying mass effect, differential diagnosis must include degenerative processes, inflammatory processes, and chronic processes of vascular origin.

When evaluating the CSF spaces, especially those in the basal region, ventricles, spinal canal, and resection cavities, one must consider the possibility of artifactual signal changes induced by pulsatile movements of the CSF. The prominence of these artifacts varies with the particular imaging sequence used (see Sect. 5.3).

6. The *blood supply* of the tumor and its *relation to the large intracranial vessels* often can be accurately assessed with MR, obviating the need for conventional angiography. Examples are tumors enveloping the carotid artery and its branches and tumor ingrowth into the venous sinuses. Arterial flow and rapid venous flow appear dark. Slow-moving venous blood can appear bright because of paradoxical enhancement. The vascularity of a tumor can be defined by the use of flow-sensitive sequences, i.e., by varying the TR and slice thickness such that maximum flow-related enhancement is obtained at the prevailing flow velocity ([34]; see also Sect. 5.3). Arteries also may appear bright when fast sequences (e.g., FFE, FISP, FLASH) are employed (see Sect. 1.3).

7. *Enhancement* of a tumor with contrast material is helpful in detecting the lesion, defining its margins, and assessing its behavior. The original hope that multiecho sequences (e.g., Carr-Purcell-Gill-Meyboom) could eliminate the need for contrast material has not been fulfilled. The mechanism of action of MR contrast agents is discussed in Sect. 5.5.

T2-weighted sequences are the most sensitive for detecting intracerebral lesions, and the use of contrast agents in these cases is essentially adjunctive. With extra-axial tumors, however, contrast agents substantially increase the reliability of tumor detection. It is our view that contrast agents should be administered only if a lesion cannot be adequately detected and evaluated by the use of conventional SE and IR sequences.

As in CT imaging, the enhancement of an intracranial tumor beyond the vascular phase signifies absence or disruption of the blood-brain barrier. It is important to note that the limit of contrast enhancement in the early phase corresponds as little to the actual tumor boundary as does the diffuse spread of the contrast agent in the late phase [16]. A blood-brain barrier is absent in mesenchymal tumors, such as meningiomas, with the result that benign meningiomas as well as those undergoing sarcomatous change show equal enhancement. With neuroepithelial brain tumors, however, evidence of disruption of the blood-brain barrier signifies the presence of pathologic vessels and thus a higher grade of malignancy. Rare exceptions are pilocytic astrocytomas, plexus papillomas, and other tumors that have fenestrated vessels [23].

T1-weighted images are necessary for demonstrating contrast enhancement. On these scans the bright tumor stands out clearly in relation to the dark peritumoral edema or surrounding structures.

Information useful in making a pathologic diagnosis can be derived from the course of the time-signal intensity curve in dynamic studies. As in comparable CT studies, the steep initial signal rise indicates a rich tumor blood supply. The contrast material escapes at a variable rate into the perivascular interstitial tissue, depending on the degree of disruption of the blood-brain barrier, where it becomes diffusely distributed or undergoes a gradual washout. Studies using a gradient echo sequence in a small number of tumors showed a very rapid signal rise flattening to a plateau in pituitary adenomas, a rapid rise with a gradual fall in meningiomas, a less rapid rise with a peak signal at 3–5 min in acoustic neuromas, a gradual rise in gliomas, and a moderately steep rise followed by a gradual signal increase in metastases [31]. The most pronounced signal increases relative to noncontrast scans were seen in acoustic neuromas (approximately 360%) and meningiomas (approximately 180%); smaller increases were seen in neurofibromas and pituitary adenomas [10].

A pathologic diagnosis can be made with varying degrees of confidence from the MR features of intracranial tumors, although proof of the diagnosis must be obtained directly. Tumors of the neuroepithelial tissues are particularly apt to show structural diversity, and a pathologic diagnosis might well prove difficult even with the benefit of histologic specimens. In MR imaging as in CT, familiarity with the history and clinical presentation is very often essential for the evaluation of findings.

The quantitative determination of relaxation times does not contribute significantly to pathologic diagnosis. Because tumor tissue is permeated by blood vessels, connective tissue, edema, and regressive changes, the values measured in vivo overlap to such a degree that they are practically useless for purposes of differentiation. Changes in relaxation times in response to radiation and chemotherapy show potential value as a means of evaluating treatment response at an early stage. Further studies are needed, however, before such information can be evaluated in detail.

10.2 Tumors of Neuroepithelial Tissue

10.2.1 Astrocytic Tumors

Astrocytomas

The astrocytomas, arising from the astroglia, include several subtypes which vary in their gross and microscopic features. They are classified as "semibenign" (grade 2) in the WHO system.

Incidence: In the series of Zülch [66], astrocytomas accounted for 6.6% of the 9000 tumors reviewed. One-fourth to one-third of all gliomas were astrocytomas. The peak incidence of astrocytomas occurs between 35 and 45 years of age.

Sites: Astrocytomas occur most frequently at the convexity of the hemispheres, where they involve both the cortex and the white matter. The frontotemporal and frontoparietal regions are sites of predilection (Fig. 10.2), but the tumors may involve all other brain regions, including the temporal, parietal, occipital, and basal ganglia, the pons, and the spinal cord (Fig. 10.3, see Fig. 10.24 c). The tumors spread slowly beyond the white matter and invade the corpus callosum and septum pellucidum.

Pathology: Astrocytomas are classified as fibrillary, protoplasmic, or gemistocytic according to the predominant cell type. *Fibrillary* astrocytomas are the most common histologic type and occur at various sites in the CNS. They contain abundant intracyto-

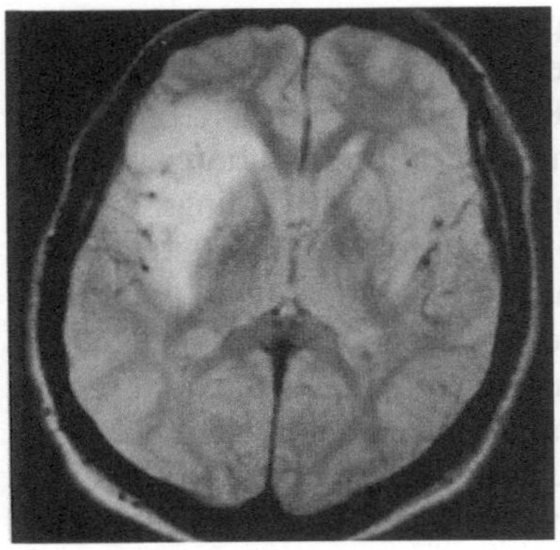

10.2

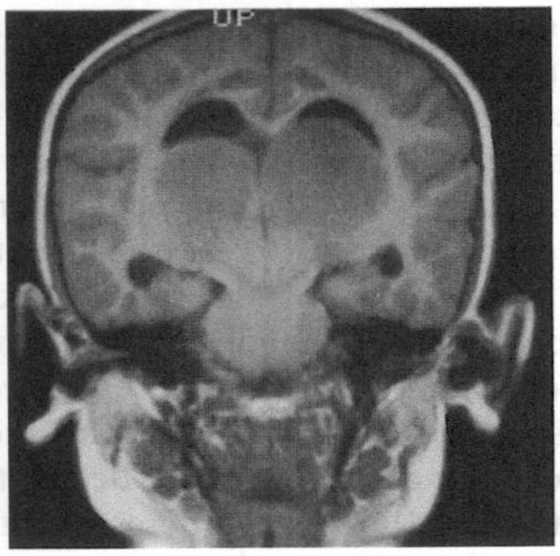

10.3

Fig. 10.2. Low-grade astrocytoma in a 56-year-old man with cerebral seizures. Frequent location and shape of low-grade frontotemporal gliomas. This diagnosis is supported by the fact that the tumor has been observed for several years with only very little increase in size. Axial scan, SE 3.0 s/45 ms, (1.0 T)

Fig. 10.3. Bilateral symmetric astrocytoma (WHO grade 2) of the basal ganglia, the upper brainstem (biopsy) and cerebellum in a 4-year-old girl with unsteady gait, nausea, and vomiting. Coronal scan, SE 0.6 s/15 ms, (1.5 T)

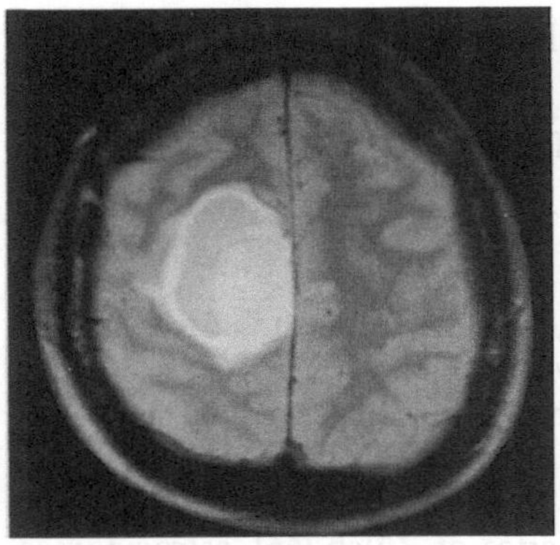

10.4

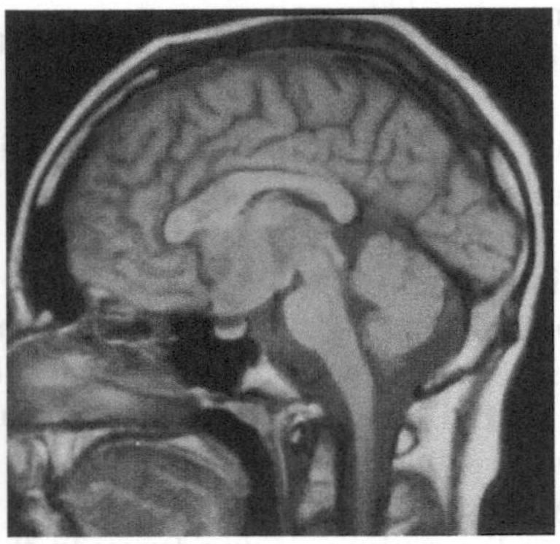

10.5

Fig. 10.4. Fibrillary astrocytoma (WHO grade 2) in a 27-year-old man with focal seizures of the left leg for 4 years and now presenting with hemihypesthesia. At surgery a firm solid tumor with small pseudocystic regressive changes was found. Well-outlined lesion with prolonged relaxation times. Axial scan, SE 3.0 s/45 ms, (1.0 T)

Fig. 10.5. Mixed glioma, mainly astrocytoma (WHO grade 2), in a 12-year-old boy with recurrent visual disturbances, papilledema, and occlusive hydrocephalus. Biopsy revealed a spongy, mucoid structure of the tumor with astrocytic elements containing isomorphic nuclei, little cytoplasm, and varying amounts of glial fibrils. Also cells of ependyma and densely packed small round cells with small nuclei and a honeycomb-shaped rim of cytoplasm were found. The ill-defined tumor has prolonged T1 and T2 and involves the corpus callosum, the septum pellucidum and the chiasm. Sagittal scan, SE 0.7 s/3 ms (1.0 T)

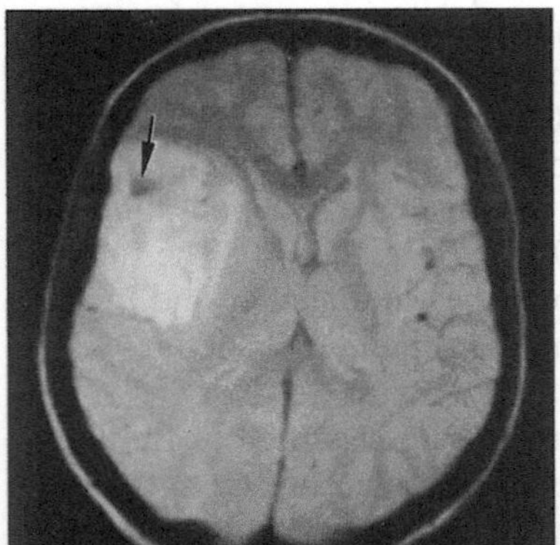

10.6

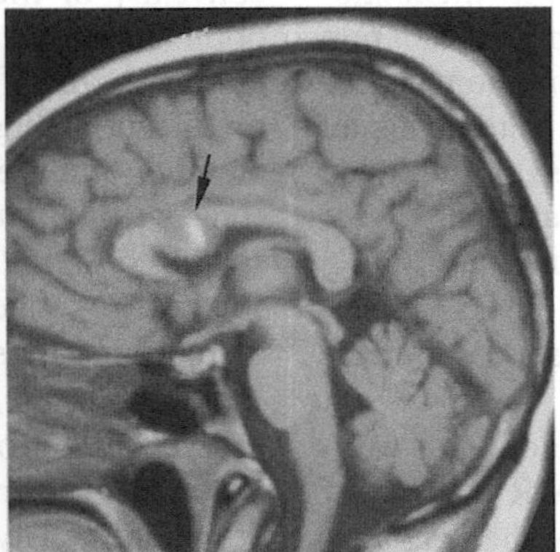

10.7

Fig. 10.6. Mixed glioma (oligoastrocytoma, WHO grade 2-3) in a 49-year-old woman with focal seizures. The hypointense focus *(arrow)* does not correspond to calcifications seen on CT; it was hyperintense on T2-weighted images indicating cystic fluid. Axial scan, SE 2.5 s/40 ms (1.0 T)

Fig. 10.7. Mixed glioma (WHO grade 2) in a 27-year-old woman with sudden headache. Small hemorrhage *(arrow)* in small, fairly well delineated tumor of the anterior corpus callosum. The tumor tissue also contained hemosiderin-laden macrophages and small calcifications. Midsagittal scan, SE 0.5 s/17 ms (1.0 T)

plasmic glial fibrils and few capillary vessels (Fig. 10.4). Next most frequent are the *gemistocytic* tumors, which usually involve the frontal lobe and consist of cytoplasm-rich cells with fibrils and often with highly tortuous vessels. The *protoplasmic* astrocytomas, which occur mostly in the temporal region, contain abundant cytoplasm with very few fibrils and a somewhat greater number of vessels. Mixed forms are much more common than the pure histologic types (Figs. 10.5, 10.7). The consistency of the astrocytoma depends on its content of intracytoplasmic fibrils.

The margins of circumscribed astrocytomas show both infiltrative and expansive modes of growth. The diffuse forms, which are difficult at first to distinguish from mild brain swelling, produce only a uniform expansion of the brain tissue. These tumors appear as hypodense areas on noncontrast CT scans, and they show no enhancement after the administration of intravenous contrast material.

Except for the diffuse growths, all astrocytomas show an early tendency toward mucoid change, with the formation of solitary large cysts or multiple smaller cysts, especially in fibrillary and gemistocytic lesions (Fig. 10.6). Hemorrhage and necrosis in the low-grade tumors are extremely rare, as are calcifications [66] (Fig. 10.7; see also Fig. 14.24).

Initial symptoms vary with the site of occurrence and include focal seizures (with temporal or central involvement), personality change (with frontal involvement), or signs of increased intracranial pressure.

CT and MR findings: see p. 239-240.

Pilocytic Astrocytomas

Pilocytic astrocytomas are a special form of astrocytoma with a better prognosis (WHO grade 1). Distinction is made between pilocytic astrocytomas of the cerebellum ("cerebellar astrocytoma") and those of the optic chiasm.

Incidence: Pilocytic astrocytomas account for about 6% of all intracranial tumors and are most common in younger patients. They account for 30% of gliomas in children [66].

Sites: The tumors mostly arise at the center of the cerebellum, whence they spread into the hemispheres. Less commonly they occur in the optic nerve or chiasm, in the hypothalamus (Fig. 10.8), or in the outer wall of the lateral ventricles, where they grow as large hemispheric tumors. Finally they may occur in the pons, medulla oblongata, and spinal cord, where they frequently display a cystic type of growth and may be mistaken for syringomyelia.

Pathology: Pilocytic astrocytomas are well demarcated and usually grow by expansion, although infiltrative growth can occur at the periphery. The tumors form solitary or multiple cysts of variable size. They may fill the third ventricle and obstruct the foramen of Monro. They are moderately cellular with an irregular stroma containing few vessels that sometimes show angioma-like tortuosity. The tumors tend toward hyalination. They may appear solid, partially solid with multiple small cysts, or large and cystic with a rim of irregularly thick tumor tissue (see also p. 279, Figs. 11.7-11.9). Calcifications and internal hemorrhage are also described [1].

MR findings: see p. 239-240.

Anaplastic Astrocytomas and Glioblastomas

As the signs of anaplasia become apparent, the prognosis of the astrocytomas worsens to WHO grade 3.

These signs of anaplasia are as follows [66]:

- Increased cellularity
- Pleomorphism with degeneration of the cells
- High mitotic rate and rapid growth
- Abnormal stroma with proliferation of pathologic vessels (sinusoidal vessels and fistulas) and disruption of the blood-brain barrier

Any astrocytoma may undergo anaplastic or glioblastomatous transformation as the disease progresses. Anaplastic astrocytoma differs from glioblastoma in the degree of anaplasia. The degeneration may involve only part of the tumor, and different grades of malignancy can coexist in the same lesion. For (stereotactic) biopsies it is important to take the specimen from anaplastic areas, as these will determine the diagnosis and thus the prognosis.

Incidence: Glioblastomas constitute about 12%-17% of all intracranial tumors and are most prevalent in the middle-aged and elderly, showing a slight preponderance in males [66].

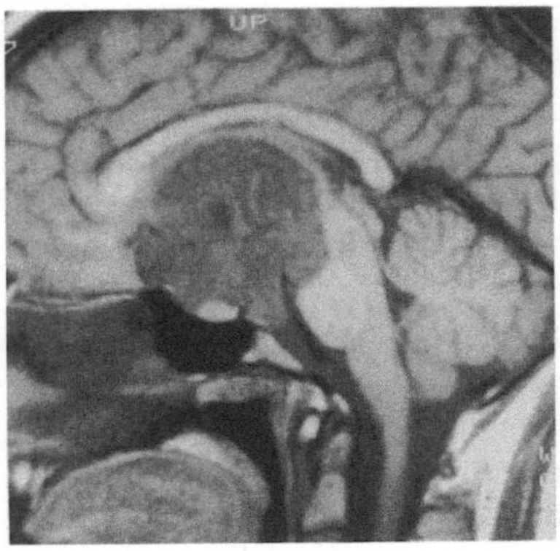

10.8

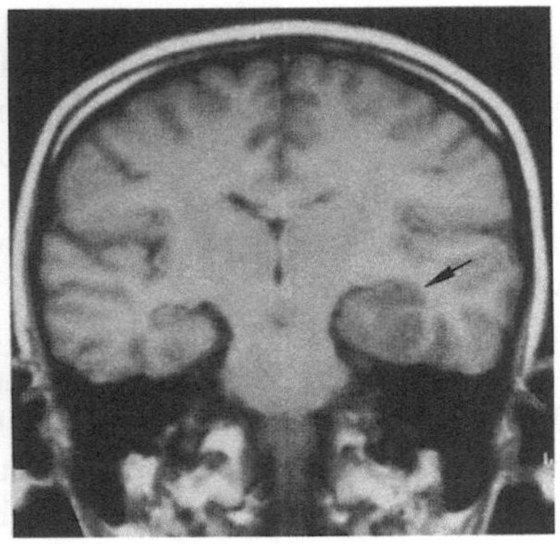

10.9

Fig. 10.8. Pilocytic astrocytoma of the optic chiasm and hypothalamus (WHO grade 1) in a 17-year-old almost blind girl. Huge, well-delineated, quite homogeneous mass. Sagittal scan, SE 0.5 s/ 17 ms (1.0 T)

Fig. 10.9. Astrocytic glioblastoma (WHO grade 3-4) in a 29-year-old man with complex partial seizures. Thickening of gyri *(arrow)* and large ill-defined area of prolonged T1 and T2. Coronal scan, SE 0.4 s/17 ms (1.0 T)

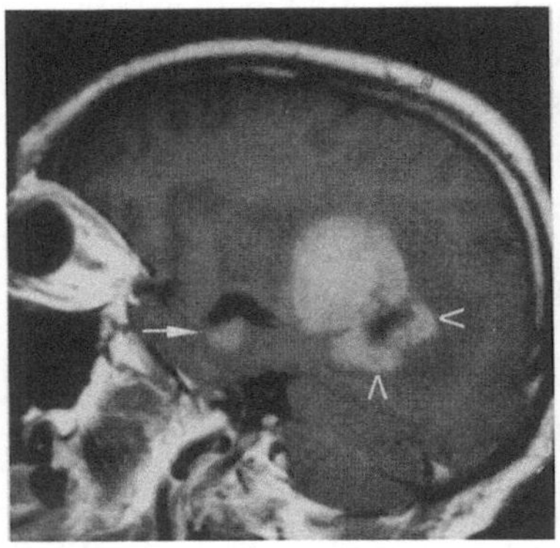

10.10

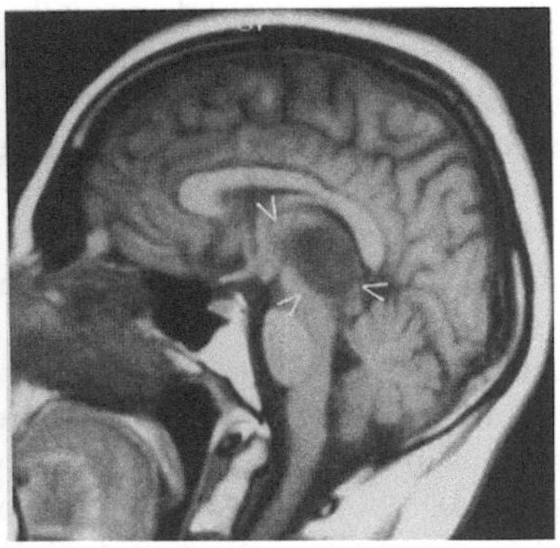

10.11

Fig. 10.10. Glioblastoma (WHO grade 4) in a 65-year-old man with a short history of headache, hemiparesis on the right, and speech disturbances. After i.v. gadolinium-DTPA enhancement occurs in the area of blood-brain barrier disruption, indicating malignant tumor. The tumor grows around the ventricle *(arrowheads)* and seems to have a seperate portion on the floor of the temporal horn *(arrow)*. Sagittal scan SE 0.6 s/15 ms; (1.5 T)

Fig. 10.11. Glioblastoma multiforme in a 37-year-old woman with double vision and increasing headache. Ill-defined partly cystic tumor *(arrowheads)* of the pineal region invading the thalami, with perifocal edema. Diagnosis derived from stereotaxic biopsy. Sagittal scan SE 0.4 s/17 ms (1.0 T)

Sites: Like astrocytomas, glioblastomas can occur anywhere in the brain and show a predominantly subcortical pattern of spread. They may be relatively circumscribed or may cross the commissures to infiltrate the opposite side ("butterfly pattern"). Occurrence in the quadrigeminal zone, cerebellum, pons, or spinal cord is unusual (Fig. 10.11).

Pathology: The wide variety of cell forms in glioblastoma, compared with astrocytoma, stems from the changes of anaplasia and especially from necrosis, fatty degeneration, and hemorrhage, which are encountered in varying degrees and stages. In most cases these changes, combined with the disrupted blood-brain barrier in the pathologic vessels, incite a perifocal edema of variable extent (Figs. 10.9-10.11).

When the stroma contains numerous mesodermal elements showing malignant degeneration, the tumor is called a "glioblastoma with sarcomatous elements."

MR findings: see p. 239-240.

Gliomatosis cerebri refers to a diffuse infiltration of extensive brain areas by glial cells. There may be sites of focal involvement, as in glioblastoma. These should be distinguished from diffuse and multicentric gliomas (Fig. 10.14).

In this very uncommon disease the entire brain or large portions of it are enlarged. Gray and white matter are involved, the underlying anatomical structure usually being preserved. Areas of demyelination of the white matter correlate with the extent of the neoplastic growth.

Besides a diffuse and more or less symmetric thickening of midline structures, MR reveals marked prolongation of T1 and T2 relaxation times of the regions affected by the disease [56].

Fig. 10.12. Oligodendroglioma (WHO grade 2, stereotaxic biopsy) in a 19-year-old man with spastic tetraparesis. Butterfly glioma of the corpus callosum. Coronal scan, IR 2.5 s/400 ms/35 ms (0.5 T). (Courtesy of Drs. Kuhn, Steen, and Terwey, Oldenburg FRG)

Fig. 10.13. Oligodendroglioma (WHO grade 2) in a 7-year-old girl with cerebral seizures. Nodular tumor with small calcification *(arrow)*. No perifocal edema. Axial scan: SE 3.0 s/120 ms (1.0 T)

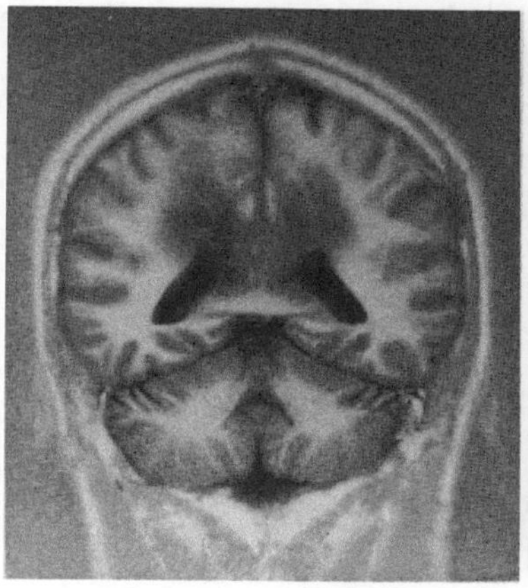

10.12

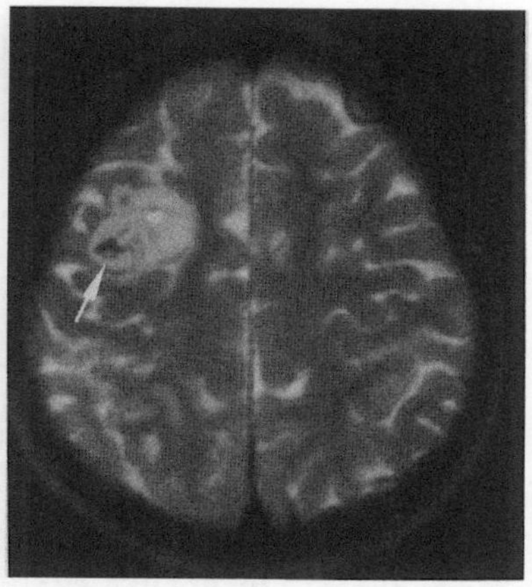

10.13

10.2.2 Oligodendroglial Tumors

These tumors arise from the oligodendroglia. Besides the true oligodendroglioma (WHO grade 2), a mixed oligoastrocytic form (grade 2) and an anaplastic form (grade 3) are recognized.

Oligodendrogliomas

Incidence: Oligodendrogliomas comprise about 4% of intracranial tumors and 18% of gliomas. They are slightly more common in males than females.

Sites: These tumors can occur anywhere in the cerebrum but show a predilection for the frontal and temporal regions. The thalamus is most commonly affected in children. They are less often found in the parietal and occipital lobes, seldom within the spinal cord, and very rarely in the cerebellum [66].

Pathology: Oligodendrogliomas have a homogeneous structure (Fig. 10.12), and their cells show a characteristic honeycomb pattern or may resemble plant cells. They grow from the white matter toward the cortex and have a tendency to undergo mucoid and cystic degeneration in small or large areas; fatty degeneration is less common. Areas of necrosis may also be present. The vessel walls as well as the parenchyma often show calcifications, which are visualized with CT in over 70% of cases. In contradistinction to the disseminated, small, patchy calcific areas in ependymomas, the calcifications of oligodendrogliomas are composed of larger conglomerates (Fig. 10.13). The blood vessels break easily, and hemorrhages of variable size are not uncommon ("apoplectic glioma") (Fig. 10.7, see also Fig. 10.15 and Fig. 14.24).

The borders of the tumor may be ill-defined (Fig. 10.12), but often the lesions are sharply demarcated from surrounding brain and show a multifocal distribution. Infiltration of the meninges can occur. The rate of growth is very slow. Metastasis by the cerebrospinal pathway does occur, and even extracranial seeding has been described [66].

Mixed Oligoastrocytomas

By definition, mixed oligoastrocytomas consist of oligodendroglial and astrocytic elements, which are indistinguishable from each other on MR images (Fig. 10.14; see also Figs. 10.5–10.7).

Anaplastic (Malignant) Oligodendrogliomas

Anaplastic oligodendrogliomas differ from the more benign form by virtue of the typical signs of anaplasia (see above), with a predominance either of cellular pleomorphism (with increased cell density, mitoses, giant cells) or of anaplasia of the tumor tissue (with necrosis, vascular proliferation, irregular stroma), as in glioblastoma. The biologic behavior of the lesion does not depend on the type of anaplasia and corresponds to grade 3 of the WHO classification. A low-grade glioma can undergo very rapid malignant transformation.

MR findings: see p. 239–240.

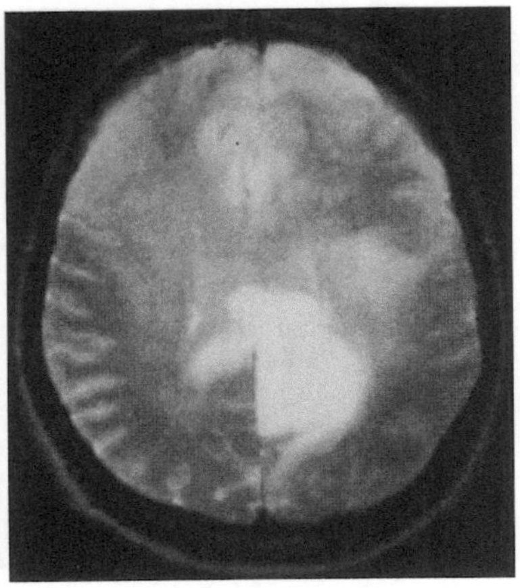

Fig. 10.14. Anaplastic mixed glioma (WHO grade 3) in a 35-year-old man with progressive headache. Diffuse glioma of both hemispheres, probably low grade except for the right parietal hyperintense area, where a grade 3 glioma was found by stereotaxic biopsy. Axial scan SE 3.0 s/120 ms (1.0 T)

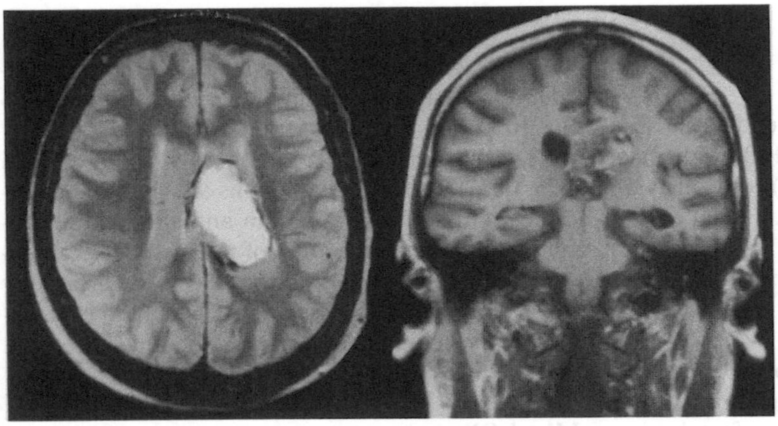

a b

Fig. 10.15 a, b. Ependymoma (WHO grade 1, stereotaxic biopsy) in a 29-year-old woman with cerebral seizures since childhood after sudden loss of consciousness and subsequent weakness of right side. **a** Initial MR showed hemorrhage in the corpus callosum suggesting vascular malformation. **b** Ten weeks later, after resorption of major portions of the hematoma, a tumor was suspected. Axial scans (**a**), coronal scan (**b**) SE 4.0 s/17 ms (1.0 T)

10.2.3 Poorly Differentiated and Embryonal Tumors

See p. 279 and Sect. 11.1

10.2.4 Ependymal and Choroid Plexus Tumors

Ependymomas and plexus papillomas are derived from the ependyma. Ependymomas are recognized as having myxopapillary, papillary, subependymal (all WHO grade 1), and anaplastic (grades 2 and 3) forms. Plexus papillomas are described below.

Ependymomas

Incidence: Ependymomas account for 4%-9% of intracranial tumors [66] and 60% of spinal gliomas [29]. Males are predominantly affected. Cerebral ependymomas are the most common hemispheric tumors in children and adolescents. They are usually anaplastic (WHO grade 3-4). The other forms tend to occur between the 2nd and 4th decades [66].

Sites: The tumors are found in the vicinity of the ependyma of the ventricular system, in the spinal canal, and in extraventricular portions of the hemispheres. In the latter case they lie against the lateral ventricle at the trigone. The tumors exhibit a surface resembling that of a cauliflower, and they can grow very large. Less frequent sites of occurrence are the lateral ventricle, the third ventricle, the quadrigeminal region, and the cerebellopontine angle (see also Sect. 11.1.2, p. 280.) (Figs. 10.15, 10.16).

Pathology: Because the normal ependyma and remnants of ependymal cells within the parenchyma serve as the matrix for these tumors, we can understand why the tumors have both intraventricular

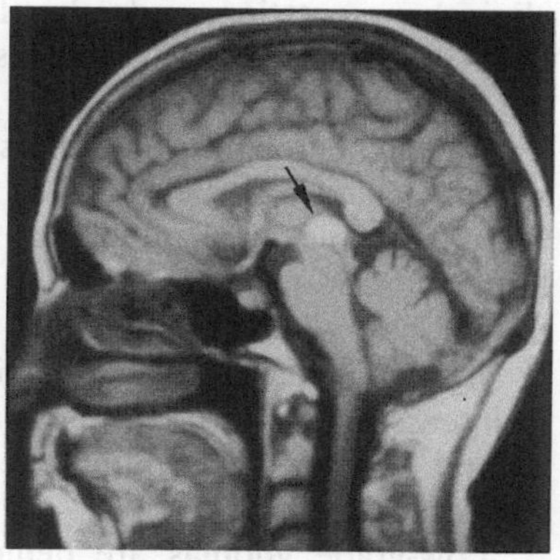

Fig. 10.16. Ependymoma (WHO grade 1) in a 52-year-old woman with episodes of headache and incipient occlusive hydrocephalus. The well delineated, homogeneous tumor of the pineal region *(arrow)* contained densely packed cells arranged in rosettes. The signal is isointense or slightly hyperintense to white matter. Midsagittal scan, SE 0.5 s/30 ms (1.0 T)

and extraventricular sites of occurrence. Benign ependymomas grow purely by expansion and adapt in shape and size to their surroundings. Their histopathology varies with their localization [66]. The densely packed cells of the tumors are isomorphic and poor in cytoplasm. Cystic changes are very common, necrotic and fatty degeneration less so. Small, round, scattered calcifications are found especially in the cerebral ependymomas [66]. The tumors appear slightly hyperdense on noncontrast CT scans, and moderate enhancement is seen after the administration of contrast medium.

Myxopapillary ependymomas occur in the region of the cauda equina (see Sect. 17.2). *Papillary ependymomas* and *subependymal forms* are very rare histologic subtypes that do not require further discussion here (see Fig. 11.10).

Anaplastic Ependymomas

Like all other types of glioma, *anaplastic ependymomas* show the classic signs of anaplasia (see above), with a disordered structure and irregular stroma. Transformation to glioblastoma has been postulated. The prognosis of the tumors is less favorable in children than in adults. Spontaneous metastases are rare but are more common after surgery [66] (see also Sects. 11.1.2 and 17.2).

MR findings: see below.

Plexus Papillomas

Incidence: Neoplasms derived from the epithelium of the choroid plexus account for 0.6% of all intracranial tumors and 3.9% of tumors in children under 12 years of age [66]. They are slightly more common in females. Their benign behavior classifies them as WHO grade 1.

Sites: The tumors occur mostly in the trigone of the lateral ventricles, in the third and fourth ventricles, and in the cerebellopontine angle (see Fig. 14.25).

Pathology: Plexus papillomas are well demarcated, but tufts of tumor may project into the surrounding brain tissue. The growth expands the ventricle locally and in children may be associated with an overproduction of CSF.

The tumor has a papillary structure. The connective tissue stroma shows edematous, mucoid, and hyaline changes and occasionally contains calcified foci. Other regressive changes do not occur [66].

Anaplastic Plexus Papillomas

Anaplastic papillomas of the choroid plexus are rare subtypes in which the typical histologic structure of the papillomas is lost, although individual papillae and psammomatous bodies may be retained. These tumors are classified as WHO grade 3–4 [66].

Differentiation must be made from metastatic carcinoma in the choroid plexus.

MR Features of the Neuroepithelial Tumors Described in Sects. 10.2.1–10.2.4; see also Sect. 10.1

The MR features of the various gliogenic tumors may be discussed under one heading because of their close similarities. Thus, differential diagnostic criteria are derived less from absolute signal patterns than from peculiarities of location, structure, clinical presentation, and other features that have been described generally and also specifically for the individual tumor types.

Benign neuroepithelial tumors that consist of essentially mature tissues, such as hamartomas (see Sect. 10.8), plexus papillomas, and pinealomas, have relaxation times similar or equal to those of normal brain. Plexus papillomas, which display only slightly increased relaxation times, may appear isointense in newborns owing to the normally long T1 and T2 values of the immature white matter [37]; see Sect. 6.2).

Low-grade gliomas are demonstrable on MR and CT images only when the increase in the volume of intracellular and extracellular water that accompanies tumor growth (e.g., formation of minute vacuoles) is sufficient to prolong T1 and T2 significantly. In vitro studies of intracranial tumor specimens have shown that an increase in cell density and the formation of microcysts contribute to the prolongation of T1 and T2 [12], resulting in a high signal on the sensitive T2-weighted sequences and a low signal on T1-weighted images. In this early stage the tumors are not easily distinguished from edema. Often they are well demarcated, and their mass effect is small compared with their extent. Because edema rarely crosses the corpus callosum to the opposite side, and then only as a late event, involvement of the corpus callosum by low-grade gliomas is suggestive of infiltration. Intravenous contrast material (e.g., gadolinium chelate) does not significantly shorten T1, because the blood-brain barrier is intact. Areas of microcystic change produce a slight heterogeneity of signal within the tumor boundaries.

With further dedifferentiation of the lesion, possibly to glioblastoma, the density of the cells, now pleomorphic, increases, and the vascularity becomes more abnormal, leading to compromise of the blood-brain barrier. The result is a supervening vasogenic edema which forms a uniform halo in the white matter surrounding the more heterogeneous, lower-intensity structures of the tumor itself. The tumor tissue may display a nodular, ringlike, or patchy structure as a result of regressive changes. Often it is possible to differentiate tumor and edema and identify regressive changes by using T2-weighted or multiecho sequences. Intravenous contrast material leads to a marked shortening of T1 in the undifferentiated vital portions of the tumor. Less malignant, diffusely growing parts of the tumor show no contrast enhancement and are not easily distinguished from edema.

With few exceptions, these considerations apply to all neuroepithelial brain tumors. Some brain regions (tuber cinereum, choroid plexus, pineal body, pituitary, area postrema, and median eminence) contain fenestrated vessels that lack a blood-brain barrier [23]. As a result, benign tumors in these areas, such as pilocytic astrocytomas, craniopharyngiomas, and plexus papillomas, show contrast enhancement, which must not be interpreted as evidence of anaplasia (Stochdorph 1981, personal communication). Radionecrotic areas also may contain fenestrated vessels, a circumstance which may cause them to be mistaken for sites of tumor recurrence.

Axial MR scans using proton-density and T2-weighted sequences (e.g., SE long TR, short and long TE) generally are adequate for the visualization of neuroepithelial tumors. If an exact description of the site of the tumor or its precursory edema is required for preoperative planning, additional views may be taken in the sagittal and coronal projections using T1-weighted parameters. If needle biopsy is proposed, it is necessary to identify the tumor areas with the highest degree of anaplasia, as they will determine the diagnosis, prognosis, and therapeutic approach. The use of contrast material is essential in identifying these tumor regions.

10.2.5 Pineal Cell Tumors

The classification of pineal cell tumors is still a subject of research. The description that follows is based on the classification of Zülch [66]. Data on the incidence of these tumors are highly questionable due to inconsistencies of nomenclature.

Pineocytomas

The definition of pineocytomas is still open to question. The lesions contain abundant isomorphic cells in a roughly papillary arrangement and have a sparse stroma. Assessments of their biologic behavior vary widely (WHO grades 1-3) (Fig. 10.17).

Pineoblastomas

Pineoblastomas are rare, highly cellular tumors of variable size that arise in the quadrigeminal region and infiltrate the surrounding tissue. They are very similar histologically to medulloblastomas (see

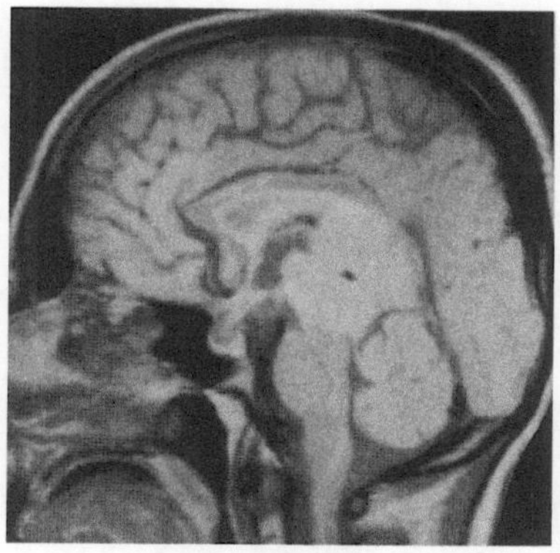

Fig. 10.17. Anisomorphic pineocytoma in a 23-year-old man with nausea, vomiting, loss of weight, and papilledema. Homogeneous tumor of slightly increased signal intensity compared to gray matter. Diagnosis confirmed by stereotaxic biopsy. Midsagittal section, SE 1.6 s/35 ms, (0.35 T)

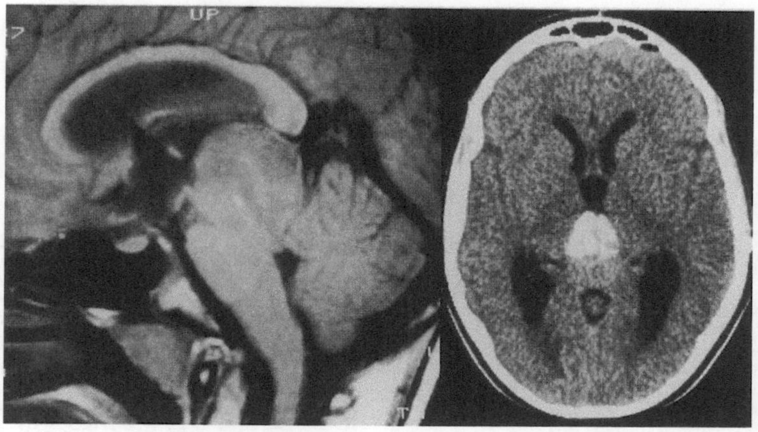

Fig. 10.18 a, b. Pineoblastoma in a 13-year-old girl with headache, nausea, and unsteady gait. The calcifications seen on CT (**b**) appear as irregular hypointensities on MR. Poor delineation of border between tumor and brainstem. Midsagittal scan (**a**) SE 0.6 s/15 ms (1.5 T); CT (**b**) without, contrast enhancement.

Sect. 11.2), and like the latter are classified as WHO grade 4. They may contain calcifications of various degree and extent (Fig. 10.18).

Pinealomas, Germinomas

Pinealomas

Incidence: Pinealomas, a common type of pineal neoplasm, predominantly affect males between 10 and 30 years of age. Assessments of their behavior vary from WHO grade 1 to grade 3.

Sites: Pinealomas lie in the quadrigeminal region and grow mainly by expansion, except for infiltration in the marginal zone. Suprasellar occurrence is possible as a result of seeding (suprasellar ectopic pinealoma/germinoma) and may lead to infiltration of the optic chiasm.

Pathology: Pinealomas are relatively firm tumors. Histologic examination shows a mixture of large clear cells and small lymphoid cells that form nests. The tumors have a relatively homogeneous structure and often show calcification. Small areas of necrosis may be seen. Metastases to other body regions have been described [66].

Germinomas

Incidence: Germinomas are common tumors of the pineal region, but also grow elsewhere. They show a much lower incidence in Western populations (0.5%-0.7%) than in Asiatics (4%-4.5%) [66]. They closely resemble pinealomas but can be distinguished from them histologically. They are classified as WHO grade 2 and 3.

Sites: The tumors usually occur in the pineal and suprasellar regions, although other sites are possible (Figs. 10.19-10.20).

Pathology: Germinomas grow mainly by expansion, but they also infiltrate their surroundings. They

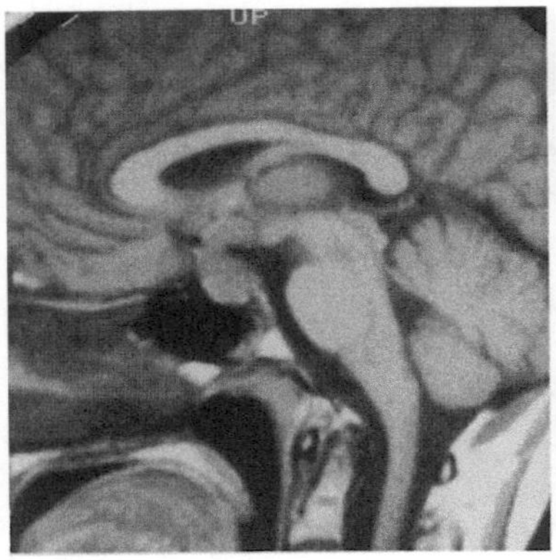

10.19

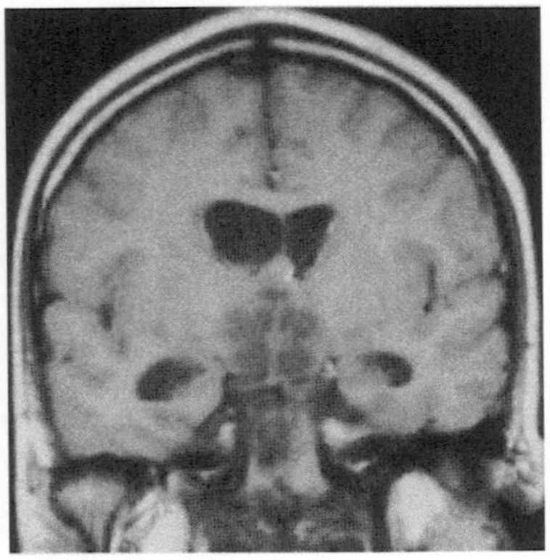

10.20

Fig. 10.19. Germinoma in a 15-year-old girl with pituitary insufficiency. Homogeneous thickening of pituitary and stalk. Sagittal scan, SE 0.4 s/17 ms; (1.0 T)

Fig. 10.20. Germinoma of the hypothalamus in a 21-year-old man with pituitary insufficiency, electrolyte disturbances, and impaired vision. Ill-defined, septated, multicystic tumor with prolonged relaxation times. Coronal scan SE 0.5 s/30 ms; (1.0 T)

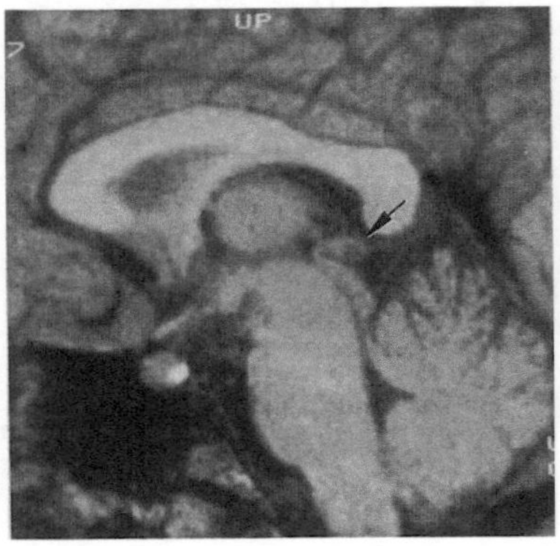

10.21

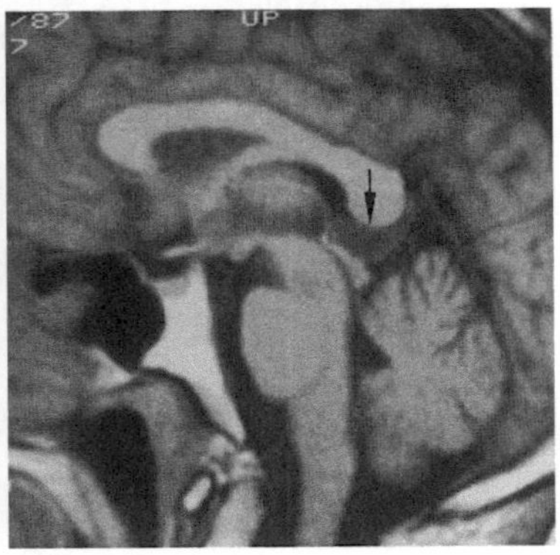

10.22

Fig. 10.21. Normal pineal gland in a 21-year-old woman. The hypointensity in the center *(arrow)* is probably caused by calcifications. Midsagittal scan, FLASH 40° 0.3 s/12 ms 3D acquisition (1.5 T)

Fig. 10.22. Pineal cyst *(arrow):* incidental finding in a 23-year-old man. The cyst has long relaxation times similar to CSF. Midsagittal scan, SE 0.4 s/17 ms, (1.0 T)

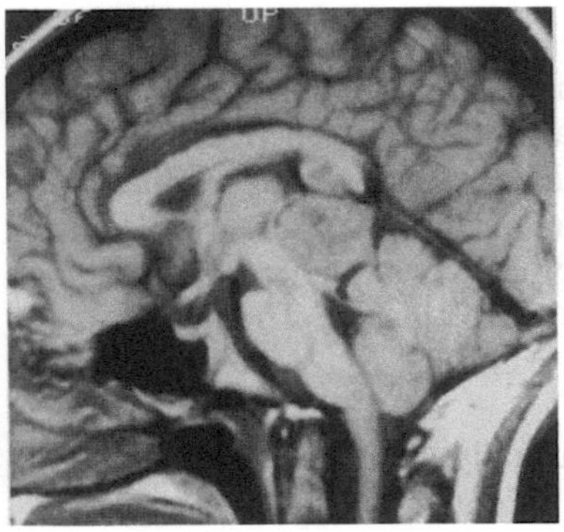

Fig. 10.23. Neuroepithelial mixed tumor (WHO grade 1-3) in a 15-year-old boy with known von Recklinghausen's disease and long-standing cerebral seizures, now presenting with headache, occasional vomiting, and lack of drive. Isointense tumor with patchy areas of decreased signal intensity, well demarcated along most of its periphery but invading the corpus callosum and thalamus. Pathology revealed a mixed neuroepithelial tumor consisting predominantly of pilocytic astrocytoma but with areas of giant cell astrocytoma and gangliocytoma. Signs of anaplasia (grade 3) were present in the portion of the tumor invading the corpus callosum. Sagittal scan, SE 0.7 s/30 ms (1.0 T)

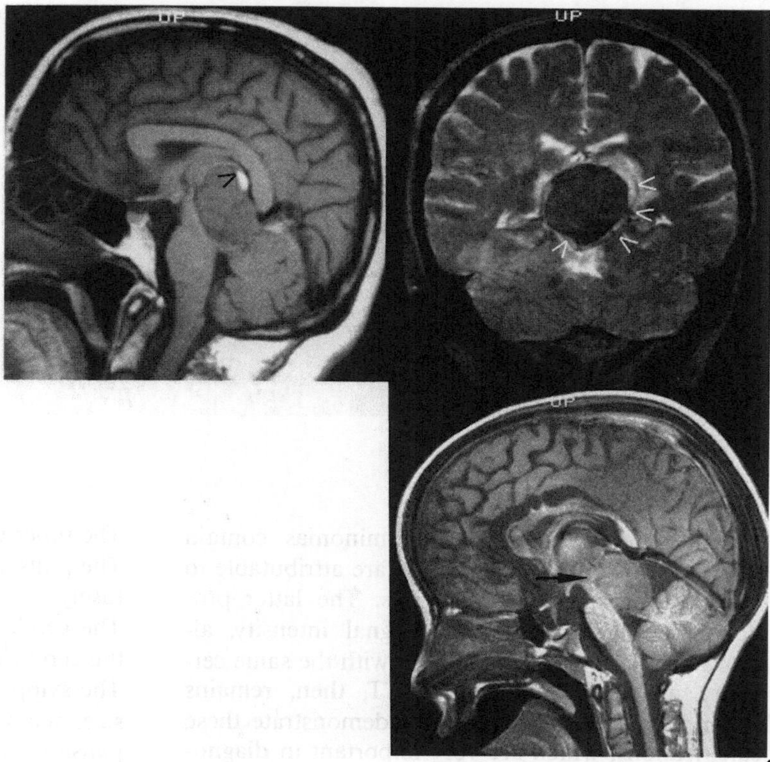

a b c

Fig. 10.24. a, b Metastasis of the pineal region in a 37-year-old woman with blurred and double vision, papilledema, and a history of carcinoma of the breast. Round tumor, for the most part well delineated, with small peripheral hemorrhages *(arrowheads)*. The tumor appears isointense to gray matter in T1-weighted and proton-density images, and hypointense with a T2-weighted sequence. Slight perifocal edema. Midsagittal scan (**a**), SE 0.6 s/15 ms; coronal scan (**b**) SE 3.0 s/120 ms. **c** Astrocytoma (biopsy: WHO grade II) of the quadrigeminal plate *(arrow)* in a 7-year-old girl with occlusive hydrocephalus and double vision. **c** Sagittal scan, SE 0.5 s/15 ms; (1.5 T)

usually show calcifications. Histologically they consist of large tumor cells in addition to polynuclear giant cells and small lymphoid cells. They can seed through the cerebrospinal pathway and can also metastasize to other body regions.

Embryonal Carcinomas

The very rare embryonal carcinomas probably arise from parenchymal cells of the pineal body. Their peak occurrence is at 15 years of age, and they show a marked predilection for males [66]. Because of their malignant, invasive growth, the prognosis is very grave.

MR Findings in Pineal Cell Tumors

Sagittal and coronal scans are excellent for the evaluation of these midline neoplasms. They clearly demonstrate the origin, size, and location of these usually well-demarcated tumors, although most pineal tumors show little contrast with the surrounding brain.

Calcifications of the pineal body (Fig. 10.21) are very rare in children under 6½ years of age and are seen in fewer than 11% of children between the ages of 11 and 14. Consequently, the finding of pineal calcifications in children should always arouse suspicion of a pineal neoplasm [62].

MR quite often reveals small pineal cysts [38]. These are thin-walled with smooth borderlines and slightly hyperintense fluid contents compared to CSF. The latter feature may be due to a higher amount of protein or, more likely, to a lack of flow effects, lowering the signal, in the CSF of the adjacent ventricle. These cysts seem to be of no clinical relevance when there is no mass effect and when another etiology (e.g., tumor cyst, parasitic cyst) can be ruled out. The etiology of these cysts is still not completely understood (Fig. 10.22).

Noncontrast CT scans usually display pineal tumors as isodense or slightly hyperdense areas that show marked enhancement following contrast infusion. The margins of the tumors are more or less well-defined.

On MR scans, benign pinealomas and germinomas are often well demarcated, and their relaxation times are equal to or only slightly longer than those

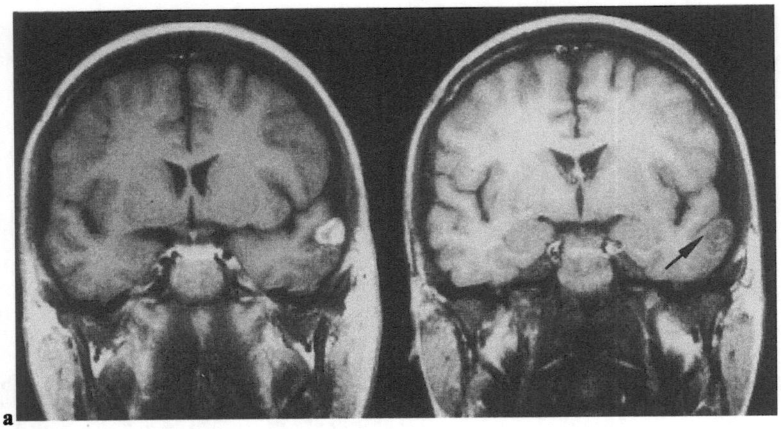
a b

Fig. 10.25 a, b. Ganglioglioma (WHO grade 1) in a 25-year-old man with focal seizures. **a** Contrast enhancement reveals a well-delineated, nodular lesion. **b** Circumscribed hypointense thickening of the middle temporal gyrus *(arrow)*. T1-weighted images: **a, b** coronal scans (**a** with, **b** without gadolinium-DTPA); (1.0 T)

of surrounding brain [26]. Germinomas contain scattered low-intensity areas that are attributable to cystic changes and calcifications. The latter produce irregular areas of low signal intensity, although they cannot be identified with the same certainty as on CT scans [30]. CT, then, remains superior to MR in its ability to demonstrate these calcifications, which are very important in diagnosis.

Malignant growth forms (pineoblastomas, embryonal carcinomas) have prolonged T1 and T2 relaxation times, and their infiltrative growth incites a perifocal edema.

By analogy with CT, tumors of the pineal region would be expected to show an increase of signal intensity on T1-weighted sequences following the intravenous administration of contrast material.

With regard to differential diagnosis, the tumors that most closely resemble pineal neoplasms are meningiomas of the quadrigeminal region (see Fig. 10.31). The neuroepithelial mixed tumor shown in Fig. 10.23, the metastasis and astrocytoma (grade II) shown in Fig. 10.24 are also similar in appearance to pineal tumors.

10.2.6 Neuronal Tumors

Incidence: Neuronal tumors are rare, showing an incidence of only 0.4% in the series of Zülch [66].

Sites: The tumors occur in the following locations:

- The cerebral hemispheres, where they form large cysts and calcifications and show a marked tendency toward nodular growth into the leptomeninges
- The tuber cinereum and third ventricle
- The pons and medulla, where they permeate diffusely
- The cerebellum, where they cause expansion of the cerebellar folia
- The sympathetic trunk, where tumors of varying size, necrotic at their centers and growing by expansion, can arise.

Pathology: These tumors lead to enlargement of the infiltrated region and produce nodular surface changes. Their center may be cystic. In the growing head, they can produce a bulge in the calvarium much like arachnoid cysts.

Gangliocytomas

Gangliocytomas of the hemispheres contain mature nerve cells. Calcifications have been seen only in temporobasal lesions. The lesions have a tough consistency and are often cystic (WHO grade 1).

Gangliogliomas

Gangliogliomas contain additional glial elements. They are predominantly cystic with a small nub of tumor (WHO grades 1 and 2). The glial component may undergo anaplastic transformation to grade 3 (Figs. 10.25-10.26).

Ganglioneuroblastomas

Ganglioneuroblastomas consist of a mixture of neurons of varying degrees of maturity and undifferentiated neuroblasts (WHO grade 3 or 4) [66].

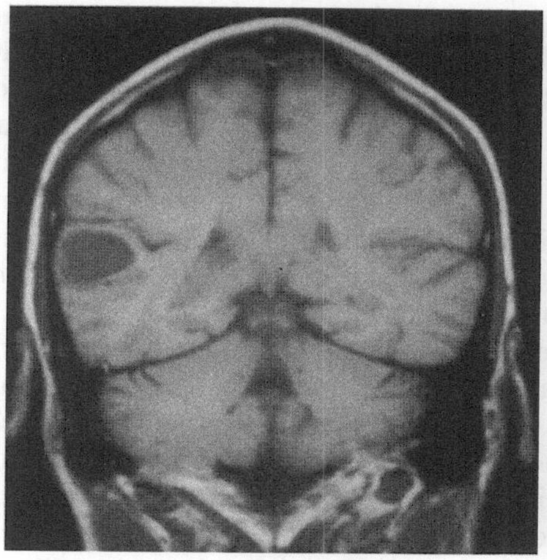

10.26

Fig. 10.26. Ganglioglioma (WHO grade 2–3) in a 33-year-old man with acoustic aura and short-term amnesia. Well-delineated tumor consisting of gangliocytic elements with anaplasia of glial components. Coronal scan SE 0.5 s/30 ms, (1.0 T)

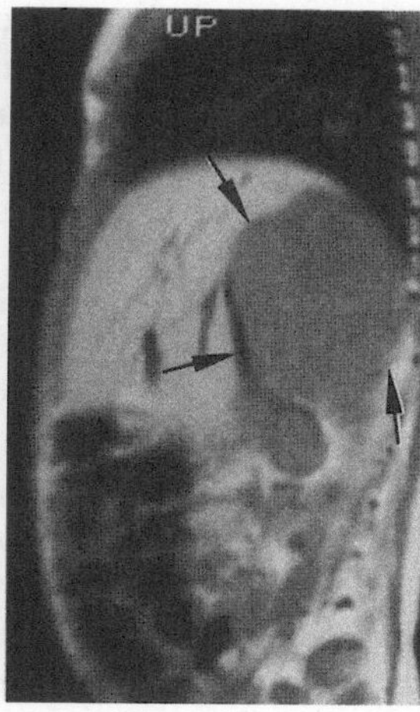

10.27

Fig. 10.27. Neuroblastoma in a 9-month-old girl with abdominal pain. Large, homogeneous paravertebral mass *(arrows)*. Sagittal scan, SE 0.4 s/17 ms (1.0 T)

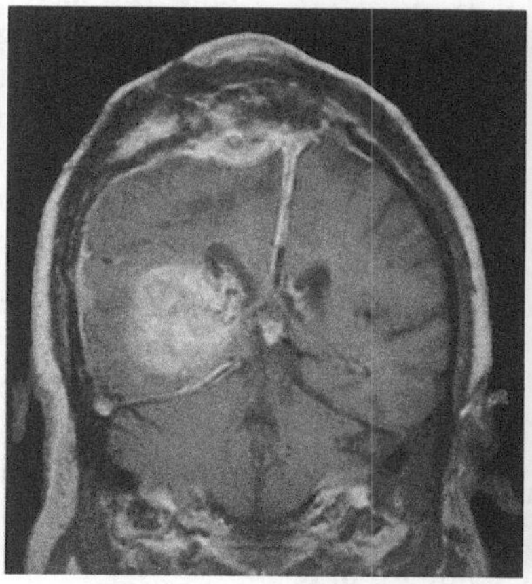

10.28

Fig. 10.28. Extensive meningiomatosis in a 52-year-old man, involving large areas of the dura, the skull with extracranial growth, and the lateral ventricle. Coronal scan after i.v. gadolinium-DTPA, SE 0.8 s/30 ms (1.5 T)

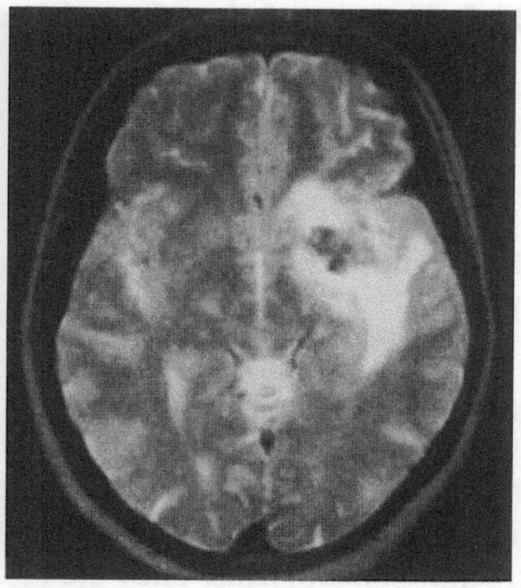

10.29

Fig. 10.29. Intraparenchymal meningioma in a 26-year-old woman with partial seizures. An unspecific, irregular, inhomogeneous, mainly hypointense mass in the left temporal lobe with perifocal edema is seen on MR. The diagnosis of meningioma is more reliable on CT, which revealed a well-delineated, nodular tumor with marked contrast enhancement and small calcifications. Axial scan, SE 2.5 s/112 ms (1.0 T)

Anaplastic (Malignant) Gangliocytoma/Ganglioglioma

See “Gangliogliomas” above.

Neuroblastomas

Grouped together with the neuroblastomas are retinoblastomas and sympathoblastomas.

Incidence: The tumors are mainly found in the first 3 years of life, rarely in older children. Data on prevalence vary widely.

Pathology: These are highly cellular tumors with a largely homogeneous structure that grow rapidly and form metastases (WHO grade 4) (Fig. 10.27). They may show spontaneous regression or may mature to differentiated neuronal tumors.

MR Findings in Neuronal Tumors

Larger, solid neuronal tumors have relaxation times equal to or slightly greater than those of brain tissue. Cystic areas display a marked increase in T1 and T2 due to their homogeneous, fluid contents. With smaller tumors, attention must be given to the initially subtle expansion of the involved region (e.g., the widening of a gyrus). Regressive changes make the tumor structure heterogeneous. Perifocal edema is seen with malignant, infiltrative growths.

Primitive Neuroectodermal Tumors

Primitive neuroectodermal tumors, described by Becker et al. [7], have microscopic features similar to medulloblastoma and pineoblastoma. They present irregular and in some cases ill-defined margins, frequently surrounded by a thin halo of edema. The tumors display cystic changes and calcifications and can grow very large. Except in isolated cases [2], the prognosis is poor.

CT and MR Findings. Primitive neuroectodermal tumors resemble neuroblastomas on CT scans, appearing isodense to slightly hyperdense, nonhomogeneous, and showing marked enhancement after the administration of contrast material. To date, MR findings for these lesions have not been reported. Presumably the appearance would be that of a malignant tumor with regressive changes, including calcification, and would be nonspecific.

10.3 Tumors of the Nerve Sheath Cells

See Chap. 11.

10.4 Tumors of Meningeal and Related Tissues

10.4.1 Meningiomas

Incidence: Meningiomas, mesodermal tumors of meningeal origin, comprise about 16%-20% of intracranial neoplasms. They are more common in females and occur chiefly in the middle and later decades of life, but represent also 1%-2% of primary intracranial tumors in children.

Sites: Meningiomas can occur anywhere in the craniospinal space, but they show definite sites of predilection. In order of frequency, these are [66]: the sagittal sinus and falx, the convexity, the olfactory groove, the tuberculum sellae, the sphenoid wing, the middle fossa and Meckel's cave, the cerebellopontine angle, the tentorium, the lateral ventricles, and the craniocervical junction.

Pathology: Meningiomas, which are multiple in about 1%-2% of cases [66], generally appear as smooth, globular tumors that grow purely by expansion. A few send fingerlike projections into the surrounding brain and present a rough or finely nodular surface that is more solidly fused to the brain tissue. Especially in the middle fossa, meningiomas can grow en plaque or form a sheet of growth spreading out from a nodular mass, as on the medial sphenoid wing or at the attachment of the tentorium to the petrous pyramid. Meningiomas at some sites can invade the dural sinuses (e.g., the sagittal sinus, confluence of sinuses, cavernous sinuses). The tumors are also prone to invade the adjacent bone and can greatly expand it (Fig. 10.28). Sometimes in these cases only a thin layer of tumor tissue is visible on the surface. The attachments of nodular tumors commonly show a hyperostosis from which fibrous tissue extends radially into the tumor (Fig. 10.33). Primary intraparenchymal growth has also been reported. The stromal cell of the pia-arachnoid that invests the perforating blood vessels as they enter the surface of the brain has been postulated as the cell of origin of these tumors, which do not have a dural site of attachment [52]. The histologic type (see below) of intraparenchymal meningiomas does not appear to be uniform. However, a higher incidence of the sarcomatous [51] or the angioblastic [49] type has been discussed (Fig. 10.29).

The following subtypes of meningioma are recognized on the basis of tissue architecture [66]:

1. Meningotheliomatous (endotheliomatous) meningiomas (WHO grade 1) (Figs. 10.32-10.35)
2. Fibrous (fibroblastic) meningiomas (grade 1) (Fig. 10.31)
3. Transitional (mixed) meningiomas (grade 1) (Fig. 10.36)
4. Psammomatous meningiomas (grade 1) (Fig. 10.38)
5. a) Angiomatous meningiomas (grade 1) (Fig. 10.39)
   b) Hemangioblastic meningiomas (grade 1)
   c) Hemangiopericytic meningiomas (grades 2 and 3)
6. Papillary meningiomas (grade 2 or 3)
7. Anaplastic (malignant) meningiomas (grades 2-4)

The highly cellular *meningotheliomatous* meningiomas (Figs. 10.32-10.35) and the fiber-rich *fibrous* meningiomas (Fig. 10.31) show a largely homogeneous structure. They tend to form concentric calcifications called psammomatous bodies. These calcifications are predominant in *psammomatous* meningiomas (Fig. 10.38). *Endotheliomatous* meningiomas tend to undergo mucoid-hydropic degeneration with the formation of large or small cysts. Fatty degeneration is less common.

Angiomatous meningiomas contain a network of many capillaries and veins interspersed with large

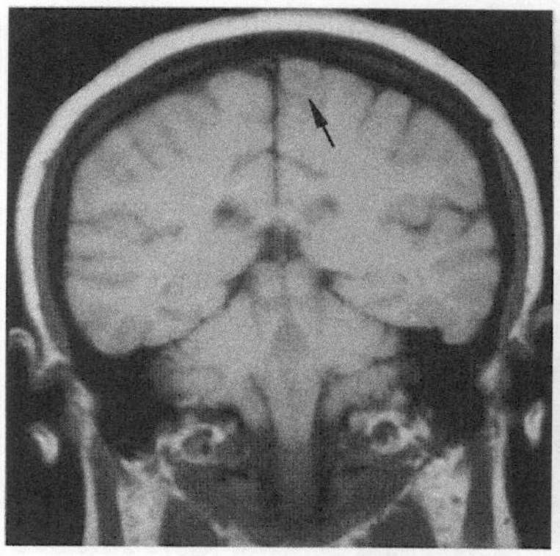

10.30

Fig. 10.30. Meningioma in a 40-year-old woman with syncopes. Small parietal meningioma *(arrow)* with slightly prolonged relaxation times. Coronal scan, SE 0.7 s/30 ms, (1.0 T)

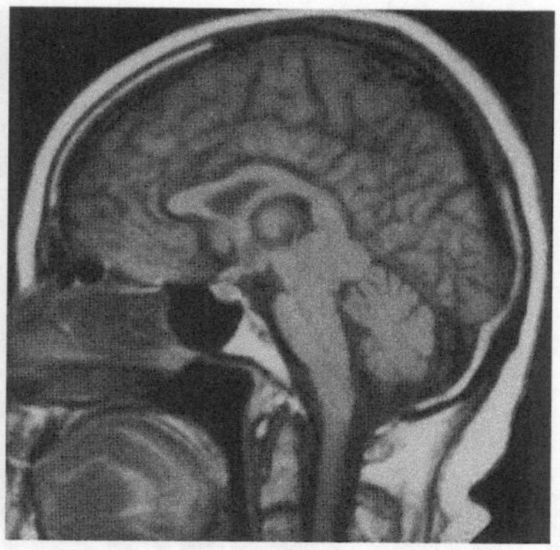

10.31

Fig. 10.31. Fibrous meningioma of the quadrigeminal region in a 57-year-old woman with progressive gait disturbances. Nodular, homogeneous, fairly well delineated tumor with slightly prolonged relaxation times. Midsagittal scan, SE 0.7 s/30 ms (1.0 T)

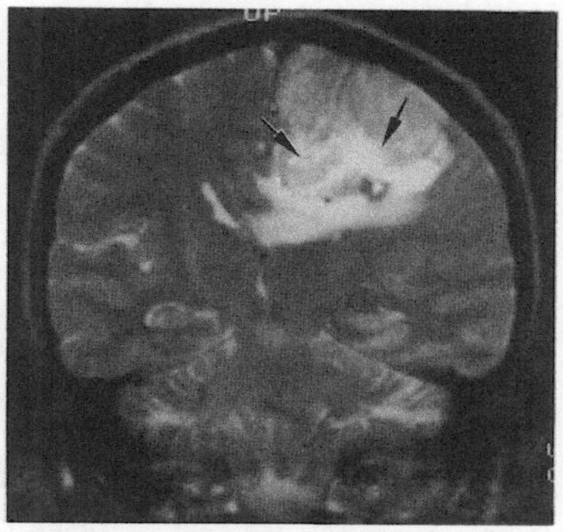

Fig. 10.32. Meningotheliomatous meningioma, partly necrotic, in a 52-year-old woman with focal seizures and slight hemiparesis. Large, well-defined parietal tumor with typical brushlike vasculature and incomplete dark border of displaced vessels. The irregular hyperintense areas within the tumor *(arrows)* represent necrosis. Moderate perifocal edema. Coronal scan, SE 2.5 s/120 ms (1.0 T)

cells or nests of cells (Fig. 10.39). *Hemangioblastic* meningiomas are rare. Because of their greater propensity for recurrence and metastasis, hemangiopericytic meningiomas are classified as WHO grade 2 or 3. The same is true of the *papillary* form, which also is rare.

Large meningiomas may be found without perifocal edema, while small tumors may be associated with pronounced *edema.* No reliable correlation is evident among the size, location, type, and malignancy of the tumor. According to Stochdorph (1981, personal communication), edema develops when the tumor has displaced the cortex and come in contact with the white matter.

10.4.2 Meningeal Sarcomas

The group of meningeal sarcomas includes *fibrosarcoma, polymorphic cell sarcoma,* and *primary meningeal sarcomatosis,* all assigned to WHO grade 3 or 4 [66]. These tumors, which grossly resemble meningiomas and metastases or spread diffusely in the subarachnoid space, show the invasive behavior of a malignancy with early edema formation.

10.4.3 Primary Melanotic Tumors

The category of primary melanotic tumors includes circumscribed primary melanomas of the CNS as well as the diffuse form, melanomatosis. The tumors arise from the chromatophores of the leptomeninges.

Incidence: Primary melanomas are rare; prevalence data are not available.

Sites: The lesions can occur anywhere in the CNS, showing no predilection for specific sites.

Pathology: The tumors show a uniform structure. They invade the brain tissue along blood vessels and are considered highly malignant (Fig. 10.42).

MR Findings in Meningiomas and Related Tumors

Most meningiomas show little or no signal contrast with brain tissue (Fig. 10.30). On T1-weighted se-

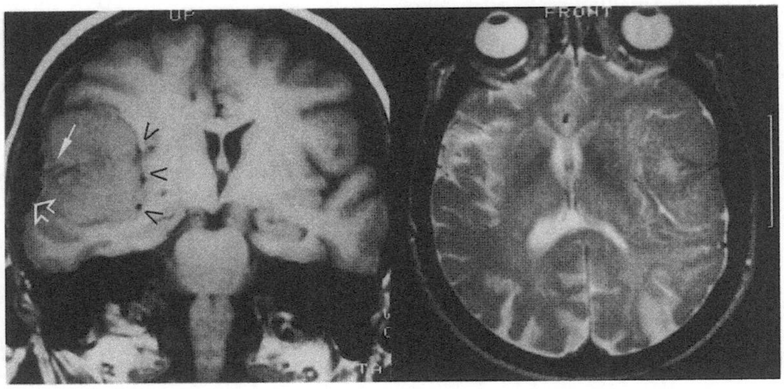

a b

Fig. 10.33 a, b. Meningotheliomatous meningioma (WHO grade 1) in a 63-year-old woman with a focal seizure and latent hemiparesis. A vascular hilus *(arrow)* and, at the border of the tumor, branches of the middle cerebral artery *(arrowheads)* are seen. In **b** a thin layer of CSF seems to surround the tumor. No perifocal edema. Thickening of the adjacent bone *(open arrow)*. Coronal scan (**a**), SE 0.6 s/15 ms; axial scan (**b**), SE 2.5 s/90 ms (1.0 T)

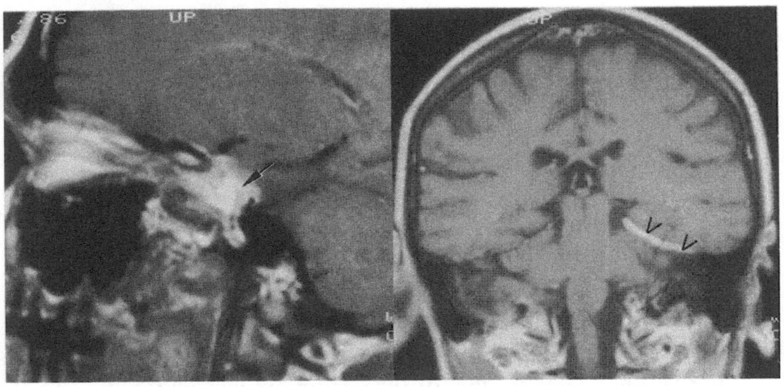

a b

Fig. 10.34 a, b. Parasellar meningotheliomatous meningioma after intravenous injection of contrast medium (gadolinium-DTPA) in a 42-year-old woman with lateral deviation of the right eye and progressive visual loss. Tumor growth in the cavernous sinus and the carotid canal with compression of the carotid artery *(arrow)*, and en plaque growth along the tentorium *(arrowheads)*. **a** Parasagittal, **b** coronal scan through the tentorium (SE 0.7 s/30, 17 ms; 1.0 T)

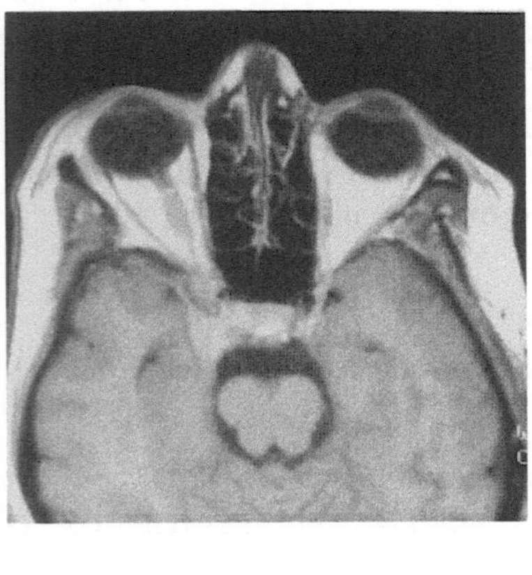

Fig. 10.35. Meningotheliomatous meningioma in a 39-year-old woman with papilledema and visual impairment of the left eye. The tumor is growing within the cavernous sinus and invading the sella encasing the optic nerve. The thickening of the optic nerve is due to chronic venous congestion; tumor invasion of the intraorbital dural sheet was not seen at operation. Axial scan, SE 0.6 s/15 ms after i.v. gadolinium-DTPA, (1.5 T). In the plain scan the tumor appeared isointense to grey matter.

quences fibromatous meningiomas (Fig. 10.31) give a slightly lower signal than the cerebral cortex, while endotheliomatous meningiomas (Figs. 10.32 u. 10.33) may be isointense with the cortex. Spagnoli et al. [55] deny that a significant correlation exists between the pathologic classification of a meningioma and its MR appearance. With isointense tumors, attention must be given to indirect tumor signs (see p. 232), which may be quite subtle when the lesion is small (Fig. 10.30). On T2-weighted images, meningiomas are usually slightly hyperintense but occasionally isointense, in which case perifocal edema, if present, can be a helpful localizing sign. Zimmermann et al. [63] state that the incomplete, hypointense rim produced by a venous or arterial capsule is a common feature of meningiomas (Figs. 10.32, 10.33).

The structure of most meningiomas is homogeneous; less often the lesion is patchy and displays cystic components. The tumor margins are well-defined except in cases of infiltrative growth. In larger tumors a characteristic vascular hilus can occasionally be recognized (Figs. 10.32–10.33).

Intravenous contrast material (e.g., gadolinium chelate) leads to a marked signal increase in T1-weighted sequences. In dynamic studies the signal intensity initially rises sharply to about 180% compared with the signal on noncontrast scans before slowly falling again [31]. This causes the tumor and its flat extensions to stand out clearly on the image (Fig. 10.34). The latter are poorly demonstrated with noncontrast MR. Their detection is important, however, as they can form a nidus for recurrence if left behind at operation. The same is true of en plaque growths. With very small meningiomas located, say, on the wall of the cavernous sinus (Figs. 10.35, 10.36), good contrast is seen between the tumor and the hypointense dura in a later phase (e.g., 45 min after administration of contrast material) owing to the longer retention of enhancement by the neoplasm [8]. Contrast material should always be administered for the evaluation of multiple meningiomas, and the examination should be performed in several planes. The intraorbital portion of a meningioma of the sphenoid wing is visualized with less clarity after i.v. gadolinium-DTPA injection due to the reduced contrast between the orbital fat and the enhanced tumor tissue (Fig. 10.37). When marked regressive changes exist, meningiomas are indistinguishable from other tumor types following contrast injection, because even calcifications cannot be identified with certainty (Fig. 10.40).

Like CT, MR is unable to differentiate between benign and malignant growths [55].

Tumor ingrowth into the venous sinuses, and thus the patency of those channels, can be evaluated by analyzing flow effects on sagittal and coronal images. The usually fast-moving blood in the patent sinus will appear dark in the first echo (flow void) and will produce a signal in the second echo (even-echo rephasing). Phase mapping and cine studies are also useful in these cases. Thrombosis and tumor tissue give a signal in both echoes, because their spins are stationary. The tumor, finally, shows a signal increase on T1-weighted images after the administration of gadolinium-DTPA.

Differentiation is required from pituitary adenoma, neurinoma, plexus papilloma, plasmocytoma (Fig. 10.40), metastases (Fig. 10.41), and neuroepithelial tumors with nodular growth. Difficulties can arise with adenoma or neurinoma. The finding of a normal-size sella, a pituitary stalk dorsal to the tumor, and enostosis of the tuberculum sellae is consistent with the diagnosis of meningioma. In the cerebellopontine angle, meningiomas generally do not show involvement or expansion of the porus acusticus internus, although exceptions do occur (see Fig. 11.24) [41]. Coronal scans often demonstrate a close relation to the tentorium. Neurinomas show greater contrast enhancement than meningiomas and appear markedly brighter. Differentiation from metastases and neuroepithelial tumors can be difficult for meningiomas that show pronounced regressive changes. In these cases the above-mentioned vascular rim sign, a CSF cleft (Fig. 10.33 b), and an intervening dural margin can provide evidence of an extra-axial tumor [55].

Primary melanotic tumors may closely resemble meningiomas (Fig. 10.42)

10.5 Primary Malignant Lymphomas

The group of primary malignancies of the lymphoreticular system encompasses the following tumors [66]:

- Reticulum cell sarcoma
- Adventitial cell sarcoma
- Hodgkin's disease (Fig. 10.45)
- Plasmocytoma (see Fig. 10.40)
- Histiocytosis (hypothalamic granuloma)

These lesions may also represent secondary growth (metastasis or invasion). The following description is limited to the more common forms.

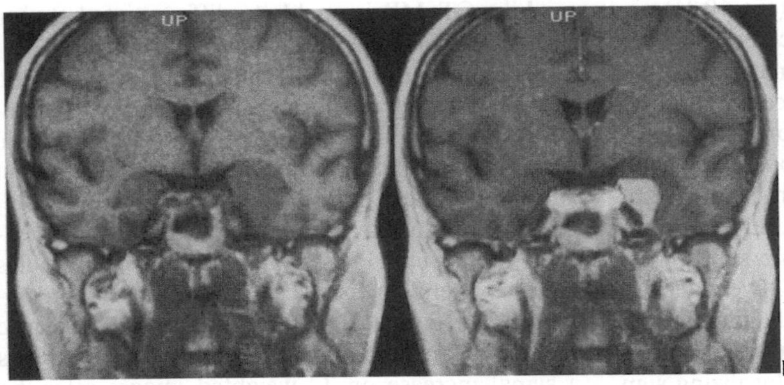

Fig. 10.36 a, b. Transitional parasellar meningioma in a 50-year-old woman with a complex partial seizure. Nodular, homogeneous tumor, isointense to gray matter, attached to the wall of the cavernous sinus. Coronal scans, SE 0.7 s/30 ms (1.0 T); **a** without, **b** with gadolinium-DTPA

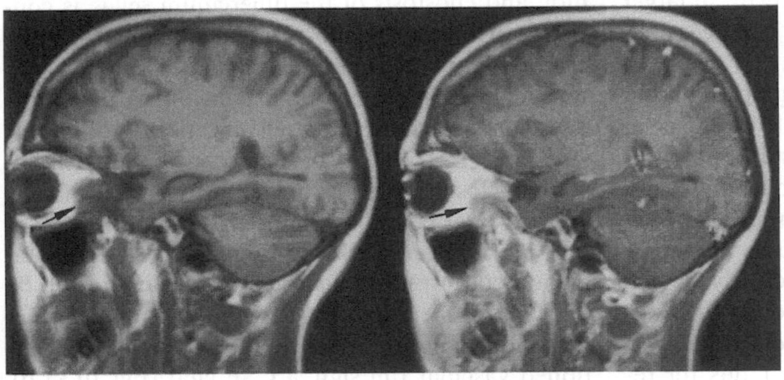

Fig. 10.37 a, b. Meningioma of the sphenoid wing in a 41-year old woman with exophthalmos and double vision. Intraorbital tumor growth *(arrow)*. **a** without, **b** with contrast enhancement (gadolinium-DTPA). Gadolinium-DTPA reduces contrast between tumor and fat-containing tissue. Parasagittal scan, SE 0.4 s/17 ms (1.0 T)

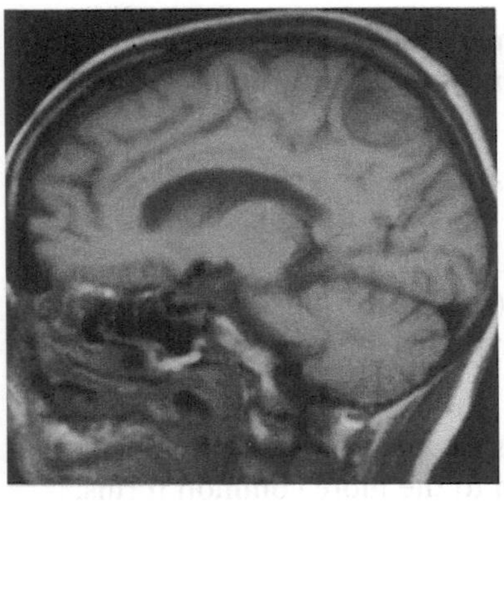

Fig. 10.38. Psammomatous meningioma in a 69-year-old woman with one focal seizure. Sagittal scan, SE 0.7 s/30 ms (1.0 T)

Fig. 10.39. Angiomatous meningioma in a 42-year-old woman with focal seizures and hemiparesis. The tumor consists of multiple cysts and solid tissue with extensive deposition of hemosiderin. Large perifocal edema. Axial scan, SE 1.5 s/100 ms (1.0 T)

Fig. 10.40. Well-differentiated plasmacytoma in a 60-year-old woman with hypoesthesia of the left side of the face and the left forearm, and pain projecting into the right orbit. Large, well-delineated tumor with hyperostosis and hypointense borderline very similar to a meningioma. Coronal scan, SE 2.5 s/120 ms (1.0 T)

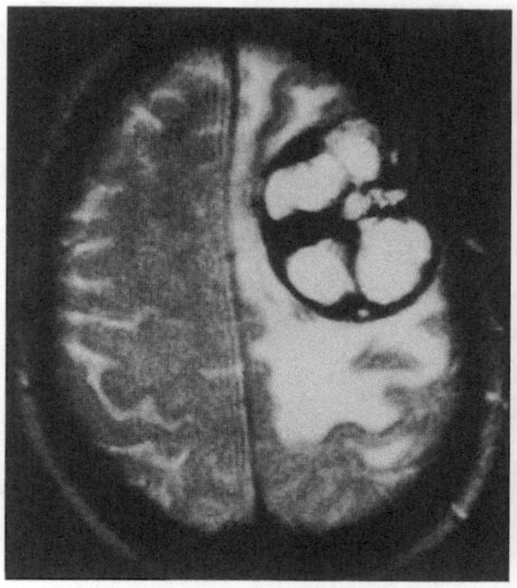

10.39

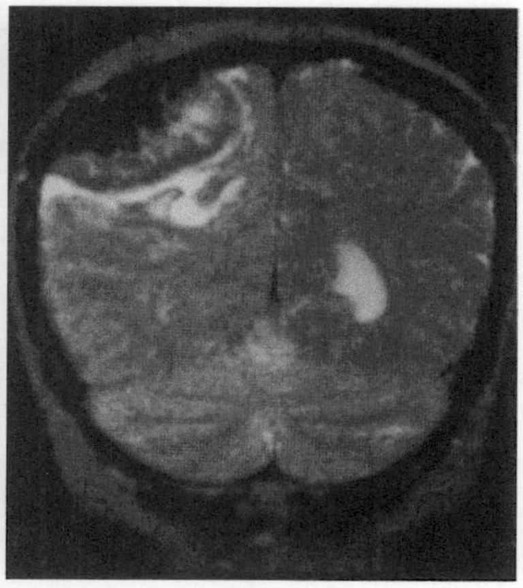

10.40

Fig. 10.41. Cylindroma of the lacrimal gland simulating meningioma in a 44-year-old female presenting with double vision after surgery. Coronal scan after i.v. gadolinium-DTPA, SE 0.4 s/30 ms (1.5 T)

Fig. 10.42. Primary malignant melanoma of the craniocervical junction in a 51-year-old man with proggressive quadriplegia. Isointense, exophytic tumor without clear demarcation from the cord. Coronal scan, SE 0.7 s/30 ms (1.0 T)

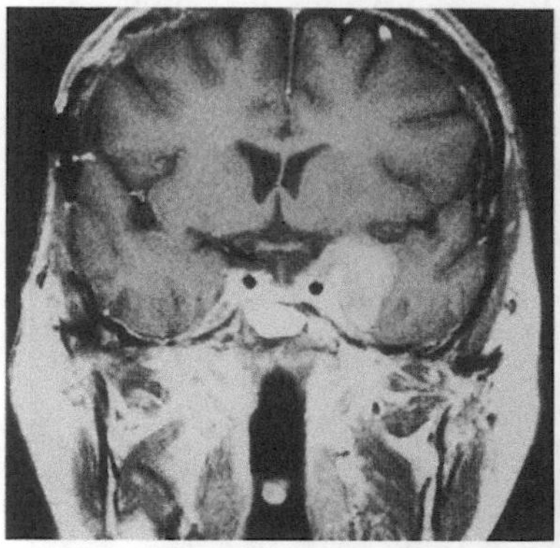

10.41

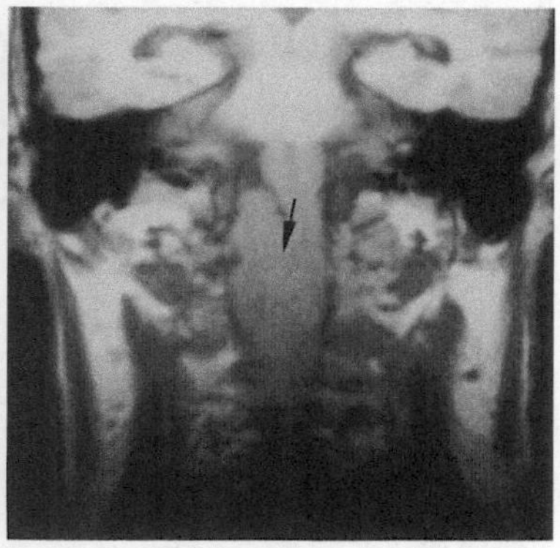

10.42

Incidence: These tumors account for about 1% of intracranial growths [66] and chiefly affect older individuals. The major primary malignant lymphomas are adventitial cell sarcoma and the reticulum cell sarcoma, known also as perithelial sarcoma or microglioma.

Sites: Adventitial cell sarcoma may be solitary or multiple and can occur anywhere in the CNS with no obvious areas of predilection, although it appears to favor periventricular structures.

Pathology: Histologic examination shows perivascular infiltrations of lymphocytes and histiocytes in the white matter, which may coalesce and exhibit only a relatively small mass effect. The tumors usually have a homogeneous structure.

CT and MR Findings

Lymphomas appear isodense to slightly hyperdense on CT scans, present a homogeneous structure, and show moderate contrast enhancement.

On MR scans they show slightly prolonged T1 and T2 times, irregular margins, and a narrow band of perifocal edema. Analogous to contrast CT, a shortening of T1 is noted after i.v. administration of contrast material (Figs. 10.43–10.44). When cortisone is administered the tumor structure may become nonhomogeneous and the tumor may diminish in size.

Fig. 10.45 shows a case of Hodgkin's lymphoma with extradural growth of the tumor before and after radiotherapy.

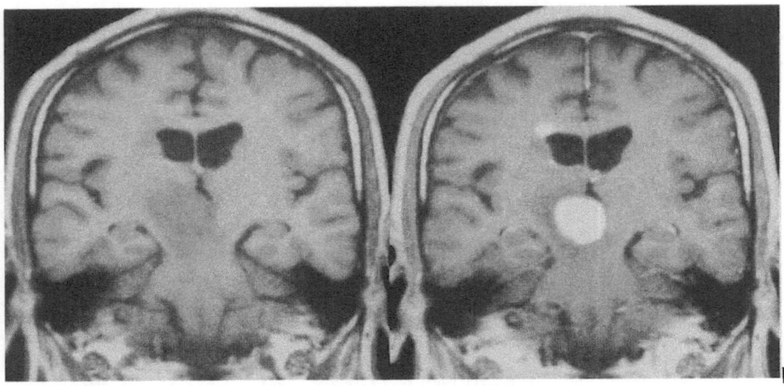

a b

Fig. 10.43. a, b. Malignant non-Hodgkin's lymphoma in a 47-year-old man with double vision and gait disturbances. A lymphoma was suspected because the lesions dissolved after treatment with cortisone and radiotherapy. Coronal scans (**a, b**) SE 0.4 s/17 ms; (**b**) with gadolinium-DTPA) (1.0 T)

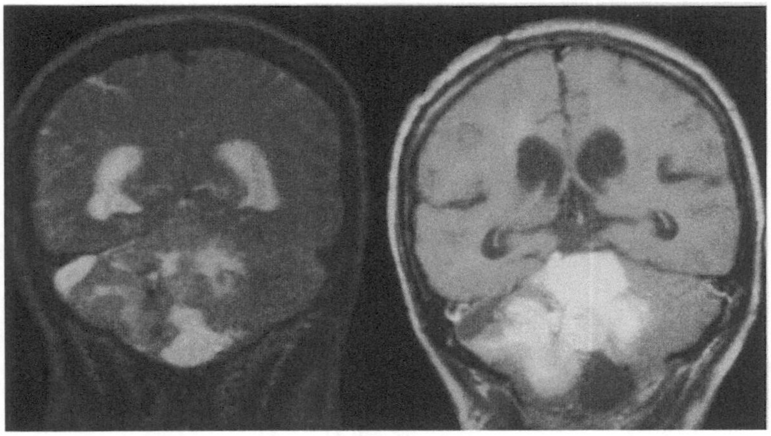

a b

Fig. 10.44 a, b. Histiocytic reticulum cell sarcoma in a 58-year-old woman with rotatory vertigo, nausea, and repeated vomiting. **a** In the native scan the ill-defined lesion shows prolonged relaxation times, mainly of the white matter of the cerebellum. **b** With i.v. gadolinium-DTPA a large irregular area of blood-brain barrier disruption involving gray and white matter is obvious, demonstrating the extension of the tumor more reliably. Coronal scans: (**a**) SE 2.5 s/120 ms, (**b**) SE 0.7 s/45 ms (1.0 T)

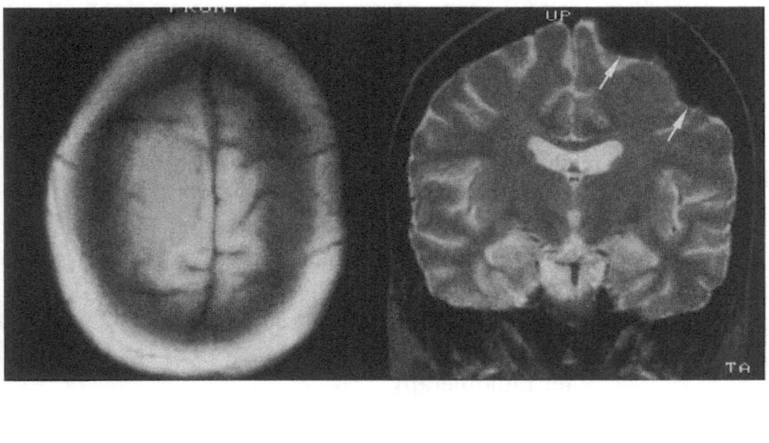

a b

Fig. 10.45 a, b. Hodgkin's disease in a 16-year-old girl with known systemic Hodgkin's disease. The granuloma is confined to the leptomeninges *(arrows)*. Homogeneous tumor tissue isointense with gray matter on T1 weighting (**a**) and hypointense on proton-density and T2-weighting (**b**). Axial scan before radiotherapy: **a** SE 0.6 s/15 ms; coronal scan after radiotherapy: **b** SE 3.0 s/90 ms (1.5 T)

Fig. 10.46. Histiocytosis X in a 30-year-old man with a solitary right parietal lesion. Sagittal scan, SE 0.6 s/15 ms, (1.5 T)

Fig. 10.47. Histiocytosis X (biopsy) in a 2½-year-old girl with persistent back pain. Vertebra L2 is collapsed. A dorsal part with prolonged T2 *(arrow)* is displaced into the spinal canal. The intervertebral discs seem intact. Midsagittal scan, SE 3.0 s/90 ms (1.5 T)

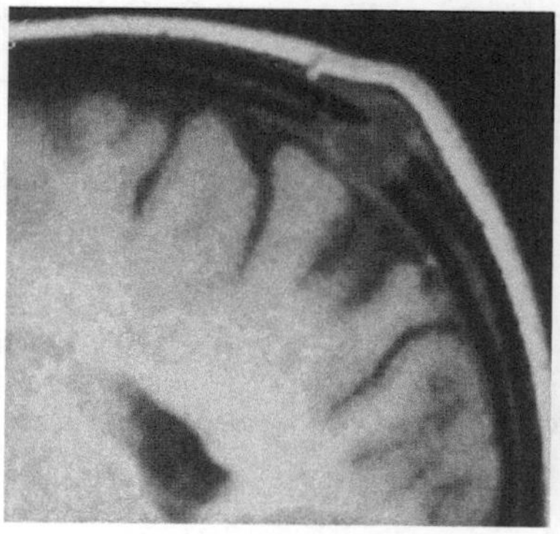

10.46

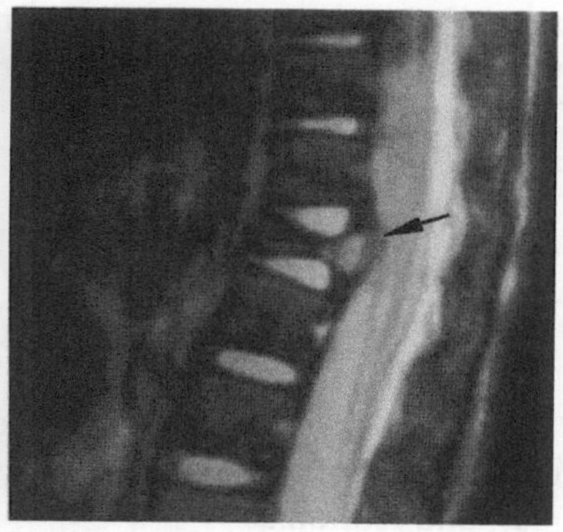

10.47

10.5.1 Histiocytosis X

Histiocytosis X of the CNS consists of granulomatous tissue of unexplained origin in the region of the infundibulum. The tissue contains histiocytes, plasma cells, and reactive glia. Rarely, lesions develop in the hemispheres, the cerebellum, the optic chiasm, and the spinal cord. The clinical picture is usually dominated by diabetes insipidus and deficiency of growth hormone as a sign of pituitary insufficiency.

Other forms of this reticuloendothelial disease are eosinophilic granuloma - the mildest - and disseminated granulomas in the bone and soft tissues - the most severe [20] (Figs. 10.46, 10.47).

MR Findings

The lesions of histiocytosis X show prolonged T1 and T2 relaxation times and present a patchy, nonhomogeneous structure. Especially with an intracerebral focus, perifocal edema is readily distinguished from the lower-intensity tumor with its irregular margins.

In chronic cases where there is necrosis and fibrotic replacement of the foam cells (lipoid, i.e., cholesterol deposits) in the tumor, the nonspecific prolongation of T1 and T2 is less pronounced [20]. Metastases should be considered in differential diagnosis, especially in older patients.

10.6 Tumors of Blood Vessel Origin

The group of tumors originating from blood vessels includes hemangioblastoma (Lindau's tumor) and monstrocellular sarcoma.

10.6.1 Hemangioblastoma

See Sect. 11.1.2

10.6.2 Monstrocellular Sarcoma

Incidence: Monstrocellular sarcomas are seen in patients of all age groups, with no peak incidence. Prevalence data are uncertain because of confusion about nomenclature, but [66] cites an incidence of 1.5% of intracranial growths. The malignant behavior and rapid growth of the tumors classify them as WHO grade 4 lesions.

Sites: Monstrocellular sarcomas have no sites of predilection and are found in all regions of the brain.

Pathology: The tumors are relatively homogeneous, fleshy, and frequently contain cysts of variable size. Necrosis, fatty degeneration, and hemorrhage are less commonly seen. Calcifications do not occur. The tumors can infiltrate the leptomeninges and dura and lead to intracranial seeding. Histologically there are giant tumor cells with inclusion bodies. Among the cells is a dense network of reticular fibers, which impart a firm consistency to the tumor. Pathologic vessels with fistulae and shunts, as in glioblastoma, are not described [66].

MR Findings

At this writing we have no observations of our own or reports from the literature on the MR appearance of monstrocellular sarcomas. From the pathologic features of these tumors, we would expect to find a nonhomogeneous signal with increased relaxation times in the solid components, which would contain homogeneous cysts with long T1 and T2 relaxation times and areas of hemorrhage with short T1 and long T2.

10.7 Germ Cell Tumors

The group of germ cell tumors encompasses germinomas, embryonal carcinomas, choriocarcinomas, and teratomas.

10.7.1 Germinomas

See Sect. 10.2.5.

10.7.2 Embryonal Carcinomas

See Sect. 10.2.5.

10.7.3 Teratomas

Incidence: Teratomas are tumors that arise from multiple germ layers. They are very rare among intracranial growths, constituting about 0.3% of the total according to Zülch [66]. They are considered to be benign (WHO grade 1).

Sites: The pineal region is the commonest site for these growths within the skull, although other brain areas may be involved. Males are predominantly affected.

Pathology: The tumors are well demarcated and encapsulated. Most are hard like cartilage, many have cysts on their surface, and some are permeated by calcifications and bony spicules. They grow extremely slowly by expansion.

CT and MR Findings

On CT scans the tumors present sharp margins and a heterogeneous structure due to the presence of radiopaque calcific foci, bone, and hypodense fat-containing substances.

The MR pattern is marked by a combination of fat-containing elements, which have short relaxation times, and low-signal-intensity calcifications [9].

10.8 Other Malformative Tumors and Tumor-Like Lesions

10.8.1 Craniopharyngiomas

See Sect. 10.9.3

10.8.2 Rathke's Cleft Cysts

See Sect. 10.9.3

10.8.3 Epidermoid and Dermoid Cysts

These cystic lesions can occur anywhere in the CNS; however, because of their predilection for the posterior fossa they are described in detail in Sect. 11.2.3. Figure 10.48 shows a large epidermoid cyst in the frontotemporal region in a young woman.

10.8.4 Colloid Cysts

Colloid cysts are included in the larger group of neurepithelial cysts, together with the noncolloid ependymal and choroidal epithelial cysts.

Incidence: No data are available on the prevalence of colloid cysts. Clinical manifestations, especially paroxysmal headaches, ataxia, gait disturbances, fainting spells, and mental disorders due to CSF stasis, are commonly reported between 20 and 60 years of age.

Site: Colloid cysts occur in the third ventricle between the foramina of Monro, where they can block CSF flow and incite an obstructive hydrocephalus.

Pathology: The origin of these cysts remains controversial. The primitive neuroepithelium, which forms the roof plate of the tela choroidea, and the epithelium of the choroid plexus are considered the possible matrix of the cysts, which are smooth and spherical and can reach a size of 3–4 cm. The cysts usually contain mucous material, and may calcify.

Noncolloid neuroepithelial cysts have also been reported elsewhere in the hemispheres, in the ventricles, the subarachnoid space, the brainstem, and the posterior fossa. They have to be distinguished from cystic tumors and epidermoid or dermoid cysts [44].

Fig. 10.48. Epidermoid cyst in a 26-year-old woman with headache. Asymmetric skull and middle cerebral fossa. Large, well-defined, irregular mass with inhomogeneous structure and prolonged relaxation times. Parasagittal scan, SE 0.7 s/30 ms (1.0 T)

Fig. 10.49. Colloid cyst: incidental finding in a 47-year-old woman with known multiple sclerosis. Round homogeneous tumor in the area of the foramen of Monro with increased signal intensity due to short relaxation times. Axial scan, SE 0.4 s/35 ms (0.5 T). (Courtesy of Drs. Kuhn, Steen, and Terwey, Oldenburg, FRG)

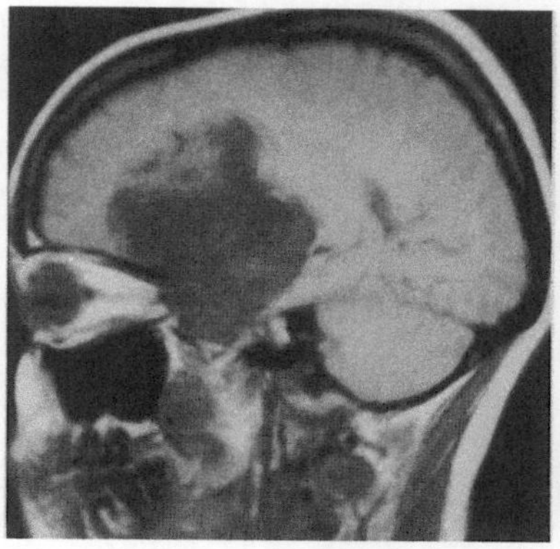

10.48

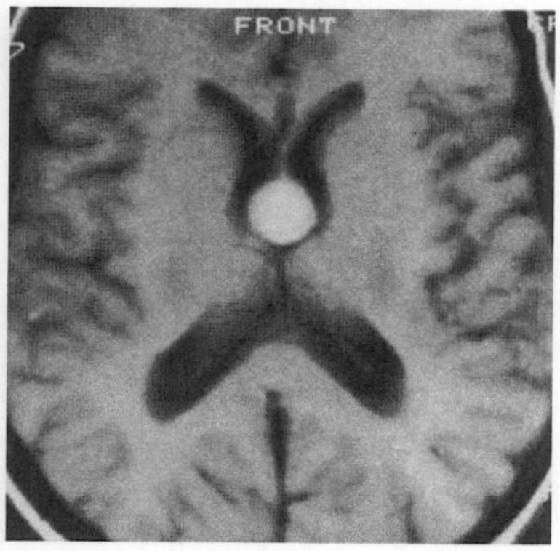

10.49

Fig. 10.50. Colloid cyst in a 54-year-old woman with frequent syncopes, headache, and nausea. The bright ring probably is caused by mucoid substrate and the epithelial secreting tissue; the low signal (in all sequences) of the center *(arrow)* is secondary to deposits of paramagnetic ions. Midsagittal scan SE 0.6 s/35 ms (0.5 T). (Courtesy of Drs. Kuhn, Steen and Terwey, Oldenburg, FRG)

Fig. 10.51. Ependymal cyst in a 20-year-old woman with large head and hydrocephalus. Huge intraventricular cyst containing CSF-like fluid. Sagittal scan, SE 0.5 s/30 ms; (1.0 T)

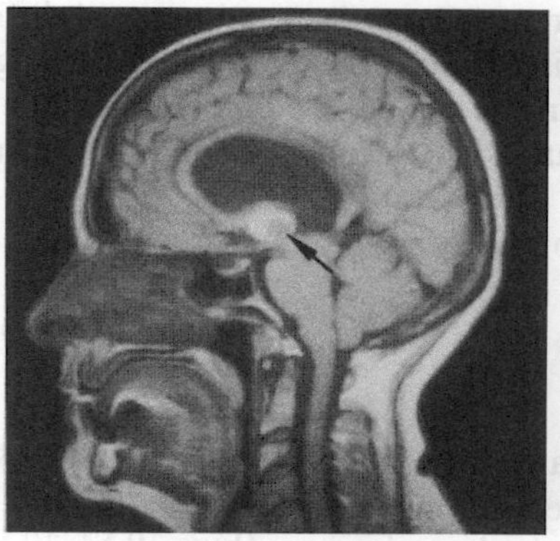

10.50

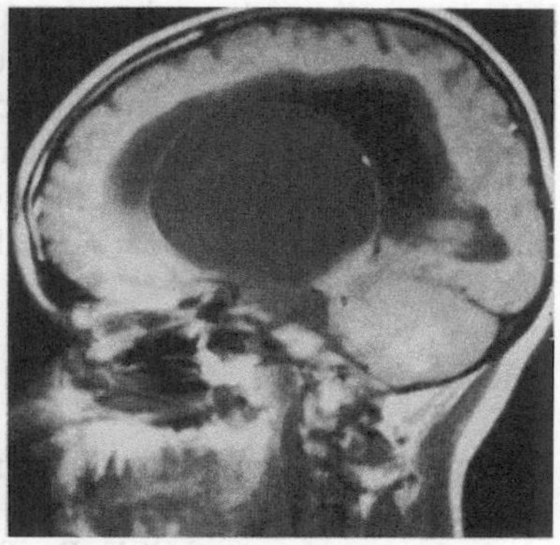

10.51

CT and MR Findings

Colloid cysts may appear isodense, hyperdense, or clearly calcified on CT images. Contrast enhancement occurs in 90% of lesions [41].

On MR scans the cysts may appear hypointense or isointense with brain, or their relaxation times may be prolonged to varying degrees. An increased protein content shortens the relaxation times (hydration effect) (Figs. 10.49–10.50).

Spectroscopic studies of the mucinous content of a colloid cyst revealed mainly sodium, calcium, and magnesium, trace amounts of silicon, copper, iron, and phosphorus, and a slight trace of aluminum [15]; calcium is not considered to be responsible for the high attenuation values in CT [25]. In Fig. 10.50 a ring-shaped lesion is seen with an outer ring of high signal intensity in T1-weighted, proton-density and T2-weighted images, and a central portion of low signal intensity suggesting short T2 or low proton density. The prolonged relaxation times of the capsule are thought to be due to the pathologic epithelial secreting tissue. The low signal of the center most likely represents a high concentration of those ions mentioned above with paramagnetic properties. The mucoid substrate of the central contents probably causes the high signal described in IR images [53].

Differentiation is required from subependymomas, which likewise appear isointense to slightly hyperintense on T2-weighted images.

10.8.5 Enterogenous Cysts

See p. 162.

10.8.6 Ependymal Cysts

The very rare ependymal cysts are lined with ependyma and contain CSF. They are believed to repre-

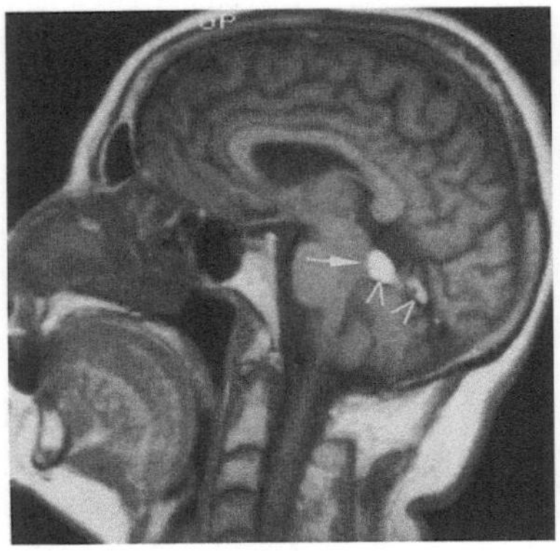

10.52

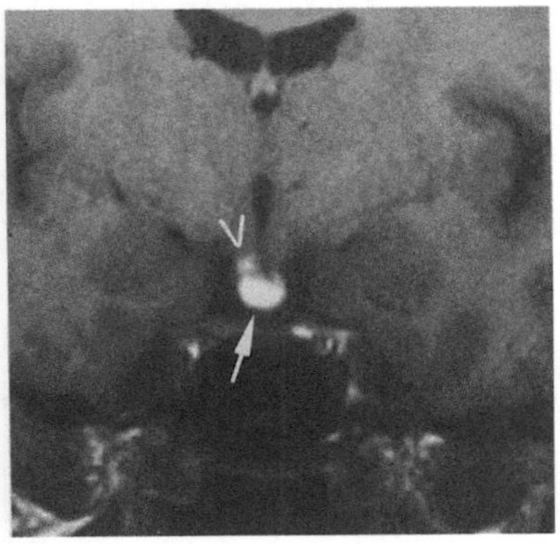

10.53

Fig. 10.52. Lipoma of the vermis cistern: incidental finding in a 53-year-old woman with headache. Nodular lesion *(arrow)* with short relaxation times and small marginal calcifications of low signal intensity *(arrowheads)*. Parasagittal scan, SE 0.5 s/17 ms (1.0 T)

Fig. 10.53. Small lipoma *(arrow)* of the tuber cinereum in a 28-year-old woman with anorexia. The infiltration of the hypothalamus *(arrowhead)* renders a complete removal impossible. Coronal scan, SE 0,6 s/15 ms (1.5 T)

sent a separation of parts of the ventricular system [66]. A growth tendency is not apparent.

Here we should mention the existence of other ependymal cysts which are found in the region of the mesencephalon, diencephalon, and spinal canal and show a tendency to enlarge. The nature of these cysts remains unclear (see also p. 292).

MR Findings

Ependymal cysts present smooth margins and a homogeneous structure with long relaxation times equivalent to those of CSF. Perifocal edema is not demonstrated (Figs. 10.51).

10.8.7 Lipomas

Lipomas are tumors of maldevelopmental origin. Their biologic behavior is classified as WHO grade 1.

Incidence: Lipomas are very rare, and their incidence is estimated to be less than 1%.

Sites: Sites of predilection for lipomas are the corpus callosum, infundibulum, quadrigeminal region, cerebellopontine angle, and spinal canal.

Pathology: As a rule, lipomas are well-demarcated tumors composed of homogeneous fatty tissue, sometimes containing an abundance of vessels, similar to angioma (angiolipoma). Usually they are firmly adherent to adjacent tissue (Fig. 10.53). Scaly calcifications are often found on the tumor surface.

Lipomas of the cerebellopontine angle have a tendency to infiltrate cranial nerve roots, including the fascicles of the trigeminal nerve. This makes total removal difficult and causes remarkable postoperative neurologic deficits when attempted. The tumors follow the trigeminal pathways (into Meckel's cavity) and usually cause progressive symptoms [61].

CT and MR Findings

The fatty tissue of lipoma displays the typical short relaxation times of fat, causing it to appear bright and sharply marginated on T1-weighted sequences (Figs. 10.52–10.53). The scaly calcifications produce a low signal; they are easier to identify on CT scans and more easily distinguished from blood vessels (flow void).

On CT images the differential diagnosis includes hypodense lesions such as epidermoid cysts (see p. 288), arachnoid cysts, metastases, abscesses. etc. However, only in Lipomas negative Hounsfield units can be measured.

On MR images epidermoid tumors usually have prolonged relaxation times. In contrast to cholesteatomas, which may be hyperintense on both T1-weighted and T2-weighted images, bony destruction of the petrous ridge is not seen in lipomas [61].

10.8.8 Hypothalamic Neuronal Hamartomas

Hypothalamic neuronal hamartomas, classified as WHO grade 1, produce clinical symptoms in childhood including seizures, obesity, dwarfism, and pubertas praecox.

Incidence: Hamartomas are extremely rare. Prevalence data are not available.

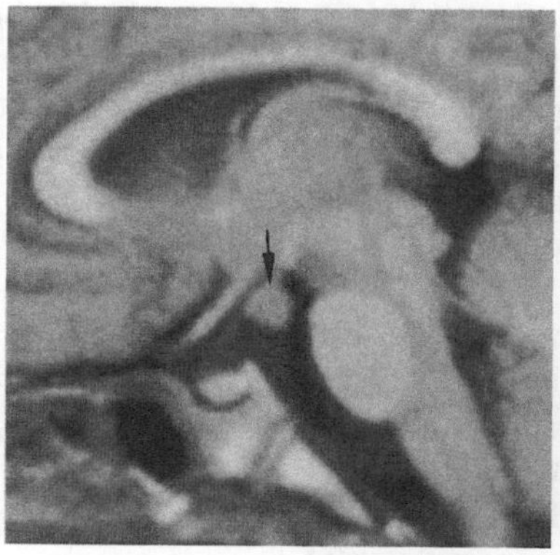

10.54

Fig. 10.54. Hamartoma of the tuber cinereum in a 4-year-old girl with pubertas praecox. The small lesion *(arrow)* is isointense with gray matter. Sagittal scan, SE 0.4 s/17 ms (1.0 T)

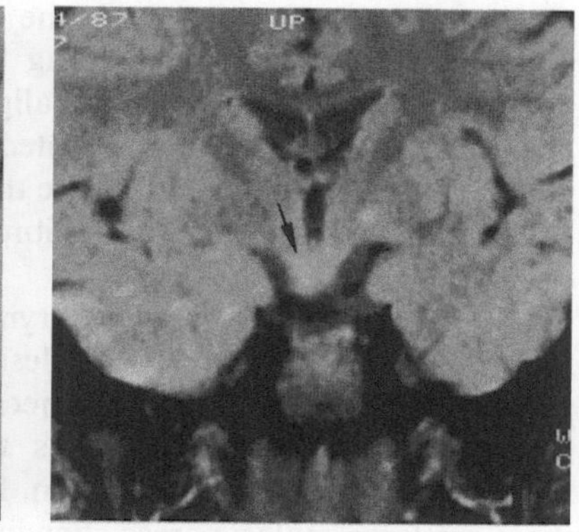

10.55

Fig. 10.55. Hamartoma of the tuber cinereum in an 8-year-old boy with pubertas praecox. The small tumor *(arrow)* is isointense with gray matter. Coronal scan, SE 2.5 s/35 ms (1.0 T)

Sites: These tumors are found mostly in the tuber cinereum between the pituitary stalk and mamillary bodies, but they have also been found in the temporal lobe [37] and in other regions of the brain.

Pathology: Neuronal hamartomas of the hypothalamus are composed of mature neuronal elements that terminate irregularly in nerve fibers. Recurrence and anaplasia are unknown.

CT and MR Findings

As mature neuronal structures, hamartomas appear isodense on CT scans.

They are isointense with the gray matter on MR scans [37] (Fig. 10.54–10.55), but have also been reported to display a slightly increased signal on T2-weighted sequences [46]. Figure 10.55 shows an isointense hamartoma of the tuber cinereum in a 8-year-old girl with pubertas praecox. The lesion did not show enhancement on CT after the intravenous administration of contrast material.

10.9 Tumors of the Pituitary

10.9.1 Tumors of the Anterior Lobe

Pituitary Adenomas

Pituitary adenomas comprise between 8% and 15% of all intracranial tumors. They arise from cells of the anterior lobe of the pituitary and almost invariably lead to excessive hormone production or to anterior pituitary insufficiency. The secretion of all anterior lobe hormones may be increased by the tumor. Eventually the growth may expand beyond the sella, encroaching on the optic chiasm about 1.5 cm above the sellar inlet plane and causing visual disturbances (visual field defects, vision loss, optic atrophy). Parasellar expansion toward the cavernous sinus can cause oculomotor paralysis with diplopia.

Pituitary adenomas can occur at any age, though they are rare before 10 years of age. They are most common from 30 to 60 years, with a peak incidence between 45 and 50 years. Adenomas are very rarely seen in persons over 60 years of age.

General neuropathologic aspects of adenomas: These epithelial tumors of the pituitary have a soft or friable consistency compared with the normally firm tissue of the anterior lobe. Microadenomas lack a fibrous capsule, often making it difficult to identify the boundary between the tumors and surrounding tissue. Pressure effects can cause the adjacent glandular tissue to become thinned, leaving behind a "pseudocapsule" of interstitial fibrous tissue. Macroadenomas, which reach and expand the normal boundaries of the gland, have a firm capsule. The capsular contents are usually soft. These tumors have a globular shape and grow by expansion; most can be surgically removed through a transsphenoidal approach. If the tumor lacks a firm capsule, its extensions may insinuate between the nerves and vessels of the sellar region, project behind the sella or toward the anterior skull base, or invade the third ventricle and burrow into the adjacent brain. These invasive components are not accessible through the transsphenoidal route and must be exposed through a craniotomy (Fig. 10.66, 10.67).

The tumors can also invade the dura and medullary cavities of the surrounding bone and thus mimic the invasive growth of a malignancy. The *architecture* of adenomas may be medullary, stroma-poor, or alveolar; in the latter type the lesion is permeated by septa-like bands of fibrous tissue with capillaries.

Regressive changes occur in varying patterns and frequencies. It is common for the lesion to acquire a pseudopapillary structure due to necrosis and liquefaction. Chromophobe adenomas are particularly apt to undergo cystic degeneration. Less commonly there are large malacic areas showing pseudocystic change, probably due to a deficiency of blood flow. Hemorrhages of varying size (see Fig. 10.60, 10.62 and 10.64), which are most frequent in eosinophil adenomas, leave behind iron deposits in the pericapillary stroma. Adenomas also may contain calcium deposits and, less frequently, areas of fibrosis and hyalination.

The foregoing histologic structural features may be found with varying frequency in almost all types of adenoma. However, the immunohistologic features of the different types of pituitary adenoma are distinctive and thus form the basis for classification [3].

The *classification* of pituitary adenomas has undergone a fundamental change in recent years. The traditional division into eosinophil, basophil, and chromophobe types based on histologic staining properties (using hematoxylin-eosin) has been replaced by a functional classification based on endocrinologic factors. The two classifications are compared in Table 10.2.

Table 10.2. Pituitary adenomas: histologic staining properties and hormonal activity

Secreted hormones	Staining properties
HGH (human growth hormone)	Eosinophilic
PRL (prolactin)	Eosinophilic and chromophobic
ACTH (adrenocorticotropic hormone)	Basophilic
TSH (thyroid-stimulating hormone)	Basophilic
FSH (follicle-stimulating hormone)	Chromophobic, also eosinophilic
LH (luteotropic hormone)	Chromophobic, also eosinophilic
Hormonally inactive tumors	Chromophobic

Figure 10.56 shows the *size* of the various tumor types at the time of diagnosis. Tumors associated with excess hormone production are generally diagnosed earlier than nonfunctioning adenomas.

HGH-Producing Adenomas

Growth-hormone-producing adenomas cause acromegaly in adults (enlargement of facial features, enlargement of the hands and feet, hirsutism, etc.) and gigantism in children and adolescents (excessive body growth before closure of the epiphyseal plates).

Prolactinomas

Prolactinomas cause hyperprolactinemia in females, which is manifested clinically by galactorrhea and primary or secondary amenorrhea.

More than 60% of prolactin-secreting adenomas are diagnosed in women as microadenomas (i.e., tumors smaller than 10 mm in diameter) because of their marked clinical symptoms (see Fig. 10.56). The earliest symptom in males is loss of libido and impotence. Especially in older males, who pay little attention to the early hormonal symptoms, the tumors can grow quite large and compress the optic chiasm. Locally invasive growth is also possible (see Fig. 10.59, 10.63).

It is fairly common for prolactinomas to contain calcifications, psammomatous bodies, and amyloid deposits. Cystic changes and hemorrhages are also common. The latter can cause acute clinical deterioration.

ACTH-Producing Adenomas

The overproduction of ACTH by these tumors leads to hyperadrenocorticism (Cushing's syndrome) with truncal obesity, striae atrophicae, buffalo neck, hirsutism, hypertension, muscular weakness, osteoporosis, and other symptoms.

A large percentage of these tumors (90% of the 112 cases in the series of Fahlbusch et al. [17]) are microadenomas, and many go undiagnosed until surgical exploration. Because they are the smallest of the pituitary adenomas and very often show diffuse or even extraglandular extension, they may escape detection by imaging procedures (Fig. 10.57).

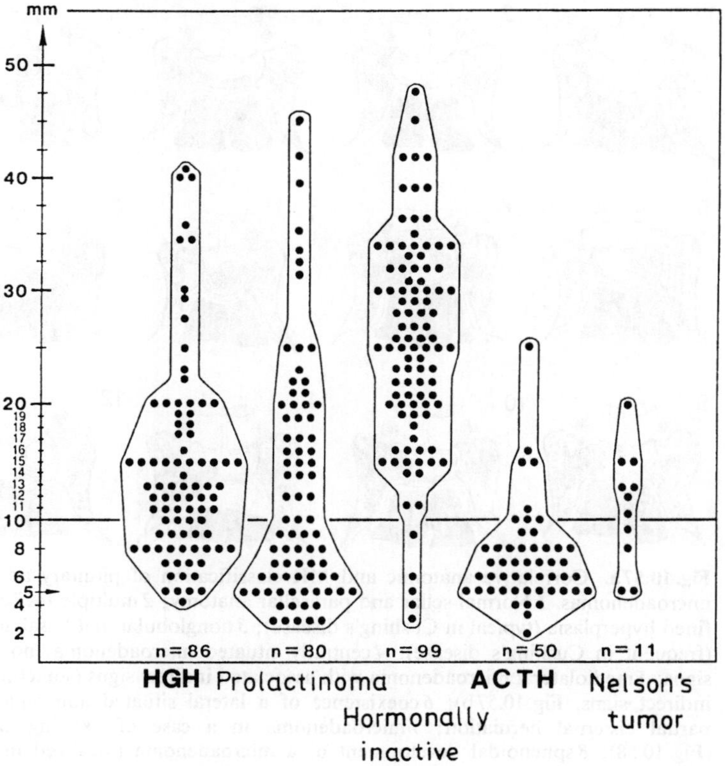

Fig. 10.56. Size of 326 pituitary adenomas at diagnosis

TSH-, FSH- and LH-Producing Adenomas

Because of their extreme rarity, adenomas producing TSH, FSH, and LH will not be described in detail. The general histologic criteria relevant in diagnostic imaging apply to these lesions.

Hormonally Inactive Adenomas

The hormonally inactive adenomas are relatively common, accounting for about 30% of all adenomas. Often they go undetected until they have expanded sufficiently to encroach upon adjacent brain structures, producing symptoms (optic chiasm syndrome, oculomotor disturbances, CSF obstruction).

Pituitary Adenocarinomas

Primary carcinomas of anterior lobe cells are very rare. They may secrete ACTH and prolactin, and they are difficult to distinguish histologically from adenomas. The diagnosis of carcinoma cannot be considered proven until distant metastases are demonstrated [3].

MR and CT Findings

Technique: The sellar region is most effectively examined using a head coil. Surface coils are not advantageous because of the distance of the sella from the cranial surface. Coronal projections are more useful than sagittal for detecting microadenomas, as they facilitate bilateral comparison of the glands and sellar floor. Sagittal scans are also indicated for macroadenomas so that the full extent of the tumors can be ascertained.
From the standpoint of *diagnostic imaging criteria,* it is appropriate to treat microadenomas and macroadenomas separately.

Microadenomas

The diagnosis of microadenomas (tumors less than 10 mm in diameter as defined by Hardy [21]) is established by clinical and endocrinologic methods. Imaging procedures serve to support the diagnosis, exclude a different type of process, and demonstrate the anatomy that will be encountered in the surgical approach.

Because hormone-secreting microadenomas often measure only a few millimeters in size (e.g.,

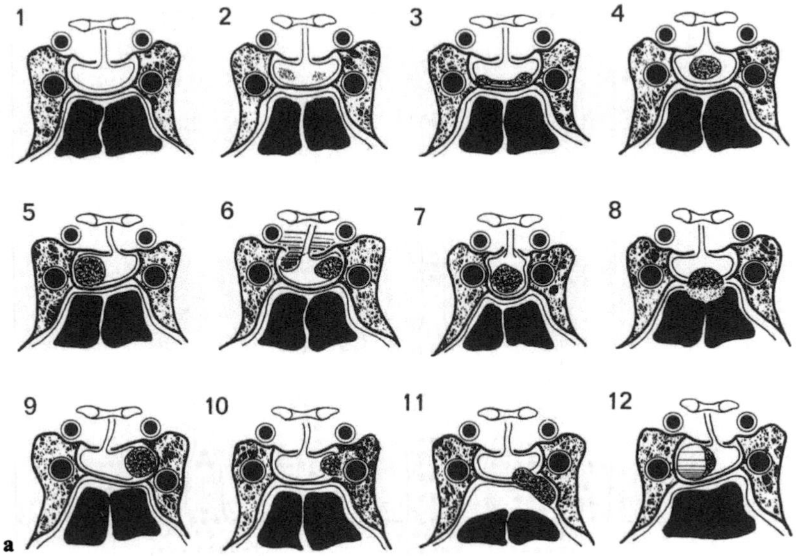

a

Fig. 10.57 a. Correlative anatomic and MR classification of pituitary adenomas: microadenomas. *1* Normal sellar and parasellar anatomy; *2* multiple foci of ill-defined hyperplasia (typical in Cushing's disease); *3* nonglobular, flat basal adenoma (frequent in Cushing's disease); *4* centrally situated microadenoma: no indirect signs; *5* mediolateral microadenoma with associated indirect signs (sometimes only indirect signs, Fig. 10.57 b); *6* coexistence of a lateral situated adenoma with a partial cisternal herniation; *7* microadenoma in a case of "kissing carotids" (Fig. 10.58); *8* sphenoidal development of a microadenoma (localized invasion); *9* extraglandular parasellar development with compression of the cavernous sinus; *10* parasellar microadenoma with perforation of the medial wall of the cavernous sinus (Fig. 10.59); *11* parasellar subcavernous microadenoma; *12* regressive changes (cyst, older hemorrhage, necrosis) in a microadenoma (Figs. 10.60). (Modified from [43])

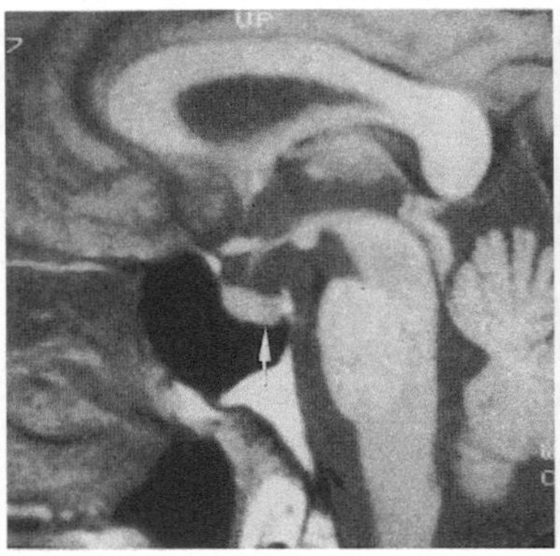
b

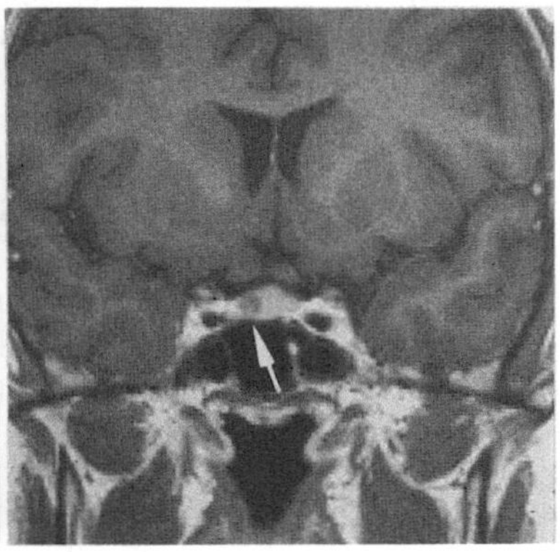
c

Fig. 10.57 b, c. Cushing's disease **b.** in a 35-year-old man with a microadenoma in the dorsal portion of the pituitary (arrow). Sagittal scan, SE 0,6 s/15 ms (1.5 T). **c.** in a 21-year-old woman with a microadenoma in the lateral portion of the gland (arrow). Coronal scan after iv. gd-DTPA, SE 0,5 s/15 ms (1.5 T)

ACTH-producing adenomas), their detection places very great demands on the resolving power of the imaging equipment. Consequently, the indirect signs of microadenoma are just as important as direct signal changes in the detection of the lesion.

The *indirect signs of microadenoma* are as follows:

- A superiorly convex diaphragma sellae. (Normally the diaphragm is flat or concave. In young women and during pregnancy, the gland may temporarily increase in height to 10 mm and become convex, but it should present a symmetric contour and a centered infundibulum.)
- An oblique sellar floor
- An oblique pituitary stalk

The contours of the upper sellar border and pituitary stalk contrast sharply with the dark CSF of the

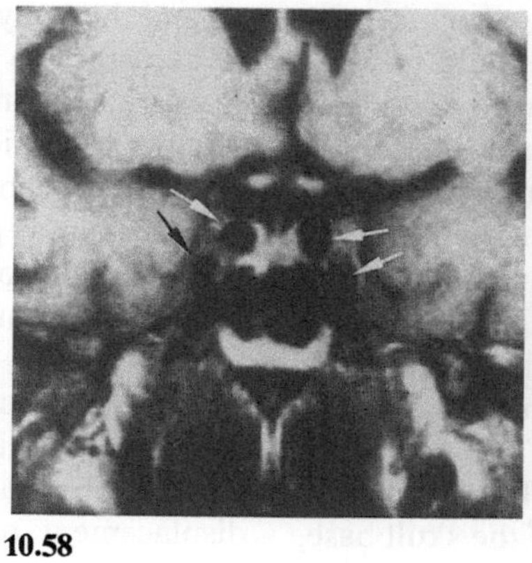

10.58

Fig. 10.58. "Kissing" carotid arteries (see Fig. 10.57). This anatomic situation complicates transsphenoidal surgery. Coronal scan, SE 0.6 s/25 ms (1.0 T)

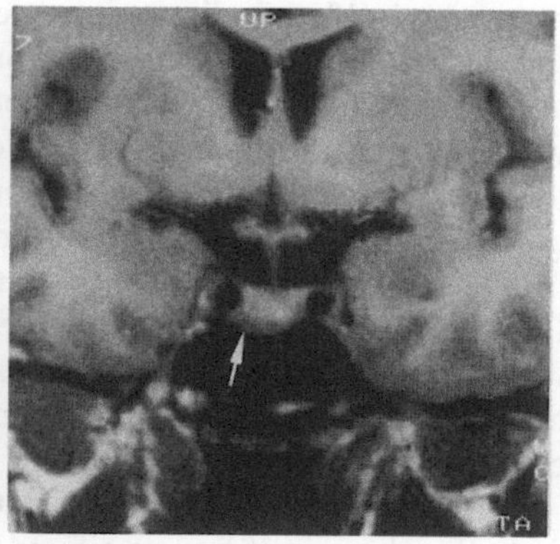

10.59

Fig. 10.59. Parasellar microprolactinoma *(arrow)* invading the cavernous sinus (see Fig. 10.57). 20-year-old woman. Coronal scan, SE 0.5 s/15 ms (1.5 T)

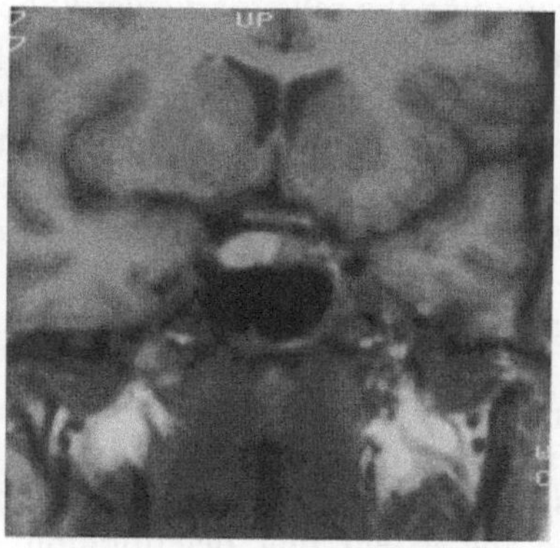

Fig. 10.60. Microadenoma with recent hemorrhage in a 32-year-old woman with secondary amenorrhea. Hyperintense hematoma due to the paramagnetic effect of methemoglobin. Coronal scan, SE 0.5 s/30 ms (1.0 T)

chiasmatic cistern on T1-weighted sequences. The diaphragma sellae, also hypointense, is more easily recognized on proton-density images (SE long TR, short TE) than on T1-weighted or T2-weighted scans, where it is obscured by partial volume effects of the CSF. The floor of the sella, which usually consists of a thin sheet of compact bone, is delineated by the higher signal intensity of the gland. The low-signal compact bone itself is indistinguishable from the dark air in the sphenoid sinus [24].

Direct signs of microadenomas: CT scans usually show microadenomas as low-density area within the gland. Limiting factors for direct detection are the size of the tumor, its configuration, and its localization within the gland. The smallest tumors of our series demonstrated by CT were 3-4 mm in diameter and of central location (see Fig. 10.57). Laterally growing tumors apposed to the cavernous sinus, poorly circumscribed, nonglobular adenomas, and ill-defined hyperplasias can hardly be identified by CT. Coexisting cisternal herniation also impairs detection. These factors account for the high percentage of false-negative findings in Cushing's disease, which is caused by tumors of less than 5 mm in diameter in the majority of cases.

On MR scans, the normal gland and pituitary stalk have a homogeneous structure and a signal intensity close to that of the white matter. In most cases microadenomas display prolonged relaxation times, appearing dark on T1-weighted sequences, isointense on proton-density images, and light on T2-weighted images. These signal differences can be subtle. T2-weighted images appear to be less sensitive on the whole than T1-weighted sequences, and superimposition of the high-signal CSF of the adjacent cistern hinders the differentiation of anatomic structures. Hemorrhage is recognized in both T1-weighted and T2-weighted images by the pathognomonic appearance of a very high signal intensity, whereas cysts are hypointense on T1-weighted images and hyperintense on T2-weighted images.

As demonstrated in a series of 30 surgically resected microadenomas, the sensitivity of CT and MR in the direct detection of microadenomas is almost equal. When indirect signs were also taken into consideration, 22 of these tumors could be visualized by MR, 20 by CT. The undetected adenomas were 2–4 mm in diameter and belonged mainly to the group of Cushing's disease. Hemorrhagic and cystic components could be differentiated by MR in all four cases of this series, but in only one by CT, where all these tumors appeared hypodense. As with CT, non-neoplastic changes in the gland, especially pars intermedia cysts and pituitary infarcts, can mimic an adenoma.

The advantages of MR over CT arise mainly from the absence of bone artifacts of the skull base, the clear delineation of the anatomic structures surrounding the sella, particularly the cavernous sinus and the carotid artery, and the superior display of the indirect signs of microadenomas without the need for contrast medium. Volume averaging in parasagittal sections close to the carotid artery can cause artifacts mimicking microadenoma.

Fig. 10.57 shows the various types of tumor growth in microadenomas (Fig. 10.57–10.60).

Direct coronal and sagittal projections are best suited for the detection of adenomas. A slice thickness of 6 mm may be sufficient, although thinner sections are more favorable for smaller adenomas, to the extent that deterioration of the signal-to-noise ratio permits. Three-dimensional data acquisition can be helpful here for the resolution of fine details.

The intravenous administration of *contrast material* (e.g., gadolinium chelate) leads to a marked shortening of T1 in the normal gland. Much as in dynamic studies using contrast CT, a microadenoma displays little or no enhancement in the initial phase (Fig. 10.57c). Acquisitions at 3 s, 30 s, and 5 min showed "delayed" enhancement of the adenoma in 50% of the lesions; a reduction or reversal of contrast was noted on later images [14]. Whether these dynamic studies will improve the sensitivity in detecting microadenomas still has to be ascertained. It is hoped, however, that further improvements in the spatial resolution of MR will entirely obviate the need for intravenous contrast material in most cases.

Macroadenomas

Macroadenomas can be directly visualized without difficulty. The main concern is to define the position of the lesion in relation to the optic chiasm, the internal carotid artery (see Fig. 10.61) and cavernous sinus, the third ventricle and foramen of Monro, and the bony structures of the skull base. It is also necessary to determine whether the growth can be extirpated through a transsphenoidal approach or whether a craniotomy will be required (Fig. 10.61).

Transsphenoidal surgery is appropriate for *suprasellar* tumor growth when:

1. The tumor possesses a capsule
2. The sella is sufficiently enlarged with a wide aperture

It may be assumed that the tumor has a *capsule* when its margins are well defined and approximately spherical and the lesion is causing upward displacement of the A1 segment of the anterior cerebral artery, which is easily resolved with MR. The slightly elevated diaphragm cannot be visualized directly, except in rare cases [13, 35]. If the expanding tumor is covered by a thickened diaphragm forming a "real" capsule, this can be depicted by MR as the borderline of the tumor. Tumor extensions insinuating among the nerves and vessels of the sellar region (optic chiasm, optic nerve, carotid syphon, posterior communicating artery, basilar artery), as well as retrosellar and subfrontal projections, imply absence of a tumor capsule (Fig. 10.65–10.69). If a well-defined upper convexity is not seen, tumor invasion of the brain has to be considered. These extensions are not accessible to transsphenoidal surgery. Suprasellar growth can be distinguished from the slightly higher intensity optic chiasm better than on CT scans. The *sella* should ideally show a bowel-shaped expansion so that suprasellar tumor components can easily enter the sella during the transsphenoidal extirpation. Tumor tissue that is more remote from the sellar inlet plane cannot be removed by this route. This also applies to hourglass-shaped tumors, which indicate a narrow sellar inlet.

When there is *parasellar extension* toward the cavernous sinus the following types can be distinguished:

1. Tumors displacing the cavernous sinus. It usually cannot be determined whether the tumor has merely displaced the medial wall of the sinus or has invaded it. Even with the use of contrast medium (gadolinium chelate) this question cannot be resolved.
2. Subcavernous growth.
3. Supracavernous and supraclinoidal extension. This differentiation is of major importance for the operative approach; while in types 1 and 2 the transsphenoidal route is indicated, in type 3 the adenoma has to be removed via the transcranial approach (see also Fig. 10.61).

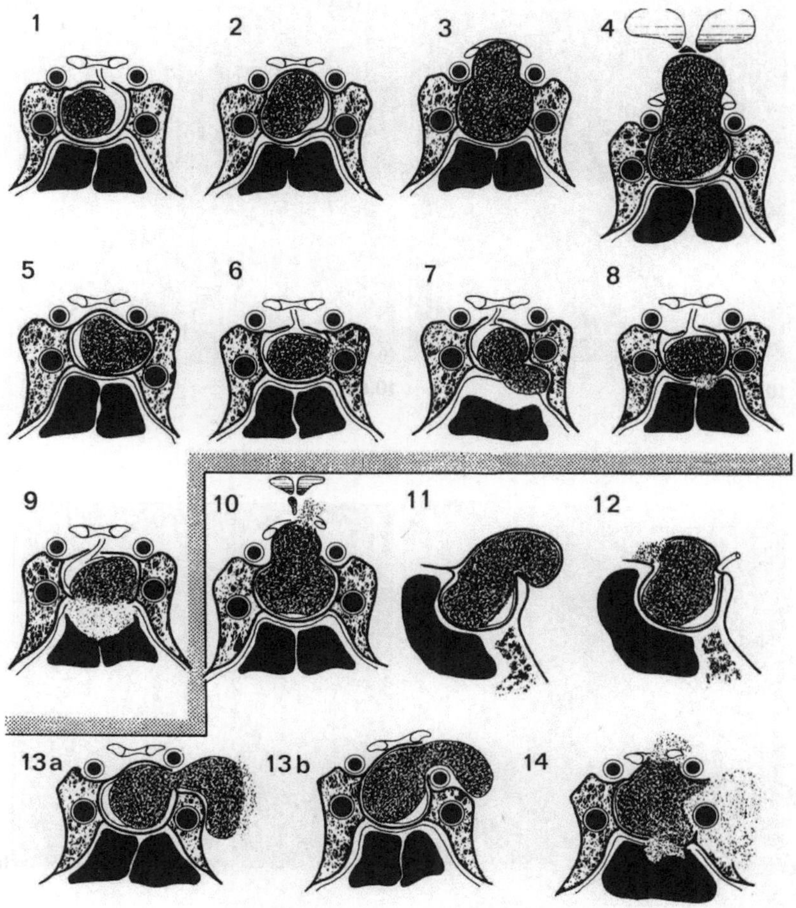

Fig. 10.61. Correlative anatomical and MR classification of pituitary adenomas: macroadenomas. *1* Intrasellar macroadenoma; *2* intra- und suprasellar development without visual compromise; *3* intra- and suprasellar development with visual compromise (Fig. 10.62, Fig. 10.65); *4* suprasellar extension with obstructive hydrocephalus; *5* parasellar development with compression of the cavernous sinus and engulfment of the internal carotid artery; *6* parasellar development with perforation and invasion of the cavernous sinus (Fig. 10.63); *7* parasellar extradural subcavernous macroadenoma (Fig. 10.68); *8* localized sphenoidal invasion; *9* diffuse sphenoidal invasion (Fig. 10.70); *10* suprasellar development with brain invasion (no adequate chiasm syndrome); *11* retrosellar development (enclosed or invasive) (Fig. 10.73); *12* subfrontal extension with invasion (or without) of the basal frontal lobe (Fig. 10.66); *13a* parasellar intradural supraclinoidal development between the superior margin of the cavernous sinus and supraclinoidal internal carotid artery (Fig. 10.68); *13b* parasellar intradural supraclinoidal development between the supraclinoidal internal carotid artery and optic chiasm; *14* "giant adenoma" (Fig. 10.69). (Modified from [43])

Frequently the carotid syphon is displaced, deformed, and enveloped; in contrast to the situation with parasellar meningiomas (see Fig. 10.34), it is rarely compressed. The carotid artery is easily traced within the tumor as a dark band (flow void), and angiography may be dispensed with if the vessels around the sella are well displayed (see Fig. 10.58 and 10.59).

With invasive growth into the skull base, the tumor can be readily distinguished from the fat-containing bone marrow (e.g., in the clivus) on T1-weighted images owing to its longer relaxation times. In the region of the paranasal sinuses, however, MR is inferior to CT in its ability to detect and evaluate destruction of the delicate bony structures (Fig. 10.70).

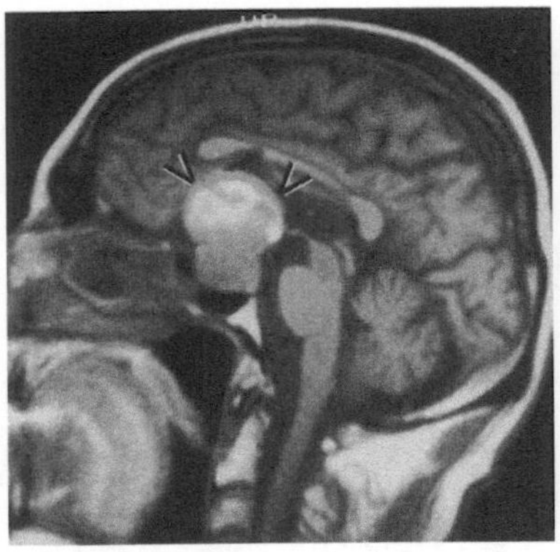

10.62

Fig. 10.62. Macroadenoma in a 64-year-old man with sudden loss of vision. Large adenoma with acute hemorrhage. The tumor has a firm capsule *(arrowheads)*. Midsagittal scan (**a**) SE 0.4 s/17 ms; (1.0 T)

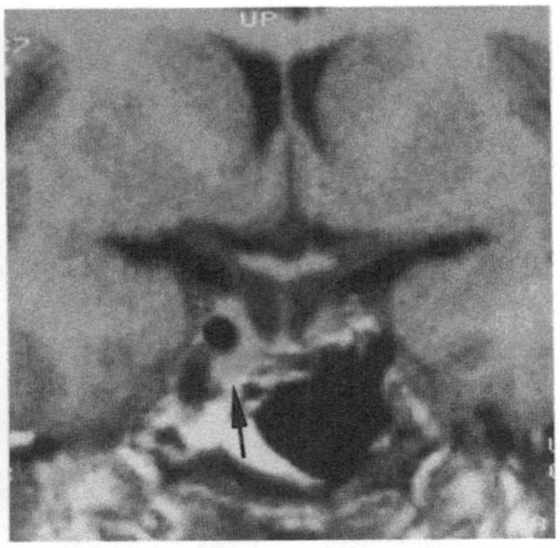

10.63

Fig. 10.63. Prolactinoma *(arrow)* invading the cavernous sinus in a 34-year-old woman presenting with severe pain in the territory of the second division of the fifth cranial nerve after incomplete surgical removal of the tumor. Coronal scan, SE 0.45 s/15 ms (1.5 T)

a

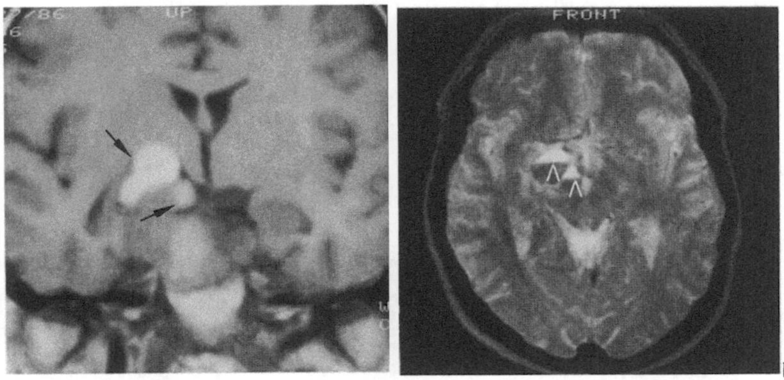

b

Fig. 10.64 a, b. Macroprolactinoma with hemorrhagic cysts *(arrows)*. Fluid level in **b** *(arrowheads)*. **a** Coronal scan, SE 0.7 s/17 ms; **b** axial scan, SE 3.0 s/120 ms (1.0 T)

Most macroadenomas have prolonged relaxation times and appear darker than the normal gland on T1-weighted images. The different types of adenoma do not show significant differences in their signal intensities. In our series, no close interindividual correlation of MR signal intensity and tumor consistency was found during surgery, in contrast to the results of Snow et al. [54], who found isointense signals in T1-weighted and T2-weighted images in all three firm tumors of their series. However, our analysis of 14 tumors with mainly intrasellar and parasellar extension showed a predominance of low signal intensities for soft tumors in both T1-weighted and T2-weighted sequences. This pattern was not seen in 36 tumors with predominantly extrasellar and suprasellar growth; in this group isointense signal on T1-weighted images was commonly found. Eight firm tumors had different signal intensities in both sequences.

The injection of intravenous contrast material (e.g., gadolinium chelate) is followed by a rapid and pronounced rise in the signal intensity of solid tumor components on T1-weighted scans. Differences in contrast enhancement are not apparent among the different types of adenoma. This is also true for other non-neoplastic lesions, such as granulomatous inflammation, as shown in Fig. 10.71–10.72).

The question of *tumor recurrence* is very difficult to resolve without benefit of comparative preoperative and postoperative scans. Because of anatomic changes and uncharacteristic signal values, foreign material introduced at operation to seal the sellar floor (e.g., muscle, fascia, lyophilized dura, fat) can be indistinguishable from recurrent tumor growth at an atypical site. With hormone-secreting adenomas, endocrinologic criteria such as a renewed increase in hormone production can be helpful in evaluating for recurrence.

Fig. 10.65. Prolactinoma in a 16-year-old boy with visual disturbances. Macroadenoma with suprasellar growth without tumor capsule. Midsagittal scan, SE 0.7 s/30 ms (1.0 T)

Fig. 10.66. Macroadenoma in a 35-year-old man with visual disturbances. The tumor grows anteriorly over the planum sphenoidale, making the transcranial approach necessary. Sagittal scan, SE 0.4 s/17 ms (1.0 T)

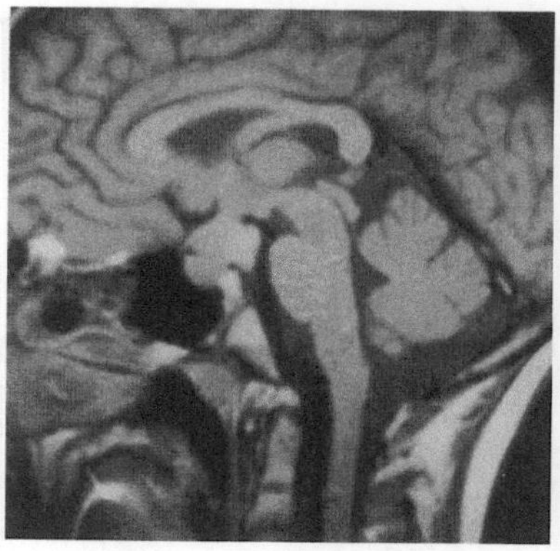

10.65

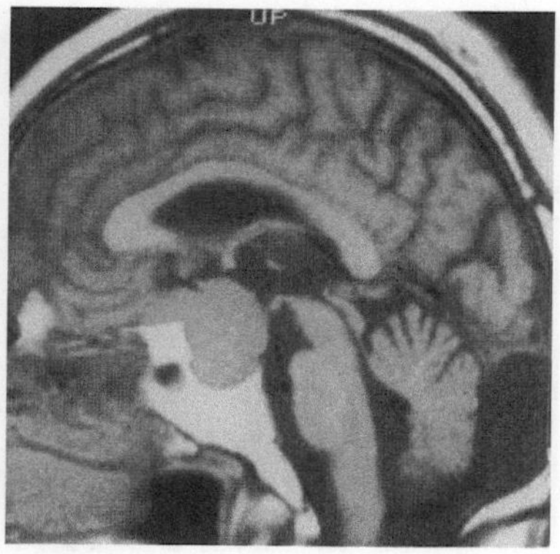

10.66

Fig. 10.67. Inactive chromophobic adenoma in a 34-year-old woman with oculomotor palsy. Parasellar, intradural, supraclinoidal extension of the adenoma with invasion of the temporal lobe *(arrowheads)*. Coronal scan, SE 0.5 s/30 ms, (1.0 T)

Fig. 10.68. STH-producing macroadenoma with supraclinoidal intradural and subcavernous extradural growth (see Fig. 57.61, *7* and *13*) in a 44-year-old woman with acromegaly. Coronal scan, SE 0.5 s/15 ms (1.5 T)

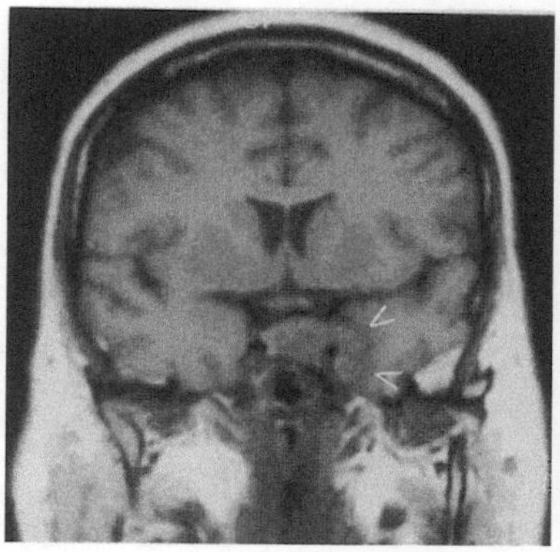

10.67

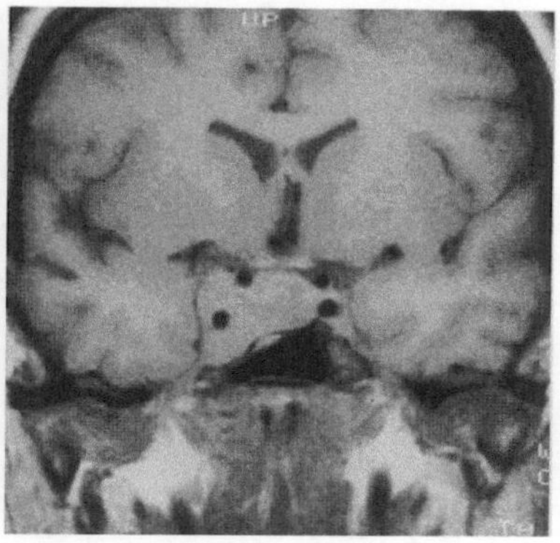

10.68

The *medical treatment of prolactinomas with bromocriptine* is prescribed for the purpose of reducing the tumor size and hormone excess (Fig. 10.73). Approximately 60% of prolactinomas respond to this therapy. Weissbuch [59] describes MR signal changes during bromocriptine therapy which point to a shortening of T1 and a shortening or lengthening of T2. The effect of bromocriptine initially consists in an involution of the tumor cells with a reduction in cell size, particularly involving the organelles of protein synthesis. Later effects consist of edematous cell changes, necrosis, and fibrosis. As a result, prolactinomas treated with short-term bromocriptine are softer and more fluid, while firm, fibrotic areas are encountered after long-term therapy [36]. In six cases of our own series, after short-term treatment the tumors were found to be of inhomogeneous consistency with predominance of medium and firmer areas, although their original consistency prior to therapy is unknown. Pojunas et al. [47] describe a shortening of T2 with and without shortening of T1 in two patients treated with bromocriptine.

A *postoperative abscess* in the sellar region appears on CT scans as an enhancing, ringlike structure with a central zone of lower density. So far this complication has not been evaluated with MR. By analogy with CT and with MR findings in brain abscess, MR presumably would demonstrate a ringlike structure that shows contrast enhancement on T1-weighted scans and whose center gives a slightly lower signal because of the longer relaxation times of pus.

10.9.2 Lesions of the Posterior Lobe

Lesions of the posterior lobe of the pituitary, which is part of the hypothalamohypophyseal system, are the cause of diabetes insipidus.

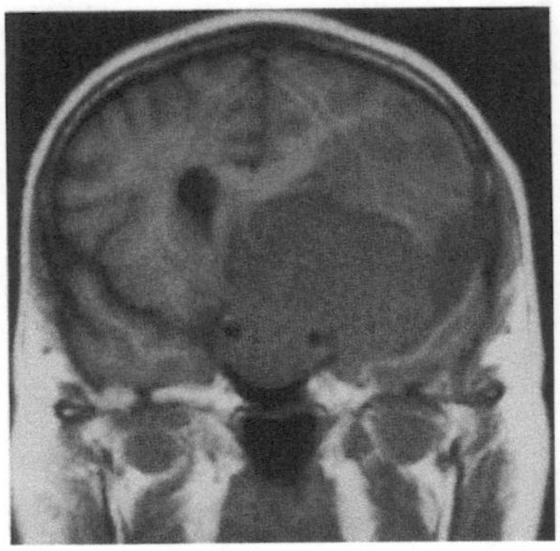

10.69

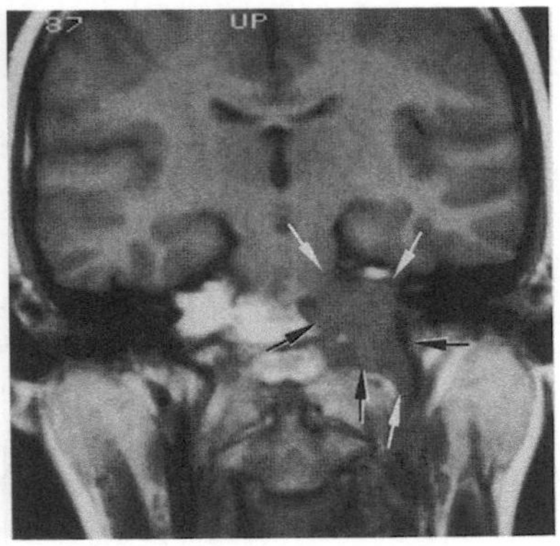

10.70

Fig. 10.69. Giant adenoma in a 52-year-old woman with visual disturbances and mental changes. Huge, homogeneous, solid tumor with prolonged relaxation times growing from the sella into the anterior cerebral fossa. Coronal scan, SE 0.4 s/17 ms; (1.0 T)

Fig. 10.70. Pituitary adenoma with Nelson's syndrome in a 27-year-old woman with palsy of the twelfth cranial nerve (after central Cushing's syndrome with primary adrenalectomy in 1975 and known pituitary tumor since 1980). Large, invasive tumor with homogeneous structure *(arrows)* and with signal intensity similar to that of gray matter. Coronal scan, SE 0.4 s/17 ms (1.0 T)

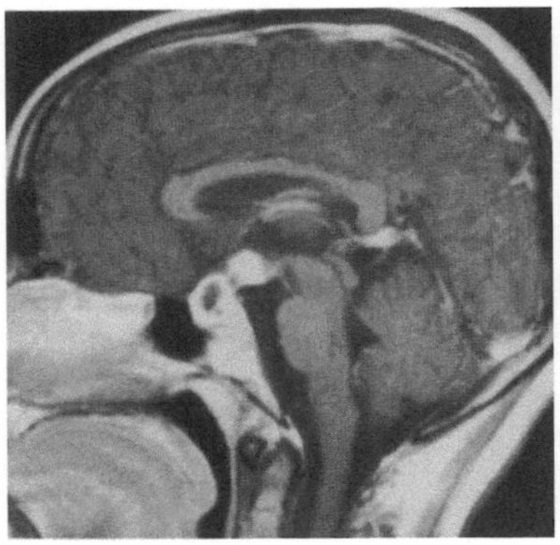

10.71

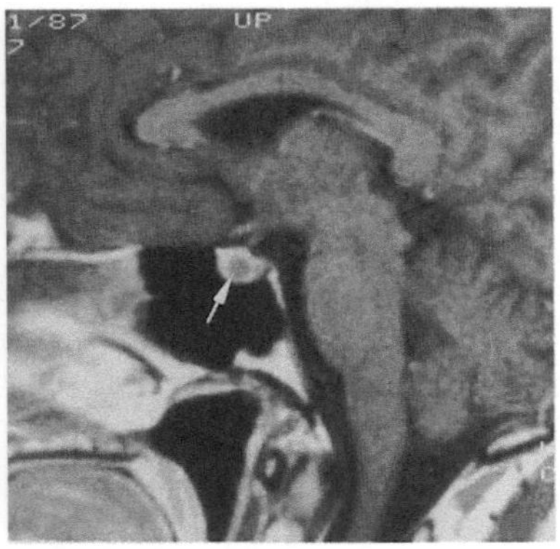

10.72

Fig. 10.71. Granulomatous inflammation in a 16-year-old girl with endocrinological disturbances. Tumorlike lesion isointense to gray matter involving the pituitary and infundibulum with distinct contrast enhancement. Midsagittal scan, SE 0.4 s/17 ms with i.v. gadolinium-DTPA (1.0 T)

Fig. 10.72. Scar tissue *(arrow)* of chronic, unspecific intrasellar inflammatory process in a 42-year-old woman with pituitary insufficiency and suspected microadenoma. Sagittal scan, after i.v. gadolinium-DTPA, SE 0.3 s/17 ms (1.0 T)

Randell et al. [48] have described a primary and a secondary type of this disease. The primary type includes both familial and idiopathic diabetes insipidus, whereas the secondary type may be induced by trauma, vascular disease, infections, systemic conditions, and tumors such as metastases, teratomas, germinomas, hamartomas, and histiocytosis X.

MR Findings

Frequently, midsagittal T1-weighted scans of this region will demonstrate an intrasellar structure of high signal intensity apposed to the dorsum sellae (Fig. 10.74). This signal is markedly reduced on T2-weighted scans. Mark et al. [39] attributed the signal to an extraglandular "fat pad," but more than 500 transsphenoidal pituitary operations [17, 18] performed from 1982 to 1987 have failed to demonstrate this structure. Kucharczyk [32] believes that the signal comes from intracellular fat of the neurohypophysis, but Nishimura et al. [42] deny that this can account for the high signal intensity. These authors state that the posterior lobe is composed of intrinsic pituicytes and a large bundle of unmyelinated nerve fibres [48] whose T1 values are longer than those of myelinated fibers. The question of whether membrane-bound neurosecretory granules that contain the hormones of the posterior lobe (vasopressin and oxytocin) are responsible for the high signal intensity remains unanswered.

Fugisawa et al. [19] demonstrated the posterior lobe and pituitary stalk as a hyperintense structure in T1-weighted and proton-density images in a series of 60 normal volunteers. The high signal within the posterior lobe, could not be detected, however, in five cases of diabetes insipidus.

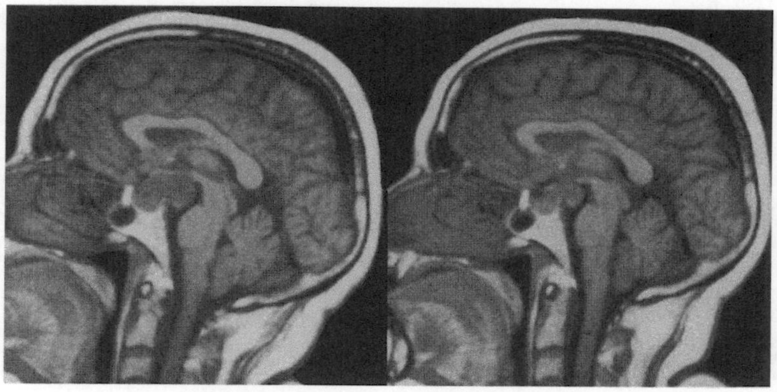

Fig. 10.73 a, b. Macroprolactinoma in a 37-year-old woman with amenorrhea. Large tumor with supra- and retrosellar growth. Before (**a**) and after (**b**) 8 weeks of treatment with bromocriptine. Midsagittal scans, SE 0.4 s/17 ms (1.0 T)

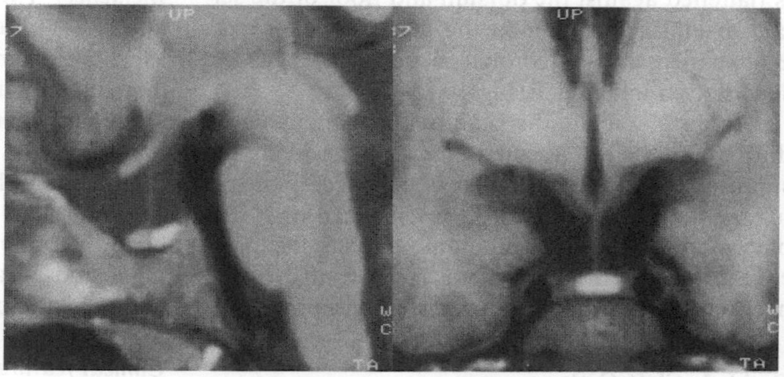

Fig. 10.74 a, b. Normal pituitary in an 8-year-old boy. The hyperintense dorsal portion corresponds to the normal posterior lobe of the pituitary. **a** Sagittal, **b** coronal scans, SE 0.6 s/15 ms (1.5 T)

10.9.3 Other Lesions Related to the Pituitary

Empty Sella Syndrome

The diaphragma sellae is formed by a layer of dura stretching from the dorsum to the tuberculum sellae and between the medial dural walls of the cavernous sinuses. It forms the roof of the sellar groove and contains a central aperture of quite variable size [11] through which the pituitary stalk passes from the hypothalamus to the pituitary.

If a natural or acquired defect exists in the diaphragma sellae, the intracranial pressure can cause the chiasmatic cistern to bulge into the sella (cisternal herniation) and impinge upon the bony structures of the sella. This results in a progressive enlargement of the sella, which appears "empty" on radiographs. Although the anterior lobe of the pituitary is compressed by the increased intrasellar pressure and is pushed against the wall of the sella, hormonal disturbances are rare.

Besides the primary form, "empty sella" can also be secondary to operations and irradiation [18].

If the optic chiasm becomes displaced into the sella, varying degrees of optic chiasm syndrome can result (see Fig. 10.77).

Differentiation is required from space-occupying intrasellar arachnoid cysts that result from cystic dilatation of the supradiaphragmatic cistern with blockage of the intrasellar CSF circulation.

MR Findings

On T1-weighted images the slightly enlarged sella appears as dark as the CSF of the suprasellar cistern. The pituitary stalk is apposed centrally to the dorsum sellae and communicates with a gland that

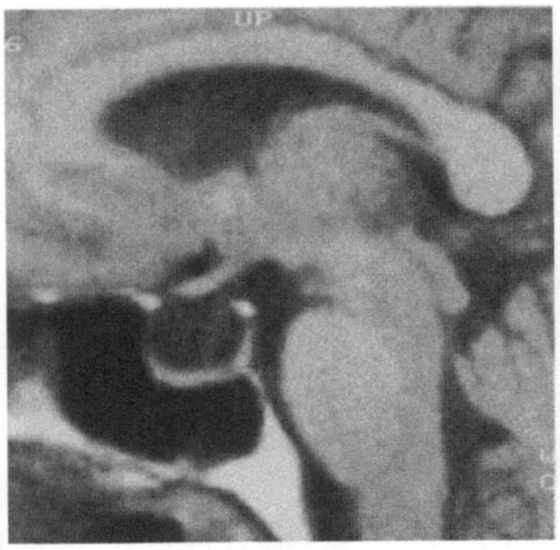

10.75

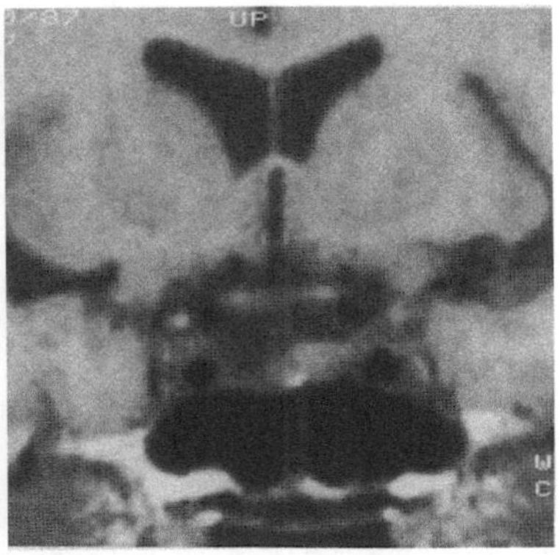

10.76

Fig. 10.75. Empty sella: incidental finding in a 57-year-old woman. Sagittal scan, SE 0.4 s/17 ms (1.0 T)

Fig. 10.76. Unilateral cisternal herniation in a 56-year-old woman with minor pituitary insufficiency. Coronal scan of the anterior part of sella, SE 0.5 s/17 ms (1.0 T)

is flattened against the dorsum and floor of the sella. On midsagittal section the gland appears crescent-shaped, and on coronal section it presents the shape of an inverted T (Fig. 10.75–10.77).

Because arachnoid septa are not seen, it can be difficult to detect a communication between the suprasellar and the intrasellar CSF space. If the pituitary stalk cannot be directly visualized or if displacement of the infundibulum suggests the presence of a closed, cystic mass, it generally will be necessary to perform contrast cisternography.

Rathke's Cleft Cysts

Rathke's cleft cysts are intrasellar epithelial, serous, or mucous cysts lined with remnants of Rathke's pouch, which forms the anterior lobe of the pituitary and the pars intermedia. These cysts can occasionally become quite large. Their epithelium is distinct histologically from other cystic lesions of the sellar region associated, for example, with hemorrhages or infarcts [66].

MR Findings

The homogeneous cystic contents of Rathke's cleft cysts may correspond in intensity to CSF (serous contents), or they may give a high signal on T1-weighted and T2-weighted scans (mucous contents) (Fig. 10.78) [33]. A cyst with serous contents requires differentiation from an "empty sella" (see above).

Craniopharyngiomas

Craniopharyngiomas arise from remnants of the craniopharyngeal canal (Rathke's pouch).

Incidence: These congenital tumors are relatively rare (1.2% of all tumors in the series of Zülch [66]). Most are diagnosed in childhood and adolescence, though some are detected in later life. The tumors are slightly more common in males than females.

Sites: Craniopharyngiomas may be intrasellar and/or suprasellar. They grow entirely by expansion toward the optic chiasm or third ventricle, and retrosellar and parasellar extension is possible into the middle, anterior, and posterior cranial fossae.

Clinical features: Signs of pituitary insufficiency are commonly seen. If cholesterol within the cyst enters the CSF, a recurring meningeal reaction with fever can result. Large tumors expanding into the cranium produce symptoms of a local mass lesion with visual disturbances, oculomotor paralysis, and hypothalamic insufficiency.

Pathology: Craniopharyngiomas consist of solid and encapsulated cystic components. The solid portions, formed by wide bands of squamous epithelium surrounded by vascular connective tissue, are permeated by numerous cystic cavities. Calcifications give these a hard consistency. The cysts contain a turbid brownish fluid, resembling machine oil, that is rich in cholesterol crystals. The blood vessels of the connective tissue are fenestrated [23].

The floor of the adjacent third ventricle may show an extensive reactive gliosis that can resemble a pilocytic astrocytoma [66]. Craniopharyngiomas grow very slowly and are classified as WHO grade 1 tumors. Nevertheless, the prognosis varies because the tumors often cannot be totally removed due to fusion with adjacent structures (optic chiasm, hypothalamus).

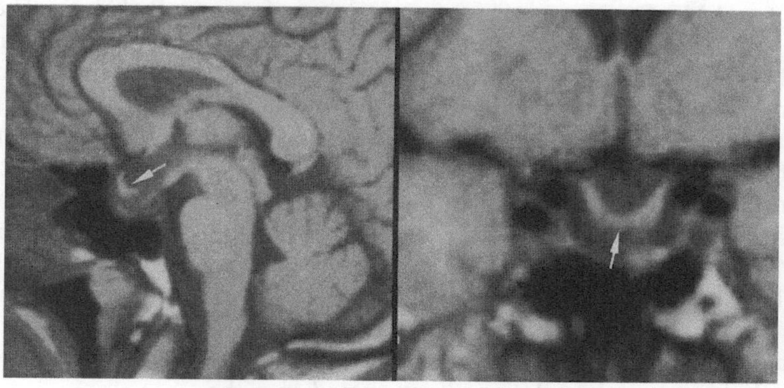

a b

Fig. 10.77 a, b. Empty sella with herniation of chiasm in a 46-year-old woman with complete pituitary insufficiency. Normal vision. The chiasm *(arrows)* is herniated into the empty sella. (**a**) Midsagittal, (**b**) coronal scans, SE 0.6 s/30 ms (1.0 T)

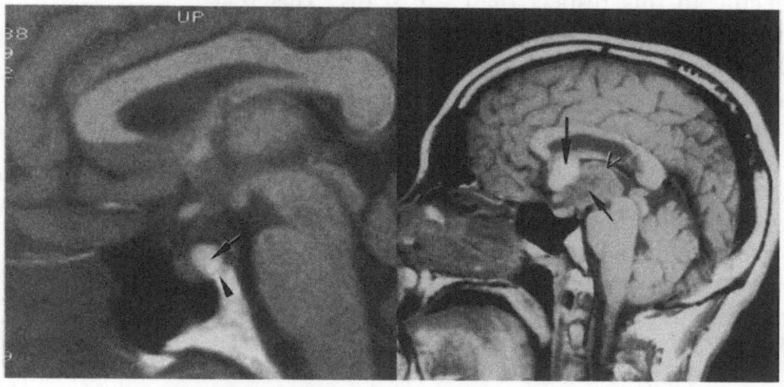

a b

Fig. 10.78. a Rathke's cleft cyst in a 45-year old woman presenting with diabetes insipidus. The high signal intensity (arrow) was caused by mucous contents of the cyst found at surgery. Between the cyst and the floor of the sella the posterior lobe *(short arrow)* can be suspected. Sagittal scan, SE 0.45 s/15 ms (1.5 T). **b** Craniopharyngioma in a 33-year-old man with visual disturbances and pituitary insufficiency. Suprasellar tumor with cystic *(arrow)*, and solid *(arrowhead)* compartments containing calcifications *(small arrow)* which could be indentified only by CT. Sagittal scan, SE 0.6 s/15 ms; (1.5 T)

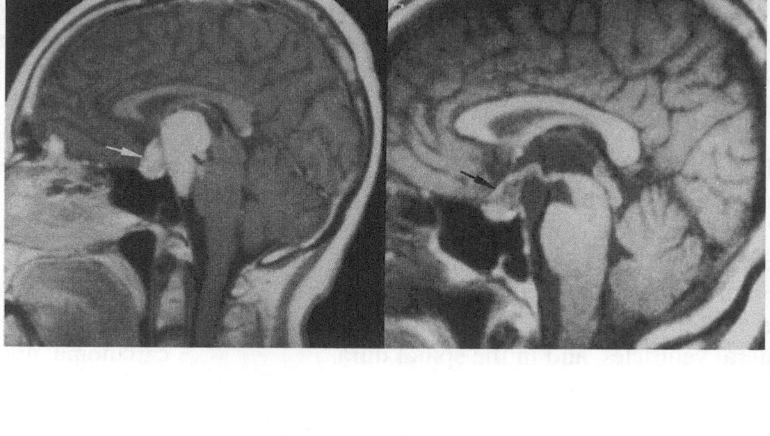

a b

Fig. 10.79 a, b. Craniopharyngioma in a 54-year old woman with deterioration of vision. A small suprasellar solid tumor *(arrow)* is associated with a large retrosellar cyst of cholesterin-containing fluid. After drainage of the cyst **(b)** the cholesterin content is significantly lower. Midsagittal scans (SE 0.4 s/17 ms), **(a)** with gd-DTPA showing enhancement of the solid tumor, **(b)** 7 month after stereotaxic drainage (1.0 T)

CT and MR Findings

The CT detection of craniopharyngiomas is based on the presence of calcifications and cysts. The same is true of MR imaging. The relaxation times of the cysts may be markedly shortened, depending on their cholesterol content or recent hemorrhage. The cysts produce a high, uniform signal on T1-weighted images, which usually is seen even when the lesions appear isodence or hypodense on CT scans (Figs. 10.78, 10.79). Thus MR is more reliable than CT in the detection of these cysts, especially in cases where lesions have spread into the bone and pneumatized spaces of the skull base. Cysts with a low cholesterol content and no calcifications are indistinguishable from cysts of other etiology.

Calcifications in craniopharyngiomas always produce low signals on MR images, which are less specific in this respect than CT scans. This reaffirms the general superiority of CT over MR in the identification of calcifications. Calcifications are very rare in adenomas but can form as a sequela to hemorrhage.

Solid tumor components present a less homogeneous structure and less well-defined margins than are seen in pituitary adenomas. They have slightly prolonged relaxation times. A marked rise of signal intensity is seen on T1-weighted scans after the intravenous administration of contrast material (Fig. 10.79).

10.10 Local Extensions from Regional Tumors

10.10.1 Glomus Jugulare Tumors, Chordomas

Because of their predilection for the posterior fossa, glomus jugulare tumors and chordomas are described in Sects. 11.2.4, 11.2.5.

10.10.2 Chondromas

Chondromas are very rare tumors that usually arise in the dura close to synchondroses but may also be found on the falx, in the parasellar region, in the cerebellopontine angle, in the choroid plexus of the lateral ventricles, and in the spinal dura.

Pathology: The tumors are encapsulated by dura and grow mainly by expansion, although they can infiltrate the adjacent bone. Their surface is knobby and lobulated, their consistency soft to rubbery. The tumor tissue shows an irregular structure composed of hyaline cartilage with myxomatous changes and microcysts, calcifications, and occasionally areas of true ossification. Chondromas may take a benign course, but they may also undergo malignant change and infiltrate the brain, muscle, skin, and bone.

MR Findings

Small chondromas may present as homogeneous masses with increased T1 and T2 relaxation times. With larger lesions, the nonhomogeneous structure of the tumor may be expressed in a somewhat more irregular signal pattern. The sharp intracranial border of the nodular tumors is formed by the dura, which may be infiltrated by the anaplastic forms (Fig. 10.80).

10.10.3 Chondrosarcomas

Chondrosarcomas may form as primary malignancies or may develop from a chondroma. They are gelatinous or hard, lobular, infiltrating tumors that form chondroid substances but not bone. The tumor tissue is highly cellular. The prognosis is poor.

MR findings are as for chondromas (see above).

10.10.4 Olfactory Neuroblastomas

Olfactory neuroblastomas, rare tumors of the middle decades of life known also as esthesioneuroblastomas, probably arise from the olfactory mucosa and grow in the region of the paranasal sinuses (Fig. 10.81).

Pathology: The tumors are composed of long cells or lymphoid cells arranged in the form of rosettes or showing no particular architectural arrangement. They grow invasively in all directions, even invading the orbit, anterior fossa, and brain (WHO grade 4) [66]. Metastases are possible. Differentiation is required from lymphosarcoma, anaplastic carcinoma, and other malignancies.

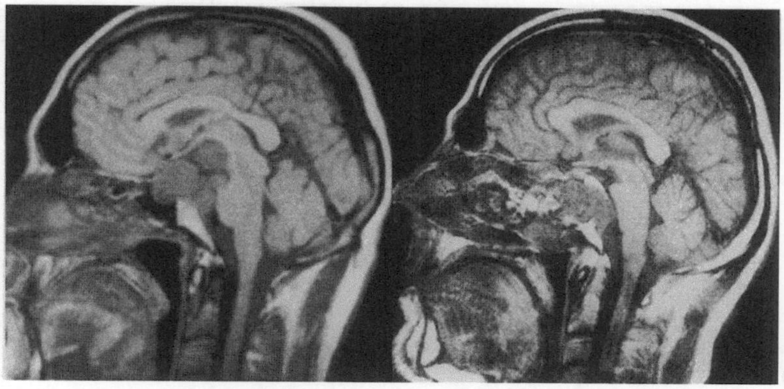

a b

Fig. 10.80. **a** Chondroma in a 28-year-old man with complete ophthalmoplegia and visual field defects. Well-delineated, nodular tumor with prolonged T1 and T2 in the parasellar and retrosellar region. Histology revealed moderate degree of anaplasia. Midsagittal scan, SE 0.7 s/30 ms (1.0 T). **b** Chondrosarcoma (recurrent tumor of a primary lesion of the sphenoid sinus) in a 34-year-old man with amaurosis of the left eye. Destruction of the clivus by a large, quite homogeneous mass which displaces the pons and grows down to the epipharynx. Sagittal scan, SE 0.5 s/30 ms (1.5 T)

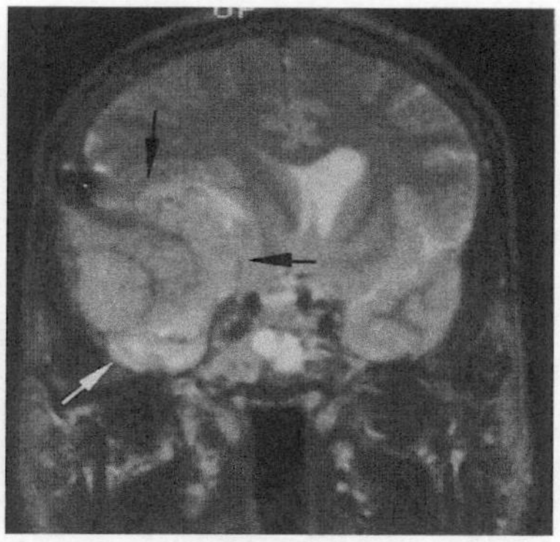

Fig. 10.81. Olfactory neuroblastoma *(arrows)*, recurrent tumor, in a 35-year-old man with hemiparesis. Coronal scan, 2.5 s/120 ms (1.0 T); after i.v. gadolinium-DTPA the tumor showed marked enhancement.

MR Findings

Experience with these rare tumors is limited. They destroy the bone of the paranasal sinuses and invade the neighboring structures, e.g., orbit, dura, and brain. The relaxation times may be slightly prolonged, and the structure of the lesion may be more or less homogeneous. Moderate enhancement may be seen with i.v. gadolinium-DTPA.

10.10.5 Adenoid Cystic Carcinomas

The rare adenoid cystic carcinomas (also known as cylindromas) arise from the columnar epithelium of the paranasal sinuses or eustachian tube. They can extend upward into the anterior fossa by eroding through the bony skull base and displace the brain like a meningioma. More commonly, however, they expand back toward the gasserian ganglion and middle fossa and may invade the cerebellopontine angle.

Pathology: These cellular epithelial tumors show regressive changes consisting of a colloid-filled network of small cysts. Anaplasia is rare, and invasion of the brain is unknown. The lesions are classified as semibenign (WHO grade 2).

MR Findings

Experience with these rare lesions is still limited. The few cases among our own material showed a signal hypointense to that of brain tissue in all sequences, similar to connective tissue; with i.v. gadolinium-DTPA marked enhancement was seen. The structure was slightly irregular, and in the case

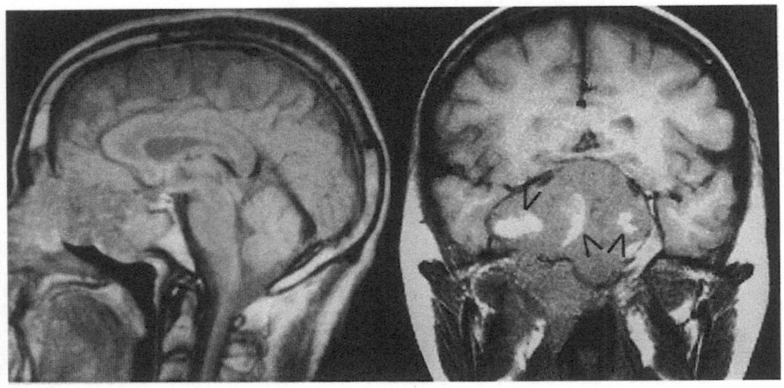

a b

Fig. 10.82 a, b. Adenoid cystic carcinoma. **a** In a 50-year-old man with repeated nosebleed. Ill-defined, solid tumor destroying the frontal skull base and paranasal bony structures, with irregularly low signal intensity in all sequences, **a** Midsagittal scan, SE 2.5 s/30 ms; (1.0 T). **b** in a 33-year-old woman with headache and bilateral exophthalmos. Huge mass invading the orbits and cranial cavity without penetrating the dura mater. Intratumoral hemorrhages *(arrowheads)* and cystic regressive changes are seen. There was marked tumor enhancement with i.v. gadolinium-DTPA. **b** Coronal scan, SE 0.7 s/30 ms, (1.0 T)

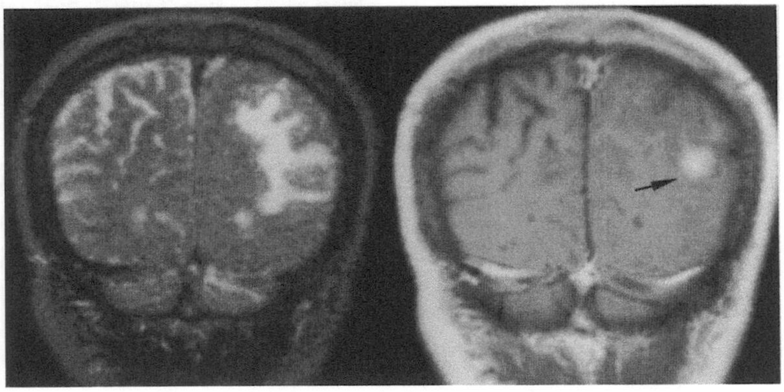

a b

Fig. 10.83 a, b. Metastasis of primary tumor of unknown site in a 57-year-old man with headache and slight hemiparesis. An occipital lesion *(arrow)* can only be identified on contrast enhancement (**b**); in the T2-weighted image (**a**) only the edema is seen. Coronal scans: **a** SE 2.5 s/120 ms, **b** SE 0.7 s/30 ms (1.0 T)

shown in Fig. 10.82b cystic regressive changes and tumor hemorrhages have occurred. The lesions have destroyed the bony membranes of the paranasal sinuses and invaded the orbits and the cranial cavity without penetrating the dura. See also Fig. 10.41.

10.11 Metastatic Tumors

Primary tumors that metastasize intracranially through hematogenous seeding are, in decreasing order of frequency, bronchial carcinomas, breast carcinomas, hypernephromas, malignant melanomas, and tumors of the gastrointestinal tract.

Incidence: Data on the incidence of solitary or multiple metastases range from 4% to 20%. Reports indicate that metastatic carcinoma, which occurs predominantly in the middle and higher decades, is more prevalent than sarcoma, which can develop in children and adolescents.

Sites: Metastatic tumors occur mostly in subcortical areas of the brain but are also found in the white matter, the CSF spaces, the suprasellar and parasellar regions, the quadrigeminal region, and the cerebellopontine angle.

Pathology: The histologic features of metastatic tumors are extremely variable. The metastasis may resemble the primary tumor, or it may be so anaplastic that it is difficult even for the pathologist to classify. Metastases usually present as sharply demarcated nodules or as cystic masses with ill-defined borders, but any intermediate state may be observed. The lesions may lie adjacent to the dura or form expansive, plaquelike growths in the CSF

Fig. 10.84. Metastasis of thyroid carcinoma in a 74-year-old woman who noticed a soft bulge on the back of her head. Midsagittal scan, SE 0.4 s/35 ms; (0.5 T). (Courtesy of Drs. Kuhn, Steen, and Terwey, Oldenburg, FRG)

Fig. 10.85. Metastasis of malignant peripheral neuroepithelioma in a 10-year-old boy with initial lesion of the scapula, now presenting with metastasis to the spine, headache, weakness on the right, and aphasia. Large, partly cystic tumor with irregular structure of the solid compartments, which contain hemosiderin deposits. Moderate enhancement was seen after i. v. gadolinium-DTPA. Axial scan, SE 3.0 s/ 120 ms; (1.0 T)

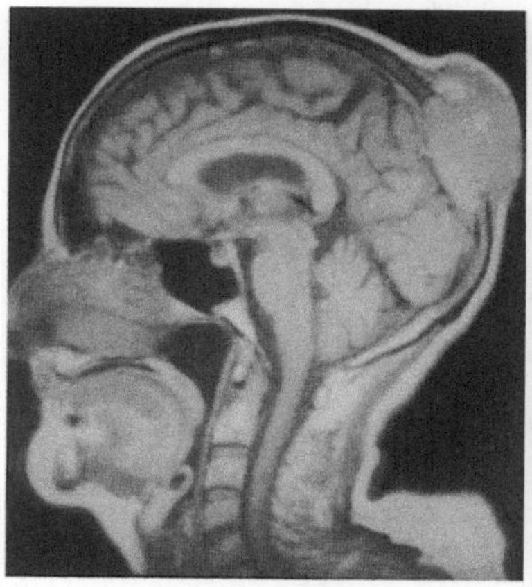

10.84

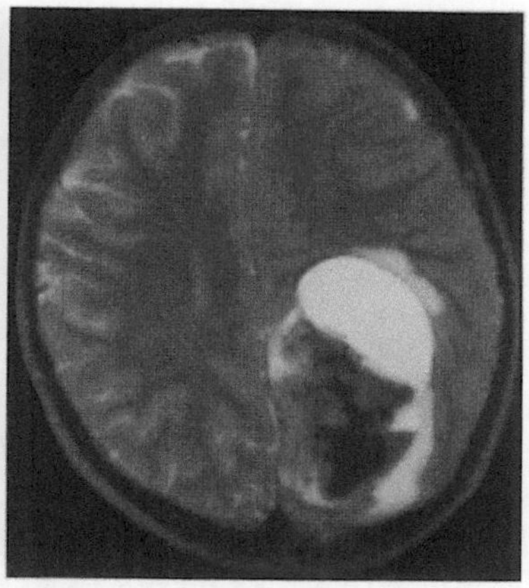

10.85

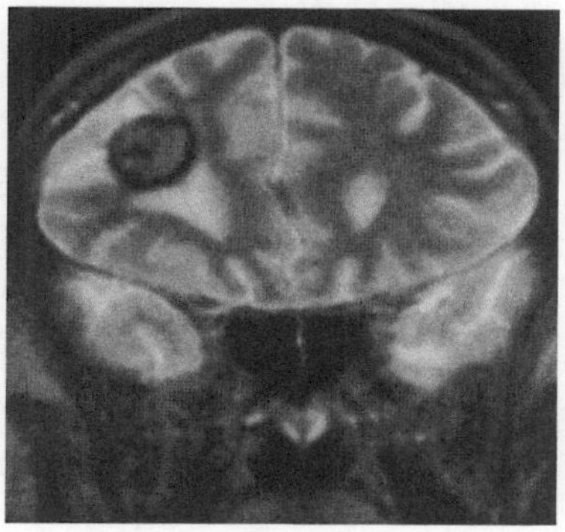

Fig. 10.86. Metastasis of primary extragonadal, embryonal carcinoma in a 27-year-old man with focal seizure. Nodular lesion of frontal lobe with dark ring of hemosiderin deposits and irregular center; slight perifocal edema. Multiple metastases of the spine were also found. Coronal scan, SE 2.5 s/ 120 ms (1.0 T)

space. Regressive changes with liquefaction can mimic the appearance of an abscess.

Hemorrhages occur mostly in metastases of hypernephromas, melanomas, and chorionic epitheliomas [66].

A striking feature of metastases is the frequent occurrence of perifocal edema that is quite extensive in relation to the size of the lesion. However, some metastases are unaccompained by an edematous zone.

MR Findings

T2-weighted MR sequences are better than CT for detecting metastases because of their ability to demonstrate even small increases in relaxation times. Small metastases are usually identified from their accompanying edema. The prolongation of relaxation times in the tumor itself is less pronounced than in the edema, often making it possible to differentiate edema and tumor on T2-weighted scans (e.g., multiecho sequences). With leptomeningeal seeding of the metastases, there is a danger that the isointense CSF signal will mask the changes on T2-weighted as well as T1-weighted images (see Fig. 11.16).

In the rare cases where edema is absent, an isointense tumor may escape detection. But because metastases lack a blood-brain barrier, contrast material generally will provide marked enhancement of the lesion on T1-weighted sequences. We feel, therefore, that *the use of contrast material is essential for the exclusion of cerebral metastases* (Fig. 10.83). After the administration of contrast material, metastases will present a nodular, ringlike, or garlandlike structure. Usually, multiple sites of occurrence must be demonstrated before a confident

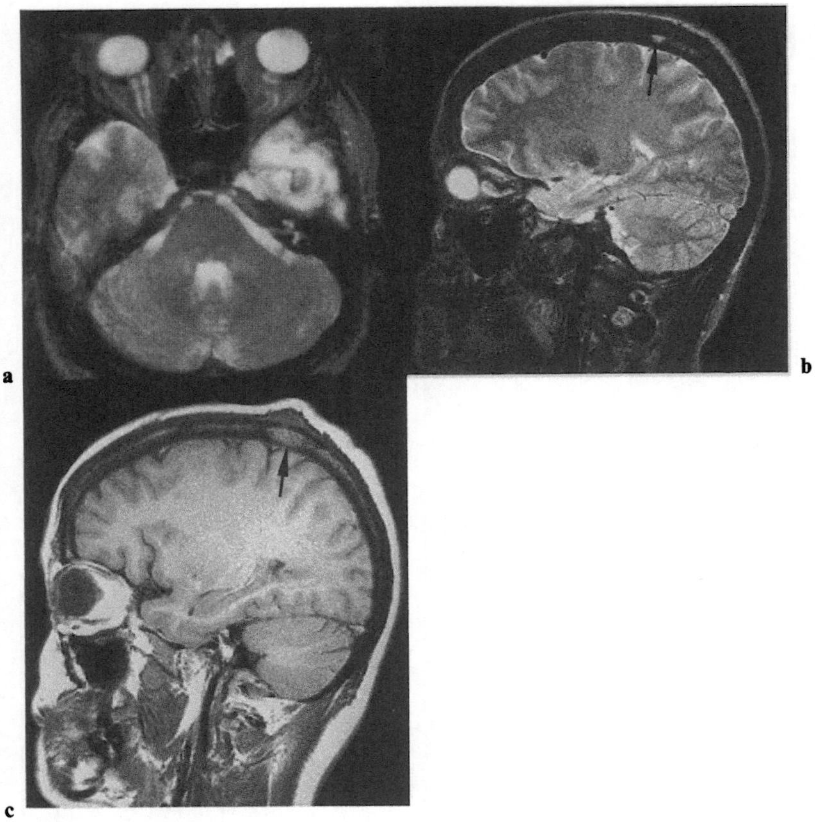

Fig. 10.87 a–c. Metastasis of malignant melanoma in a 52-year-old man with headache and one seizure. Nodular lesion in the temporal lobe with moderate edema. Axial scan: **a** SE 3.0 s/120 ms (1.0 T). **b, c** Malignant melanoma in a 33-year-old woman with a right parietal bump (*arrow in* **c**). Two months earlier only a small, unspecific hyperintensity of the diploe was seen (*arrow* in **b**). Sagittal scans: **b** SE 3.0 s/90 ms, **c** SE 0.6 s/15 ms (1.5 T)

diagnosis of metastases can be made. The multifocal occurrence of neuroepithelial brain tumors (e.g., glioblastomas) is far less common.

Hemorrhages (subacute to chronic) are recognized by their high signal intensity in T1-weighted sequences (see Sect. 5.2).

In the case of larger hemorrhages, it is possible for the metastasis to be obscured by hematoma. If doubt exists, follow-up scans should be performed with use of contrast material. Because old blood and enhancing metastases both give high signals on T1-weighted scans, evaluation can be difficult. It may be helpful in these cases to perform contrast CT in the hypodense phase of a hemorrhage, although the picture is somewhat confused by enhancing, hyperemic granulation tissue at the periphery of the hematoma.

When metastases are suspected, differentiation is required from other types of multifocal lesion, such as glioblastomas, sarcomas, meningiomas, abscesses, granulomas, and parasitic cysts.

Metastatic melanomas can have an MR appearance that differs from the metastases of other primaries. (Fig. 10.87) Paramagnetic, stable free radicals in the melanin can shorten the T1 and T2 relaxation times, causing the lesions to appear dark on the conventional T2-weighted sequence and light on T1-weighted sequences [4, 60]. This can cause uncertainty in the differentiation of fatty tissue, e.g., in the orbit.

In dural carcinomatosis, which occurs predominantly with carcinoma of the breast, small cell cancer of the lung, or lymphoma, a crescent-shaped lesion of intermediate signal intensity on both T1-weighted and T2-weighted images has been described [57]. This is not characteristic of either subdural hematoma or empyema (see Fig. 11.16).

10.12 Pseudotumor Cerebri

The term pseudotumor cerebri denotes a rise of intracranial pressure due not to the presence of a tumor but to a general expansion of the brain volume. The pathogenic mechanism is not yet understood. Possible causes are sinus thrombosis, intoxication, and endocrine or metabolic disorders, especially after prolonged steroid therapy and its sudden withdrawal. Contraceptive use also has been implicated.

MR Findings

So far there are no reports of MR imaging of pseudotumor cerebri. Given the pathology of the condition, one would expect to find diffuse, fairly pronounced increases in T1 and T2 with compression of the internal and external CSF spaces.

References

1. Afra D, Müller W, Slowik F, Firsching R (1986) Supratentorial lobar pilocytic astrocytoma: report of 45 operated cases, including 9 recurrences. Acta Neurochir (Wien) 81: 90-93
2. Altman N, Fitz CR, Chuang S, Harwood-Nash D, Coffer C, Armstrong D (1985) Radiological characteristics of primitive neuroectodermal tumors in children. AJNR 6: 15-18
3. Asa SL, Kovacs K (1983) Histological classification of pituitary disease. Clin Endocrinol Metab 12 (3): 567-596
4. Atlas SW, Grossman RI, Hackney DB, Goldberg HI, Bilaniuk LT, Zimmerman RA (1986) MR imaging in intracranial metastatic melanoma. Presented at the RSNA '86, Chicago
5. Baily O, Cushing H (1926) A classification of tumors of the glioma group. Lippincott, Philadelphia
6. Baily O, Cushing H (1930)
7. Becker LE, Hinto D (1983) Primitive neuroectodermal tumours of the central nervous system. Hum Pathol 16: 538-550
8. Berry I, Brant-Zawadzki M, Osaki L, Brasch R, Murovic J, Newton TH (1986) Gd-DTPA in clinical MR of the brain: 2. Extraaxial lesions and normal structures. AJNR 7: 789-793
9. Brant-Zawadzki M, Kelly W (1986) Brain tumors. In: Brant-Zawadzki M, Norman D (eds) Magnetic resonance imaging of the central nervous system. Raven, New York, pp 151-186
10. Breger RK, Papke RA, Haughton VM, Williams AL, Daniels DL, Pojunas KW (1986) Gadolinium enhancement of extraaxial neoplasms. Presented at the RSNA '86, Chicago
11. Busch W (1951) Die Morphologie der Sella turcica und ihre Beziehungen zur Hypophyse. Virchows Arch 320: 437-458
12. Chatel M, Darcel F, de Certaines J, Benoist L, Bernard AM (1986) T1 and T2 proton nuclear magnetic resonance (NMR) relaxation times in vitro and in human intracranial tumors. J Neurooncol 3: 315-321
13. Daniels DL, Pojunas KW, Kilgore DP, Pech P, Meyer GA, Williams AL, Haughton VM (1986) MR of the diaphragma sellae. AJNR 7: 765-769
14. Dwyer AJ, Frank JA, Oldfield EH, Hickey AM, Cutler GB, Loriaux DL, Schiable TF, Doppman JL (1986) Gd-DTPA-enhanced MR imaging in the evaluation of pituitary adenomas. Presented at the RSNA '86, Chicago
15. Donaldson JO, Simon RH (1980) Radiodense ions within a third ventricle colloid cyst. Arch Neurol 37: 246-248
16. Earnest F IV, Kelly PJ, Scheithauer B, Kall B, Cascino TL, Ehman EL, Forbes G (1986) Pathologic contrast enhancement of cerebral lesions: a comparative study using stereotactic CT, stereotactic MR imaging, and stereotactic biopsy. Presented at the RSNA '86, Chicago
17. Fahlbusch R, Buchfelder M, Schrell U (1985) Neurochirurgische Therapie neuroendokrinologischer Störungen. Internist (Berlin) 26: 293-301
18. Fahlbusch R, Schrell U, Buchfelder M (1985) Neurochirurgische Behandlung von Adenomen der Hypophyse. Ein Bericht über 200 Patienten an der Neurochirurgischen Klinik der Universität Erlangen in den Jahren 1983/84. Nervenheilkunde 4: 7-16
19. Fujisawa I, Nishimura K, Asato R, Tagashi K, Itoh K, Noma S, Kawamura Y, Sago T, Minami S, Nakano Y, Itoh H, Torizuka K (1987) Posterior lobe of the pituitary in diabetes insipidus: MR findings. J Comput Assist Tomogr 11 (2): 221-225
20. Graif M, Pennock JM (1986) MR imaging of histiocytosis X in the central nervous system. AJNR 7: 21-23
21. Hardy J (1969) Transsphenoidal microsurgery of the normal and pathological pituitary. Clin Neurosurg 16: 185-217
22. Hilal SK, Ra BJ, Silver AJ, Mun IK (1985) In vivo sodium imaging using a very short echo time: potential for selective imaging in intracellular sodium and extracellular space. Radiology 157: 188
23. Hirano A (1983) Praktischer Leitfaden der Neuropathologie. Springer, Berlin Heidelberg New York
24. Huk WJ, Fahlbusch R (1985) Nuclear magnetic resonance imaging of the region of the sella turcica. Neurosurg Rev 8: 141-150
25. Isherwood I, Pullan BR, Rutherford RA, Strang FA (1977) Electron density and atomic number determination by computed tomography. Br J Radiol 50: 613-619
26. Karnaze MG, Sartor K, Winthrop JD, Gado MH, Hodges FJ (1986) Suprasellar lesions: evaluation with MR imaging. Radiology 161: 77-82
27. Kelly PJ, Daumas-Duport C, Kispert DB, Kall BA, Scheithauer BW, Illig JJ (1987) Imaging-based stereotaxic serial biopsies in untreated intracranial glial neoplasms. J Neurosurg 66: 865-874
28. Kernohan JW, Mabon RF, Svien HJ, Adson AW (1949) A simplified classification of the gliomas. Symposium on a new simplified concept of gliomas. Proc Staff Meet Mayo Clin 24: 71-75
29. Kernohan JW, Sayre GP (1952) Tumors of the central nervous system. Atlas of tumor pathology, section 10, fasc 35. Armed Forces Institute of Pathology, Washington DC
30. Kilgore DP, Strother CM, Starshak RJ, Haughton VM (1986) Pineal germinoma: MR imaging. Radiology 158: 435-438
31. Kornmesser W, Laniado M, Niendorf HP, Deimling M, Felix R (1986) Dynamic MR imaging of intracranial tumors: fast imaging and Gd-DTPA enhancement. Presented at the RSNA '86, Chicago
32. Kucharczyk W (1986) The pituitary gland and sella turcica. In: Brant-Zawadzki M, Norman D (eds) Magnetic resonance imaging of the central nervous system. Raven, New York, pp 187-208
33. Kucharczyk W, Davis DO, Kelly WM, Sze G, Norman D, Newton TH (1986) Pituitary adenomas: high-resolution MR imaging at 1.5 T. Radiology 161: 761-765
34. Kucharczyk W, Kelly WM, Davis DO, Norman D, Newton TH (1986) Intracranial lesions: flow-related enhance-

ment on MR images using time-of-flight effects. Radiology 161: 767-772
35. Kucharczyk W (1987) The pituitary and sella turcica. In: Brant-Zawadzki M, Norman D (eds) Magnetic resonance imaging of the central nervous system. Raven, New York, pp 187-208
36. Landolt AM, Osterwalder V (1984) Perivascular fibrosis in prolactinomas: is it increased by Bromocriptine? J Clin Endocrinol Metab 58: 1179-1183
37. MacKay IM, Bydder GM, Young IR (1985) MR imaging of central nervous system tumors that do not display increase in T1 or T2. J Comput Assist Tomogr 9 (6): 1055-1061
38. Mamourian AC, Towfighi J (1986) Pineal cysts: MR imaging. AJNR 7: 1081-1086
39. Mark L, Pech P, Daniels D, Williams A, Haughton V (1984) The pituitary fossa: a correlative anatomic and MR study. Radiology 153: 453-457
40. Mikhael MA, Ciric IS, Wolff AP (1985) Differentiation of cerebellopontine angle neuromas and meningiomas with MR imaging. J Comput Assist Tomogr 9: 852-856
41. Morrison G, Sobel DF, Kelley WM, Norman D (1984) Intraventricular mass lesions. Radiology 153: 435-442
42. Nishimura K, Fujisawa I, Togashi K, Itoh K, Nakano Y, Itoh H, Torizuka K (1986) Posterior lobe of the pituitary: identification by lack of chemical shift artefact in MR imaging. J Comput Assist Tomogr 10 (6): 899-902
43. Nistor R (1989) Diagnostische Wertigkeit und therapeutische Konsequenzen der Kernresonanztomographie in der Neuroendokrinologie. Thesis, University of Erlangen-Nürnberg
44. Numaguchi Y, Conolly ES, Kumra AK, Vargas EF, Gum GK, Mizushima A (1987) Computed tomography and MR imaging of thalamic neuroepithelial cysts. J Comput Assist Tomogr 11 (4): 583-585
45. Oot RF, New PF, Pile-Spellman J, Rosen BR, Shoukimas GM, Davis KR (1986) The detection of intracranial calcifications by MR. AJNR 7: 801-809
46. Petermann SB, Steiner RE, Bydder GM (1984) Magnetic resonance imaging of intracranial tumors in children and adolescents. AJNR 5: 703-709
47. Pojunas KW, Daniels DL, Williams AL, Haughton VM (1985) MR imaging of prolactin-secreting microadenomas. AJNR 7: 209-213
48. Randell RV, Clark RC, Bahn RC (1960) Classification of the causes of diabetes insipidus. Mayo Clin Proc 34: 299-302
49. Rubinstein LJ (1972) Tumors of the central nervous system. In: Rubinstein LJ (ed) Atlas of tumor pathology, 2nd series, fasc 6. Armed Forces Institute of Pathology, Washington DC, pp 160-198
50. Russell DS, Rubinstein LJ (1977) Pathology of tumors of the nervous system. Willimas and Wilkins, Baltimore
51. Sano K, Wakai S, Ochiai C, Takakura K (1981) Characteristics of intracranial meningiomas in childhood. Childs Brain 8: 98-106
52. Schroeder BA, Samaraweera RN, Starshak RJ, Oechler HW (1987) Intraparenchymal meningioma in a child: CT and MR findings. J Comput Assist Tomogr 11 (1): 192-200
53. Scotti G, Scialfa G, Colombo N, Landoni L (1987) MR in the diagnosis of colloid cysts of the third ventricle. AJNR 8: 370-372
54. Snow RB, Lavyne MH, Lee BCP, Morgello S, Patterson RH (1986) Craniotomy versus transsphenoidal excision of large pituitary tumors: the usefulness of MRI in guiding the operative approach. Neurosurgery 19 (1): 59-64
55. Spagnoli MV, Goldberg HI, Grossman RI, Bilaniuk LT, Gomori JM, Hackney DB, Zimmerman RA (1986) Intracranial meningiomas. Radiology 161: 369-375
56. Spagnoli MV, Grossman RI, Packer RJ, Hackney DB, Goldberg HI, Zimmerman RA, Bilaniuk LT (1987) Magnetic resonance imaging determination of gliomatosis cerebri. Neuroradiology 29: 15-18
57. Tyrvell RL, Bundschuh CV, Modic MT (1987) Dural carcinomatosis: MR demonstration. J Comput Assist Tomogr 11 (2): 329-332
58. Virchow R (1847) Zur Entwicklungsgeschichte des Krebses. Virchows Arch (A) 1: 94 (cited by Zülch KJ [66]
59. Weissbuch SS (1986) Explanation and implications of MR signal changes within pituitary adenomas after Bromocriptin therapy. AJNR 7: 214-216
60. Woodruff WW, Djang WT, McLendon RE, Heinz ER, Voorhees DR (1986) High-field MR imaging of intracranial melanoma. Presented at the RSNA '86, Chicago
61. Yuh WTC, Barloon TJ, Jacoby CG (1987) Trigeminal nerve lipomas: MR findings. J Comput Assist Tomogr 11 (3): 518-521
62. Zimmerman RA, Bilaniuk LT (1982) Age-related incidence of pineal calcifications detected by computed tomography. Radiology 142: 659-662
63. Zimmerman RA, Fleming CA, Saint-Louis LA, Lee BCP, Manning JJ, Deck MDF (1985) Magnetic resonance imaging of meningiomas. AJNR 6: 149-157
64. Zülch KJ (1957) Brain tumors. Their biology and pathology. 1st edn. Springer, New York
65. Zülch KJ (1979) Histological typing of tumors of the central nervous system. World Health Organization, Geneva (International histological classification of tumors, no 21)
66. Zülch KJ (1986) Brain tumors: their biology and pathology, 3rd edn. Springer, Berlin Heidelberg New York

11 Tumors of the Posterior Fossa

D. BALERIAUX and G. MICHELOZZI
With the collaboration of C. CHRISTOPHE, P. HAESENDONCK, M. LEMORI,
S. LOURYAN, G. RODESCH, and C. SEGEBARTH

MR imaging has a major role in the examination of central nervous structures in the posterior fossa [3, 5, 13, 23, 25, 30, 40, 42, 49, 51, 52, 65], where bone artifact seriously limits the effectiveness of CT for soft tissue evaluation. CT remains the primary modality, however, for imaging the bony structures of the petrous pyramid and skull base [26, 66].

The absence of radiation hazard makes MR imaging ideal for the examination of children, in whom 50% of brain tumors are located in the posterior fossa. In this section we shall describe the MR appearances of tumors of the brainstem and cerebellar hemispheres, extra-axial tumors, and diseases that are important in the differential diagnosis of these lesions.

11.1 Intra-axial Tumors

11.1.1 Tumors of the Brainstem

Incidence: Gliomas of the brainstem are relatively common in children, comprising 25% of all space-occupying lesions of the posterior fossa. In adults, neoplastic changes of the brainstem are far more likely to be metastatic in nature (Fig. 11.1). Brainstem gliomas are manifested clinically by progressive bilateral cranial nerve deficits, pyramidal tract signs, and cerebellar symptoms. Obstruction of CSF flow with hydrocephalus is a late event.

Sites: Gliomas of the brainstem show a predilection for the pontine region [25], from which they spread upward, downward, or possibly in both directions [40]. Isolated gliomas can occur in the mesencephalon, in the tectum mesencephali, or even at the bulbar level [30, 59]. They can also spread through the cerebral peduncles to the thalamus and hypothalamus and form exophytic lobulations.

Pathology: The gross and histologic features of brainstem gliomas correspond to those described for gliomas in general (see p. 230). Regressive changes such as calcifications and cyst formation are rare.

CT and MR Findings

Brainstem gliomas appear hypodense or, less commonly, isodense on CT scans. On postcontrast scans the tumors may show nodular, ringlike, or patchy enhancement, which generally indicates a high degree of anaplasia (see Fig. 11.3).

With MR, direct sagittal scans are excellent for evaluating the bulbomesencephalic profile and measuring the brainstem diameter [20, 23, 25, 35] in order to detect the circumscribed or diffuse expansions that are so commonly associated with tumor infiltration (91% of cases in our experience) (Fig. 11.2) [40]. Sagittal scans also give information on the status of the cerebral aqueduct [59], the fourth ventricle, and the prepontine cistern, demonstrating any compression or constriction of these spaces by exophytic tumor growth (Fig. 11.3) [30, 70, 71].

Most brainstem tumors are recognized by their increased relaxation times T1 and T2 [5, 30, 40, 42, 51]. Tumors giving an isointense signal on T1-weighted and T2-weighted images are less common [51].

Areas of tumor infiltration giving low signals on T1-weighted scans are more clearly demarcated and of smaller extent than the hyperintense areas on T2-weighted scans, which blend the tumor and edematous zone [5, 49, 61, 65]. This is especially true of tumors infiltrating the brainstem. The use of gadolinium-DTPA is helpful only in selected cases, because enhancement is not often seen [51] and indicates only zones where the blood-brain barrier is disrupted, without defining the true limits of tumor infiltration [11, 22, 32] (Fig. 11.3).

We have often (43%) seen isointense signals on T1-weighted images in cases where T2-weighted images consistently showed increased signals whose

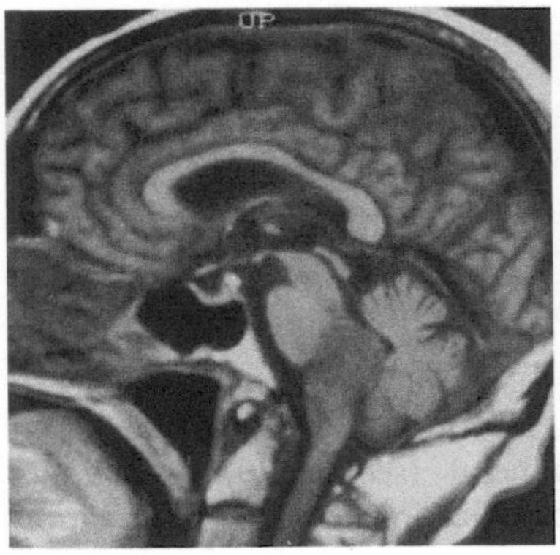

11.1

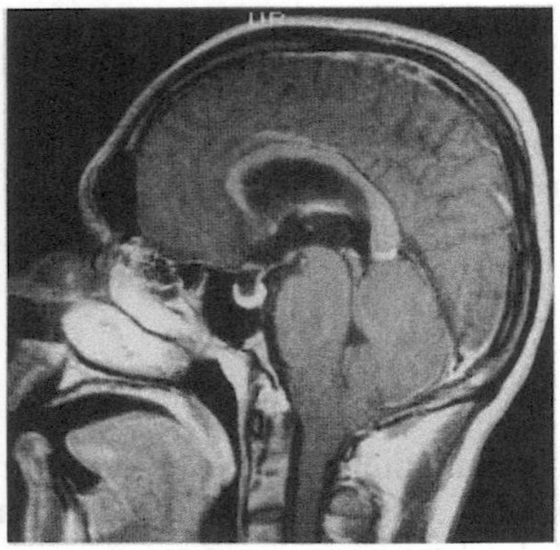

11.2

Fig. 11.1. Metastasis of the brainstem in a 76-year-old man with multiple metastases of lung cancer. Hypointense mass lesion bulging into the fourth ventricle. Midsagittal scan, SE 0.4 s/17 ms (1.0 T)

Fig. 11.2. Fibrillary astrocytoma (WHO grade 2) of the brainstem in a 25-year-old man with slowly progressive spasticity, latent cranial nerve palsy, and nausea. Diffuse swelling of the brainstem without enhancement after i.v. gadolinium. On T2-weighted images an ill-defined hyperintensity of the midbrain, pons, cerebellar peduncles, and medulla oblongata was seen. Diagnosis confirmed by stereotaxic biopsy. Midsagittal scan SE 0.6 s/15 ms; (1.5 T)

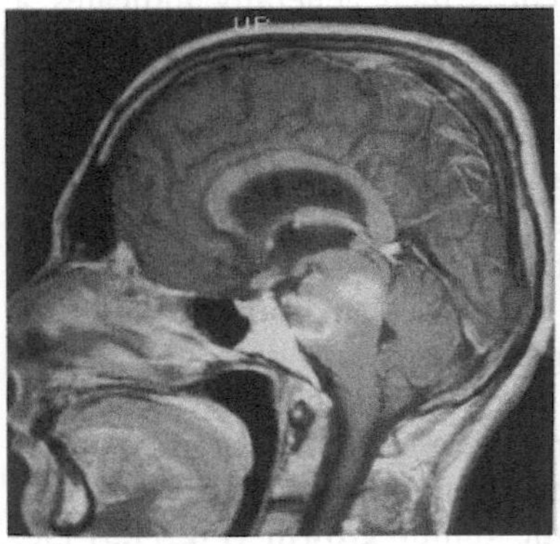

11.3

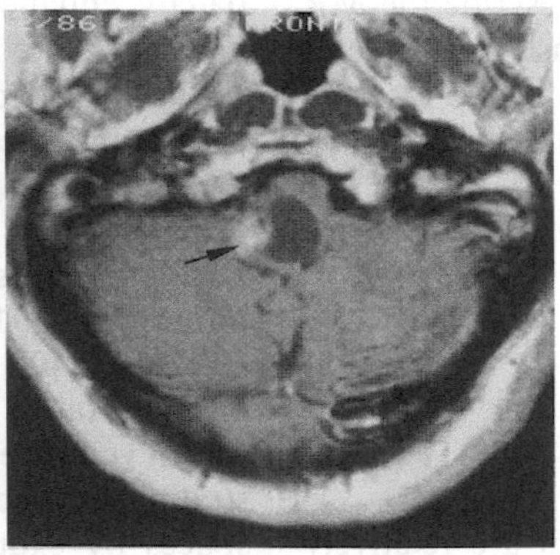

11.4

Fig. 11.3. Glioblastoma (WHO grade 4) of the brainstem (biopsy) in a 30-year-old man with rapidly progressive cranial nerve palsies, spasticity, and nausea. Diffuse enlargement of brainstem with focal enhancement after i.v. gadolinium. Sagittal scans, SE 0.6 s/15 ms (1.5 T)

Fig. 11.4. Pilocytic astrocytoma (WHO grade 1) of the brainstem with cysts. With gadolinium-DTPA the solid tumor portions enhance *(arrow)*. Axial, scan, SE 0.7 s/30 ms (1.0 T)

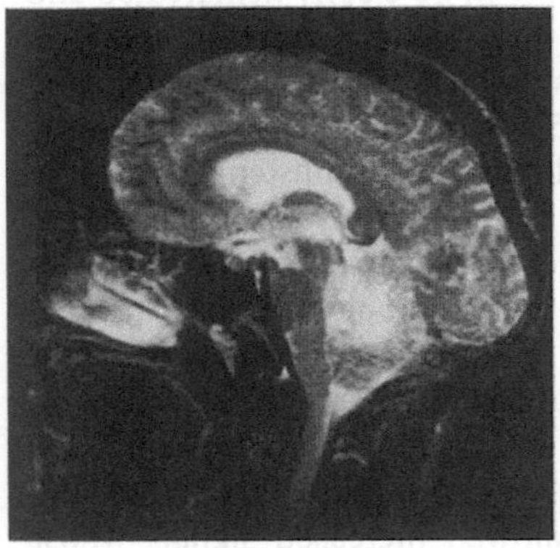

11.5

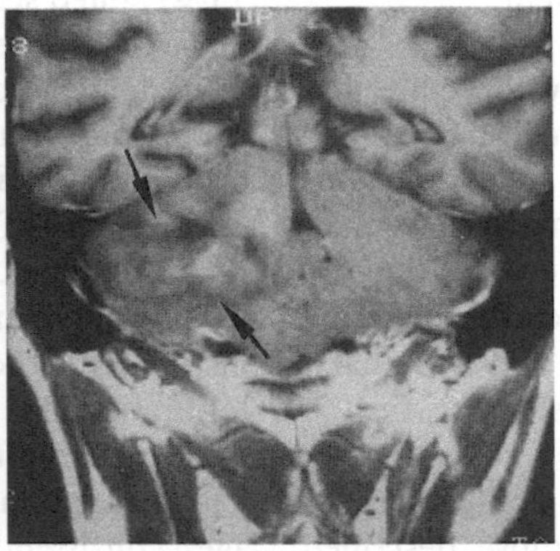

11.6

Fig. 11.5. Medulloblastoma in a 29-year-old man with unsteady gait and early signs of intracranial hypertension. Ill-defined, slightly inhomogeneous mass with prolonged T1 and T2 in the roof of the fourth ventricle. Midsagittal scan SE 1.2 s/100 ms (0.5 T)

Fig. 11.6. Medulloblastoma in a 36-year-old man with vertigo, nystagmus, and unsteady gait. Ill-defined patchy mass with only small enhancing portions after i.v. gadolinium *(arrow)*. Coronal scan, SE 0.45 s/15 ms (1.5 T)

intensity varied with the degree of T2 weighting. In 90% of cases the signal intensity was increased in the second echo compared with the first echo (50 ms); in 10% the signal increase was not pronounced or even absent (Fig. 11.2). No correlation is apparent between this variable signal pattern and the histology of the lesions.

Cystic components [34] and areas of intratumoral necrosis are characterized by prolonged T1 and T2 compared with solid tumor components (Fig. 11.4). Calcifications, which give low signals in T1-weighted and T2-weighted images, are rarely seen in infiltrating lesions of the brainstem [30, 38]. Sites of intratumoral hemorrhage [30, 51] are easily identified by their increased signal on T1-weighted and T2-weighted images (see Sect. 5.2).

11.1.2 Cerebellar Tumors

Like the brainstem, the cerebellum is a relatively common site of primary tumor involvement in children, whereas cerebellar tumors in adults are generally metastatic. Medulloblastoma, astrocytoma, ependymoma, and metastases (Figs. 11.16, 11.17) are the most common forms [27, 34, 50, 52, 65]. Lymphomas are also seen (see Figs. 10.43, 10.44).

Dermoid tumors (Fig. 11.28) [65], teratomas, lipomas, choroid plexus papillomas [58], hemangioblastomas ([53], von Hippel-Lindau disease) (see Figs. 11.14, 11.15), gangliogliomas, hamartomas [50], and histiocytosis X are less frequent, although the cerebellar fossa is a preferred site for their occurrence.

Medulloblastoma

Medulloblastoma, a poorly differentiated, primitive tumor, is the prime cerebellar malignancy of childhood and adolescence. The collective term medulloblastoma encompasses two subtypes: desmoplastic medulloblastoma and medullomyoblastoma. The biologic behavior of these tumors places them in WHO grade 4.

Incidence: Medulloblastomas comprise about 20% of all brain tumors in children and adolescents and 8.8% of tumors after 20 years of age [72].

Sites: The usual site of medulloblastoma in children is on the midline on the roof of the fourth ventricle and in the inferior vermis of the cerebellum (Fig. 11.5). From there the tumor spreads in all directions. Predominant involvement of one cerebellar hemisphere is common in older children, and eventually the tumor sends exophytic extensions into the surrounding cisterns. Desmoplastic medulloblastoma typically occurs as a nodular growth in the cerebellar hemispheres of older adolescents, but may also be ill-defined and of irregular structure (Fig. 11.6).

Pathology: Medulloblastomas are moderately demarcated tumors that show infiltrative growth at their margins. They are permeated by connective tissue to varying degrees. Histologically they are extremely cellular, relatively hypovascular, and show little tendency to undergo regressive changes. Foci of necrosis or fatty degeneration are occasionally found at the tumor core; calcification and cyst formation are uncommon. When the tumor reaches the subarachnoid space, seeding via the cerebrospinal pathway can occur within the ventricular system, in the extracerebral subarachnoid space, and throughout the spinal canal. These metastases (drop metastases) can appear as nodular, or plaquelike growths. Metastasis to other body organs has also been described [72].

Desmoplastic medulloblastoma consists of islets of cells surrounded by a network of reticulin fibers.

Medullomyoblastomas contain cellular elements of nonstriated and striated muscle.

Pilocytic Astrocytoma

Incidence: Pilocytic astrocytoma of the cerebellum (see p. 235) is the most common cerebellar neoplasm, accounting for about 6% of all brain tumors and 30% of pediatric gliomas. Its peak incidence occurs between 8 and 15 years of age. It is classified as WHO grade 1 because of its slow rate of growth.

Sites: These tumors arise in the middle vermis region of the cerebellum (Figs. 11.7, 11.8), whence they spread into the hemispheres, infiltrate the pons and medulla (see Fig. 11.4), and finally invade the upper cervical cord.

Pathology: Most pilocytic astrocytomas are encapsulated and grow mainly by expansion, with some infiltration peripherally (Fig. 11.8). They very often contain multiple small cysts or a few large cysts with protein-rich contents which, unlike angioblastoma, may be enclosed by only a narrow rim of tumor (Fig. 11.9). Solid forms are less common. Calcifications and residues of small hemorrhages are

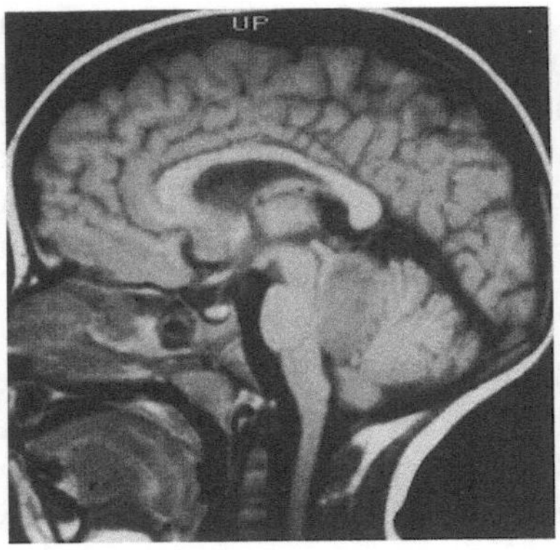

11.7

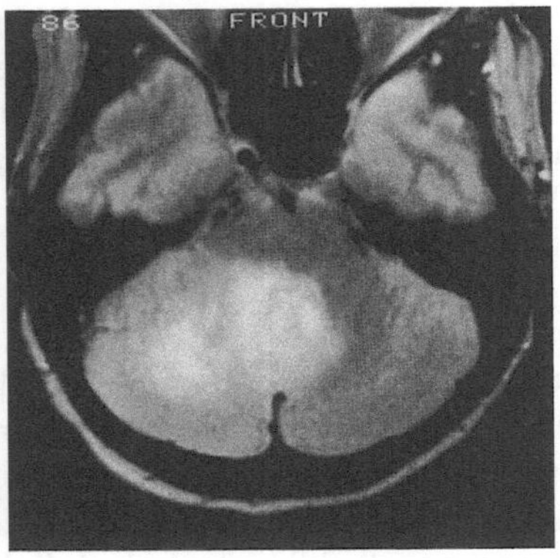

11.8

Fig. 11.7. Pilocytic astrocytoma (WHO grade 1) in a 6-year-old girl with vertigo and gait disturbances. Well-delineated, homogeneous lesion with prolonged relaxation times in the upper vermis and roof of the fourth ventricle. Midsagittal scan SE 0.7 s/30 ms (1.0 T)

Fig. 11.8. Pilocytic astrocytoma with localized areas of anaplastic astrocytoma (WHO grade 2–3) in a 53-year-old woman with vertigo, gait disturbances, weakness of right side, occasional double vision, and hydrocephalus. Large, ill-defined area of prolonged relaxation times in the lower vermis, lingula, and the central lobe of the upper vermis, and in the left cerebellar hemisphere. Axial scan, SE 3.0 s/45 ms, (1.0 T)

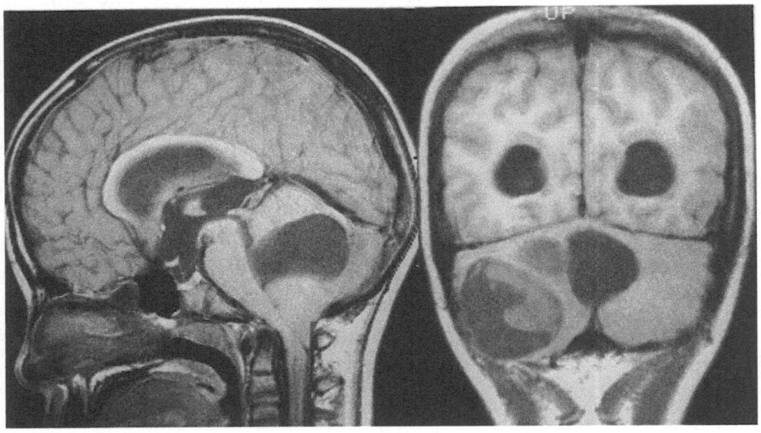

a b

Fig. 11.9 a, b. Cystic pilocytic astrocytoma (WHO grade 1) in a 13-year-old boy with headache and unsteady gait. Low position of cerebellar tonsils and compression of the outflow of the aqueduct. Midsagittal (**a**) and coronal (**b**) scans, SE 0.6 s/15 ms (1.5 T)

occasionally seen. Histologically the tumor consists of strands of isomorphic piloid cells that are permeated by an irregular stroma. Blood vessels are generally rare and may form angiomalike tangles. The tumor is not known to metastasize [72].

Ependymoma

Incidence: Ependymoma (see p. 238) is among the most common tumors of the posterior fossa, especially in childhood and adolescence.

Sites: Ependymomas arise in the vicinity of the ependyma, their major sites of occurrence being the fourth ventricle, the aqueduct, and the spinal cord. In the fourth ventricle the tumors are fused to the caudal portion of the rhomboid fossa, from which they expand into the fourth ventricle and surrounding cisterns and downward to the cervical cord.

Pathology: The benign form of ependymoma grows purely by expansion and presents a nodular surface (Figs. 11.10–11.12). Most ependymomas are extremely cellular and have a relatively homogeneous structure, although their histopathology shows some variations depending on the site of occurrence. Regressive changes are rare, cystic changes being somewhat more common than calcification, necrosis, or fatty degeneration.

The biologic behavior of ependymomas is variable and ranges from WHO grade 1 to grade 4, depending on the degree of anaplasia (Fig. 11.13). Spontaneous metastases are rare but are more common following surgery, in which case any part of the CNS may be affected.

Fig. 11.10. Ependymoma, subependymal form (WHO grade 1), in a 42-year-old woman with neck pain and flickering in front of both eyes. Nodular, enhancing, exophytic tumor; occlusive hydrocephalus. Sagittal scan SE 0.45 s/30 ms with i.v. gadolinium (1.5 T)

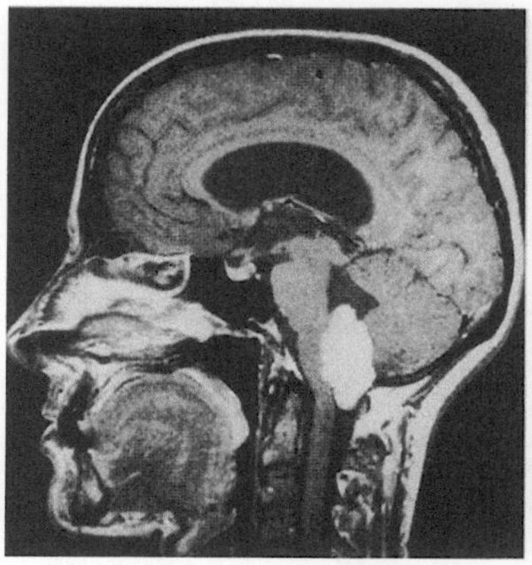

11.10

Fig. 11.11. Ependymoma (WHO grade 2) in a 2-year-old girl with unsteady gait, nausea, and vomiting. Recurrent tumor after partial removal, now infiltrating also the medulla and the cervical cord. Sagittal scan SE 0.6 s/26 ms (1.0 T)

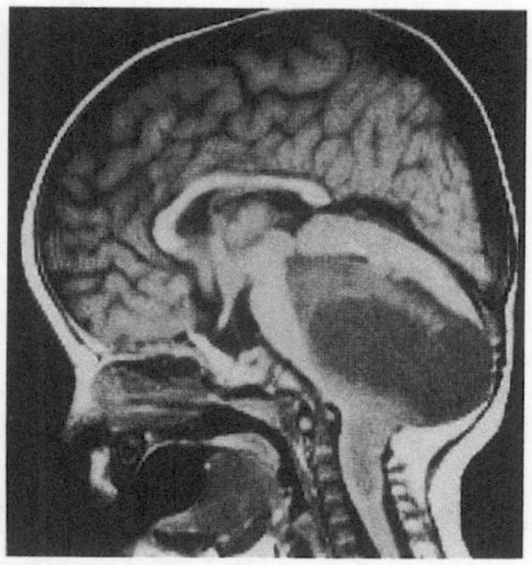

11.11

Fig. 11.12. Ependymoma (WHO grade 2) in a 4-year-old boy with unsteady gait, headache, and swallowing difficulties after partial removal of the tumor 1 year previously. Tumor recurrence in the floor of the brainstem invading the right cerebellar hemisphere *(arrow)*; hypointense lesion on T1-weighted images. Marked enhancement with i.v. gadolinium-DTPA. Coronal scan, SE 0.4 s/17 ms (1.0 T)

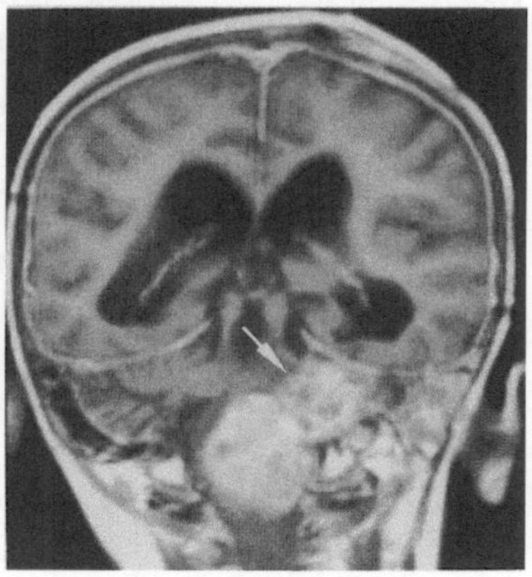

Fig. 11.13 a, b. Anaplastic ependymoma (WHO grade 3–4) in a 60-year-old man with progressive gait disturbances, double vision, vertigo, and nausea for 2 months. After i.v. gadolinium (**b**) the tumor and its structure are depicted more clearly. Coronal scans: **a** SE 2.5 s/120 ms, **b** 0.7 s/30 ms (1.0 T)

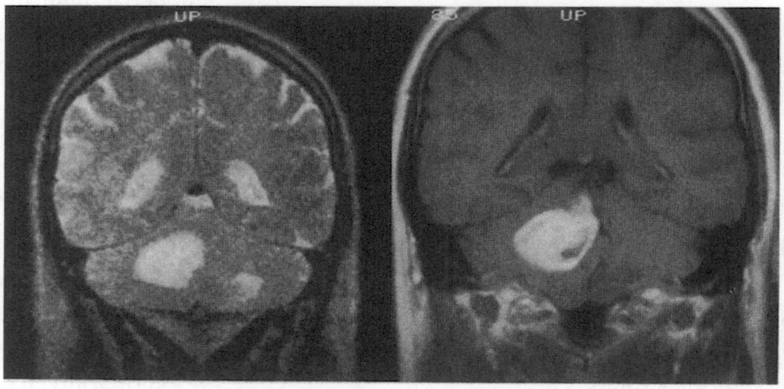

a b

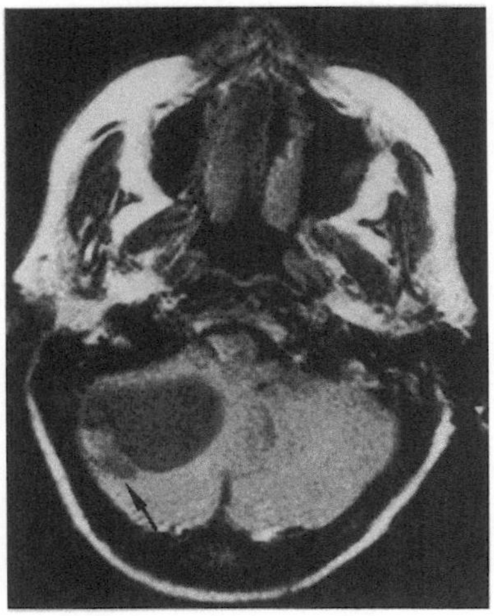

Fig. 11.14. Hemangioblastoma (Lindau's tumor) in a 59-year-old man with nausea, vomiting, and ataxic gait. Large cyst with tumor nodule *(arrow)* at its dorsolateral aspect. Axial scan, SE 0.6 s/50 ms (1.5 T)

a 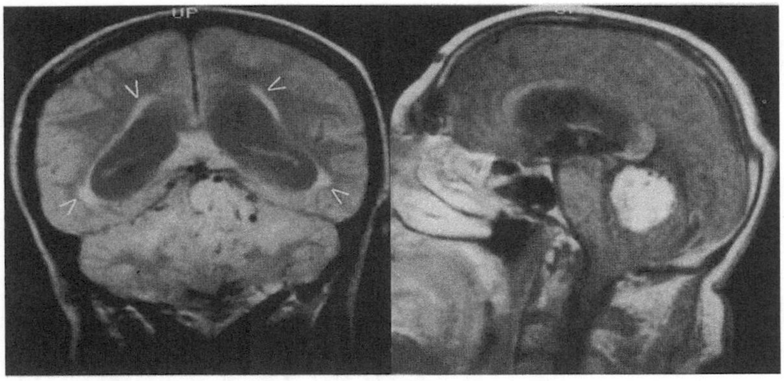 b

Fig. 11.15 a, b. Angioblastoma (WHO grade 1) in a 61-year-old man with disorder of balance and organic psychosyndrome. **a** Native scan: highly vascular tumor of the upper vermis which cannot be differentiated from its perifocal edema. **b** With i.v. gadolinium, marked enhancement of a solid, well-delineated tumor. Interstitial edema *(arrowheads)* is best seen in the proton-density image (**a**). Coronal scan, **a** SE 2.5 s/35 ms, midsagittal scan, **b** SE 0.7 s/30 ms (1.0 T)

Hemangioblastoma

The following forms of hemangioblastoma are recognized according to [72]:

1. Hemangioblastomas or Lindau's tumor as a solitary or multiple growth
2. Lindau's syndrome, involving a hemangioblastoma of the brain in association with renal and pancreatic cysts
3. Lindau's disease, an isolated, hereditary cerebellar angioblastoma
4. Von Hippel's disease, involving hereditary angiomatosis of the retina
5. Von Hippel-Lindau disease, a hereditary combination of angiomas of the retina and cerebellar angioblastomas

Incidence: Hemangioblastomas form about 1% of all intracranial tumors. They show a peak incidence between 35 and 45 years of age.

Sites: Sites in the posterior fossa include the cerebellar hemispheres, the cerebellar vermis, and the roof of the fourth ventricle. Spinal cord involvement is possible. Cerebral occurrence is less common.

Hemangioblastomas of the cerebellar hemispheres are usually cystic (Fig. 11.14), with a small, solid nub of tumor usually attached to the wall of a large, solitary cyst. Purely solid forms are rare (Fig. 11.15). In the fourth ventricle the tumor lies at the ventricular outlet, where it may be mistaken for a large tumor of the medulla. Tumors of the spinal cord may form elongated cysts that can mimic syringomyelia [72].

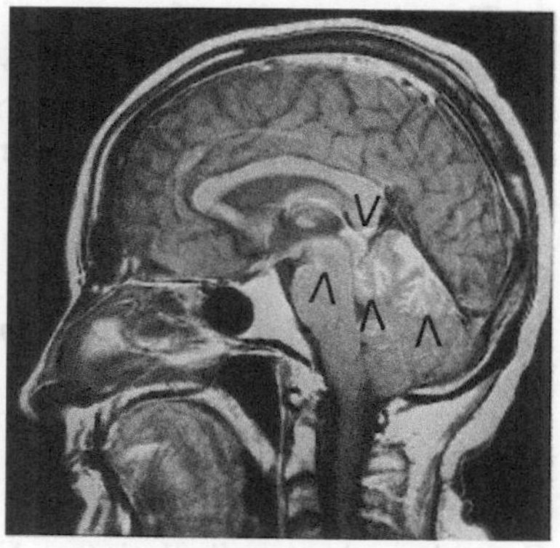

Fig. 11.16. Cerebellar metastasis and meningiomatosis carcinomatosa of the posterior fossa from an unknown primary tumor (CSF cytology: probably carcinoma of the colon) in a 56-year-old woman with dizziness, nausea, and unsteady gait. Only with i.v. gadolinium-DTPA can the spreading tumor in the subarachnoid space *(arrowheads)* be clearly demonstrated. Sagittal scan, SE 0.6 s/15 ms, (1.5 T)

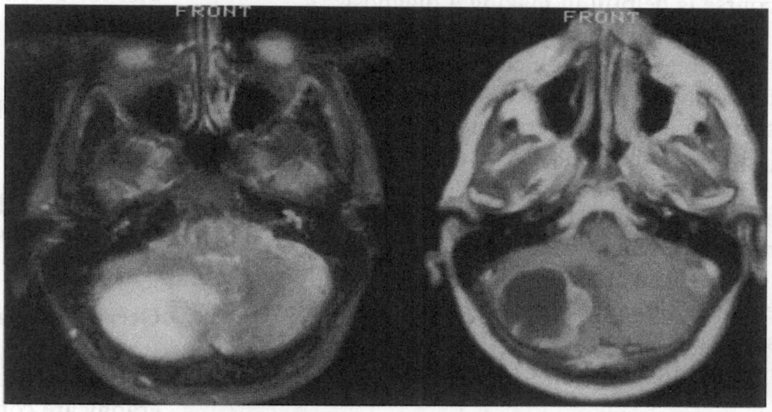

Fig. 11.17 a, b. Multiple metastases of the cerebellum in a 49-year-old man with bronchial carcinoma. With i.v. gadolinium (b) the structure of the lesions is revealed clearly. Axial scans: **a** SE 3.0 s/120 ms, **b** SE 0.4 s/17 ms (1.0 T)

Pathology: The contents of the large cysts are protein-rich and usually show traces of hemorrhage. The solid, nodular tumor component consists of a dense capillary network of large cavernous vessels (see Fig. 11.15). The growth rate is very slow, but the solid tumor infiltrates adjacent tissues. Calcification does not occur. The tumor is classified as WHO grade 1; anaplastic forms are unknown. Purely solid tumors imply a less favorable prognosis (Fig. 11.15) [72].

MR Findings in Cerebellar Tumors

Both direct and indirect signs contribute to the diagnosis of cerebellar tumors. Among the indirect signs, an obstruction of CSF flow, especially at the level of the fourth ventricle, is seen with greater frequency than with tumors of the brainstem. Involvement of the cerebellar tonsils or transtentorial extension is readily identified on sagittal and coronal T1-weighted MR images.

As a direct sign, cerebellar tumors usually produce an increase in T1 and T2, although the signal pattern is not specific enough for differential diagnosis. However, the morphologic features of the tumors permit an etiologic diagnosis to be made with some confidence based on the presence of cystic components, solid tumor nodules, calcification, fatty inclusions [41], and vascular elements, which are readily identified on the MR image. These features are described fully for the specific tumor types, and the reader is referred to the appropriate sections of the text (Sect. 11.1.2). As in CT, the sites of occurrence (e.g., vermis, hemisphere, fourth ventricle) and the enhancement that occurs after contrast injection are useful only as suggestive signs.

The characteristic features of hemangioblastoma are well demonstrated with MR [53]. Primitive neoplasms and metastatic tumors are difficult to differentiate. Both may be surrounded by extensive edema.

11.1.3 Differential Diagnosis of Intra-axial Expansive Lesions

Demyelinating Diseases

Central pontine myelinolysis (see Figs. 8.30, 8.31) appears as symmetric, oval-shaped areas of low signal intensity on T1-weighted images and as a somewhat more extensive zone of high signal intensity on T2-weighted images. Knowledge of the clinical course is helpful in making a diagnosis.

Multiple sclerosis may occur in the brainstem, in the cerebellar peduncles, and in the cerebellar hemispheres. It produces rounded areas of varying size that appear hyperintense on T2-weighted scans (see also Figs. 8.8, 8.11).

The multiple occurrence of comparable lesions above and below the tentorium facilitates the diagnosis and makes it easier to distinguish the patchy lesions from tumors. Usually a mass effect is not evident, although demyelinating diseases can assume a space-occupying, tumorlike character during the course of their progression.

Abscess of the Cerebral Trunk and Cerebellar Hemispheres

Abscesses of the cerebral trunk and cerebellar hemispheres appear as conspicious mass lesions with associated perifocal edema. They show prolonged T1 and T2 relaxation times on MR images. In doubtful cases a diagnosis can be made from the clinical course (see Figs. 15.1-15.4).

Ischemic Lesions

Ischemic lesions (see p. 307) can produce signal changes resembling tumors and abscesses. Usually a diagnosis can be made by relating the affected areas to vascular territories and by referral to the clinical history. During the phase of ischemic swelling, these lesions may be associated with a pronounced mass effect leading to acute CSF stasis. In rare cases it is possible to define the causative thrombosis in the basal vascular segments or within the distal segment of the basilar artery (Fig. 11.18, see Figs. 5.15, 5.16).

Intraparenchymatous Hematomas

Regardless of their cause [45], the MR features of intraparenchymatous hematomas depend on the age of the hemorrhage (acute, subacute, chronic) and the field strength of the MR imager [19, 24, 60, 69]. These relationships are described in detail in Sect. 5.2.

Because the high-intensity signal on T1-weighted images of subacute and chronic hemorrhages may persist for several months, MR is able to distinguish hemorrhagic lesions from other types of cyst for a considerably longer period than CT (see Sect. 5.2).

Arteriovenous Malformations

Arteriovenous angiomas [36, 39, 55] and venous angiomas [1, 57] have a very characteristic MR appearance, which is described fully in Sect. 14.1.

Occult Vascular Malformations

Vascular malformations not demonstrable by angiography are common in the brainstem and cerebellar hemispheres (see Sect. 14.2). These lesions have a known [47] but nonspecific CT appearance, producing a slightly hyperdense and usually rounded focus that occasionally shows calcific inclusions. The density of the lesion increases after contrast injection. The MR features of the malformations are fairly characteristic, making them easy to distinguish from neoplasms (see Sect. 14.2). Intravenous gadolinium-DTPA does not contribute to the diagnosis of these occult vascular malformations [9].

11.2 Extra-axial Tumors

11.2.1 Neurinomas

Neurinomas (schwannomas) arise from the neurilemma (Schwann's sheath).

Incidence: Neurinomas are the most common extra-axial tumors of the posterior fossa and account for

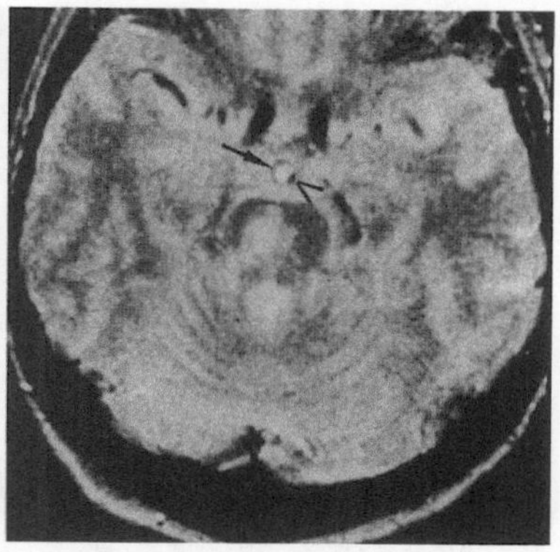

Fig. 11.18. Ischemic lesion of the upper brainstem. The nonspecific finding of a hyperintense area can be interpreted as an ischemic lesion in association with the incomplete hyperintense thrombosis of the basilar artery *(arrow)*. The low signal (flow void) indicates the small residual patent lumen of the basilar artery *(arrowhead)*. Axial scan, SE 1.5 s/100 ms (0.5 T)

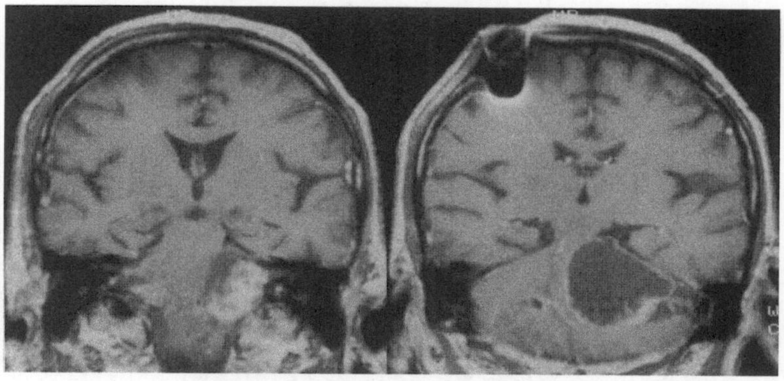

Fig. 11.19 a, b. Cystic acoustic neurinoma (WHO grade 1, Antoni type A) in a 66-year-old man with hearing loss and signs of occlusive hydrocephalus. With i.v. gadolinium, solid, inhomogeneous tumor tissue is seen in the cerebellopontine angle and outlining the cyst as a narrow tumor capsule. Coronal scans: **a** through the internal auditory canal, **b** further dorsal, both SE 0.7 s/30 ms (1.0 T)

about 5%-8% of all intracranial growths. They arise from the vestibular component of the 8th nerve or, less commonly, the trigeminal nerve, nerves 9, 10, 11, and 12, and the autonomic nervous system. The bilateral occurrence of acoustic neurinomas is very rare [14, 33] and should arouse suspicion of von Recklinghausen's disease.

Sites: The major sites of occurrence of neurinomas are the cerebellopontine angle and the internal acoustic meatus.

Pathology: Neurinomas are well-demarcated, often finely nodular tumors enclosed in an arachnoid capsule. They are often firm and fibrous at their periphery and soft at their core. Cystic degeneration is uncommon in acoustic neurinomas and can make them difficult to distinguish from angioblastoma (Fig. 11.19). The tumors usually cause erosion and cuplike expansion of the internal auditory canal. Trigeminal neurinomas cause a sharply delineated bone defect in the floor of the middle cranial fossa, erosion of the anteromedial part of the pyramid, and involvement of the superior orbital fissure, the clinoids, the optic canal, and the adjacent lateral wall of the sphenoid sinus (Fig. 11.20) [54].

Histologically, Antoni (1920) distinguishes between a fibillary type (A) and a reticular type (B) of neurinoma. Type A features moderately densely packed cells arranged in specific patterns and surrounded by fiberlike condensations [72]. In the reticular, less cellular type B, hyaline and fatty degeneration are present as signs of regressive change. Type B also is prone to cystic degeneration, which is most pronounced in spinal neurinomas [72].

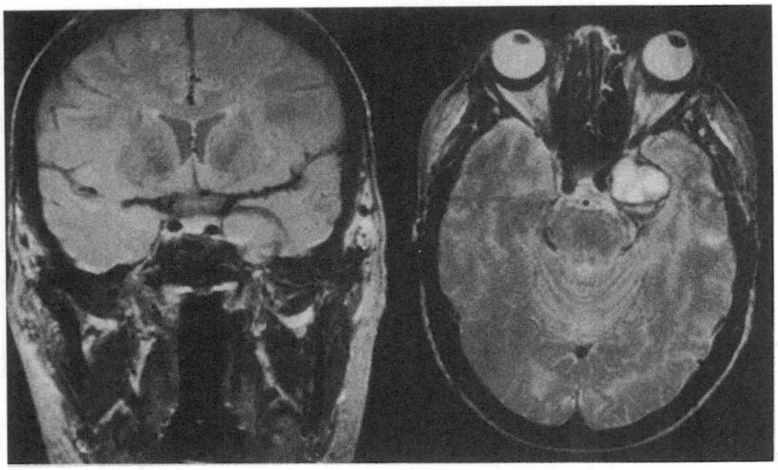

a b

Fig. 11.20 a, b. Parasellar neurinoma, probably related to the trigeminal nerve, in a 52-year-old woman with double vision for 4 weeks. Nodular and cystic mass in the parasellar region surrounded by a dark capsule of dura. **a** Coronal scan, SE 1.2 s/50 ms; **b** axial scan, SE 1.2 s/100 ms (1.5 T)

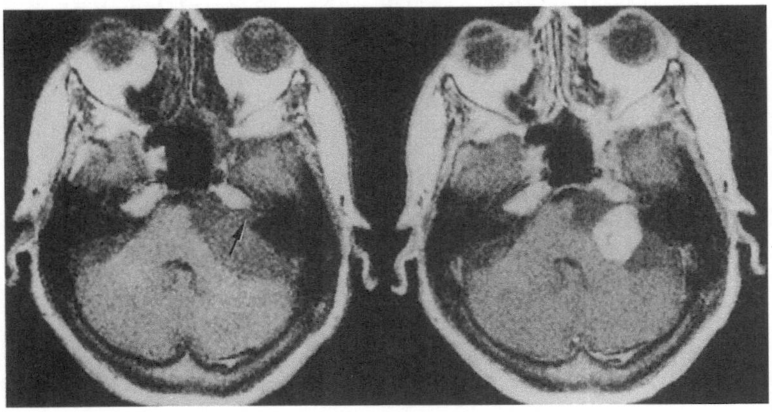

a b

Fig. 11.21 a, b. Acoustic neurinoma in a 65-year-old woman with hearing loss in left ear. Large nodular tumor with prolonged relaxation times in the cerebellopontine angle with dilatation of internal auditory canal *(arrow)*. The tumor borders are clearly depicted only with i.v. gadolinium. Axial scans **(a, b)** SE 0.25 s/30 ms (0.5 T)

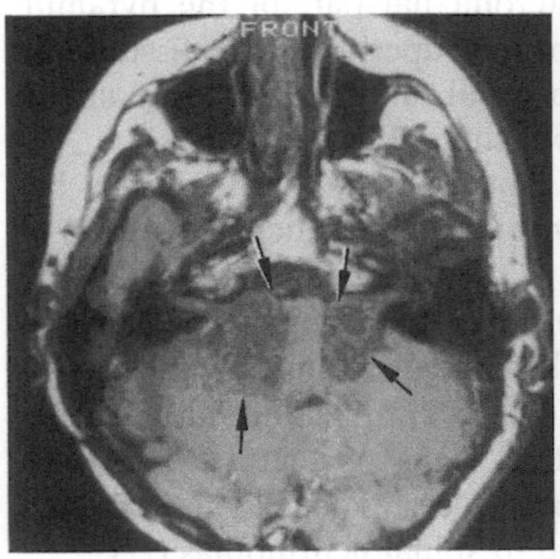

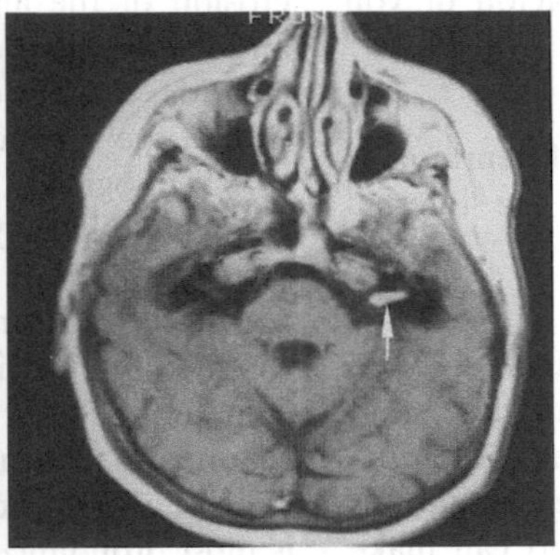

11.22 **11.23**

Fig. 11.22. Bilateral acoustic neurinoma in a 30-year-old woman with von Recklinghausen's disease. Axial scan, SE 0.35 s/22 ms (1.5 T)

Fig. 11.23. Small acoustic neurinoma in a 66-year-old woman with progressive hypacousis. The hypointense, intracanalicular tumor shows marked enhancement with i.v. gadolinium *(arrow)*. Axial scan, SE 0.7 s/30 ms (1.0 T)

MR Findings

T1-weighted images, T2-weighted images with cisternographic effect, images in oblique planes, and images made with special surface coils can provide excellent anatomic definition of the acousticofacial bundle both inside and outside the auditory canal [4, 17, 33, 46, 68].

MR also provides atraumatic visualization of other cerebellopontine angle structures including bony elements, blood vessels, fluids, and nervous tissues [13, 15, 21, 66].

Besides showing indirect tumor signs (see p. 232), MR is excellent for demonstrating the direct features of small tumors, including the often subtle edema that forms in the adjacent nervous tissue. Associated bony changes can also be subtle and are seen with greater clarity on CT scans.

Acoustic neurinomas generally appear isointense or hypointense to adjacent brain tissue on T1-weighted images (Figs. 11.21–11.23). This low signal intensity makes it difficult to distinguish small tumors from the similarly hypointense CSF of the pontine angle cistern. But proton-density and T2-weighted images cause the tumor to appear hyperintense relative to the brain parenchyma and to the CSF. Enzmann and O'Donoghue [21] consider a TR of 800 ms (with TE of 25 ms, 1.0 T) optimal for the detection of small tumors of the cerebellopontine angle and the internal auditory canal.

When necrotic and cystic components appear, the structure of the tumor becomes nonhomogeneous. With their long relaxation times, these regressive changes appear dark on T1-weighted images and bright on T2-weighted images. Fine, low-signal calcifications are less commonly observed.

Neurinomas show very rapid and pronounced enhancement with paramagnetic contrast material (e.g., gadolinium-DTPA; see Sect. 5.5), similar to their behavior on postcontrast CT [2, 14, 43].

Very small neurinomas produce a segmental expansion of the acousticofacial bundle [14, 15, 21], which is apparent even on noncontrast images. However, the intensive uptake of paramagnetic contrast material permits a more reliable identification, especially of intracanalicular growths. It is important to obtain the images immediately after injection of the contrast agent, for maximal enhancement is seen after only 5 min, and very little enhancement may remain after 15 min (Fig. 11.21, 11.23).

Neurinomas of the trigeminal nerve are reported to display an unspecific prolongation of T1 and T2 relaxation times, but have a typical hourglass appearance when they extend across the petroclinoid ligament into Meckel's cavity [31, 54].

11.2.2 Meningiomas

The most common sites for meningiomas (see p. 246) in the posterior fossa are the cerebellopontine angle, the tentorial region, and the area about the foramen magnum [2, 38, 62]. Generally their secondary symptoms are the result of a mass effect on neighboring structures (Fig. 11.25).

Intratumoral calcifications are relatively common in meningiomas, while zones of necrosis are rare. The internal auditory canal, though usually not affected, is not excluded from involvement (Fig. 11.24). Because the classic bony changes associated with meningiomas (osteocondensation) are poorly displayed on MR images, CT is an important adjunctive study.

MR Findings

The appearance of meningiomas on T1-weighted images is variable, but the tumors usually appear isointense or hypointense relative to brain (Figs. 11.24–11.26). On T2-weighted images meningiomas may appear hypointense, isointense, or hyperintense; the T2 of meningiomas may be shorter than that of neurinomas [2]. The signal intensity of meningiomas is sometimes very similar to that of brain tissue, especially the gray matter, and this can be a useful criterion for differential diagnosis. The latter is further aided by analyzing the tumor morphology: neurinomas occur mostly at the level of the porus acusticus internus and envelop the acousticofacial bundle, while meningiomas lie eccentric to the porus on a broad area of attachment to the petrous bone and usually are distinctly separate from the acousticofacial bundle (Fig. 11.26) [44].

Meningiomas often produce a heterogeneous signal (Fig. 11.27). This is explained by the presence of coarse calcifications, blood vessels, and also cystic degeneration in some instances. The absence of a blood-brain barrier within the meningioma and the vascularity of the tumor account for its rapid enhancement with gadolinium-DTPA (Fig. 11.24), analogous to CT [2, 56]. The nature of the enhancement is comparable to that of neurinomas, although contrast uptake in meningiomas is even more rapid and direct (see Sect. 5.5) [44]. In rare cases neurino-

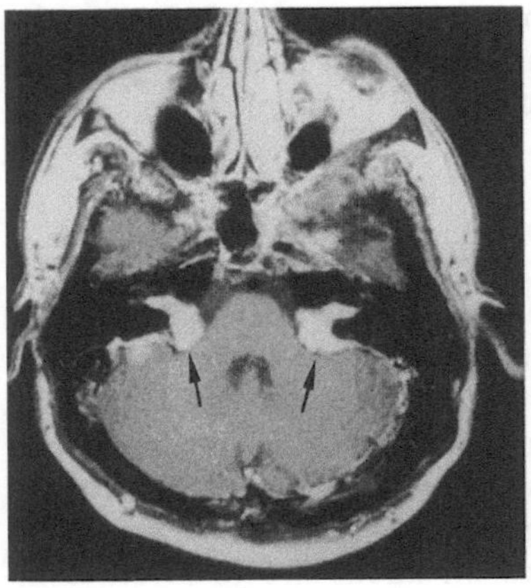
11.24

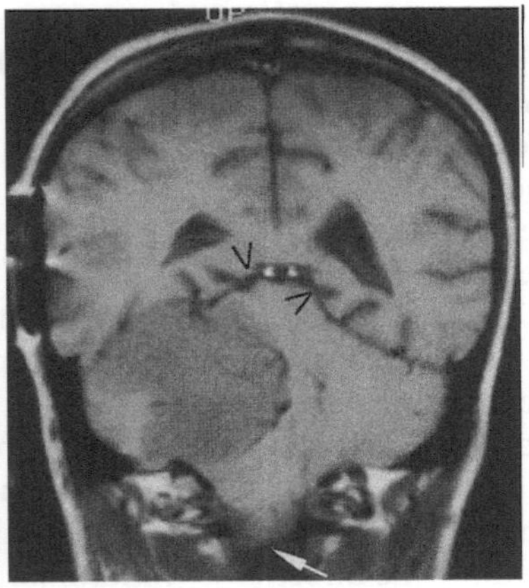
11.25

Fig. 11.24. Bilateral meningioma *(arrows)* of the cerebellopontine angle in von Recklinghausen's disease with i.v. gadolinium. Note the involvement of the internal auditory canals. Axial scan, SE 0.5 s/30 ms (1.5 T)

Fig. 11.25. Proliferating meningioma (WHO grade 2) in a 16-year-old girl with continuous headache and hypacousis. The large tumor with prolonged relaxation times originates from the tentorium and grows predominantly into the posterior fossa. Note the low level of the cerebellar tonsil *(arrow)* and the displaced vermis in the tentorial notch *(arrowheads)*. Coronal scan, SE 0.8 s/30 ms (1.0 T)

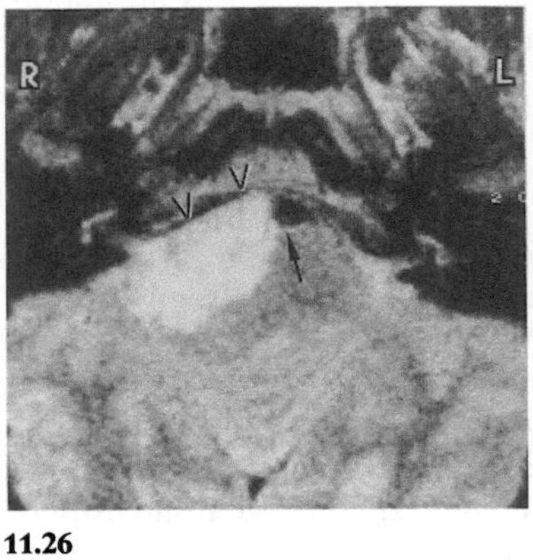

11.26

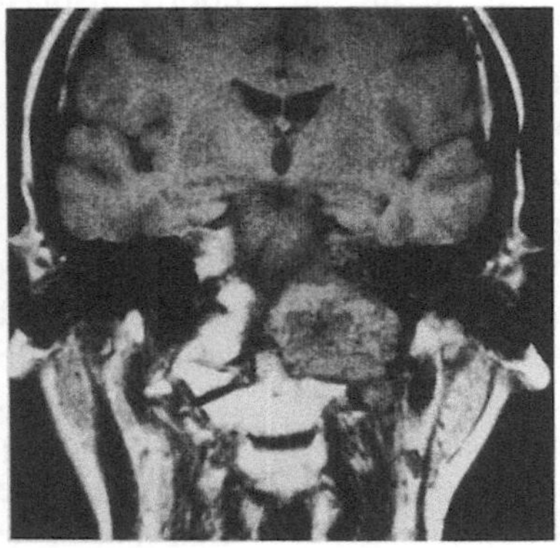
11.27

Fig. 11.26. Meningioma of the cerebellopontine angle and clivus. Mass lesion within pontocerebellar cistern *(arrowheads)* lateral to the basilar artery *(arrow)* with displacement and compression of the brainstem. The tumor appeared isointense in the T1-weighted scan, hyperintense in more T2-weighted scans. No involvement of internal auditory canal. Axial scan, SE 1.5 s/100 ms (0.5 T)

Fig. 11.27. Hemangiopericytic meningioma: tumor recurrence in a 50-year-old man with unilateral spasticity. Coronal scan, SE 0.5 s/30 ms, (1.5 T)

ma and meningioma may be found coexisting in the same patient! [7].

11.2.3 Epidermoid and Dermoid Cysts

Epidermoid and dermoid cysts develop as malformations during embryogenesis. They are distinct from other squamous epithelium-containing tumors, craniopharyngiomas, and inflammatory cholesteatomas of the middle ear [72]. They are classified as grade 1 tumors (WHO) because of their slow rate of extra-axial or extradural growth.

Incidence: These tumors form about 1.8% of intracranial growths [72], with epidermoids showing a higher incidence than dermoids. Symptoms generally appear between 25 and 45 years of age.

Sites: Epidermoids may occur in any CSF space (see Fig. 10.48), but show a preference for the cerebellopontine angle and petrous bone [8, 18, 37], the prepontine cisterns, the sellar region, the ventricular system, and the quadrigeminal region. They may extend into Meckel's cave and the tentorial incisure (Fig. 11.28). Dermoids are most apt to lie in the sellar region, around the pons, or along embryonic closure lines, e.g., between the maxilla and orbit [72].

Pathology: Epidermoids and dermoids grow very slowly. *Epidermoids* have a smooth or nodular sur-

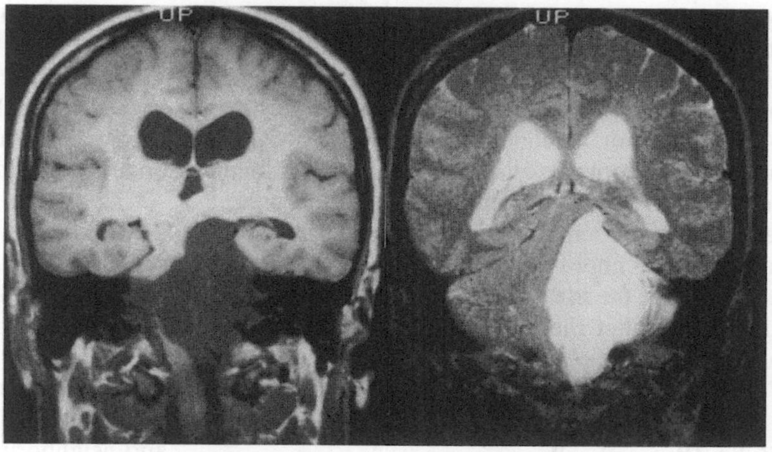

a b

Fig. 11.28 a, b. Epidermoid cyst in a 33-year-old man with facial pain and unsteady gait. Huge mass in the posterior fossa extending from the foramen magnum to the tentorial notch with displacement of the brainstem. Coronal scans: **a** SE 0.6 s/15 ms, **b** SE 3.1 s/110 ms (1.5 T)

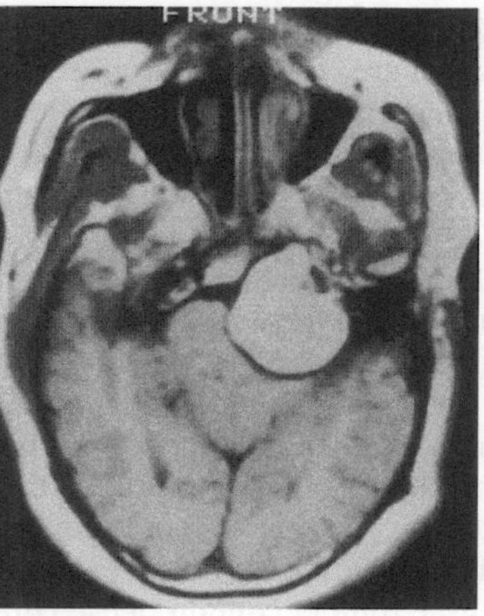

Fig. 11.29. Cholesteatoma in a 50-year-old man with hearing loss in left ear. Huge encapsulated mass extending from the petrous part of the temporal bone into the posterior fossa. High signal intensity is caused by the cholesterol content of the cyst. Axial scan, SE 0.5 s/30 ms (1.0 T). (Courtesy of Dr. Sneider, Johannesburg, SA)

face and contain desquamated, cholesterol-containing debris (disintegrating keratin lamellae). Rarely they may show peripheral calcifications. While the cysts erode adjacent bone at the apex of the petrous pyramid or in the region of the geniculate ganglion (of the facial nerve) and tympanic-mastoid cavity (also the seat of acquired inflammatory cholesteatomas; Fig. 11.29), they tend to ensheath vascular structures like the basilar artery. *Dermoids* contain structures of the skin such as hairs, sebaceous material, and sweat glands, giving them a much more heterogeneous structure than epidermoids.

Epidermoids are particularly apt to incite aseptic inflammatory reactions in the surrounding tissue, possibly leading to ependymitis, arachnoiditis, and even aqueductal stenosis [72]. The cysts can rupture, spilling their contents (cholesterol, keratin) into the CSF system and generating a meningeal reaction.

CT and MR Findings

On CT scans, epidermoids can appear more or less hypodense. They do not change their density after contrast injection.

The MR features of the cysts are variable and nonspecific. Cysts that contain little or no lipid material (i.e., cholesterol) appear dark on T1-weighted images because of their long T1 (Fig. 11.28) [42]. Cysts with greater amounts of fat-containing substances display shorter T1 and T2 times, and their high-level signal contrasts with the dark CSF. This type of presentation is illustrated by the cholesteatoma in Fig. 11.29. Lesions with prolonged relaxation times may appear completely or partially hyperintense on T2-weighted sequences, and they may be mistaken for arachnoid cysts, neurinomas, meningiomas, exophytic gliomas, or metastases of the cerebellopontine angle. Epidermoids often present less regular borders and a less homogeneous structure than arachnoid cysts.

As in CT, the use of intravenous contrast material does not alter the MR signal of the epidermoid tumor.

11.2.4 Glomus Jugulare Tumors

Glomus jugulare tumors belong to the group of neuroendocrine tumors or paragangliomas [67], which are classified into pheochromocytomas, sympathic paragangliomas, and parasympathic paragangliomas or chemodectomas. The latter include carotid body tumors, aortic body tumors, vagus body tumors, tympano-jugulare body tumors or glomus jugulare tumors, and an unclassified group. All these types of tumors may grow as a benign form or as undifferentiated malignant form.

Paragangliomas, which originate from neural crest cell derivatives, may be found in the base of the skull along the course of the carotid artery, the nodose ganglion of the vagus nerve, and the nerves supplying the middle ear and the jugular bulb. These tumors contain dense core vesicles in the tumor cells and they are highly vascular with fenestration of the tumor vessels.

Incidence: Glomus jugulare tumors represent the most frequent type of paraganglioma. However, exact data on prevalence are not available at this time.

Sites: The tumors orginate in the middle ear, usually in the hypotympanic recess, destroy the surrounding bone of the petrous pyramid, invade the mastoid, and finally reach the neck (Fig. 11.30). The main access for intracranial epidural spread is through the foramen jugulare; the extension does usually not involve the brain itself but may infiltrate the cranial nerves and venous sinuses.

Pathology: The tumors are highly vascular and consist histologically of cellular clusters surrounded by a vascular stroma. They are classified as WHO grade 2 or 3 [72].

MR and CT Findings

The neurovascular structures of the foramen jugulare are directly visible on MR images [16], while CT scans are useful for the evaluation of adjacent bone destruction.

The heterogenous signal on MR scans reflects the decidedly vascular nature of glomus tumors, described as "salt and pepper" appearance by Olson et al. [48]. Variations in signal intensity are caused by different flow velocities in the tumor vessels [6] or by the formation of thrombi (Fig. 11.31) [43]. On MR images also the extension of the tumor into the posterior fossa and its relationship to the brainstem and neighboring major vessels can be visualized directly.

Small glomus tumors located exclusively within the petrous bone seem to be displayed better on CT scans, which provide a more accurate definition of the fine bony structures of the petrous pyramid.

On the other hand, MR is preferred for evaluating the permeability of the adjacent venous sinuses when there is suspicion of tumor infiltration. This can be done without contrast material owing to the sensitivity of MR to a flowing medium (see Sect. 5.3).

11.2.5 Chordomas

Chordomas arise from remnants of the notochord. They have a benign form, which is detected incidentally in older patients, as well as an invasive form with an accompanying mass effect [72].

Incidence: Chordomas are rare (about 0.2% according to Zülch [72]). They are somewhat more common in men than women and show a peak incidence between the ages of 20 and 40 years.

Sites: Sites of predilection for chordomas are the clivus, sella, nasopharynx, dens, and the sacrococcygeal region of the spine. The tumors generally arise extradurally on the midline, eroding their way laterally into the cerebellopontine angle or anteriorly into the nasopharynx.

Clinical symptoms include headache, progressive cranial nerve palsy (the sixth nerve being most frequently involved), and long tract signs with no or only a late increase of intracranial pressure.

Pathology: Chordomas can become very large. They have a smooth, often nodular surface and a soft,

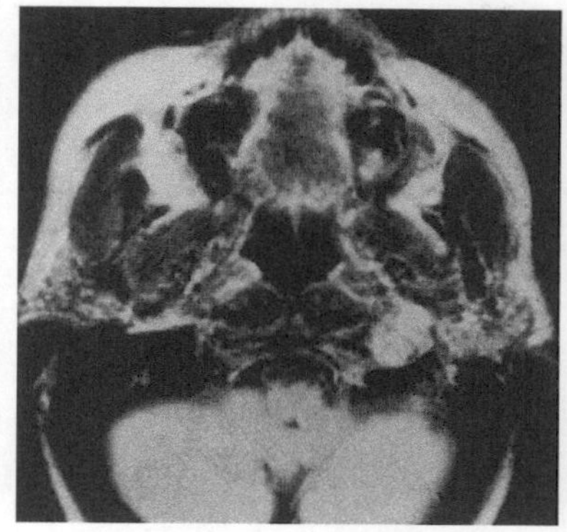

11.30

Fig. 11.30. Glomus jugulare tumor in a 61-year-old woman with tinnitus and hypacousis for 4 years and paresis of the ninth and tenth cranial nerves for 9 months. Axial scan, SE 1.5 s/50 ms (1.5 T)

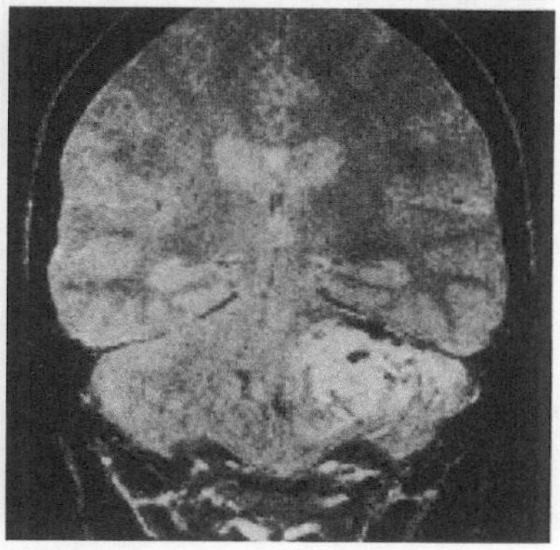

11.31

Fig. 11.31. Glomus jugulare tumor extending into the left cerebellar hemisphere. Highly vascular tumor. Coronal scan, T2-weighted.

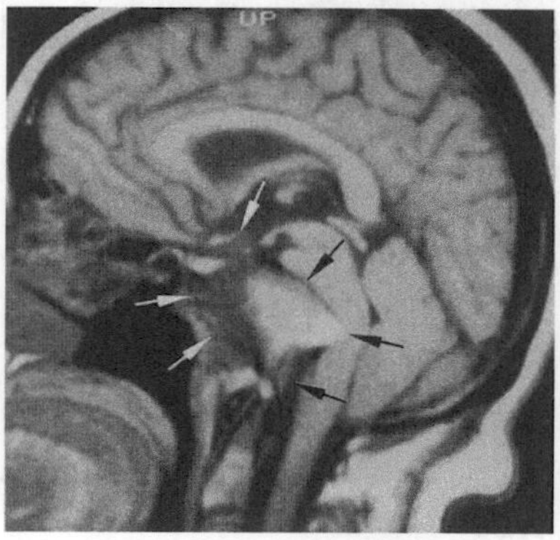

11.32

Fig. 11.32. Chordoma in a 50-year-old woman with vertigo, pressure sensation behind right eye, progressive spasticity, and cerebellar ataxia. Large exophytic tumor of the clivus *(arrows)* with short and long relaxation times displacing the pons. At surgery a soft, partly cystic tumor with hemorrhage was found. Midsagittal scan, SE 0.7 s/17 ms (1.0 T)

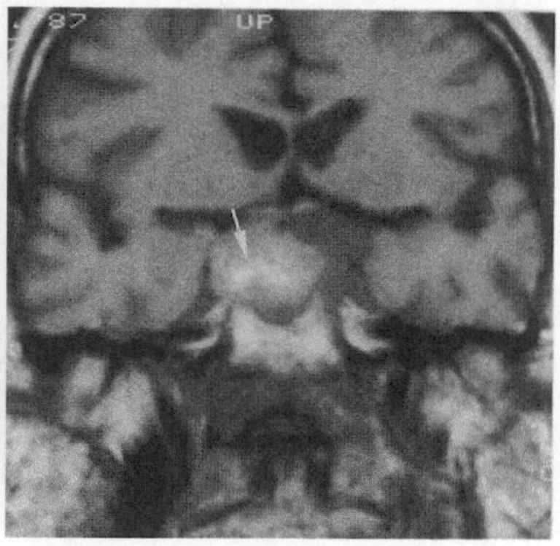

11.33

Fig. 11.33. Chordoma in a 68-year-old man with headache, palsy of abducens nerve, pituitary insufficiency, and visual disturbances. Large nodular tumor with compartments of different signal intensity (*arrow:* recent hemorrhage), with destruction of the sella and clivus. Coronal scan, SE 0.7 s/30 ms (1.0 T)

mucous, or elastic consistency. The tumor tissue consists of vesicular cells resembling plant cells and is permeated by connective tissue and sometimes by osteoid regions. Regressive changes in the form of mucoid degeneration and polymorphic calcifications [25, 26, 38, 42], are more common than hemorrhage and necrosis (Fig. 11.32) [72].

MR Findings

Chordomas often appear isointense with the brainstem on T1-weighted images, making it difficult to appreciate the extra-axial character of the tumor. Other chordomas may appear hyperintense due to hemorrhage as shown in Figs. 11.32, 11.33. They usually give a high signal on T2-weighted images and, unlike brainstem tumors, show marked enhancement by gadolinium chelate.

Bony involvement is appreciated best on T1-weighted midsagittal images. Osteolysis of the clivus is manifested by the partial or complete replacement of the intense signal of fat-containing bone marrow by lower-intensity tumor tissue. Osteolysis of the clivus is not observed with intra-axial growths; in doubtful cases this can facilitate differentiation of the two tumor types.

The variable and gradually increasing signal intensity in the tumor makes it possible to separate the anterior tumor margin from the adjacent mucosa of the nasopharynx, which displays an immediate and intense contrast enhancement (e.g., with gadolinium chelate).

The relation of the chordoma to the vascular structures of the cranial base, especially the basilar artery, also can be evaluated with MR.

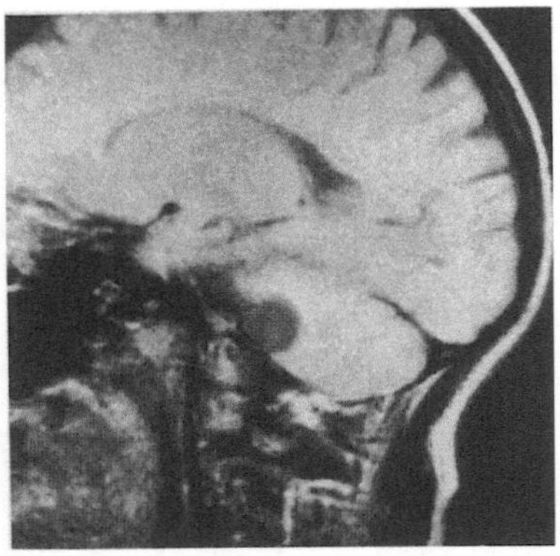

Fig. 11.34. Ependymal cyst of right cerebellopontine angle. Sagittal scan T1-weighted, clearly demonstrates a cystic lesion within the cistern but the signal within the cyst is very similar to that of CSF. CT metrizamide cisternography showed absence of communication between cyst and CSF. (Courtesy of Prof. Baert and Dr. Wilm, University of Leuven, Belgium)

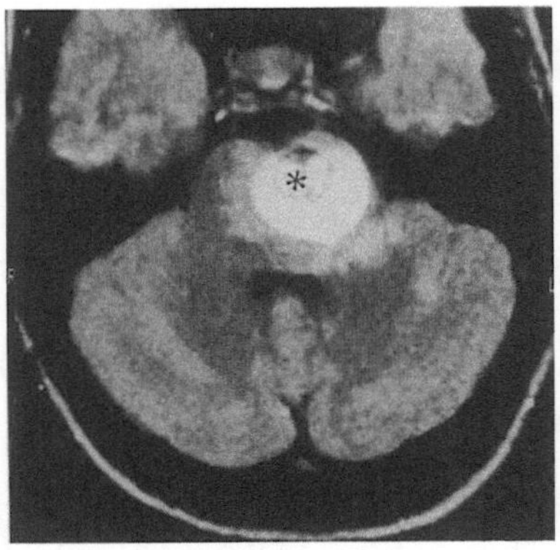

11.35

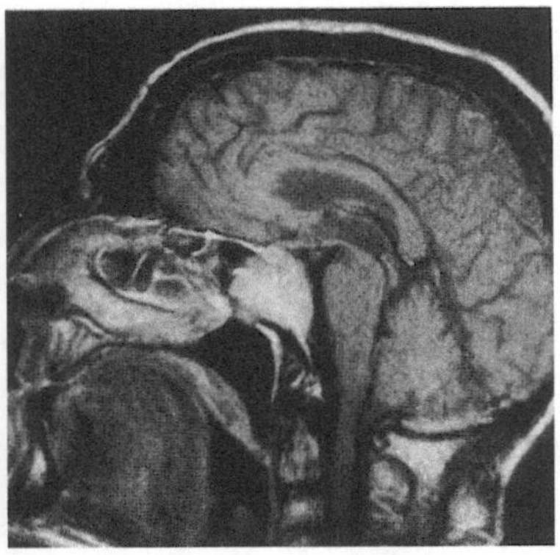

11.36

Fig. 11.35. Thrombosed giant aneurysm of the basilar artery. Hyperintense recent hemorrhage surrounds a partially thrombosed aneurysm *(asterisk)* with hypointense annular rim. Axial scan, SE 1.5 s/50 ms (0.5 T)

Fig. 11.36. Plasmocytoma of the skull base in a 71-year-old man with palsy of the sixth cranial nerve and visual impairment. Homogeneous enhancing tumor mass with distension of the clivus. Sagittal scan, SE 0.65 s/50 ms with i.v. gadolinium (1.5 T)

11.2.6 Differential Diagnosis of Expansive Extra-axial Lesions of the Posterior Fossa

Arachnoid Cysts

Arachnoid cysts are commonly found in the lateral or medial portion of the retrocerebellar area, from which they can expand into the cerebellopontine angle. Less frequently they may lie behind the clivus or level with the quadrigeminal cistern [27, 34, 71]. The MR signal pattern of the cystic contents closely resembles CSF (see Figs. 7.10, 7.13).

MR provides excellent anatomic delineation of arachnoid cysts, although it cannot confirm or exclude communication of the cyst with the CSF space. For that we must rely on CT scans taken after intrathecal contrast injection [12]. This study also makes it possible to differentiate arachnoid cysts from epidermoid tumors, which may have similar MR features. Because arachnoid cysts may show greatly delayed enhancement after intrathecal contrast injection, the CT study should be repeated several hours after administration of the contrast medium. This type of contrast enhancement is not seen in epidermoid tumors.

Ependymal Cysts

Extra-axial ependymal cysts (see p. 192) are a rarity (Fig. 11.34). Their signal resembles that of CSF, making them difficult to identify within the cisterns on T1-weighted images. With T2 weighting, the cystic fluid can give a somewhat higher signal than CSF, whose signal intensity is decreased by pulsatile movements (see Sect. 5.3). As the protein content of the cyst increases, the relaxation times become shorter. The cyst does not enhance on CT scans after intrathecal contrast injection.

Other cystic lesions are found in the setting of congenital malformations such as Dandy-Walker syndrome, Blake's pouch, etc. (see Sect. 7.2).

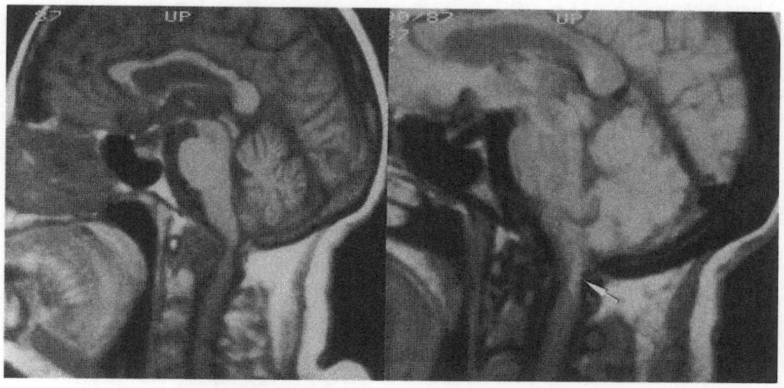

Fig. 11.37 a, b. Primary chronic polyarthritis in a 77-year-old woman with perception disorder of right arm and subluxation of atlanto-occipital joint. Tumor-like hypointense mass of the dens compressing the cord, which shows signs of gliosis *(arrow)*. Midsagittal scans: **a** SE 0.4 s/17 ms, **b** SE 1.8 s/35 ms, (1.0 T)

Basilar Artery Aneurysms

A giant aneurysm of the basilar artery [25, 38] also can present as a space-occupying lesion of the posterior fossa. Typically these aneurysms produce no signal on MR images (flow void sign). They are difficult to identify within the equally low-signal cisterns on T1-weighted scans, but T2-weighted scans show them as dark areas that contrast sharply with the bright CSF.

Caution is advised when interpreting images made with a high field (1.5 T), for the CSF pulsations in the prepontine and lateropontine cisterns can produce artifacts with low signal intensity (see Sect. 5.3) [10]. Thrombotic and hemorrhagic complications (Fig. 11.35) in large basilar artery aneurysms produce a signal increase that must be distinguished from the hyperintense zones of slow-moving blood within the aneurysm (see Sect. 5.3).

Other Extra-axial Neoplastic Lesions

Other, primitive tumors of the skull base occurring in the posterior fossa are chondromas [26, 29, 52] and chondrosarcomas [46], which are described in Sect. 10.10.

More commonly, neoplastic lesions of the skull base are secondary to the spread of tumors from the rhinopharynx or inner ear or represent distant metastases [43], many of which may remain confined to the dura.

Tumor involvement of the compact bone of the skull base can be difficult to recognize on T1-weighted images in areas where the hypointense lesion blends with the low-signal compact bone. By contrast, neoplastic changes within the bone give a high signal on T2-weighted images, while the bone itself remains hypointense in the absence of osteolysis.

Tumor invasion of the clivus is characterized on T1-weighted images by a disappearance of the typical high signal of the bone marrow. These images are therefore excellent for detecting this involvement [25] (Fig. 11.36).

MR also can delineate the arteriovenous vascular system at the skull base, which may be involved by infiltrating lesions.

Expansive Lesions of the Craniovertebral Junction

MR imaging is the most important modality for evaluating diseases about the foramen magnum. Typical tumors of this region are meningiomas, metastases, and chordomas, whose MR features have been described above.

It should be noted that deformation of the skull base, whether congenital (basilar invagination or impression, Fig. 11.39) or acquired as a result of Paget's disease, can cause severe displacements of the protuberance and medulla and thus exert a significant mass effect in the occipital region [3, 64]. These deformities are most clearly demonstrated with MR, making it possible to avoid the misdiagnoses (e.g., multiple sclerosis, amyotrophic lateral sclerosis) that are so common in these patients.

Pseudotumors composed of fibrous or granular tissue, e.g. rheumatic granulomas and inflammatory masses (Figs. 11.37, 11.38), and associated with atlantoaxial subluxation can simulate real tumors impinging on the medulla oblongata and upper cervical cord. They give a low signal on T1-weighted and T2-weighted images, which serves to distinguish them from meningioma and chordoma [28, 63].

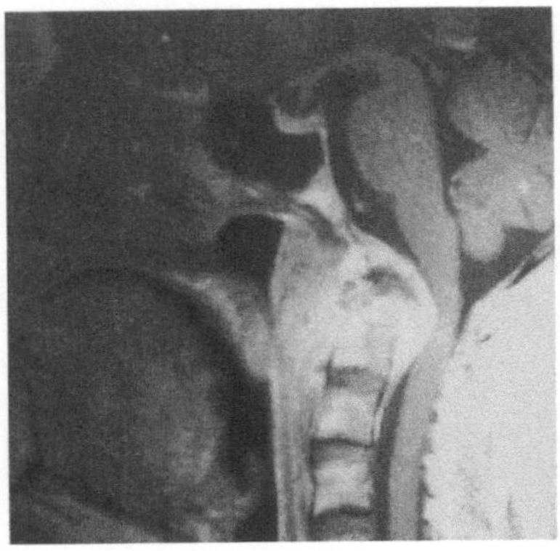

Fig. 11.38. Inflammatory granuloma in a 62-year-old man with slight spasticity. Large tumorlike mass involving the clivus, dens, and atlas, with destruction of bone and infiltration of adjacent soft tissue. Compression of the cord. Marked enhancement after i.v. gadolinium-DTPA. Midsagittal scan, SE 0.5 s/15 ms (1.5 T)

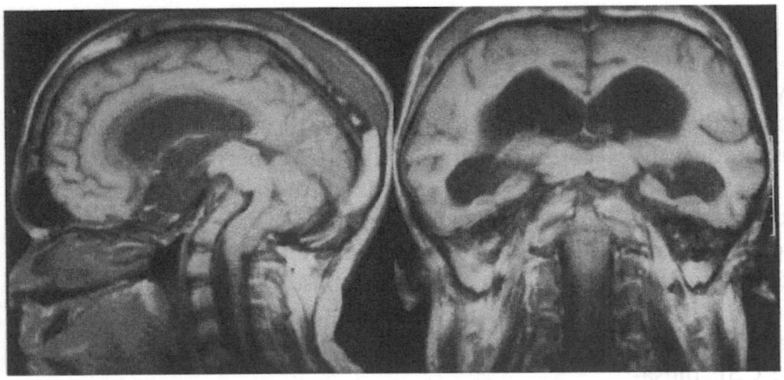

a b

Fig. 11.39 a, b. Basilar impression in a 20-year-old man with extreme deformity of the skull base. The posterior fossa is small, giving the elongated medulla and cerebellar tonsils an Arnold-Chiari type I aspect. The deformed pons overrides the tip of the dens and rudimentary clivus and is covered by the crus of the cerebrum. Large head, enlarged cervical canal. Arrested hydrocephalus with the corpus callosum thinned out. Midsagittal (**a**) and coronal (**b**) scans, SE 0.6 s/26 ms (1.0 T)

References

1. Augustyn GT, Scott JA, Olson E, Gilmor RL, Edwards MK (1985) Cerebral venous angiomas: MR imaging. Radiology 156: 391-395
2. Berry I, Brant-Zawadzki M, Osaki L, Brasch R, Murovic J, Newton TH (1986) Gd-DTPA in clinical MR of the brain: 2. Extraaxial lesions and normal structures. AJNR 7: 789-793
3. Bewermeyer H, Dreesbach HA, Hunermann B, Heiss WD (1984) MR imaging of familial basilar impression. J Comput Assist Tomogr 8: 953-956
4. Bocquet J, Vignaud J et al. (1984) IRM du neurinome de l'acoustique. J Neuroradiol 11: 263-273
5. Bradac GB, Schorner W, Bender A, Felix R (1985) MRI (NMR) in the diagnosis of brain-stem tumors. Neuroradiology 27: 208-213
6. Bradley WG Jr, Waluch V (1985) Blood flow: magnetic resonance imaging. Radiology 154: 443-450
7. Bradley WG Jr, Waluch V, Yadley RA, Wycoff RR (1984) Comparison of CT and MR in 400 patients with suspected disease of the brain and cervical spinal cord. Radiology 152: 695-702
8. Brant-Zawadzki M, Badami JP, Mills CM, Norman D, Newton TH (1984) Primary intracranial tumor imaging: a comparison of magnetic resonance and CT. Radiology 150: 435-440
9. Brant-Zawadzki M, Berry I, Osaki L, Brasch R, Murovic J, Norman D (1986) GD-DTPA in clinical MR of the brain: 1. Intraaxial lesions. AJNR 7: 781-788
10. Burt TB (1987) MR of CSF flow. Phenomenon mimicking basilar artery aneurysm. AJNR 8: 55-58
11. Claussen C, Laniado M, Schorner W, Niendorf HP, Weinmann HJ, Fiegler W, Felix R (1985) Gadolinium-DTPA in MR imaging of glioblastomas and intracranial metastases. AJNR 6: 669-674
12. Crisi G, Calo M, De Santis M, Angiari P, Merli GA (1984) Metrizamide-enhanced computed tomography of intracranial arachnoid cysts. J Comput Assist Tomogr 8 (5): 928-935
13. Curati WL, Graif M, Kingsley DPE, King T, Scholtz CL, Steiner RE (1986) MRI in acoustic neuroma: a review of 35 patients. Neuroradiology 28: 208-214
14. Curati WL, Graif M, Kingsley DPE, Niendorf HP, Young IR (1986) Acoustic neuromas: Gd-DTPA enhancement in MR imaging. Radiology 158: 447-451
15. Daniels DL, Herfkins R, Koehler PR, Millen SJ, Shaffer KA, Williams AL, Haughton VM (1984) Magnetic resonance imaging of the internal auditory canal. Radiology 151: 105-108
16. Daniels DL, Schenck JF, Foster T, Hart H, Millen JS, Meyer GA, Pech P, Haughton VM (1985) Magnetic resonance imaging of the jugular foramen. AJNR 6: 699-703
17. Daniels DL, Schenck JF, Foster T, Hart H Jr, Millen JS, Meyer GA, Pech P, Shaffer KA, Haughton VM (1985)

Surface-coil magnetic resonance imaging of the internal auditory canal. AJNR 6: 487-490
18. Davidson HD, Ouchi T, Steiner RE (1985) NMR imaging of congenital intracranial germinal layer neoplasms. Neuroradiology 27: 301-303
19. Delapaz RL, New PFJ, Buonanno FS, Kistler JP, Oot RF, Rosen BR, Taveras JM, Brady TJ (1984) NMR imaging of intracranial hemorrhage. J Comput Assist Tomogr 8 (4): 599-607
20. Drayer B, Burger P, Darwin R, Riederer S, Herfkens R, Johnson GA (1986) Magnetic resonance imaging of brain iron. AJNR 1986; 7: 373-380
21. Enzmann DR, O'Donohue J (1987) Optimizing MR imaging for detecting small tumors in the cerebellopontine angle and internal auditory canal. AJNR 8: 99-106
22. Felix R, Schorner W, Laniado M, Niendorf HP, Claussen C, Fiegler W, Speck U (1985) Brain tumors: MR imaging with gadolinium-DTPA. Radiology 156: 681-688
23. Flannigan BD, Bradley WG Jr, Mazziotta JC, Rauschning W, Bentson RB, Lufkin RB, Hieshima GB (1985) Magnetic resonance imaging of the brainstem: normal structure and basic functional anatomy. Radiology 154: 375-383
24. Gomori JM, Grossman RI, Goldberg HI, Zimmerman RA, Bilaniuk LT (1985) Intracranial hematomas: imaging by high-field MR. Radiology 157: 87-93
25. Han JS, Bonstelle CT, Kaufman B, Benson JE, Alfidi RJ, Clampitt M, Van Dyke C, Huss RG (1984) Magnetic resonance imaging in the evaluation of the brainstem. Radiology 150: 705-712
26. Han JS, Huss RG, Benson JE, Kaufman B, Yoon YS, Morrison SC, Alfidi RJ, Rekate HL, Ratcheson RA (1984) MR imaging of the skull base. J Comput Assist Tomogr 8: 944-952
27. Han JS, Benson JE, Kaufman B, Rekate HL, Alfidi RJ, Huss RG, Sacco D, Yoon YS, Morrison SC (1985) MR imaging of pediatric cerebral abnormalities. J Comput Assist Tomogr 9 (1): 103-114
28. Hawkes RC, Holland GN, Moore WS, Corston R, Kean DM, Worthington BS (1983) Craniovertebral junction pathology: assessment by NMR. AJNR 4: 232-233
29. Holland BA, Kucharcyzk W, Brant-Zawadzki M, Norman D, Haas DK, Harper PS (1985) MR imaging of calcified intracranial lesions. Radiology 157: 353-356
30. Hueftle MG, Han JS, Kaufman B, Benson JE (1985) MR imaging of brain stem gliomas. J Comput Assist Tomogr 9 (2): 263-267
31. Jefferson G (1955) The trigeminal neurinomas with some remarks on malignant invasion of the gasserian ganglion. Clin Neurosurg 1: 11-54
32. Kilgore DP, Breger RK, Daniels DL, Pojunas KW, Williams AL, Haughton VM (1986) Cranial tissues: normal MR appearance after intravenous injection of Gd-DTPA. Radiology 160: 757-761
33. Kingsley PE, Brooks GB, Leung A W-L, Johnson MA (1985) Acoustic neuromas: evaluation of magnetic resonance imaging. AJNR 6: 1-5
34. Kjos BO, Brant-Zawadzki M, Kucharczyk W, Kelly WM, Norman D, Newton TH (1985) Cystic intracranial lesions: magnetic resonance imaging. Radiology 155: 363-369
35. Koehler PR, Haughton VM, Daniels DL, Williams AL, Yetkin Z, Charles HC, Shutts D (1985) MR measurements of normal and pathologic brainstem diameters. AJNR 6: 425-427
36. Kucharczyk W, Lemme-Plaghos L, Uske A, Brant-Zawadzki M, Dooms G, Norman D (1985) Intracranial vascular malformation: MR and CT imaging. Radiology 156: 363-389
37. Latack JT, Kartush JM, Kemink JL, Graham MD, Knake JE (1985) Epidermoidomas of the cerebellopontine angle and temporal bone: CT and MR aspects. Radiology 157: 361-366
38. Lee BCP, Kneeland JB, Deck MDF, Cahill PT (1984) Posterior fossa lesions: magnetic resonance imaging. Radiology 153: 137-143
39. Lee BCP, Herzberg L, Zimmerman R, Deck MDF (1985) MR imaging of cerebral vascular malformations. AJNR 6: 863-870
40. Lee BCP, Kneeland JB, Walker RW, Posner JB, Cahill PT, Deck MDF (1985) MR imaging of brainstem tumors. AJNR 6: 159-163
41. Mackay IM, Bydder GM, Young IR (1985) MR imaging of central nervous system tumors that do not display increase in T1 or T2. J Comput Assist Tomogr 9: 1055-1061
42. McGinnis BD, Brady TJ, New PFJ, Buonanno FS, Pykett IL, Delapaz RL, Kistler JP, Taveras JM (1983) Nuclear magnetic resonance (NMR) imaging of tumors in the posterior fossa. J Comput Assist Tomogr 7 (4): 575-584
43. McMurdo SK Jr, Brant-Zawadzki M, Bradley WG Jr, Chang GY, O Berg B (1986) Dural sinus thrombosis: study using intermediate field strength MR imaging. Radiology 161: 83-86
44. Mikhael MA, Ciric IS, Wolff AP (1985) Differentiation of cerebellopontine angle neuromas and meningiomas with MR imaging. J Comput Tomogr 9 (5): 852-856
45. Naseem M, Zacharias SB, Stone J, Russell E (1986) Cervicomedullary hematoma: diagnosis by MR. AJNR 7: 1096-1098
46. New PFJ, Bachow TB, Wismer GL, Rosen BR, Brady TJ (1985) MR imaging of the acoustic nerves and small acoustic neuromas at 0.6 T: prospective study. AJNR 6: 165-170
47. New PFJ, Ojemann RG, Davis KR, Rosen BR, Haros R, Kjellberg RN, Adams RD, Richardson EP (1986) MR and CT of occult vascular malformations of the brain. AJNR 7: 771-779
48. Olson WL, Dillon WP, Kelly WM, Norman D, Brant-Zawadzki M, Newton TH (1987) MR imaging of paragangliomas. AJR 148: 201-204
49. Pennock JM, Bydder GM, Dubowitz LMS, Johnson MA (1986) Magnetic resonance imaging of the brain in children. Magn Reson Imaging 4: 1-9
50. Peterman SB, Steiner BE, Bydder GM (1984) Magnetic resonance imaging of intracranial tumors in children and adolescents. AJNR 5: 703-709
51. Peterman SB, Steiner RE, Bydder GM, Thomas DJ, Tobias JS, Young IR (1985) Nuclear magnetic resonance imaging (NMR, MRI) of brain stem tumours. Neuroradiology 27: 202-207
52. Randell CP, Collins AG, Young IR, Haywood R, Thomas DJ, McDonnell MJ, Orr JS, Bydder GM, Steiner RE (1983) Nuclear magnetic resonance imaging of posterior fossa tumors. AJNR 4: 1027-1034
53. Rebner M, Gebarski SS (1985) Magnetic resonance imaging of spinal-cord hemangioblastoma. AJNR 6: 287-289
54. Rigamonti D, Spetzler RF, Shetter A, Drayer BP (1987) Magnetic resonance imaging and trigeminal schwannoma. Surg Neurol 28: 67-70

55. Schörner W, Bradac GB, Treisch J, Bender A, Felix R (1986) Magnetic resonance imaging (MRI) in the diagnosis of cerebral arteriovenous angiomas. Neuroradiology 28: 313-318
56. Schörner W, Laniado M, Niendorf HP, Schubert C, Felix R (1986) Time-dependent changes in image conrast in brain tumors after gadolinium-DTPA. AJNR 7: 1013-1020
57. Scott JA, Augustyn GT, Gilmor RL, Maeley J Jr, Olson EW (1985) Magnetic resonance imaging of a venous angioma. AJNR 6: 284-286
58. Sherman JL, Citrin CM, Bowen BJ, Gangarosa RE (1986) MR demonstration of altered cerebrospinal fluid flow by obstructive lesions. AJNR 7: 571-579
59. Sherman JL, Citrin CM, Barkovich AJ, Bowen BJ (1987) MR imaging of the mesencephalic tectum: normal and pathologic variations. AJNR 8: 59-64
60. Sipponen JT, Sepponen RE, Sivula A (1984) Chronic subdural hematoma demonstration by magnetic resonance. Radiology 150: 79-85
61. Smith AS, Weinstein MA, Modic MT, Pavlicek W, Rogers LR, Budd TG, Bukowski RM, Purvis JD, Weick JK, Duchesneau PM (1985) Magnetic resonance with marked T2-weighted images: improved demonstration of brain lesions, tumor, and edema. AJNR 6: 691-697
62. Spagnoli MV, Goldberg HI, Grossman RI, Bilaniuk LT, Gomori JM, Hackney DB, Zimmerman RA (1986) Intracranial meningiomas: high-field MR imaging. Radiology 161: 369-375
63. Sze G, Brant-Zawadzki MN, Wilson CR, Norman D, Newton TH (1986) Pseudotumor of the craniovertebral junction associated with chronic subluxation: MR imaging studies. Radiology 161: 391-394
64. Tjon-A-Tham RTO, Bloem JL, Falke THM, Bijvoet OLM, Gohel VK, Harinck BI, Ziedses Des Plantes GB Jr (1985) Magnetic resonance imaging in Paget disease of the skull. AJNR 6: 879-881
65. Vignaud J, Bocquet M, Aubin ML, Iba-Zizen MT, Stoffels C (1984) NMR imaging of intra-axial tumours of the posterior fossa. J Neuroradiol 11: 249-261
66. Vignaud J, Jardin C, Rosen L (1986) The ear. Diagnostic imaging: CT scanner, tomography and magnetic resonance. Masson, Paris
67. Williams ED (1980) Histological typing of endocrine tumors. International histological classification of tumors, no 23. WHO, Geneva
68. Young IR, Bydder GM, Hall AS, Steiner RE, Worthington BS, Hawkes RC, Holland GN, Moore WS (1983) The role of NMR imaging in the diagnosis and management of acoustic neuroma. AJNR 4: 223-224
69. Zimmerman RA, Bilaniuk LT, Grossman RI, Levine RS, Lynch R, Goldberg HI, Samuel L, Edelstein W, Bottomley P, Redington RW (1985) Resistive NMR of intracranial hematomas. Neuroradiology 27: 16-20
70. Zimmerman RA, Bilaniuk LT, Packer R, Sutton L, Johnson MH, Grossman RI, Goldberg HI (1985) Resistive NMR of brain stem gliomas. Neuroradiology 27: 21-25
71. Zimmerman RA, Fleming CA, Lee BCP, Saint-Louis LA, Deck MDF (1986) Periventricular hyperintensity as seen by magnetic resonance: prevalence and significance. AJNR 7: 13-20
72. Zülch KJ (1986) Brain tumors. Their biology and pathology, 3rd edn. Springer, Berlin Heidelberg New York

12 Diseases of the Eyeball, Orbit, and Accessory Structures

U. MÖDDER and F. E. ZANELLA

Magnetic resonance imaging, like computed tomography, is becoming an important modality for evaluations of the orbit, because conventional survey radiographs, X-ray tomograms, and contrast studies of the orbital blood vessels often furnish only indirect evidence of desease and are unable to portray the actual pathologic changes in soft tissues. The orbit contains a number of complex structures within a very confined space, including the globe with its proton-poor lens and proton-rich vitreous body, muscles, nerves, fat, blood vessels, and bone.

12.1 Technical Requirements

An effective imaging system for this region must offer good spatial resolution with multiplanar capabilities and an optimum signal-to-noise ratio with high contrast resolution. These requirements are satisfied best by MR imaging with surface coils [16]. The advantage of high spatial resolution is partially offset by the small field of view, whose size varies with the design of the coil. Often the field "cuts off" the orbital apex, which cannot be evaluated. Moreover, the MR signals close to the antenna show a relatively higher intensity than those distant from it, resulting in a nonhomogeneous signal intensity profile [15]. Comparison of the T1 and T2 relaxation times within the image plane is made difficult by the inherent positional variation of signal intensities. The high spatial resolution of surface coils is utilized most effectively for examining lesions that involve the globe or are close to it. For lesions of the orbital apex or diseases that have spread to the optic chiasm or middle cranial fossa, the use of a head coil may be advantageous or necessary.

Artifacts

Because a knowledge of artifacts is important for evaluating and interpreting MR images of the orbit, we shall discuss this aspect briefly [19] (see also Sect. 1.3.5).

Motion artifacts are not uncommon in examinations of the orbit. They are caused by arrhythmic movements which often are hard to suppress and cannot be eliminated by triggering. Spontaneous eye movements during the examination lead to significant structural blurring in the direction of the phase gradient [15]. The higher the field strength of the imaging system, the more sensitive it is to motion-related artifacts. T2-weighted images in particular are seldom free of artifacts because of the long acquisition times. Fast imaging with gradient echoes (fast field imaging or "flash" images) would seem to offer a solution, but this technique is highly sensitive to even the smallest ocular movements.

Flow artifacts caused by moving blood or pulsating vessels generally are inconsequential in the orbital region, because the majority of orbital vascular diseases involve "low-flow" processes. The major exception to this rule is the rare carotid-cavernous fistula.

Susceptibility artifacts are caused by the presence of materials with different magnetic susceptibilities in the imaging volume. Even the suspicion of an intraocular or intraorbital metallic foreign body is a strict contraindication to MR imaging, because uncontrolled movements of ferromagnetic metal fragments can cause further injury to the visual apparatus. In addition, mascara or cosmetic eye shadow may contain ferromagnetic particles that suppress the MR signal by distorting the main field.

The *chemical shift* of the resonance frequency at interfaces between fat-containing and water-containing structures in the direction of the readout gradient can result in faulty spatial resolution with a shift of image structures by 1–2 mm. This effect varies with the field strength and is already pronounced at a gradient strength of 30 gauss/m and a static field of 1.5 T, producing a 1.8-mm geometric shift of fat relative to water [5]. The symmetry of the chemical shift artifact makes it fairly easy to identify, although it can be mistaken for widening of the globe or expansion of the subarachnoid space of the optic nerve if images are hastily interpreted (Fig. 12.1).

12.2 Examination Technique

The orbit is portrayed most effectively on T1-weighted images using a small slice thickness (3-5 mm) and the multislice technique. We favor sequences with early echoes (TE 30 ms) and short repetition times (TR 0.5 s). Pathologic structures can be further characterized by using a single-slice multiecho technique with a TE of 50/100/150/200 ms and a TR of 0.9 s. Alternatively, T2 weighting can be achieved by using a multislice double-echo technique with TE of 50/100 ms and a TR of 1.5-2 s.

In MR, as in CT, the basic view for evaluating the orbits is the axial projection. This projection permits a direct comparison of both globes and correlation of MR images with axial CT images. It is also excellent for evaluating the optic nerve, the cavernous sinus, and the basal cistern. One or more other planes, the coronal and/or the sagittal, should be added, bearing in mind that angulated planes (e.g., along the long axis of the optic nerve) may be needed to define the extent of a lesion with accuracy.

The intravascular infusion of a paramagnetic contrast agent can shorten the T1 (and T2) values of the tissue. For orbital lesions it is recommended that the contrast agent be administered after first obtaining a noncontrast series of T1-weighted multislice images, especially if there is suspicion of an optic nerve sheath meningioma or sphenoid meningioma. Paramagnetic agents also heighten the contrast of malignant choroidal melanomas relative to the globe (see Figs. 12.3, 12.6).

T1-weighted images show good spatial resolution, display the vitreous and retrobulbar fat with very good contrast, and are less susceptible to artifacts than T2-weighted images. Tissue with a short T1 (fatty tissue) appears bright, while tissue with a long T1 (vitreous) appears dark. Muscle and nervous tissue have moderate signal intensities that contrast well with the high-signal orbital fat. Bony structures and air-filled paranasal sinuses do not yield a signal, so the bony laminae of the frontal sinuses and ethmoid cells and the actual paranasal sinuses normally cannot be separated from one another. The crystalline lens of the eye contains relatively few protons, and its dark appearance on T2-weighted images contrast sharply with the vitreous, which appears bright.

12.3 Eyeball

Today A-mode sonography is the primary modality for evaluation of the eyeball and can furnish a definitive diagnosis for the majority of ocular diseases. For further evaluation, the next study is CT. The role of MR imaging in ocular diseases appears to be that of providing supplementary, more detailed information on malignant melanomas of the choroid and on the retroretinal and retrochoroidal hemorrhages that may accompany those lesions.

12.3.1 Malignant Melanoma

Malignant melanomas usually occur in adulthood and are composed of melanocytes. The great majority, 75%, arise from the choroid and the rest from the uvea-iris, ciliary body, and optic nerve.

MR Findings

The paramagnetic properties of melanin lead to a shortening of T1 and T2, similar to the effect of the contrast agent gadolinium-DTPA ($T1 = 594\ \text{ms} \pm 10\%$, $T2 = 52\ \text{ms} \pm 7\%$ according to Sobel et al. 1984). Thus, melanomas appear bright on T1-weighted images and contrast sharply with the dark vitreous body and ocular wall (Fig. 12.2). T2 weighting increases the signal intensities relative to brain and muscle but not in relation to the vitreous. The melanoma remains hypointense relative to the vitreous and therefore appears dark [20].

Initial results indicate that MR imaging is more sensitive than CT in the detection of malignant melanomas. The capabilities of MR can be further enhanced by the intravenous injection of gadolinium-DTPA, which heightens the contrast between the tumor and vitreous (Fig. 12.3). With larger melanomas, it is not unusual to find areas of hemorrhage within the vitreous and sites of collateral retinal detachment in proximity to the tumor. Besides demonstrating the extent of the melanoma, MR can distinguish a subretinal hemorrhage from tumor, especially with a subacute hemorrhage. This type of hemorrhage has a short T1 and long T2 and there-

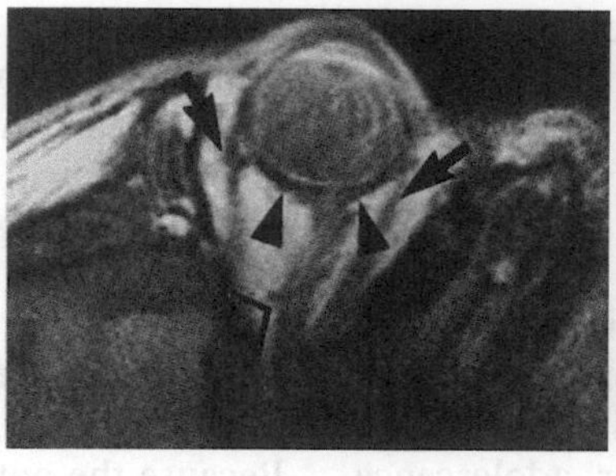

12.1

Fig. 12.1. Normal eye of a 35-year-old man with chemical shift artifact. Medial and lateral rectus muscle *(arrows)*, optic nerve *(open arrow)*, superior ophthalmic vein. The dark rim around the orbit is caused by chemical shift artifacts *(arrowheads)*. Surface coil, axial scan, SE 0.65 s/50 ms (1.5 T)

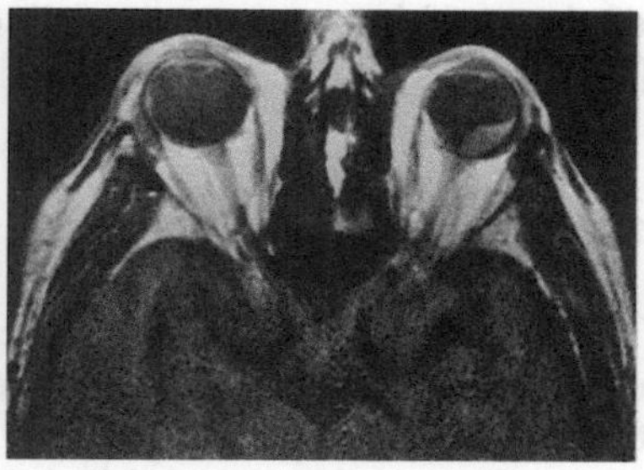

12.2

Fig. 12.2. Malignant melanoma in a 55-year-old man causing slowly progressive visual impairment for 3 months. Biconvex mass lesion of moderate to high signal intensity contrasts well with the hypointense vitreous body. No invasion of the retrobulbar space. Axial scan, SE 0.25 s/30 ms (1.5 T)

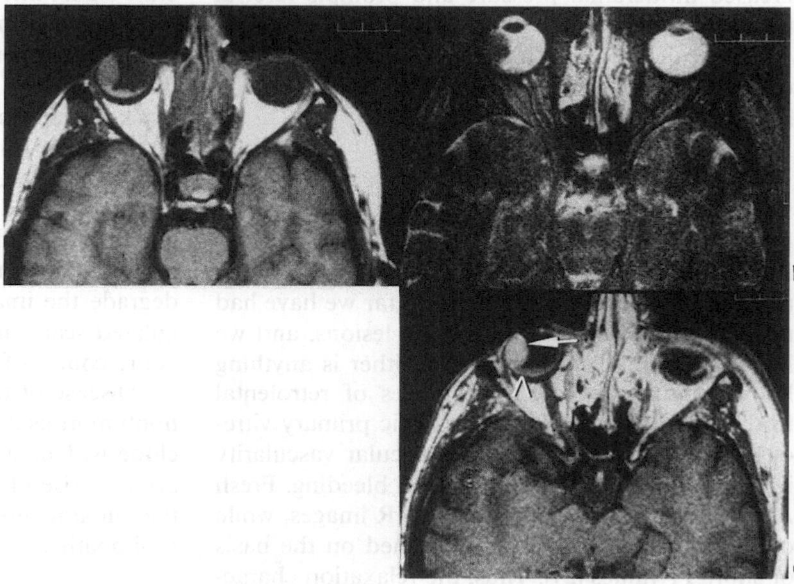

Fig. 12.3 a–c. Malignant melanoma with hemorrhage in a 50-year-old woman, causing progressive loss of vision in the right eye. Biconvex mass lesion hyperintense in **a**, hypointense in **b**. With i.v. gadolinium-DTPA **(c)**, enhancement of the tumor *(arrow)* but not of the sickle-shaped hematoma *(arrowhead)*. Sinusitis of the ethmoid cells. Axial scans: **a** SE 0.4 s/90 ms, **b** SE 0.9 s/200 ms, **c** SE 0.4 s/30 ms (1.5 T)

fore is easily distinguished from melanoma and the ocular wall on T2-weighted images. An accurate diagnosis, however, relies on the absence of significant artifacts.

So far it has not been possible to differentiate ocular melanomas into histologic types – the relatively benign spindle cell form versus the malignant epitheloid cell form – by means of MR imaging. Nor does MR have the necessary spatial resolution (even with surface coils) to show tumor infiltration through Bruch's membrane into the choroidal veins, which has already occurred in 63% of patients at the time the disease is diagnosed.

12.3.2 Retinoblastoma

Retinoblastomas resemble neuroblastomas histologically and occur in early childhood. Bilateral occurrence is not unusual. Calcifications are seen in up to 95% of cases.

MR Findings

Calcifications are not clearly displayed as separate structures on MR images, so differential diagnosis is far more difficult than with CT. Sobel et al. [18] state that the relaxation characteristics of retinoblastoma are similar to those of other nonmelanotic, nonhemorrhagic malignances.

12.3.3 Choroidal Osteoma

Choroidal osteoma is a rare ossifying tumor of the choroid that predominantly affects young women. As with retinoblastoma, only the soft-tissue portion of the ossifying osteoma is visible on MR images [20].

12.3.4 Drusen of the Optic Disk

The major sign of papillary drusen is the presence of calcium deposits within hyaline excressences on the optic disk. Patients present clinically with a visual field defect in childhood or adolescence. Prominence of the optic disk raises suspicion of increased intracranial pressure and prompts referral for exclusion of brain tumor [23].

The calcium deposits do not produce a signal on MR images and are displayed better on CT scans.

12.3.5 Rare Diseases of the Eyeball

Retinal astrocytic hamartomas commonly occur in association with phakomatoses. So far we have had no personal experience with these lesions, and we know of no published reports. Neither is anything known about the MR appearances of retrolental fibroplasia or persistent hyperplastic primary vitreous (PHPV). The abnormal intraocular vascularity in PHPV predisposes to intravitreal bleeding. Fresh *hemorrhages* have a short T2 on MR images, while older hemorrhages may be presumed on the basis of short T1 values [21]. Thus, the relaxation characteristics of ocular wall or subretinal hemorrhages in the subacute phase usually make it possible to determine their etiology, which may relate to hypertension, anticoagulant therapy, diabetes mellitus, trauma, or surgical procedures. Experience to date indicates that MR cannot provide etiologic differentiation of posterior ocular wall thickenings caused by episcleritic inflammation, pseudotumor, leukemic or lymphatic infiltration, amyloid deposits, or tumor metastasis.

In *phthisis bulbi,* T1-weighted images demonstrate the shrunken eyeball, while T2-weighted images show retroretinal collections of fluid or blood. Not infrequently, the retina appears funnel-shaped because of its attachment to the intraocular portion of the optic nerve (Fig. 12.4) [9]. The calcifications that form in this condition are poorly displayed by MR.

Changes in the integrity of the *blood-aqueous barrier* occur in a number of systemic and ocular diseases, including diabetic and hypertensive retinopathy. By introducing gadolinium-DTPA into the bloodstream, it is possible to demonstrate leakage of the contrast agent into the vitreous [4]. At present it is unclear whether alterations of the blood-aqueous barrier will have clinical relevance comparable to that of changes in the blood-brain barrier.

12.4 Optic Nerve

Because the optic nerve is embedded in fatty tissue throughout its course in the orbital funnel, its moderate signal intensity contrasts well with the higher-level signal from the surrounding fat. At high field strengths, a chemical shift artifact can occur in the direction of the readout gradient (see Fig. 12.1). The black line accompanying the optic nerve should not be mistaken for a unilateral dilatation of the subarachnoid space or a pathologic feature. The intracanalicular and intracranial portions of the optic nerve are well displayed on MR scans, since there is no radiation hardening by the surrounding bone to degrade the image quality. Sagittal or perhaps angulated scans are advantageous for delineating the entire course of the optic nerve in one plane.

Disease of the optic nerve may be tumorous or nontumorous in nature. Nontumorous processes include widening of the subarachnoid space secondary to a rise of intracranial pressure. Expansion of the subarachnoid space is also seen in endocrine orbitopathy.

12.4.1 Optic Nerve Glioma

Optic nerve gliomas in children are usually benign and are uncommon, although they develop in 11% of cases of von Recklinghausen's disease. Optic nerve gliomas in adults are usually malignant.

MR Findings

Gliomas produce relatively weak or moderately intense signals that make them difficult to distinguish from the normal optic nerve (Fig. 12.5) [3, 6].

12.4.2 Optic Nerve/Sheath Meningioma

Optic nerve/sheath meningiomas show a low signal intensity on both T1-weighted and T2-weighted images. Separation of the tumor from the optic nerve is not possible. However, the administration of

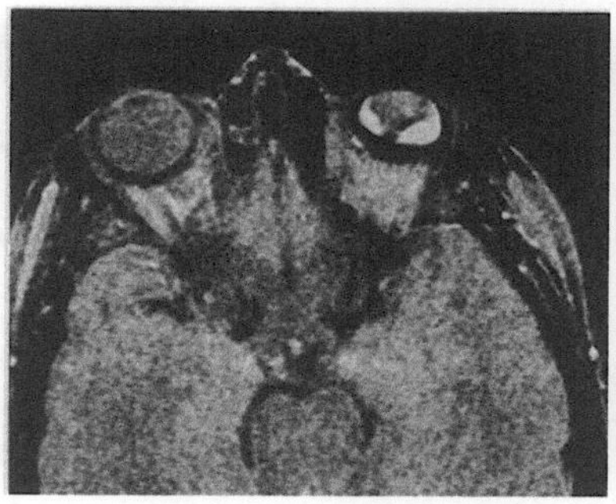

12.4

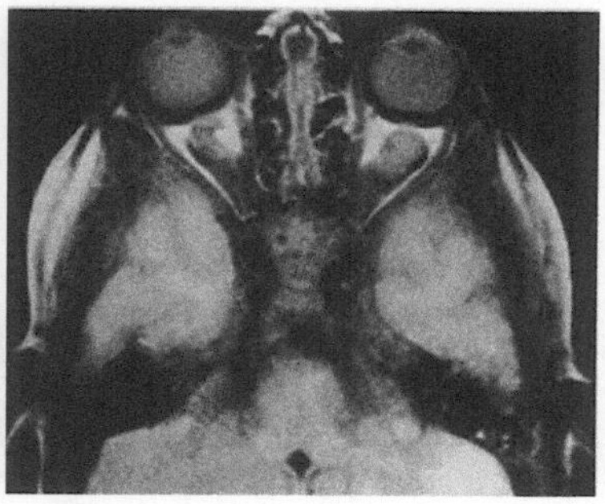

12.5

Fig. 12.4. Phthisis bulbi on the left in a 17-year-old girl secondary to operation of a glioma of the optic nerve; the optic nerve was resected. Increased signal intensity of the left vitreous body, indicating fibrosis. Funnel-shaped retinal detachment with hyperintense subretinal fluid. Axial scan SE 0.8 s/100 ms (1.5 T)

Fig. 12.5. Bilateral glioma of the optic nerves in a 3-year-old girl with von Recklinghausen's disease. Isointense thickening of both optic nerves and good contrast differentiation among nerves, muscles, and retrobulbar fat. Axial scan, SE 1.2 s/50 ms; (1.5 T)

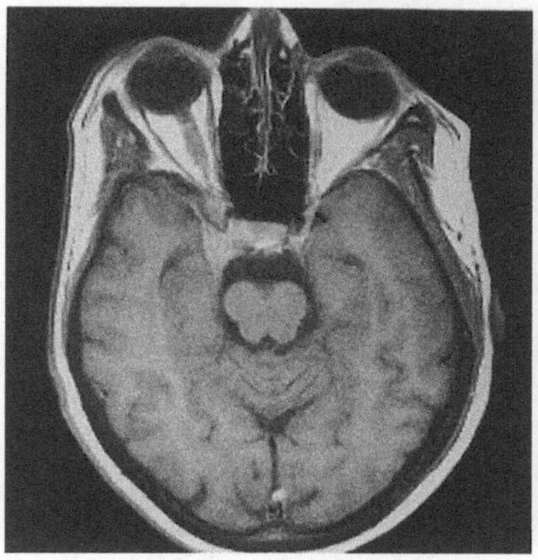

12.6

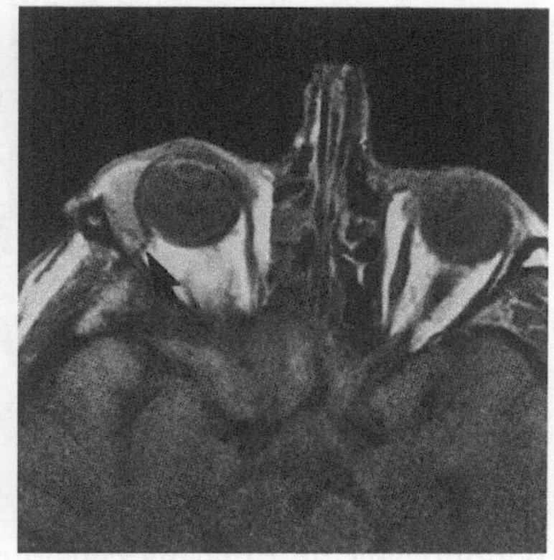

12.7

Fig. 12.6. Meningioma of the orbital apex with progressive loss of vision in the right eye in a 40-year-old woman. With i.v. gadolinium-DTPA the parasellar lesion appears hyperintense. The thickening of the ipsilateral optic nerve was not caused by tumor infiltration but probably by obstruction of the axonal flow. Axial scan, SE 0.6 s/15 ms (1.5 T)

Fig. 12.7. Lymphoma of the lacrimal gland in a 36-year-old man inhibiting mobility of the right eye for several weeks. Hyperintense enlargement of the right lacrimal gland *(arrow)* without infiltration of the wall of the dislocated eyeball or the bone. Axial scan, SE 0.55 s/30 ms (1.5 T)

paramagnetic material increases the signal intensity and thus improves contrast in the intracanalicular and intracranial regions. With this technique even small tumors or recurrent meningiomas at the orbital apex, the sphenoid, or the clinoid process can be detected with high sensitivity by MR (Fig. 12.6). Contrast is not improved in the retrobulbar space because of the high signal intensity of the fat. Calcifications in meningiomas are not detectable with MR. Also, sclerosis or expansion of the sphenoid bone, which are relatively common with sphenoid meningiomas, are demonstrated better by CT than by MR [3].

12.5 Lacrimal Glands

Enlargement of the lacrimal glands is produced by a range of diseases, such as chronic inflammation, adenoid cystic carcinoma, and lymphoma, and is characterized by moderate MR signal intensities. Consequently, the nature of the lesions cannot be established on the basis of relaxation times [2].

12.5.1 Inflammations

Acute inflammatory infiltration of the lacrimal gland is usually associated with orbital cellulitis or an orbital abscess and can be diagnosed by its external appearance. It is more difficult to classify chronic inflammatory or lymphoid infiltrations (pseudolymphoma), which form a continuum ranging to malignant lymphoma (Fig. 12.7). The value of MR in such cases is in establishing the extent of the process by means of multiplanar views.

Primary Sjögren syndrome, a systemic autoimmune disorder of the exocrine glands with infiltration of

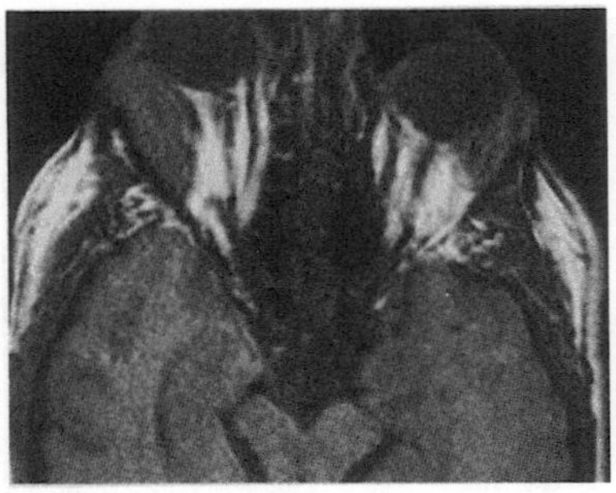

12.8

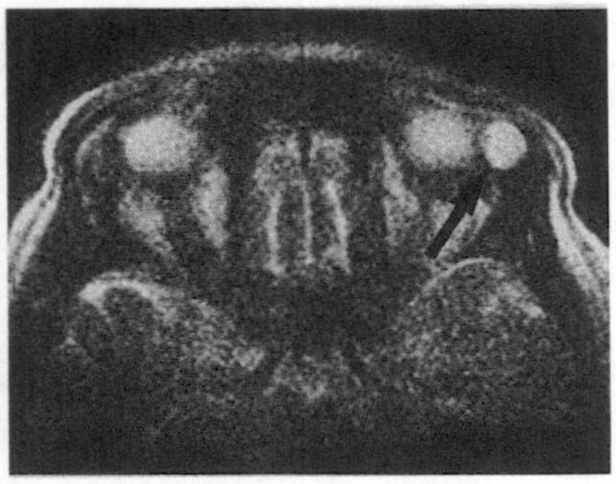

12.9

Fig. 12.8. Sjögren's syndrome in a 62-year-old man with bilateral exophthalmos due to isointense swelling of the lacrimal glands, predominantly on the right. The lateral rectus muscle is dislocated medially by the extraconal tumors. Axial scan, SE 0.5 s/30 ms (1.5 T)

Fig. 12.9. Dermoid cyst in a 20-year-old woman causing a tight nodular hyperintense mass *(arrow)* lateral to the eyeball without erosion of the adjacent bone. Axial scan, SE 0.5 s/200 ms (1.5 T)

a

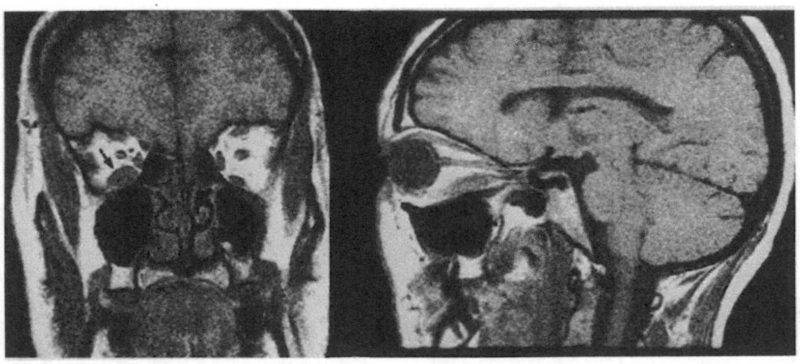

b

Fig. 12.10 a, b. Endocrine ophthalmopathy in a 50-year-old man with protrusion of the right eye. Fusiform enlargement of inferior *(arrow)* and lateral rectus muscles. **a** Coronal scan, **b** parasagittal scan parallel to the optic nerve, both SE 0.5 s/30 ms (1.5 T)

lymphocytes and plasma cells, produces a nonspecific alteration of signal intensities, like other inflammatory processes. *Secondary Sjögren syndrome* (involvement of the lacrimal glands by chronic inflammatory connective tissue diseases such as rheumatoid arthritis, lupus erythematosus, scleroderma, and mixed connective tissue diseases), has a nonspecific behavior. So far investigators have had little experience with the MR appearance of the lacrimal glands in Wegener's granulomatosis, extramedullary plasmocytoma, or circumscribed amyloid deposits. It is anticipated, however, that enlargement of the gland will be the major presenting sign of these diseases, and that biopsy will be necessary to establish the cause (Fig. 12.8).

12.5.2 Benign Tumors

The clinical hallmark of a benign lacrimal gland tumor is a long-standing (6–12 months), painless mass in the upper outer quadrant of the orbit. Other criteria of benignity are smooth contours of the lesion ánd, possibly, displacement or erosion of the orbital wall without bone destruction. About 50% of lacrimal gland tumors have an epithelial origin; half of these consist of pleomorphic adenomas.

MR Findings

Based on present knowledge [20], there are no MR signal intensities that are characteristic of benign lacrimal gland tumors. The only exception is the dermoid cyst, which is easily recognized by its high, fatlike signal intensities on both T1-weighted and T2-weighted images (Fig. 12.9). These lesions usually occur adjacent to the lacrimal glands, although other sites in the orbit are known.

12.5.3 Malignant Tumors

The major diagnostic signs of malignant lacrimal gland tumors are pain, invasive growth, and destruction of bone. Epithelial lacrimal gland malignancies tend to form calcifications [7], which are poorly depicted on MR images.

MR Findings

MR examinations of malignant lacrimal gland tumors do not show characteristic signal intensities. Sullivan and Harmo [20] found that basal cell carcinoma and adenoid cystic carcinoma had a moderate signal intensity on T1-weighted images, and that both lesions became hyperintense with increased T2 weighting.

12.6 Ocular Muscles

The coronal plane is excellent for measuring muscle diameters and for comparing both sides [10]. The axial or sagittal plane is best for imaging the long axis of a straight eye muscle.

12.6.1 Myositis

Myositis has an abrupt clincial onset and leads to painful swelling and limitation of motion. Another characteristic feature is the prompt response of the condition to steroids.

The disease produces expansion of a muscle or muscle group, which, however, cannot be distinguished by MR from enlargement due to endocrine orbitopathy. The widened ocular muscles are not known to have any pathognomonic MR relaxation characteristics; in some cases a slight increase in signal intensity has been seen.

12.6.2 Endocrine Orbitopathy

Neither the widening of the ocular muscles in endocrine orbitopathy nor expansion of the retrobulbar fat shows any definite T1 or T2 changes relative to normal values (Fig. 12.10). Edema of the retrobulbar fat would produce an attenuation of the normally high fat signal on T1-weighted images.

12.6.3 Rhabdomyosarcoma

Rhabdomyosarcomas occur predominantly in children and lead to proptosis, decreased ocular motility, and perhaps visual field defects if the lesion is extensive enough. Bone destruction is not unusual in advanced cases. T1-weighted sequences show moderate signal intensities, and T2-weighted images show higher intensities. A more detailed description is not available at the present time.

12.7 Orbit

12.7.1 Malignant Tumors

The most common malignant orbital tumors are lymphomas and metastases. Carcinomas and sarcomas (rhabdomyosarcoma, chondrosarcoma) are rare. Most orbital malignancies arise in the paranasal sinuses, nasal cavity, or nasopharynx and spread secondarily to the orbit or orbital apex. Differentiation is required from other locally destructive processes like inverted papilloma, basiloma, and esthesioneuroblastoma [12].

MR Findings

Malignant orbital tumors may appear smoothly marginated and homogeneous, or they may diffusely infiltrate adjacent tissues and become indistinguishable from muscle or from the optic nerve. Even when the primary seat of the tumor and its routes of spread are known, the proton density and the T1 and T2 relaxation times may contribute little to differential diagnosis. Because of the chemical shift phenomenon, tumor tisssue bordering directly on the orbital fat can form a "pseudoline" that may be mistaken for a displaced bony lamella. If doubt exists, a supplementary CT examination is advised.

The use of gadolinium-DTPA can produce signal shortening in the tumor, depending on the amount of blood flow through the lesion. This is especially likely to occur in extracranial meningiomas but provides insufficient information for differential diagnosis.

12.7.2 Benign Tumors

Hemangiomas

Between 9.5% and 15% of primary intraorbital tumors are vascular neoplasms. The heavily perfused *capillary hemanigomas* are predominant in infancy, while the poorly perfused, angiographically silent *cavernous hemangiomas* are more common in adults, showing a peak incidence between the second and fourth decades of life. They comprise about 80% of all angiomas. The main presenting symptom is a slowly progressive, unilateral proptosis [22].

MR Findings

Hemangiomas appear as smoothly marginated, round to oval lesions that are readily distinguished from the optic nerve and ocular muscles. Low signal intensities are measured with T1 weighting, while T2 weighting leads to high intensities as a result of the slow-moving blood (Fig. 12.11) [26, 13].

Perfused veins with varicose dilatation appear dark and are readily identified as vessels by their expanded lumen and tortuosity. A signal reversal occurs with thrombosis, because the thrombotic material leads to a relative signal increase with T1 weighting [8]. Marked dilatation of the superior ophthalmic vein and the demonstration of newly opened veins not otherwise visible are consistent with a carotid-cavernous fistula [14].

Lymphangiomas

Lymphangiomas usually occur outside the muscle cone, are not well encapsulated, and mostly affect children and adolescents. They consist of many delicate chambers filled with clear fluid, and recurrence following surgical extirpation is not uncommon.

MR Findings

Because a lymphangioma is a fluid-filled mass that is rich in protons, its signal behavior is similar to that of the eyeball. The orbital fat will appear less intense on T1-weighted images than the healthy opposite side, and T2-weighted sequences will display a brighter signal than fat because of the prolonged T2 values.

Pseudotumors

Pseudotumors are problematic in terms of differential diagnosis, because their imaging morphologies are indistinguishable from those of real tumors [17]. Diagnosis must rely on the typical, episodic course marked by remissions [1].

In the rare and extremely painful Tolosa-Hunt syndrome, the inflammatory process chiefly involves the orbital apex and spreads to the optic chiasm. It shows good response to corticosteroid therapy.

Infiltration of the retrobulbar fat prolongs T1 and thus decreases the signal intensity, while the T2 signal intensity increases slightly [18].

12.7.3 Osseous Lesions

Mass lesions originating from the bone or cartilage likewise can cause displacement or constriction of the orbital contents. These lesions include fibrous dysplasia, ossifying fibroma, osteoma, chondroma, and even sphenoid meningioma, which may be associated with sclerosis and expansion of the lateral orbital wall.

Fibrous dysplasia is a disturbance of ossification in which the bone is partially replaced by fibrous tissue.

Bony tissue appears hypointense (dark) on MR images because of its low proton content, while fibrous tissue appears somewhat more intense. On the whole, relatively low signal intensities are seen on both T1-weighted and T2-weighted images, and they vary from case to case depending on the ratio of bone to fibrous tissue components. Signal intensities may even show a nonuniform distribution within a single lesion. The extent of the ossification may be underestimated when MR imaging is performed as the primary study (Fig. 12.12).

Osteomas appear hypointense because of their low proton content. Tumor located within the paranasal sinus lumen, being surrounded by air, does not contrast with its surroundings and cannot be detected.

Mucoceles develop when paranasal sinus secretions accumulate due to obstruction of the sinus opening. Because the pathologic substrate consists of proton-rich secretions, the signal pattern resembles that of the globe, with moderate signal intensities appearing on T1-weighted images and high intensities on T2-weighted images.

12.8 Malformations

12.8.1 Neurofibromatosis

Neurofibromatosis (see also Sect. 7.7) is the major maldevelopmental disease affecting the orbit. This

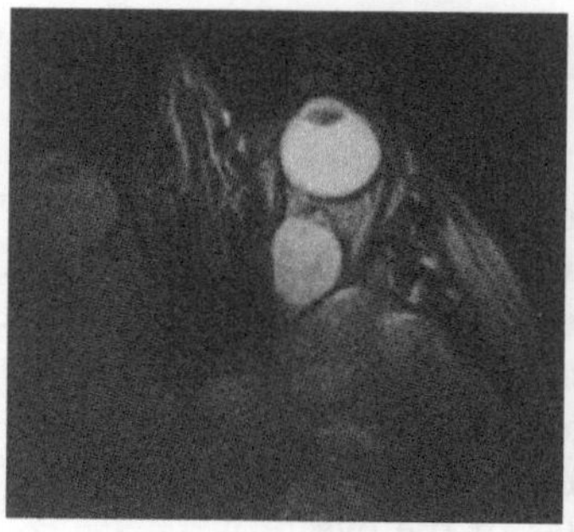

12.11

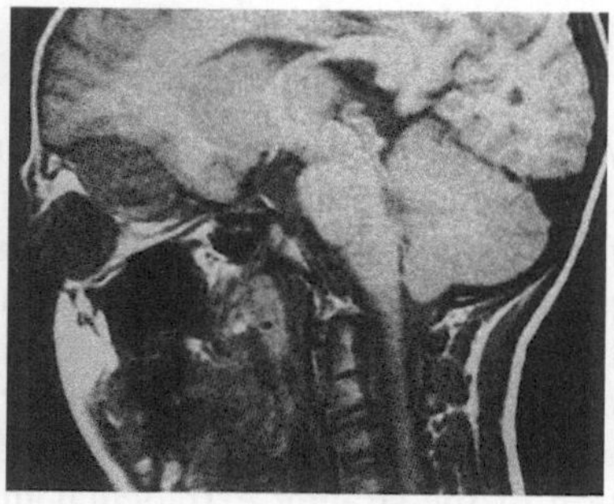

12.12

Fig. 12.11. Hemangioma of the orbit in a 41-year-old woman with protrusion of the eye for several years, now presenting with deterioration of vision. Well-delineated, smooth, slightly inhomogeneous and hyperintense mass in the retrobulbar space with slight impression of the posterior ethmoid cells. Surface coil, axial scan SE 1.0 s/200 ms (1.5 T)

Fig. 12.12. Fibrous dysplasia in a 12-year-old boy with slowly progressive asymmetry of the face and protrusion of the eye. Fusiform hypointense thickening of the roof of the orbit with smooth borderlines and without infiltrating neighboring structures. Sagittal scan, SE 0.45 s/30 ms (1.5 T). The CT scan shows a sclerosing mass with indistinct structure.

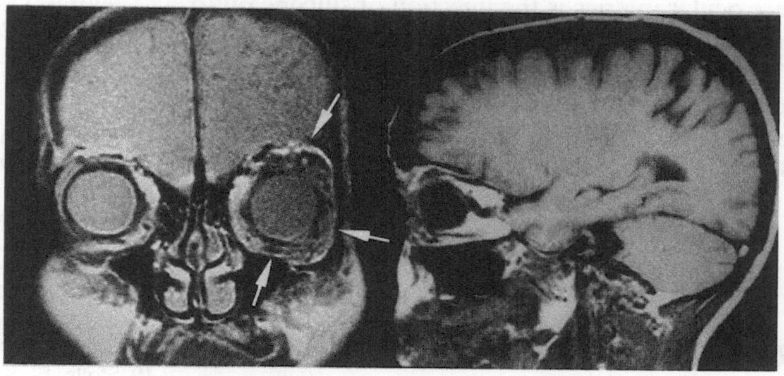

Fig. 12.13a, b. Plexiforme neurofibroma in a 36-year-old woman with von Recklinghausen's disease. **a** In the coronal scan multiple poorly delimited neurofibromas *(arrows)* are seen in the peribulbar space with secondary enlargement of the orbita. **b** In the sagittal scan the retrobulbar space and the optic nerve appear free from tumor masses. **a** SE 0.7 s/60 ms; **b** SE 0.6 s/30 ms (1.5 T)

autosomal dominant phakomatosis is associated with dysplastic defects of the sphenoid bone, optic nerve gliomas, brain tumors, neurinomas, and neurofibromas. The latter have an initially benign character, but the rate of malignant transformation increases with advancing age. With a congenital ossification defect of the sphenoid bone, the lateral bony orbital wall and possibly the floor of the middle cranial fossa are replaced by fibrous tissue. This leads to a widening of the middle fossa with herniation of the temporal lobe and orbital contents downward and forward. It is not unusual also to find a saclike dilatation of the subarachnoid space [24, 25]. Cutaneous and subcutaneous neurinomas or neurofibromatous nodules of varying size, extent, and localization often develop and cause secondary pressure erosion of adjacent bone in the midportion of the face and at the skull base.

MR Findings

The signal intensity of the soft tissue structures in neurofibromatosis is similar to that of muscle on T1-weighted images. These structures give a higher signal intensity on T2-weighted images (Fig. 12.13, see Fig. 7.57).

12.8.2 Meningocele and Meningoencephalocele

Meningocele and meningoencephalocele are rare malformations, usually detected in childhood, in which meninges or brain herniate to the outside through a congenital bony defect.

MR Findings

Large bone defects or the herniation of meningeal structures, CSF, and brain are readily appreciated on MR images. Smaller lesions may be more difficult to identify (see Figs. 7.3, 7.4).

12.9 Trauma

A sudden rise of pressure within the orbital funnel caused by external violence will fracture the orbital floor or medial orbital wall with an associated displacement of orbital fat or perimuscular fibrofatty tissue. Direct incarceration of the muscle is less common. Besides causing hemorrhage and soft tissue displacements, the trauma may alter the direction of the straight extraocular muscles of the eye. The multiplanar capabilities of MR make it ideal for demonstrating this redirection [11]. It should be added, however, that fracture lines and small displaced bone fragments are not well displayed with MR. Often the primary treatment measure for severe ocular injuries is the injection of silicone oil to prevent retinal detachment or retard its progression. The silicone oil appears hypointense on T1-weighted and T2-weighted images, showing signal characteristics very similar to those of the crystalline lens [9].

References

1. Bourjat P, Wackenheim A (1987) Röntgendiagnostisches Vorgehen bei Orbita-Tumoren. Radiologe 26: 118-122
2. Char DH, Sobel D, Kelly WM, Kjos BO, Norman D (1985) Magnetic resonance scanning in orbital tumor diagnosis. Opthalmol 92: 1305-1310
3. Edwards JH, Hyman RA, Vacira SJ, Boxer MA, Packer S, Kaufman JH, Stein HI (1985) 0.6 T magnetic resonance imaging of the orbit. AJR 144: 1015-1020
4. Frank JA, Dwyer AJ, Girton M, Knop RH, Sank VJ, Gansow OH, Magerstadt M, Brechtiel M, Doppman JL (1986) Opening of blood-ocular barrier demonstrated by constrast enhancement MR imaging. J Comput Assist Tomogr 10: 912-916
5. Grabbe E, Heller M, Maas R, Denkhaus H, Heinzerling J, Korijman H (1986) Fett-Wasser-Trennung in der MR-Tomographie: Methoden und erste klinische Anwendung. Röntgenstr 56: 34-40
6. Li KC, Poon RY, Hinton P, Willinsky R, Pavlin CJ, Hurwitz JJ, Buncic JR, Henkelman RM (1984) MR imaging of orbital tumors with CT and ultrasound correlations. J Comput Assist Tomogr 8: 1039-1047
7. Lloyd GAS (1981) Lacrimal gland tumors: the role of CT and conventional radiology. Br J Radiol 54: 1034-1038
8. Macchi PJ, Grossman RJ, Gomori JM, Goldberg HJ, Zimmerman RA, Bilaniuk LT (1986) High field MR imaging of cerebral venous thrombosis. J Comput Assist Tomogr 10: 10-15
9. Mafee MF, Peyman GA, Grisolano JE, Fletcher ME, Spigos DG, Wehrli FW, Rasouli F, Capek V (1986) Malignant uveal melanoma and simulating lesions: MR imaging evaluation. Radiology 160: 773-780
10. Markl A, Hilbertz T, Pickardt CR, Mayr B, Lissner J (1986) Computertomographie bei endokriner Orbitopathie. Digitale Bilddiagn 6: 81-85
11. McArdle CB, Amparo EG, Mirfakhrace M (1986) MR imaging of orbital blow-out fracture. J Comput Assist Tomogr 10: 116-119
12. Mödder U (1986) Orbita. In: Frommhold W, Dihlmann W, Stender AS, Thurn P (eds) Radiologische Diagnostik in Klinik und Praxis, 7th edn. Thieme, Stuttgart
13. Moseley J, Brant-Zawadski M, Mills C (1983) Nuclear magnetic resonance imaging of the orbit. Br J Ophthalmol 67: 333-342
14. Neufang KFR, Mödder U, Friedmann G (1983) Nichtinvasive Diagnostik der Karotis-Sinus cavernosus-Fisteln durch die Computertomographie. RÖFO 139: 639-643
15. Reuther G, Requardt H (1986) Kernspintomographie der Orbita mit Oberflächenspulen. RÖFO 45, 386-392
16. Schenck JF, Hart HR, Foster TH, Edelstein WA, Bottomley PA, Redington RW, Hardy CJ, Zimmerman RA, Bilaniuk LT (1986) Improved MR imaging of the orbit at 1.5 Tesla with surface coils. AJR 144: 1033-1036
17. Sobel DF, Mills C, Char D, Norman D, Brant-Zawadski M, Kaufman L, Crooks L (1984) NMR of the normal and pathologic eye and orbit. AJNR 5: 345-350
18. Sobel DF, Kelly W, Kjos BO, Char D, Brant-Zawadski M, Norman D (1985) MR imaging of orbital and ocular disease. AJNR 6: 259-264
19. Stolle E, Kühnert A, Luska G (1985) Artefakte in der bildgebenden Resonanzanalyse. In: Vogler E, Schneider GH (eds) Digitale bildgebende Verfahren-integrierte digitale Radiologie, 4 Grazer Symposium
20. Sullivan JA, Harms SE (1986) Surface-coil MR imaging of orbital neoplasms. AJNR 7: 29-34
21. terPenning BJ, Cheng HM, Barnett P, Seddon J, Sang D, Latina M, Agnayo J, Gonzales RG, Brady TJ (1986) MR imaging of enucleated human eyes at 1.4 Tesla. J Comput Assist Tomogr 10: 551-559
22. Yamasaki T, Handa H, Yamashita J, Peine JT, Tashiro Y, Uno A, Ishakawa M, Asato R (1986) Intracranial and orbital cavernous angiomas. J Neurosurg 64: 197-208
23. Zanella FE, Kirchhoff B, Mödder U (1984) Drusenverkalkungen des Sehnervenkopfes in der Computertomographie. RÖFO 141: 647-649
24. Zanella FE, Mödder U, Benz-Bohm G, Thun F (1984) Die Neurofibromatose im Kindesalter. Computertomographische Befunde im Schädel-Halsbereich. RÖFO 141: 498-504
25. Zimmerman RA, Bilaniuk LT, Metzger RA, Grossman RI, Shut L, Bruce DA (1983) Computed tomography of orbital-facial neurofibromatosis. Radiology 146: 113-116
26. Zimmerman RA, Bilaniuk LT, Yanoff M, Schenck JF, Hart HR, Foster TH, Edelstein WA, Bottomley PA, Redington RW, Hardy CJ (1984) Orbital magnetic resonance imaging. Am J Ophthalmol 100: 312-317

13 Vascular Diseases of the Brain

W. STEINBRICH and G. FRIEDMANN

Basically two types of event take place in cerebrovascular disease: hemorrhage due to vascular rupture, and tissue injury caused by an oxygen deficit [45].

A cerebral oxygen deficit is more often the result of decreased tissue perfusion than of general hypoxia (caused, for example, by respiratory difficulty, altitude sickness, anesthesia complications or anemia). Disturbances of cerebral blood flow are usually circumscribed. Generalized disturbances are uncommon and result mainly from cardiovascular disease, whereas circumscribed perfusion defects are consistently associated with vascular lesions (stenosis, occlusion, spastic contraction, traumatic vascular injury, aneurysm, angioma, "steal" syndrome). It is common for vascular lesions and circulatory disorders to coexist in the same patient. Defects of venous circulation (thromboses of the intracranial veins and sinuses) also can be a cause of cerebral hypoxic injury, usually in the form of hemorrhagic malacia.

From a clinical point of view a distinction may be drawn between cerebrovascular diseases with an acute onset ("stroke") and conditions that represent sequelae of chronic cerebrovascular insufficiency. Brain infarcts and mass bleedings have been lumped together under the heading of "stroke" because both produce similar signs and symptoms.

13.1 Disturbances of Arterial Blood Flow

13.1.1 Infarction

The leading cause of ischemic brain injury is a stroke, characterized by an acute loss of function of the affected region. If the circumscribed reduction of blood flow is severe, the area will undergo the morphologic changes of infarction. With a less severe reduction in flow, the tissue may remain viable (i.e., may not undergo necrosis), in which case the symptoms generally are reversible. In some cases of infarction the neurologic deficits are negligible and the disease remains subclinical. Cerebral ischemia can be classified as follows according to the type of presentation [24]:

1. *Subclinical infarction* usually involves smaller foci lying outside the motor and primary sensory projection areas.
2. *Transient ischemic attack* (TIA) is defined as a transient loss of focal neurologic function due to an ischemic cause that resolves completely within 24 h.
3. *Prolonged reversible ischemic neurologic deficit* (PRIND) includes all strokes that recover within 21 days.
4. *Progressing stroke* ("stroke in evolution") may correspond to a progressive infarction or multiple independent infarcts occurring in rapid succession.
5. The diagnosis of *completed stroke* is always made in retrospect, since the possibility of progression cannot be determined in the acute stage of a stroke.

Despite the availability of sophisticated diagnostic techniques, cerebral infarction generally is still diagnosed from clinical signs and typical history with acute onset of neurologic deficits [24]. So imaging procedures are useful to confirm the diagnosis, to detect complications such as hemorrhage or edema, and to provide a differential diagnosis in cases that take an atypical course. Among the imaging techniques computer tomography is a mainstay in cerebral infarction owing to its ability to demonstrate the extend of ischemic brain damage as well as edema-related mass effects or hemorrhage [5, 57]. Difficulties with CT arise only in some stages of infarct evolution [2, 4, 19, 35, 50]. Thus it is well known that CT may be negative for up to 48 h after the acute event, especially in smaller infarcts. Moreover, the so-called fogging effect can diminish the contrast between the lesion and normal brain tissue for about 14 days after the stroke event. Particular infarct locations, such as brainstem, midbrain, or lacunar (see below), may also be misleading.

Pathophysiology and Pathomorphology

While loss of function in brain tissue becomes evident when the blood flow to the tissue is reduced to about 50% of the normal perfusion (in adults about 55 ml 100 g^{-1} min^{-1}), brain damage takes place (in animal models) if blood supply is reduced to less than the critical flow of 10-15 ml 100 g^{-1} min^{-1} [3, 23, 31]. With ischemia of sudden onset, it takes only about 20 s for function to become impaired in the affected brain region, accompanied by a leakage of EEG activity. So far, reports have varied on the duration of ischemia that can be tolerated before irreversible deficits occur. The first structures to be damaged by ischemia are the neurons, followed later by swelling of the astroglia and oligodendroglia.

Three to five hours after the onset of ischemia, necrosis begins with a gradual dissolution of the myelin sheaths. By 24 h leukocyte infiltration is apparent at the periphery of the infarcted area, and by 48 h initial capillary ingrowth is seen [33]. By the end of the second day, macrophages appear about the vessels and initiate removal of the necrotic material and liquefaction (colliquation) of the infarct; this process continues over a period of months. In rare cases colliquation by macrophages does not occur, and a glial scar is formed. By the end of 2 weeks the infarcted area is walled off by gliotic tissue. Extensive glial scars often are found in the white matter adjacent to the cystic defect.

One of the earliest changes in infarction is the development of a cytotoxic (intracellular) edema [26, 32, 46] (see p. 115). The blood-brain barrier becomes disrupted (within 20 h), allowing a vasogenic (extracellular) edema to develop (see Sect. 5.1). In experimental animals, ischemic brain edema is maximal about 48 h after the vascular occlusion and takes up to 2 weeks to resolve completely.

On the pathoanatomic level, a distinction is made between "white" (anemic) infarcts and the less common "red" (hemorrhagic) infarcts. The leading cause of hemorrhagic infarcts is believed to be the resumption of blood flow (by lysis of the embolus or by the opening of collaterals) in a necrotic vascular bed [24]. They can be detected more frequently with MR (see Figs. 13.9-13.12).

Most cerebral infarctions involve both the gray matter and the white matter. Purely cortical or subcortical infarcts are rare. The term "lacunar infarct" is reserved for small, deep infarcts that are found in the lentiform nucleus, pons, thalamus, caudate nucleus, internal capsule, and centrum semiovale in hypertensive individuals [21]. Small, central infarcts can also result from the embolization of atheromatous material [35]. Circumscribed infarctions of the white matter usually occur in the "watershed" areas between the superficial and deep branches of the cerebral arteries (see Figs. 13.25, 13.26).

MR Results in Animal Models

MR imaging in experimental animals has been able to detect a signal change between 30 min and 4-6 h after a cerebral infarction [7, 10, 14, 15, 16, 33, 36, 40, 52]. This signal change is based on a rapid and striking prolongation of T1 and T2 by about 45% and in contrast, an increase in proton density by about 5%, both due to edema [15, 16, 36]. Because the permeability of the blood vessels is increased only for water at the start of edema, an excess of "free" water develops which significantly lengthens the relaxation times [7]. Later the permeability for albumin also increases, and the relaxation times shorten again slightly due to binding of the water by the albumin.

Comparison between MR parameters and measurements of regional blood flow shows no direct correlation [21a, 36]. Changes of relaxation times obviously only occur in the case of brain damage, i.e., a decrease of blood supply to below the critical level.

Imaging Methods

Keeping the experimental results in mind, T1-weighted and T2-weighted images should be of similar efficacy for the detection of cerebral infarctions. But using the SE sequence, less contrast is obtainable with T1 (TR $\leqslant$500 ms/TE $\leqslant$30 ms) than with T2 (TR $\geqslant$1800 ms/TE $\geqslant$90 ms) [8, 53]. Equivalent presentation of infarcts on T1-weighted images can be achieved only by enhancing T1 contrast using the IR sequence (Fig. 13.1) [17]. Nevertheless, SE is the most frequently used sequence in brain ischemia, for reasons of time economy and image quality [8, 11, 13, 20, 22, 34, 44, 47, 48, 53, 54, 55]. The value of fast imaging techniques (gradient echo sequences) has not yet been established.

In SE, good delineation of the infarcted areas demands TE of $\geqslant$90 ms. With such significant T2

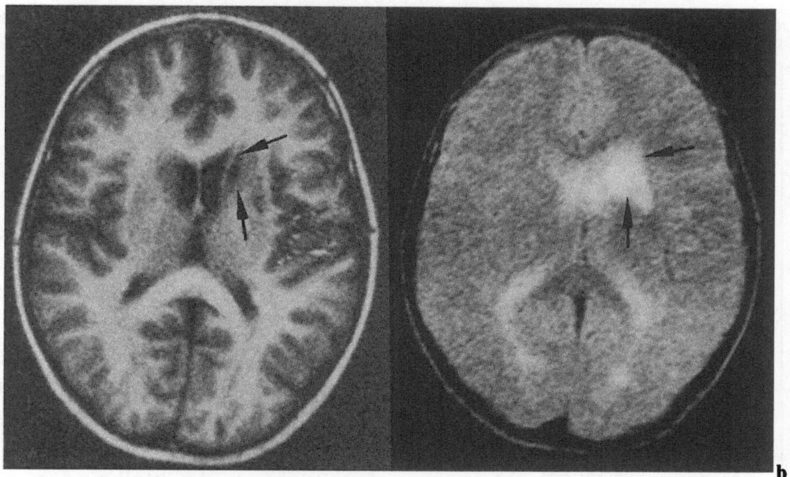

a b

Fig. 13.1 a, b. Cerebral stroke, 21 days old, with right spastic hemiparesis in a 39-year-old man. The infarct is demonstrated in the head of the left caudate nucleus and the rostral part of the internal capsule *(arrows)* in both T1-weighted images **(a)** and T2-weighted images **(b)**. Axial scans: **a** IR 1 s/0.4 s/50 ms **b** SE 0.65 s/150 ms

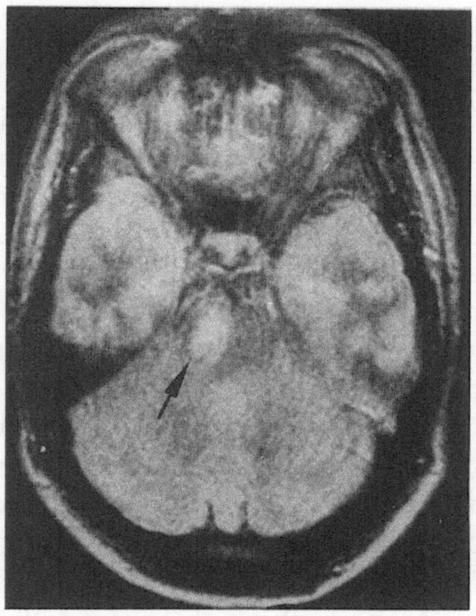

Fig. 13.2. An 8-day-old infarction of the right pons *(arrow)* in a 37-year-old man. Axial scan, SE 1.35 s/100 ms

influence one can avoid time-consuming TR of >1800 ms. T1 weighting is additionally required for the structural differentiation of cystic liquefactions from glial scars and for identifying zones of hemorrhage. SE images with a TR of 250–500 ms have been found to provide T1 weighting adequate for this purpose [27, 53].

Separation of the actual necrotic zone from the adjacent white matter edema is quite difficult in fresh infarcts but is best accomplished by proton-density weighting (SE TR ⩾1800 ms/TE ⩽50 ms). Heavier T1 weighting decreases the signal of both the necrosis and the edema.

Transverse slice orientation generally allows sufficient localization of infarcted areas to different gyri and to the segments of brain supplying vessels. For the comparison with CT slices it seems advisable to use a slice angulation parallel to the oculomeatal line. Thus patterns of vessels distribution as published in the CT literature [5] can be used. In some situations especially the distinction between the temporal and the parietal lobe and the detection of basal infarcts, additional coronal slice orientation can be helpful. Brainstem infarcts (Fig. 13.2) generally require two slice orientations - transverse and coronal or sagittal.

A slice thickness of 8 mm seems sufficient in most cases, while small lacunar infarcts are better delineated by thinner slices. Looking for brainstem or cerebellar infarcts, we generally obtain thinner (5-mm or less) slices. All these considerations lead to the recommendations laid down in Table 13.1.

Table 13.1. Recommended sequence of MR examination for cerebral infarction

First acquisition	Axial multislice series of the whole brain (12-16 slices) parallel to the oculomeatal line using a slice thickenss of 8 mm
Sequence:	SE ⩾1.8 s/⩽30 ms and ⩾90 ms (double echo, proton density and T2 weighting)
Second acquisition	Axial (as above) or coronal multislice series of the infarcted area using a slice thickness of 5-8 mm
Sequence:	SE ⩽0.5 s/⩽30 ms (T1 weighting)
Third acquisition	(for brainstem lesions) Coronal multislice series of the brainstem region using a slice thickenss of 5 mm or less
Sequence:	SE ⩾1.8 s/⩽30 ms and ⩾90 ms (double-echo technique, proton density and T2 weighting)

Detection

The high sensitivity of MR imaging found in animal studies was confirmed by a detection rate of up to 98% for cerebral infarctions in clinical studies [8, 13, 17, 20, 22, 27, 28, 29, 44, 48, 49, 53, 54, 55]. The false-negative findings with CT in certain stages of infarction do not occur with MR. It is true that the contrast between the infarct and surrounding normal brain shows some individual variations and a moderate decrease with resolution of the edema in the 2nd week, but adequate T2 weighting should give sufficient positive contrast over the whole evolution of the infarct (see "Signal Changes over Time" below).

Owing to the high contrast of MR, even smaller infarcts can be clearly visualized using the technique described (Figs. 13.2, 13.3, 13.4, 13.5). Regions of low sensitivity caused by methodologic problems, as known in the posterior fossa for CT, do not exist for MR (Figs. 13.2, 13.3, 13.4) [34].

However, motion artifacts (in restless patients) and flow artifacts (especially caused by the large basal vessels) can prevent the detection of small lesions (see Sect. 1.3.5). To eliminate these artifacts, it may be necessary to use flow compensated gradients, or apply ECG gating.

In TIA, it is common for MR to be negative even during periods when neurologic deficits are present. Blood flow disturbances are detectable with MR only in cases where the integrity of the blood-brain barrier is disrupted, leading to cerebral edema. Small infarcts associated with TIA can be identified on MR images. MR findings generally are positive in patients with a PRIND.

Extent

The exact delineation of the infarcted brain tissue obtained with MR allows clear differentiation between cortical infarcts (Fig. 13.6), subcortical infarcts (Fig. 13.7) and infarcts affecting gray and white matter. The area of increased signal intensity on T2-weighted images does not always correspond precisely to the extent of the necrotic area, because perifocal edema can have the same signal characteristics. Even in mixed sequences with more proton-density weighting, it can be very difficult to identify the margin between necrosis and edema. In some cases the edema will give a somewhat higher intensity signal on these scans; in other cases the malacic area cannot be defined until the edema has resolved, usually by the end of the 2nd week. The edema may persist for more than 14 days if the infarction is very extensive.

Complications

A *mass effect* in the edematous phase of an infarction can lead to CSF stasis (e.g., with a cerebellar infarction) and to incarceration of the uncus in the tentorial notch or herniation of the cerebellar tonsils through the foramen magnum. These anatomic distortions, and ventricular compressions (Figs. 13.8, see 13.4) can be appreciated on T1-weighted and T2-weighted images; coronal and/or sagittal T1-weighted images are especially good for detecting an impending herniation. Extensive edema leads to a decrease in blood perfusion of the whole brain, even in noninfarcted areas, but not to MR signal changes, so this phenomenon is not detectable by MR imaging.

CT and MR are complementary for the evaluation of *hemorrhages* in infarcts [27]. While CT can define the acute hemorrhage as a typical hyperdense area, MR in the subacute and chronic stage (after the 2nd-5th day) shows markedly increased signal intensities on T1-weighted images (Figs. 13.9-13.12). These are specific to hemorrhage: a short T1 is seen in infarcts only when there has been bleeding into the infarcted area. It is true that even in the acute phase of bleeding some decrease of signal intensity can be visible on T2-weighted images, but this depends on field strength and the contrast is low in low-field systems. Also in older hemorrhages, decreased signal intensities may be noted as evidence of hemosiderin deposition (see Fig. 13.20). (See Sect. 5.2 for a fuller description of the MR

Fig. 13.3. An 18-hour-old infarct of the right hemisphere of the cerebellum *(arrow)* in a 24-year-old woman. Axial scan, SE 1.2 s/100 ms

Fig. 13.4. Infarction of right cerebellum (territory of the posterior inferior cerebellar artery - PICA) in a 19-year-old woman. MR 5 days after stroke event. Axial scan, SE 1.5 s/100 ms

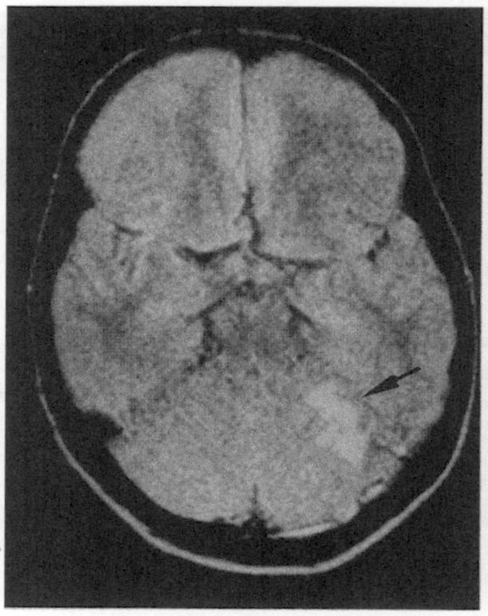

13.3

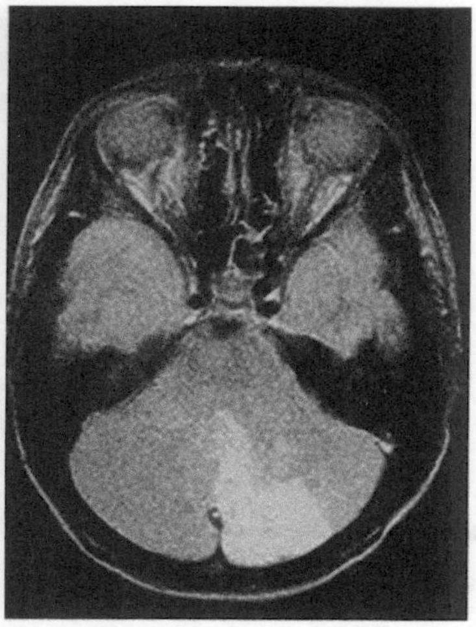

13.4

Fig. 13.5. A 16-days-old infarction of the right thalamus in a 38-year-old woman. Axial scan, SE 1.8 s/100 ms

Fig. 13.6. A 7-day-old infarction in the territory of left middle cerebral artery, predominantly involving the cortex *(arrows)*, in a 22-year-old woman. Axial scan, SE 1.35 s/100 ms

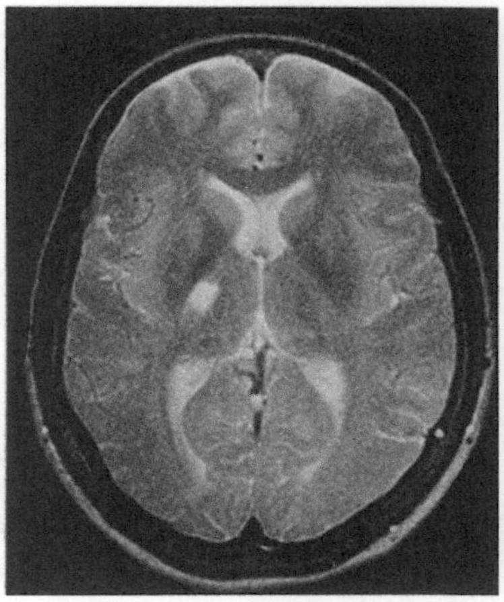

13.5

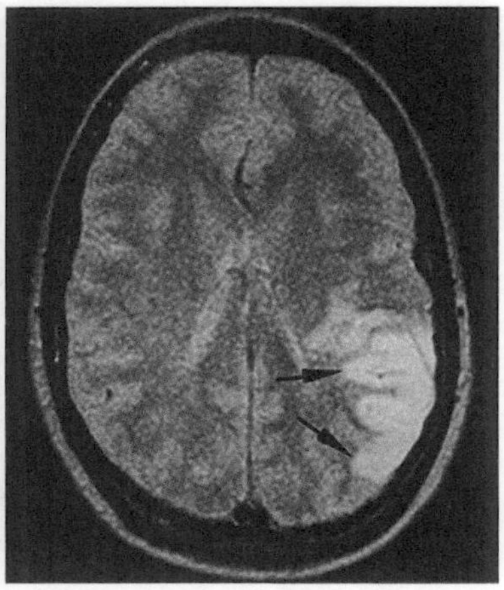

13.6

Fig. 13.7. A 23-day-old infarction in the territory of the left middle cerebral artery, predominantly involving the subcortical white matter *(arrow)*, in a 23-day-old woman. Additional small glial scar in the right frontal lobe *(long arrow)*. Axial scan, SE 1.2 s/100 ms

Fig. 13.8. Extensive infarction of the right basal ganglia *(arrows)* with compression of the ipsilateral ventricle in a 17-year-old man. Acute onset of left hemiparesis 8 days previously. Axial scan, SE 1.8 s/100 ms

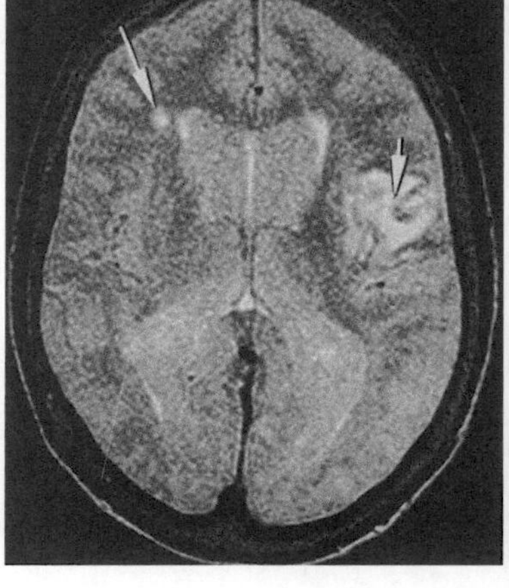

13.7

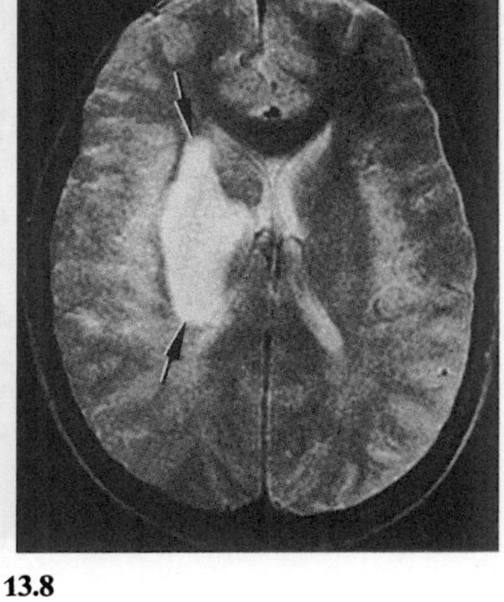

13.8

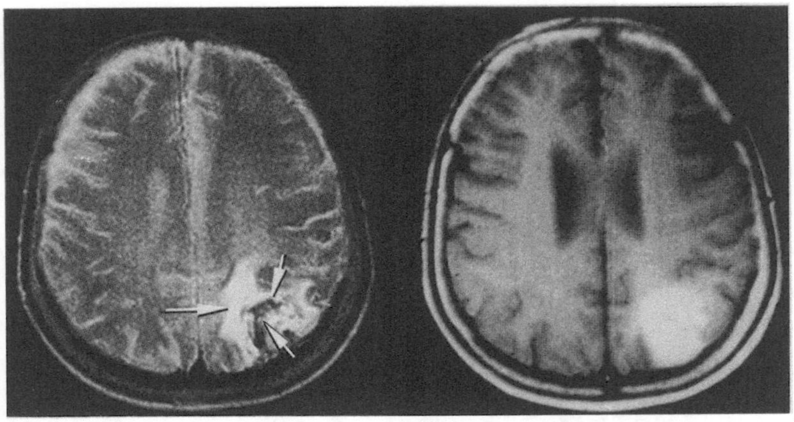

a b

Fig. 13.9 a, b. "Red" border-zone infarct between the territories of the middle and the posterior cerebral artery following carotid surgery, in a 62-year-old woman. **a** MR in the acute phase 3 days after the stroke event, using a T2-weighted sequence: signal loss in the infarcted area due to hemorrhage *(arrows)* surrounded by edema *(long arrow)*. **b** MR in the subacute phase on day 27: intense appearance of infarction in a T1-weighted image, indicating methemoglobin. Axial scans: **a** SE 1.5 s/100 ms, **b** SE 0.45 s/30 ms

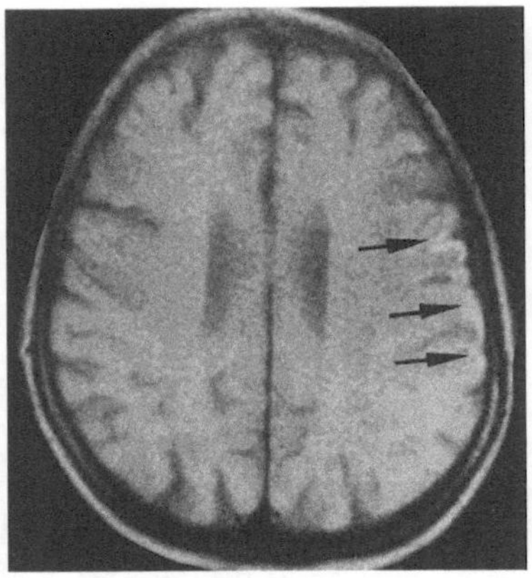

13.10

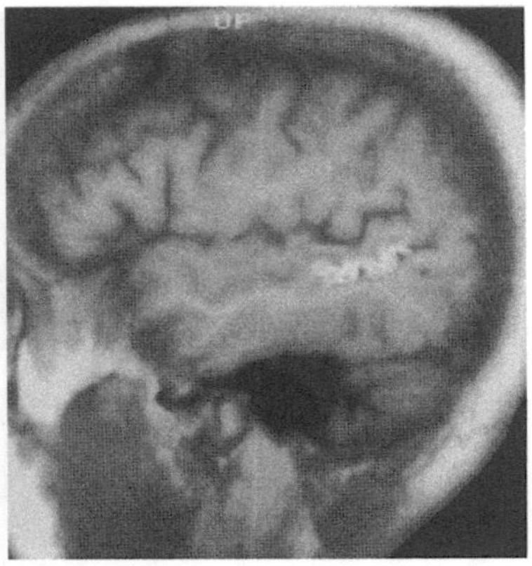

13.11

Fig. 13.10. A 22-day-old infarction in the territory of the left middle cerebral artery in a 58-year-old woman. The T1-weighted image demonstrates small cortical areas of hemorrhage *(arrows)*. Axial scan, SE 0.65 s/50 ms

Fig. 13.11. Temporal infarction in a 33-year-old woman with PRIND and a grand mal seizure. The hyperintensity of the cortical ribbon is caused by hemorrhagic infiltration, which was not detected by CT. Sagittal scan, SE 0.4 s/17 ms (1.0 T)

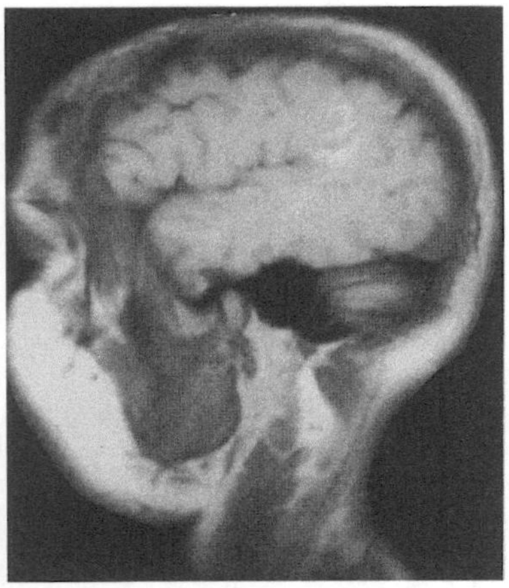

Fig. 13.12. Infarction of the territory of the parietal branch of the middle cerebral artery in a 30-year-old woman with sudden onset of global amnesia, aphasia, and one seizure 2 weeks previously. Hyperintense cortex indicates hemorrhagic infiltration. Sagittal scan, SE 0.7 s/30 ms (1.0 T)

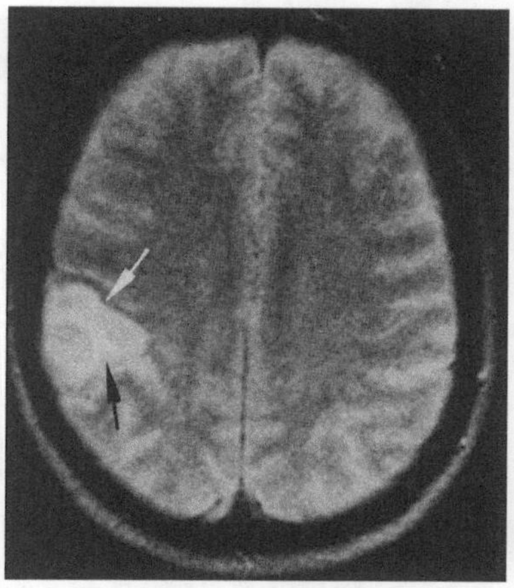

13.13

Fig. 13.13. A 22-day-old wedge-shaped infarction in the territory of the middle cerebral artery, showing a wall of glial proliferation *(arrows)*, in a 70-year-old woman. Axial scan, SE 1.5 s/100 ms

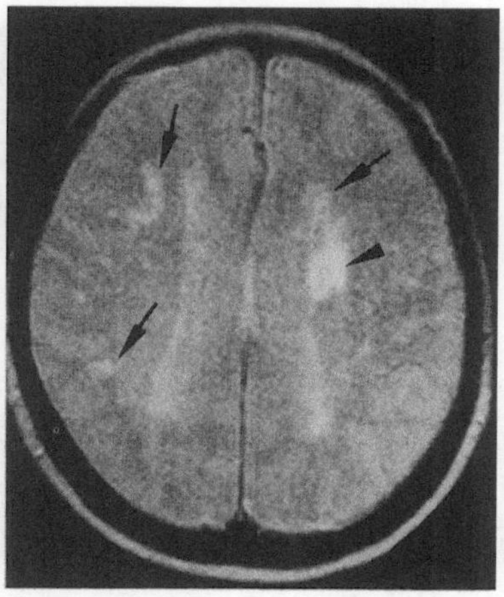

13.14

Fig. 13.14. Old lacunar infarction involving left basal ganglia *(arrowhead)*, without definite history of stroke, in a 71-year-old woman. WMLs in the deep white matter of both hemispheres *(arrows)*. Axial scan, SE 1.5 s/100 ms

characteristics of hemorrhages.) Clinically, MR seems to be significant for the detection of hemorrhagic infarcts especially in the subacute and chronic phase; CT mostly is negative in this period (Figs. 13.9–13.12).

Signal Changes over Time

T2-weighted images display a fresh infarct (the *necrotic phase* of Spatz [51]) as a smooth-margined, well-circumscribed, homogeneous area of increased signal intensity with an associated moderate to pronounced mass effect (Fig. 13.8, see Figs. 13.3, 13.4). Accompanying edema usually cannot be differentiated from the developing area of necrosis, so the extent of the edema must be calculated by means of mass effect (Fig. 13.8, see Fig. 13.5).

In the *absorption phase* [51] beginning at the end of the 2nd week, it is common for nonhomogeneities to appear in more extensive infarcts. As this occurs, signal intensity declines at the center of the lesion. This effect presumably results from a regression of edema while absorption is still in progress. Signals remain high at the periphery of the infarct, often creating a visible rim that marks the area of peripheral gliosis (Fig. 13.13, see Fig. 13.16). Areas of high signal intensity on T1-weighted scans are believed to represent hemorrhagic zones (Figs. 13.9–13.12), which occur with some frequency in the cortex [27].

Near the end of the absorption phase, the relaxation times in the infarcted area become longer again (with a corresponding signal increase on T2-weighted images and signal decrease on T1-weighted images), until final resolution of the infarct is achieved at 6–8 weeks with the formation of a cystic tissue defect (Figs. 13.14–17).

In rare cases cystic colliquation of the necrosis fails to occur, and a glial scar develops, which likewise gives a high signal on T2-weighted sequences and, unlike the cyst, is hyperintense even when shorter echo times are used (proton-density images). This serves to distinguish the cyst from a glial scar (Figs. 13.15–13.17).

Often it is not possible to determine the exact age of an infarct from the signal intensities found in a single examination. Thus, if the time of the infarction is unclear or if multiple infarctions have occurred, attention should be given to indirect signs. A pronounced mass effect suggests that the infarction has occurred within the last 14 days. As with CT, contrast enhancement (signal increase on T1-weighted images after injection of gadolinium-DTPA) is consistent with an infarct that is between 2 and 4 weeks old (Fig. 13.18) [19, 39]. Finally, reactive dilatations of the adjacent CSF spaces indicate final resolution of the infarct with substance loss (Figs. 13.19, 13.20).

The morphology of the MR signal change on postcontrast images corresponds to the pattern of contrast enhancement seen on CT scans, because both contrast materials show identical distributions within the body [39] (see also Sect. 5.5). We feel that contrast material is rarely necessary for MR studies, however, since it does not improve the detection of infarctions or the determination of their extent.

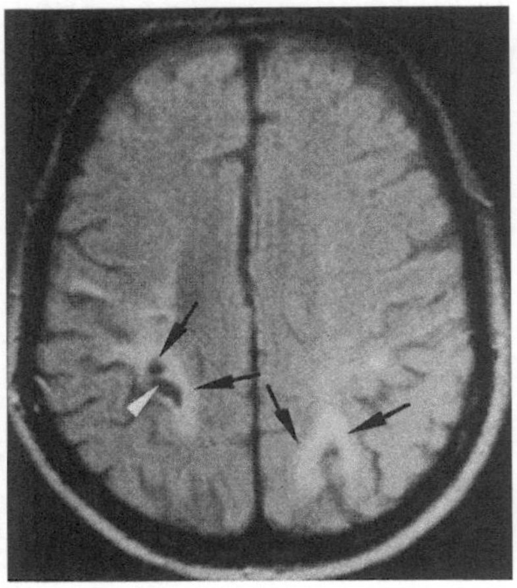

13.15

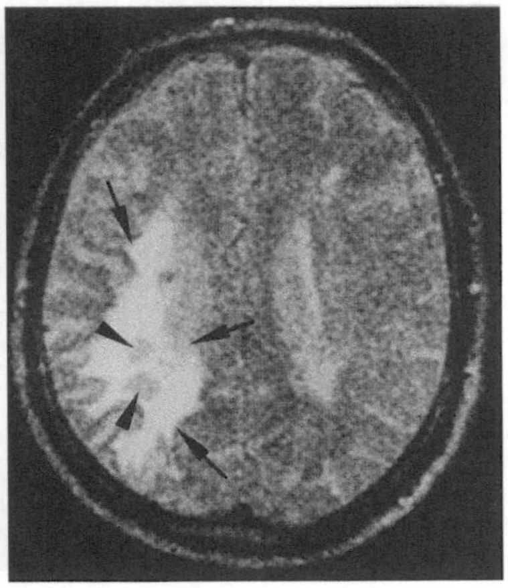

13.16

Fig. 13.15. Multi-infarct syndrome with old parieto-occipital infarctions of either glial *(arrows)* or cystic *(arrowhead)* nature. Axial scan, SE 1.2 s/50 ms

Fig. 13.16. Extensive white matter infarct in a 59-year-old man. Central cystic defects *(arrowheads)* surrounded by a broad glial scar *(arrows);* cerebral stroke after carotid surgery 2 years previously. Axial scan, SE 1.0 s/150 ms

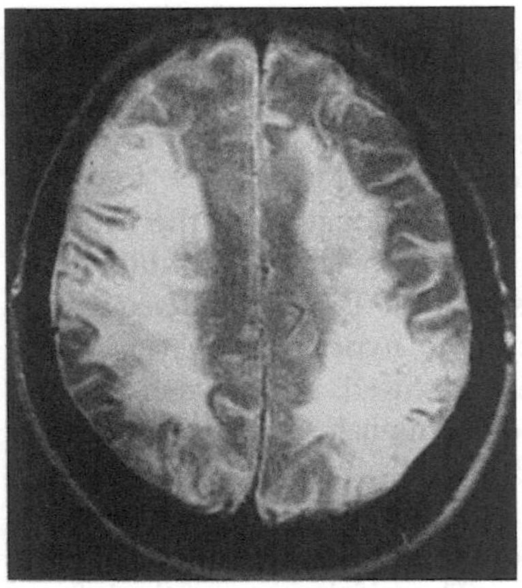

Fig. 13.17. Multi-infarct syndrome in a 49-year-old woman following right carotid occlusion and additional stenosis of left internal carotid artery. Extensive ischemic tissue defects involving cortex and white matter of both hemispheres. Axial scan, SE 1.8 s/100 ms

Evaluation

Despite its high sensitivity, MR imaging will have only a limited role in the diagnostic evaluation of stroke. In the acute phase CT is superior in the detection of hemorrhages, which are critical in terms of therapy. Exceptions are infarcts in the brainstem, midbrain, and cerebellum, which are displayed better on MR images. MR is also preferred in the subacute phase, especially when CT findings have been negative, because the infarct is not obscured by the fogging effect and because hemorrhages are accessible only to MR. The final cystic defect in the brain tissue is adequately displayed by CT, but the glial scar and its surroundings are demonstrated better by MR.

Initial clinical reports are available on the *MR imaging of nuclei other than hydrogen* [53]. The ^{23}Na nucleus is of particular interest in the diagnosis of infarctions, for the early stage of necrosis is associated with a sodium influx into the cells and thus with a rise in the total sodium concentration [30]. This technique, which is still experimental, appears to be entirely suitable for routine clinical application (Fig. 13.21).

The ^{31}P isotope is less suitable for MR imaging, but in spectroscopic analysis it provides new insights into the metabolism of the energy-rich phosphates. This metabolism is deranged early in infarctions and precedes the onset of edema formation. However, the phosphorus spectroscopy of precisely designated tissue sites [1, 37] is a costly and com-

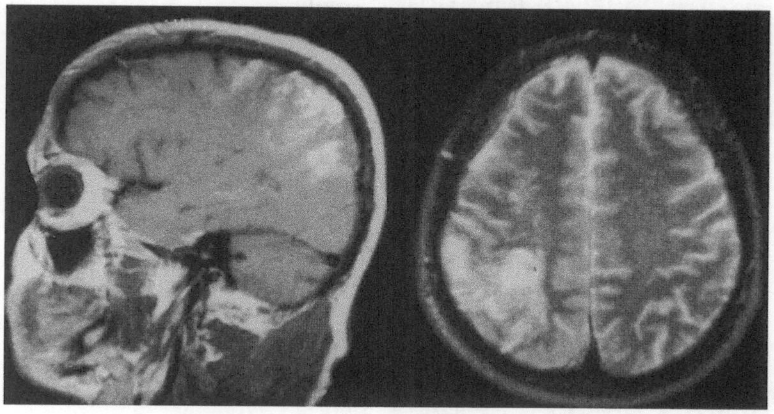

a b

Fig. 13.18 a, b. Cerebral infarction in a 47-year-old woman with left side hemiparesis. **a** with i.v.-gadolinium-DTPA the area of blood-brain barrier breakdown is depicted in the right parietal region. **b** The ischemic edema is shown as a hyperintense area. **a** Sagittal scan, SE 0.7 s/30 ms; **b** axial scan, SE 3.0 s/120 ms (1.0 T)

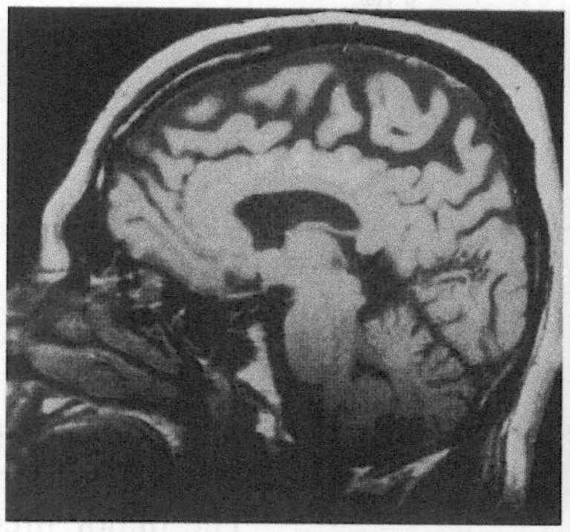

13.19

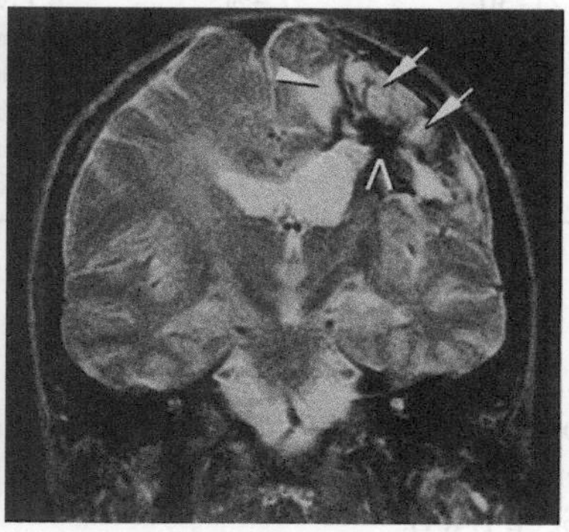

13.20

Fig. 13.19. Old bilateral infarction of the calcarine cortex in a 72-year-old man with incomplete cortical amaurosis. The paramedian sagittal scan shows the infarction of the left occipital lobe, which was almost identical on the right side SE 0.6 s/17 ms (1.0 T)

Fig. 13.20. Scan in a 19-year-old woman 3 years after "red" infarction in the territory of the middle cerebral artery. Cystic defect *(small arrows)* and perifocal glial proliferation *(arrowhead)*, areas of signal loss due to hemosiderin deposits *(open arrow)*. Coronal scan, SE 1.8 s/100 ms

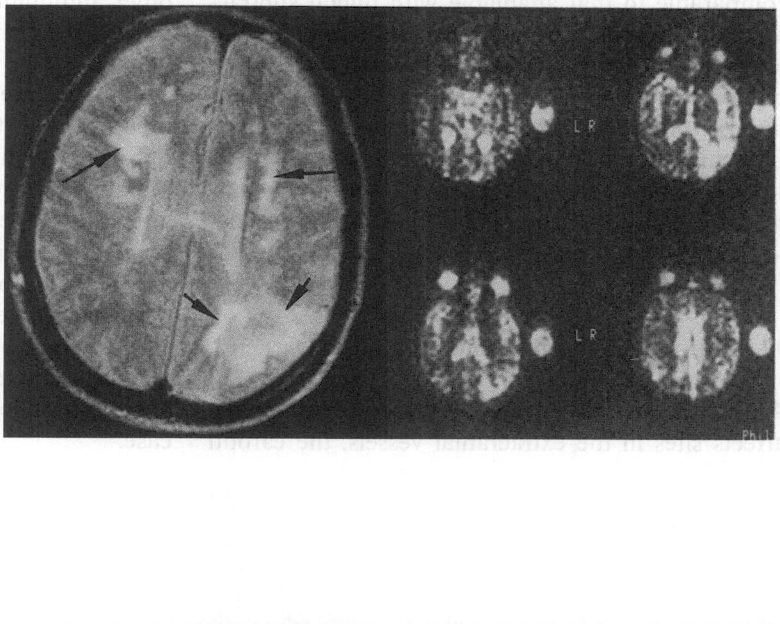

a b

Fig. 13.21 a, b. A 6-week-old infarction of the posterior territory of the left middle cerebral artery and the posterior border zone in a 65-year-old woman. Rim of glial proliferation *(arrows)*. The WMLs in the deep white matter of both hemispheres *(long arrows)* are not visible in the ^{23}Na image **(b)**. Axial scans, **a** SE 1.35 s/100 ms; **b** ^{23}Na imaging using a 3D spin-warp sequence 0.1 s/5,7 ms, 64 × 64 matrix with interpolation to 128 × 128

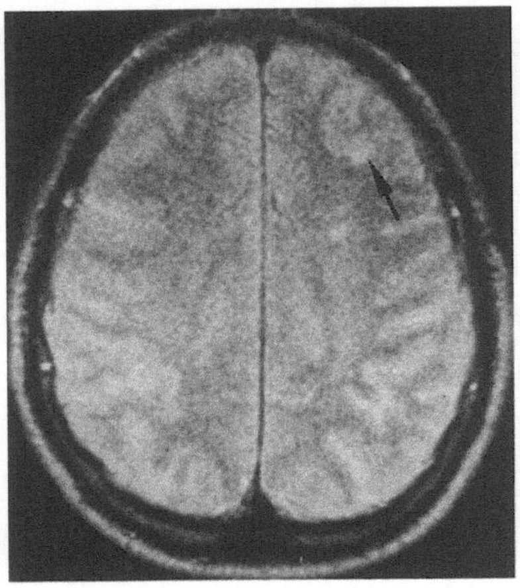

Fig. 13.22. Cerebrovascular insuffiency stage II in a 67-year-old man. MR demonstration of tiny WMLs, subcortical *(arrow)* and deep in the white matter. Axial scan, SE 1.35 s/100 ms

Age (years)	F	M	Total
0-10	-	-	-
11-20	-	-	-
21-30	7.4%	8.7%	8.0%
31-40	16.7%	16.7%	16.7%
41-50	23.1%	19.1%	20.9%
51-60	27.0%	30.2%	29.0%
61-70	43.5%	61.9%	52.3%
>70	70.0%	33.3%	56.3%

Fig. 13.23. Breakdown of patients with WMLs ($n = 91$) by age and sex as a proportion of the total collective ($n = 385$)

plex procedure that, for the time being, will be employed strictly for research purposes (see Sect. 1.4.4).

By contrast, it is expected that the imaging of extracranial vessels and segments of the intracranial vessels - *MR angiography* - will soon acquire clinical importance. Special pulse sequences, ECG triggering, and subtraction techniques in experimental systems are already providing a vascular definition comparable to that attainable with digital subtraction angiography. Complete occulusions of the internal carotid or vertebral arteries also are accessible to conventional SE imaging by the demonstration of thrombotic material in the vascular lumen. Particular attention should be given to the carotid siphon, whose constant position and bony surroundings make it especially well suited for the detection of occlusion.

13.1.2 Peripheral Angiopathies (See also Sect. 8.2)

Arteriosclerosis of the cerebral vessels preferentially affects sites in the extracranial vessels, the carotid siphon, and the basilar artery, but also frequently involves the small peripheral arteries and arterioles. The major predisposing factors for peripheral vascular occlusive disease are hypertension and diabetes mellitus [45]. Subcortical arterioslerotic encephalopathy (Binswanger's disease) may be considered a special form of peripheral cerebral arteriosclerosis of hypertensive origin [58]. Periarteritis nodosa, systemic lupus erythematosus (see also Sect. 9.4.2), and other autoimmune forms of vasculitis also tend to involve the peripheral vessels, producing microangiopathy.

Strokes are rare in the setting of peripheral blood flow disturbances. Clinically, microangiopathies are usually asscociated with generalized complaints, and severe cases may show dementia and alteration of personality [9, 18]

Pathoanatomically, general atrophic changes are accompanied by focal or diffuse demyelination of the white matter combined with microcystic necrosis and areas of glial proliferation [41]. The vessels may show sclerosis, hyalinosis (hypertension), or angiitic changes, depending on the underlying disease.

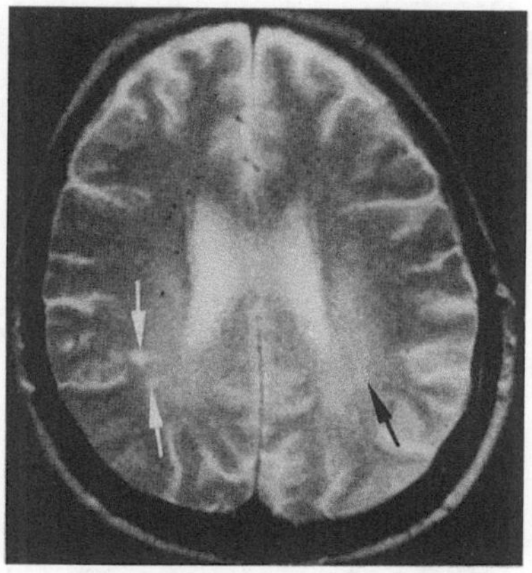

Fig. 13.24. Immunovasculitis in a 43-year-old man. WMLs in the parietal white matter *(arrows)*. Axial scan, SE 1.8 s/100 ms

The blood supply to the white matter, with watershed areas between the superficial and deep branches of the cerebral arteries, accounts for its susceptibility to injury due to microangiopathy [60].

CT and MR Findings

Cerebrovascular diseases may appear on CT scans as focal, hypodense lesions of the white matter that are most pronounced in the cerebral hemispheres. Isolated, asymmetric foci within the white matter may represent border zone infarcts secondary to occlusions of more proximal arteries, especially the internal carotid [60]. Occasionally they mark the whole borderline between the three branches of the internal carotid artery (see Fig. 13.26). These lesions have to be distinguished from largely symmetric, focal, or perhaps large and confluent hypodensities known as "white matter lesions" (WMLs), which may or may not be accompanied by general atrophic changes and are believed to result from microangiopathic disease [25].

Lesions of this type are seen much more frequently on MR images than with CT [6, 9, 43]. They are best displayed on heavily T2-weighted images (TR $\geqslant$1800 ms/TE $\geqslant$90 ms), where they show a higher signal intensity than the surrounding white matter. Usually the lesions are located deep within the white matter (Figs. 13.14–13.17, 13.22, 13.24–13.26). Less common sites are the subcortical area (see Figs. 13.14, 13.22, 13.24), the periventricular area (see Figs. 13.28–13.29) (especially in Binswanger's disease), and the internal capsule. Occasionally the lesions coexist with infarcts such as lacunar infarcts (see Fig. 13.14) or mass bleedings due to hypertension (Figs. 13.27–13.29). Differentiation from demyelinating or dysmyelinating diseases is not possible by morphologic criteria alone, and, especially in younger patients, must be derived from clinical signs and the results of CSF examinations.

The incidence of WMLs increases with age (Fig. 13.23) and rises dramatically to 30%–50% after the sixth decade of life [9, 11, 53], even in the absence of major predisposing factors - hypertension, diabetes mellitus, or autoimmune vasculitis. On the other hand, the presence of WMLs before 40 years of age is almost invariably associated with one of the foregoing conditions [53].

The extent of WMLs ranges from fine, isolated foci (see Figs. 13.22, 13.24) to extensive, more diffuse areas of heightened signal intensity (see Figs. 13.28, 13.29). If we analyze the frequency and extent of the lesions semiquantitatively according to an MR score and correlate them with the severity of stenotic changes in the carotid arteries, vertebral arteries, and basilar artery, we find that no relationship exists. This confirms the belief that WMLs must be the results of stenotic changes involving the periphery of the vessels.

Conclusions. MR is definitely superior to CT in detecting WMLs in the setting of chronic cerebrovascular insufficiency, and MR imaging is necessary in order to evaluate the lesions adequately. In younger patients, differentiation is required from demyelinating and dysmyelinating diseases, although this distinction cannot be made from morphologic criteria alone. The inability of angiography to define microangiopathic changes, plus the need to know the status of the peripheral arteries when selecting patients for surgical reconstruction of brachioce-

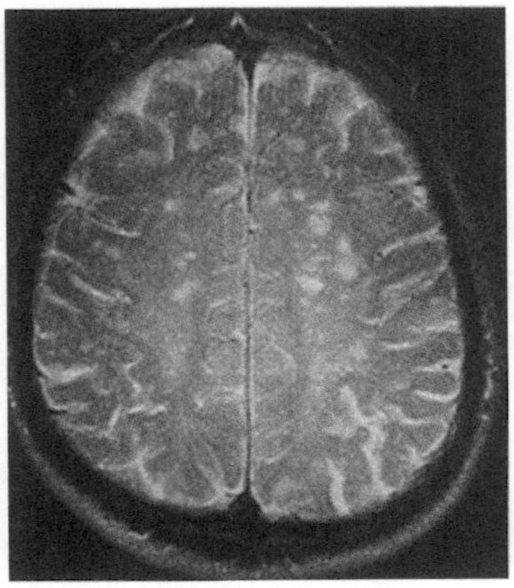

13.25

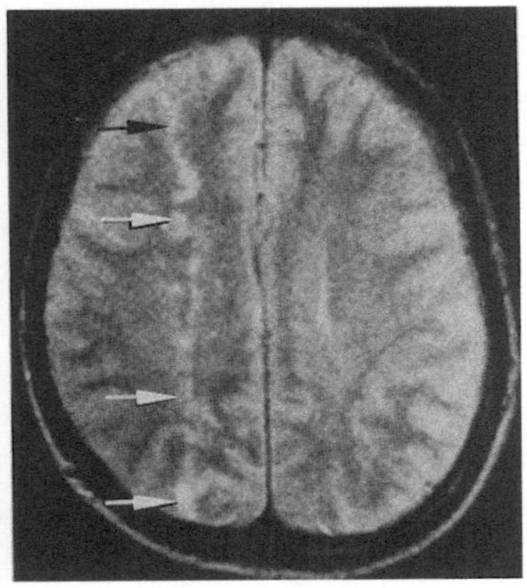

13.26

Fig. 13.25. Peripheral angiopathy due to hypertension in a 63-year-old man. Numerous WMLs in the white matter of both hemispheres. Axial scan, SE 1.8 s/100 ms

Fig. 13.26. Occlusion of right internal carotid artery in a 49-year-old man. Numerous WMLs along the border zone between anterior, middle, and posterior cerebral arteries *(arrows)*. Axial scan, SE 1.2 s/100 ms

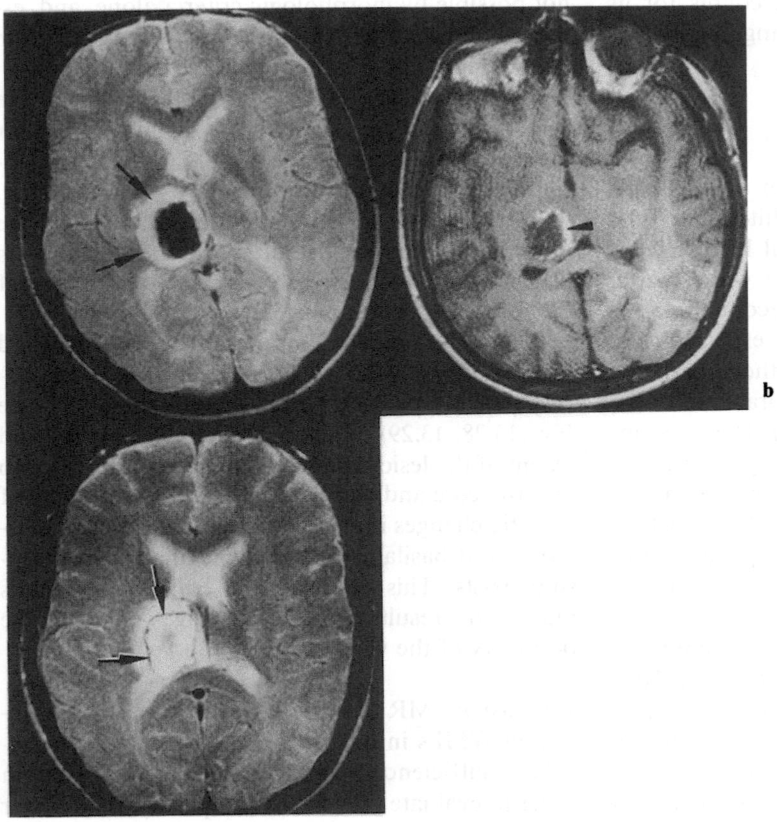

a b c

Fig. 13.27 a–c. Spontaneous bleeding in the right thalamus: observation of progress with examinations on day 2 **(a)**, day 5 **(b)** and day 11 **(c)** after the event. In the acute phase **(a)** a T2-weighted sequence demonstrates signal loss in the area of hemorrhage surrounded by perifocal edema *(arrows)*. In the early and late growing subacute phase **(b, c)** an intense ring caused by methemoglobin is seen *(arrowhead)* surrounded by a rim of low signal due to hemosiderin deposits *(arrows)*. Axial scans, **a** SE 1.8 s/100 ms; **b** SE 0.45 s/30 ms; **c** SE 1.8 s/100 ms

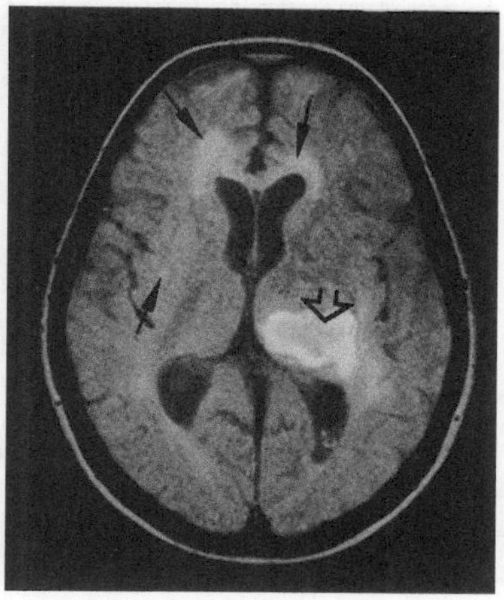

Fig. 13.28. A 3-week-old mass bleeding due to hypertension in a 46-year-old woman. Bleeding in the left thalamus *(open arrow)*, numerous partly confluent WMLs deep in the white matter and periventricular *(arrows)* caused by peripheral angiopathy due to hypertension. Axial scan, SE 1.2 s/50 ms

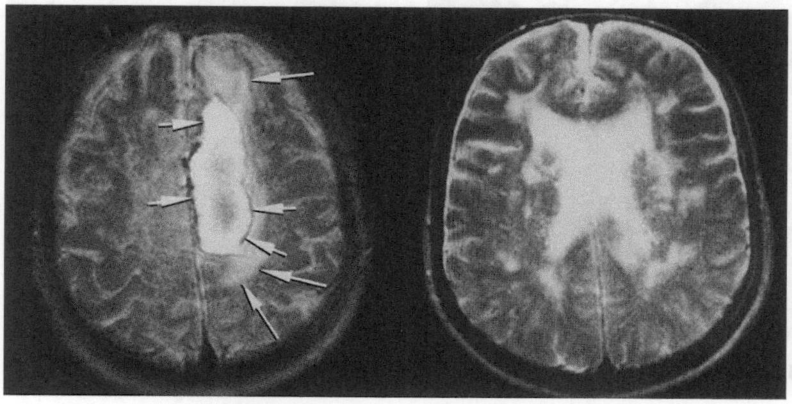

Fig. 13.29 a, b. A 10-day-old mass bleeding due to hypertension in a 56-year-old woman, involving the territory of the left anterior cerebral artery. Early signs of a rim of hemosiderin deposits *(small arrows)*, perifocal edema *(large arrows)*, numerous partly confluent WMLs deep in the white matter of both hemispheres caused by peripheral angiopathy **(b)**. Axial scans, **a, b** 1.8 s/100 ms

phalic vessels, will establish the role of MR imaging in preoperative diagnosis.

13.2 Disturbances of Venous Blood Flow

Disturbances in the venous drainage of the brain may be caused by direct external compression (edema, tumor) or by thrombotic occlusion. In the latter case a distinction is made between simple (bland) and septic thrombosis. Because the venous drainage of the brain contains extensive collaterals, circumscribed occlusions usually do not harm the tissue. More extensive thromboses of the venous sinuses and possibly of the cerebral veins lead initially to edema and later to hemorrhagic necrosis. In less severe cases the hemorrhages form a ringlike arrangement around the vessels (brain purpura), in more advanced cases mass bleedings of varying extent can be seen predominantly at the gray matter - white matter border [45, 56].

Septic thrombosis is caused by the direct spread of bacterial infection from the paranasal sinuses, ears, or facial boils. The cavernous sinus is a frequent site of occurrence. Even simple thrombosis usually can be related to head injury, pregnancy and the puerperium, inflammatory diseases of the nasopharynx, thrombophlebitis migrans, intra- or extracranial operations, or other causes.

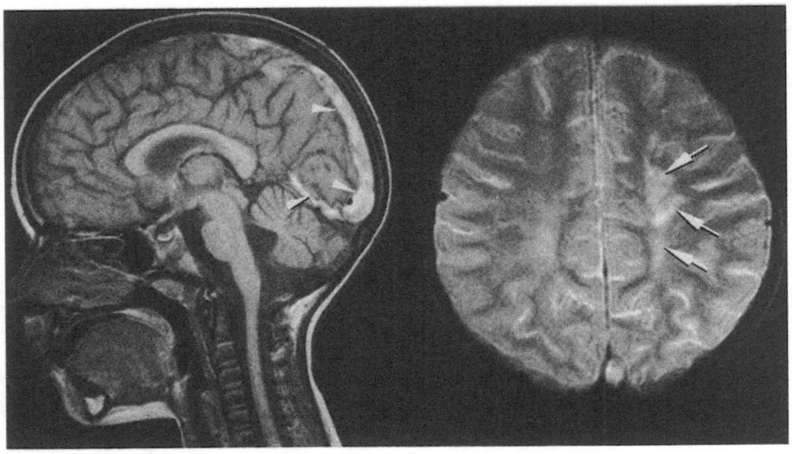

a b

Fig. 13.30 a, b. Thrombosis of the sagittal and straight sinus *(arrowheads)* in a 5-year-old boy after interstitial pneumonia with right hemiplegia and loss of vision in left eye due to fundus oculi hemorrhage. White matter edema in left hemisphere *(arrows)*. **a** Sagittal scan, SE 0.7 s/30 ms; **b** axial scan, SE 1.8 s/100 ms

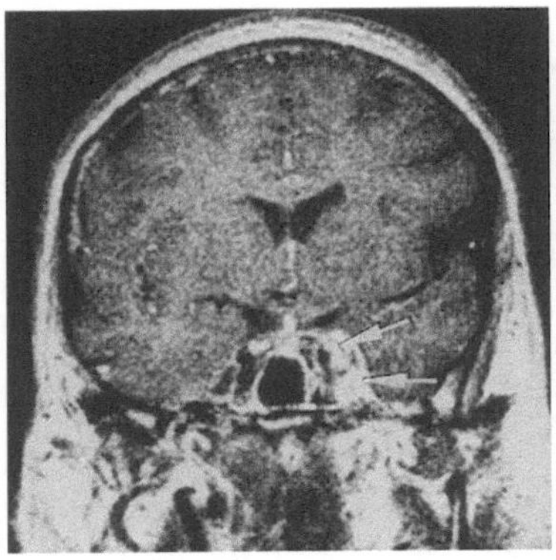

13.31

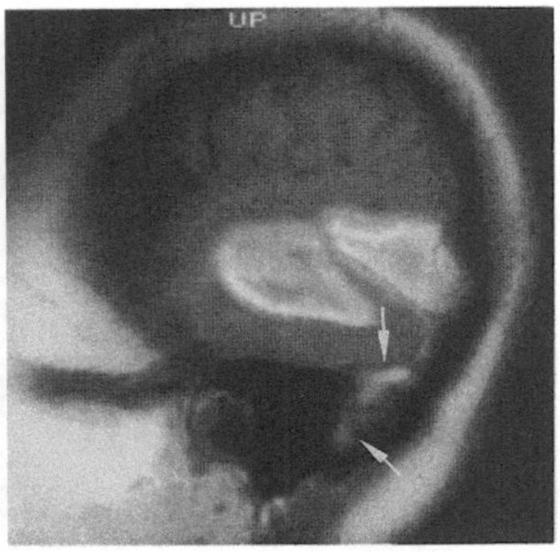

13.32

Fig. 13.31. Septic thrombosis of the left cavernous sinus in a 49-year-old woman causing enhanced signal intensities *(arrows)*. Coronal scan, SE 0.5 s/30 ms

Fig. 13.32. Thrombosis of the sigmoid sinus *(arrows)* with hemorrhagic infiltration of the temporal lobe in a 26-year-old woman with one focal seizure, no neurological deficit. Sagittal scan, SE 0.6 s/20 ms (1.5 T)

MR Findings

The intravascular signal intensity depends on a number of hemodynamic factors and their relation to the physical principles of MR, which are described in detail in Sect. 5.3.

Given the circumstances described in Chap. 5.3, a high first-echo signal in the venous channels would strongly indicate a blood flow disturbance if the vessels are coursing on the image plane. This emphasizes the importance of the midsagittal projection for the diagnosis of sinus thrombosis (Fig. 13.30). The midsagittal view should be a routine part of every MR examination of the brain, whether as an orienting view or as part of a sagittal multislice series. The reconstruction of pure phase images (phase display) [58] or the use of cine studies is recommended for more accurate differentiation between very slow flow and thrombosis (see also Sect. 5.3). When the double-echo or multiecho technique is used, it can be helpful to compare the signals of the first and second echoes, because even-echo rephasing is possible only if flow is still present. When there is total thrombotic occlusion of a vessel, the signal intensity falls with the T2 value of the thrombus material. It can also be helpful to analyze scans taken at different orientations, since the signal intensity of the thrombus remains identical on different planes when constant image parameters are used.

The signal characteristics of a thrombus depend on its age. As a rule, thrombi have relaxation times shorter than those of heparinized whole blood, although the values vary with the age of the clot. Fresh thrombi appear isointense with normal brain on T1-weighted images and hypointense on

T2-weighted images. Similar to cerebral hematomas, the signal intensities of thrombi increase over a period of several days on both T1-weighted and T2-weighted images due to the formation of methemoglobin (see Sect. 5.2). In this phase thrombosis is easily diagnosed on short TR/short TE images by virtue of its high contrast when an appropriate image plane is used (Figs. 13.30–13.32) [12, 38, 42, 56]. After the 2nd or 3rd week the lesion becomes increasingly nonhomogeneous, especially in larger vessels, presumably due to recanalization of the thrombus with associated flow effects (see Figs. 5.3, 5.5, 5.8).

The *opening of collateral channels* also can be demonstrated with MR. These present a typical vascular configuration with flow-void signs due to their higher flow velocities. The potential cerebral effects of venous insufficiency also are accessible to MR. Generalized or circumscribed edema is identified by its high signal intensities on T2-weighted images (Fig. 13.30). As in arterial infarction, it may not be possible to distinguish between edema and necrosis in the acute and subacute stage, although necrosis without hemorrhage is rare in venous blood flow disturbances. Areas of hemorrhagic malacia present high signal intensities on T1-weighted images (see Sect. 5.2) (Fig. 13.32).

Conclusions

Even the scant experience acquired to date indicates that MR will establish itself as the method of choice for detecting sinus thrombosis and for monitoring response to anticoagulant therapy. There is a danger of false-negative diagnosis due to the isointense to hypointense appearance of very fresh thrombotic occlusions. At present, then, if the MR study is negative but the patient shows clinical signs consistent with a sinus thrombosis, there is no alternative to X-ray angiography.

13.3 Hemorrhages

13.3.1 Intracerebral Hematomas Related to Vascular Disease

Intracerebral hematomas may occur in association with massive hypertensive hemorrhages, bleeding from aneurysms or arteriovenous malformations (AVMs), and hemorrhagic infarctions.

Massive hypertensive hemorrhages are due to the rupture of previously weakened small vessels during severe hypertensive episodes. The great majority of these hemorrhages occur in the putamen-claustrum region, possibly including the internal and external capsule, and thus in the territory of the lenticulostriate arteries. The causative importance of microaneurysms has frequently been stressed (see Sect. 14.1.4 and p. 210).

Massive hypertensive hemorrhages usually take the form of extensive burrowing hemorrhages, and bleeding into the ventricles is not uncommon. Spread to the subarachnoid space is less frequent. The clinical picture is always dramatic, and the mortality is about 85%. Men and women are affected equally. Massive hypertensive hemorrhages are rare before 40 years of age [45].

Massive hemorrhages due to nonhypertensive causes are grouped under the heading of *spontaneous intracerebral hematomas*. Congenital AVMs are cited as the leading cause, and accompanying subarachnoid hemorrhage is the rule.

Intracerebral hematomas are more commonly associated with angiomas than with aneurysms. Cerebral hemorrhages in patients on anticoagulant therapy can occur in the absence of a precipitating, underlying disease. Occasionally no cause is found for a spontaneous hematoma despite intensive diagnostic effort. In these cases the possibility of an occult AVM (see Sect. 14.1.2) should be considered in differential diagnosis.

The average age for spontaneous intracerebral hemorrhages is about 30 years. The clinical presentation depends strongly on the extent of the hemorrhage. The onset may be sudden, or more gradual with headache, impairment of consciousness, paralysis, and seizures.

13.3.2 Extracerebral Hematomas

Foremost among the extracerebral hematomas are the spontaneous subarachnoid hemorrhages, which are seen consistently in aneurysmatic and frequently in angiomatous hemorrhages. The spread of the hemorrhage often gives an important clue as to its source. This information can be helpful in the planning of angiography and operative treatment, which are always indicated.

MR Findings

Intracranial hemorrhages resolve by liquefaction and absorption. These processes, which produce MR signal changes, are independent of the cause and location of the hemorrhage. To avoid unnecessary repetitions, the MR features of these hemorrhages are discussed in full detail in Sect. 5.2.

References

1. Baleriaux D, Arnold L, Segebarth C, et al. (1986) ^{31}P MR evaluation of human brain tumor response to therapy. In: Book of Abstracts. Society of Magnetic Resonance in Medicine, 5th Annual Meeting, pp 41-42
2. Becker H, Desch H, Hacker H, et al. (1979) CT fogging effect with ischemic cerebral infarcts. Neuroradiology 18: 185-192
3. Betz E (1981) Physiologie und Pathophysiologie der Gehirndurchblutung. In: Diethelm L, Heuck F, Olsson D, Strnad F, Vieten H, Zuppinger A (eds) Springer, Berlin Heidelberg New York pp. 193-294 (Handbuch der medizinischen Radiologie, vol 6/1 a)
4. Bonafe A, Manelefe C, Scotto B, et al. (1985) Role of computed tomography in vertebrobasilar ischemia. Neuroradiology 27: 484-493
5. Bories J, Derhy S, Chiras J (1985) CT in hemispheric ischaemic attacks. Neuroradiology 27: 468-483
6. Bradley WG, Waluch V, Brant-Zawadzki M, et al. (1984) Patchy, periventricular white matter lesions in the elderly: a common observation during NMR imaging. Noninv Med Imag 1: 35-41
7. Brant-Zawadzki M, Bartkowski HM, Pitts LH, et al. (1984) NMR imaging of experimental and clinical cerebral edema. Noninvas Med Imag 1: 43-47
8. Brant-Zawadzki M, Solomon M, Newton TH, et al. (1985) Basic principles of magnetic resonance imaging in cerebral ischemia and initial clinical experiences. Neuroradiology 27: 517-520
9. Brant-Zawadzki M, Fein G, van Dyke C, et al. (1985) Magnetic resonance imaging of the aging brain: patchy white matter lesions and dementia. Am J Neuroradiol 6: 675-682
10. Brant-Zawadzki M, Pereira B, Weinstein P, et al. (1986) MR-imaging of acute experimental ischemia in cats. Am J Neuroradiol 7: 7-11
11. Brant-Zawadzki M, Kucharczyk W (1987) Vascular disease: ischemia. In: Brant-Zawadzki M, Norman D (eds) Magnetic resonance imaging of the central nervous system. Raven, New York, pp. 221-234
12. Braun IF, Hoffman JC, Malko JA, et al. (1985) Jugular venous thrombosis: MR imaging. Radiology 157: 357-360

12a. Brooks RA, Battocletti JH, Sances A, et al. (1975) Nuclear magnetic relaxation in blood. IEEE Trans Biomed Eng 1: 12-18

13. Bryan RN, Willcott MR, Schneiders NJ, et al. (1983) Nuclear magnetic resonance evaluation of stroke: a preliminary report. Radiology 149: 189-192
14. Bryan RN, Willcott MR, Schneiders NJ, et al. (1983) NMR evaluation of occlusive stroke in the rat. Am J Neuroradiol 4: 242-244
15. Buonanno FS, Pykett IL, Kistler JP, et al. (1982) Cranial anatomy and detection of ischemic stroke in the cat by nuclear magnetic resonance imaging. Radiology 143: 187-193
16. Buonanno FS, Pykett IL, Brady TJ, et al. (1983) Proton NMR imaging in experimental ischemic infarction. Stroke 14: 178-184
17. Bydder GM, Steiner RE, Young IR, et al. (1982) Clinical NMR imaging of the brain: 140 cases. Am J Roentgenol 139: 215-236
18. Cherryman GR, Gemmell HG, Sharp PF, et al. (1985) NMR demonstration of white matter changes in the watershed area of patients with dementia. Correlation with psychiatric evaluation and I-123-isopropylamphetamine cerebral blood flow imaging. Society of Magnetic Resonance in Medicine, 4th annual meeting, (abstract) pp 264-265
19. Davis KR, Ackerman RH, Kistler JP, Mohr JP (1977) Computed tomography of cerebral infarction: hemorrhagic, contrast enhancement and time of appearance. Comput Tomogr 1: 71-86
20. DeWitt LD, Buonanno FS, Kistler JP, et al. (1984) Nuclear magnetic resonance imaging in evaluation of clinical stroke syndromes. Ann Neurol 16: 535-545

20a. Dunn, WM, Hesselink JR, Peterson TM, et al. (1985) Correlation of regional cerebral blood flow with T1 and T2 relaxation times and brain water content in an embolic stroke model. Society of Magnetic Resonance in Medicine, 4th annual meeting, pp 269-270 (abstr.)

21. Fisher CM (1965) Lacunes: small, deep cerebral infarcts. Neurology 15: 774-784
22. Friedmann G, Steinbrich W, Heiss W-D, et al. (1985) Ischemic brain disease - comparison of MRI, CT, PET and angiography. In: Book of abstracts. Society of Magnetic Resonance in Medicine, 4th Annual Meeting, pp 271-272
23. Garcia JH (1984) Experimental ischemic stroke: a review. Stroke 15: 5-14
24. Gautier JC, Pullicino P (1985) A clinical approach to cerebrovascular disease. Neuroradiology 27: 452-459
25. Goto K, Ishi N, Gukasawa H (1981) Diffuse white-matter disease in the geriatric population. Radiology 141: 687-695
26. Gotoh O, Asano T, Koide T, Takakura K (1985) Ischemic brain edema following occlusion of middle cerebral artery in the rat. I: The time courses of the brain water, sodium and potassium contents and blood-brain barrier permeability to I-125-albumin. Stroke 16: 101-109
27. Hecht-Leavitt C, Gomori JM, Grossman RI (1986) High-field MRI of hemorrhagic cortical infarction. Am J Neuroradiol 7: 581-585
28. Heiss W-D, Friedmann G, Beil C, Steinbrich W (1985) PET-Stoffwechseluntersuchungen im Vergleich zu MRI-Befunden bei zerebrovaskulären Erkrankungen. In: Lissner J, Doppman J (eds) MR '85, Internationales Kernspintomographie-Symposium, Garmisch-Partenkirchen, Schnetztor, Konstanz, pp. 274-280
29. Heiss W-D, Herbolz K, Böcher-Schwarz HG, et al. (1986) Comparison of PET, MRI and X-ray CT in cerobrovascular disease. J Comput Assist Tomogr 10: 903-911
30. Hilal SK, Maudsley AA, Simon HE, et al. (1983) In vivo NMR imaging of tissue sodium in the intact cat before

and after acute cerebral stroke. Am J Neuroradiol 4: 245-249

31. Hossmann KA, Schuier FJ (1980) Experimental brain infarcts in cats. I. Pathophysiological observations. Stroke 11: 583-592
32. Ito U, Ohno K, Nakamura R, et al. (1979) Brain edema during ischemia and after restoration of blood flow. Measurements of water, sodium, potassium content and plasma protein permeability. Stroke 10: 542-547
33. Kato H, Kogure K, Ohtomo H, et al. (1985) Correlations between proton nuclear magnetic resonance imaging and retrospective histochemical images in experimental cerebral infarction. J Cereb Blood Flow Metab 5: 267-274
34. Kistler JP, Buonanno FS, DeWitt LD, et al. (1984) Verte bral-basilar posterior cerebral territory stroke delineation by proton nuclear magnetic resonance imaging. Stroke 15: 417-426
35. Launay M, N'Diave M, Bories J (1985) X-ray computed tomography (CT) study of small, deep and recent infarcts (SDRIs) of the cerebral hemispheres in adults. Preliminary and critical report. Neuroradiology 27: 494-508
36. Levy RM, Feustel PJ, Mills C, et al. (1985) Parallel studies of magnetic resonance imaging (MRI) and cortical blood flow in acute experimental cerebral ischemia. Society of Magnetic Resonance in Medicine, 4th annual meeting, pp 279-280 (abstract)
37. Luyten PR, Groen JP, Arnold DL, et al. (1986) ^{31}P MR localized spectroscopy of the human brain in situ at 1.5 Tesla. In: Society of Magnetic Resonance in Medicine, 5th Annual Meeting, pp 1083-1084 (abstract)
38. Macchi PJ, Grossman RI, Gomori JM, et al. (1986) High field MR imaging of cerebral venous thrombosis. J Comput Assist Tomogr 10: 10-15
39. Mancuso AA, Virapongese C, Quisling RG (1986) Early clinical experience with Gd-DTPA-enhanced magnetic resonance imaging in acute cerebral infarction and in chronic ischemic changes. In: Runge VM, Claussen C, Felix R, James AE (eds) Contrast agents in magnetic resonance; proceedings of an international workshop, SanDiego. Excerpta Medica, Amsterdam, pp 127-128
40. Mano I, Levy RM, Crooks LE, Hosobuchi Y (1983) Proton nuclear magnetic resonance imaging of acute experimental cerebral ischemia. Invest Radiol 17: 345-351
41. Marshall V, Flannigan BD, Bradley WG, et al. (1986) The MR appearance of gliosis: correlation with histopathology. Society of Magnetic Resonance in Medicine, 5th annual meeting, pp 799-800 (abstracts)
42. McMurdo SK, Brant-Zawadzki M, Bradley WG, et al. (1986) Dural sinus thrombosis: study using intermediate field strength MR imaging. Radiology 161: 83-86
43. Ormerod IEC, Du Boulay EPGH, Callanan MM, et al. (1984) NMR in multiple sclerosis and cerebral vascular disease. Lancet 8: 1334-1335
44. Pykett IL, Buonanno FS, Brady TJ, Kistler DP (1983) True threedimensional nuclear magnetic resonance neuroimaging in ischemic stroke: correlation of NMR, X-ray CT and pathology. Stroke 14: 173-177
45. Scheid W (1983) Lehrbuch der Neurologie. Thieme, Stuttgart
46. Schuier FJ, Hossmann KA (1980) Experimental brain infarcts in cats. II. Ischemic brain edema. Stroke 11: 593-601
47. Sipponen JT, Sepponen RE, Sivula A (1984) Chronic subdural hematoma: Demonstration by magnetic resonance. Radiology 150: 79-85
48. Sipponen JT, Kaste M, Ketonen L, et al. (1984) Serial nuclear magnetic resonance (NMR) imaging in patients with cerebral infarction. J Comput Assist Tomogr 8: 369-380
49. Sipponen JT (1984) Visualization of brain infarction with nuclear magnetic resonance imaging. Neuroradiology 26: 590-594
50. Skriver EB, Olsen TS (1980) Transient disappearance of cerebral infarcts in CT scan. The so called fogging effect. Neuroradiology 22: 61-65
51. Spatz H (1939) Pathologische Anatomie der Kreislaufstörungen des Gehirns. Z Ges Neurol Psychiatrie 167: 301-357
52. Spetzler RF, Zabramski JM, Kaufman B, Yeung HN (1983) Acute NMR changes during MCA occlusion: a preliminary study in primates. Stroke 14: 185-191
53. Steinbrich W, Friedmann G, Pawlik G, et al. (1986) MR bei ischämischen Hirnerkrankungen - ein Vergleich mit CT, PET (18 Fluordeoxyglukose) und angiographischen Ergebnissen. Fortschr Röntgenstr 145: 173-181
54. Steinbrich W, Friedmann G, Herholz K, Heiss W-D (1986) MR bei ischämischen Erkrankungen des Gehirns - Vergleich mit CT und PET unter Einbeziehung angiographischer Ergebnisse. In: Vogler E, Schneider GA (eds) Digitale bildgebende Verfahren, integrierte digitale Radiologie. Schering, Berlin, pp 174-179
55. Swanson RA, Schmidley JW (1985) Amnestic syndrome and vertical gaze palsy: Early detection of bilateral thalamic infarction by CT and NMR. Stroke 16: 823-827
56. Thron A, Wessel K, Linden D, et al. (1986) Superior sagittal sinus thrombosis: neuroradiological evaluation and clinical findings. J Neurol 233: 283-288
57. Thun F, Friedmann G (1981) Kopf. In: Friedmann G, Bücheler E, Thurn P (eds) Ganzkörper-Computertomographie. Thieme, Stuttgart pp 41-90
58. White EM, Edelman RR, Wedeen VJ, Brady J (1986) Intravascular signal in MR imaging: Use of phase display for differentiation of blood-flow signal from intraluminal disease. Radiology 161: 245-249
59. Zeumer H, Schonsky B, Sturm KW (1980) Predominant white matter involvement in subcortical arteriosclerotic encephalopathy (Binswanger disease). J Comput Assis Thomogr 4: 14-19
60. Zülch KJ (1985) The cerebral infarct: pathology, pathogenesis and computed tomography. Springer, Berlin Heidelberg New York

14 Vascular Malformations

W. J. Huk

Angiomatous malformations are based on a failure of the fetal blood vessels to differentiate into arteries, capillaries, and veins. In most cases the capillary network is absent, so that arteries and veins communicate directly [16]. Aneurysms are based on a congenital defect in the vessel wall.

Because angiography continues to be the primary technique for the evaluation of vascular malformations, it is convenient to subdivide these into angiographically demonstrable and angiographically occult anomalies. This division is justified by clinical, diagnostic, and therapeutic differences. MR contributes useful topographic information on the angiographically demonstrable vascular anomalies, and is becoming the method of choice for the detection of angiographically occult lesions.

14.1 Vascular Malformations of the Brain

14.1.1 Angiographically Demonstrable Vascular Anomalies

Angiography can demonstrate vascular malformations whose pathologic vessels are large enough to be visible on the angiogram and whose blood flow is rapid enough to provide adequate opacification of the anomaly during the brief period of the series of conventional angiography or digital subtraction angiography (DSA). These include the majority of *arteriovenous malformations* (AVMs), *varix or aneurysm of the vein of Galen, venous angiomas, aneurysms,* and *dural arteriovenous fistulas.*

The goal of diagnostic imaging in these vascular malformations of the brain is to demonstrate: the size of the vascular malformation; the hemodynamics within the VM (shunt volume, high-flow and low-flow compartments); the effects of the VM on the brain tissue (mass effect, hemorrhage, calcification, atrophy); and the relation of the VM to surrounding brain structures. This information is necessary to evaluate the natural risk of VMs and the risk involved in therapeutic measures (direct surgery, embolization only, combination of embolization and surgery, stereotactic radiotherapy).

Arteriovenous Malformations

Arteriovenous malformations are the most common congenital vascular anomalies. Some 93% of AVMs are supratentorial, showing a predilection for the parietal cortex [14, 35]. Eighteen percent are located in the thalamus, basal ganglia, and internal capsule [49], and 5–7% in the posterior fossa, brainstem, and spinal cord [3]. About 10% of intracranial aneurysms are associated with AVMs [49].

A review of infratentorial AVMs showed that two-thirds of the lesions were confined to the cerebellum, especially its medial portions (superior and inferior vermis, tonsils), 20% involved the medulla or pons exclusively, while the remaining 15%–20% extended into several of the foregoing regions and at least partially occupied the cerebellopontine angle [3].

Histologically, the dilated angiomatous vessels have walls of varying thickness that are composed mostly of fibrous tissue with occasional smooth muscle fibers, but without an elastic layer.

Angiomas may be associated with atrophic changes in the surrounding brain tissue, secondary thromboses of vessels, calcifications, and cerebral infarction. The veins draining the malformation show greater dilatation than the feeding arteries.

Uncertainty persists regarding the *natural risks of AVMs,* partly because experience to date is based on relatively small numbers of cases. These risks include not only the major hazards of AVMs (hemorrhage, steal effects by the AV shunt causing ischemic brain injury in adjacent and remote regions) [13], but also clinical symptoms such as headache, seizures, and neurologic deficits, which may be severe. It is important, moreover, to consider the individual characteristics of the angioma when weighing the therapeutic (especially the surgical) risk against the natural risk of the disease.

In angiographic follow-up studies performed during the first two decades of life, Luessenhop and Rosa [32] noted progressive changes in the appearance of AVMs. Initially they had a diffuse appearance with only minor alteration of the surrounding vasculature. This was followed by gradual progression toward a more compact lesion involving a larger vascular area and an increase in the shunt volume, as evidenced by enlargement of the feeding arteries and draining veins. This process has been noted by other authors during the first two decades of life [7, 53]. The changes correlate with the relative frequency and time of onset of clinical symptoms. By the end of the fourth decade, 80% of all cases will have become symptomatic [32].

Pathologic studies have shown evidence of multiple, subclinical *hemorrhages* from angiomas (indicated by hemosiderin deposits), making it apparent that only certain extravasations are large enough to produce overt signs. Based on a follow-up study of 191 untreated patients, Graf et al. [19] estimate that the probability of a clinically significant hemorrhage is 2%–3% per year for the initial bleed, with a 6% incidence of recurrent hemorrhages in the first year and 2% per year thereafter. The majority of hemorrhages occurred between 11 and 35 years of age. The authors found somewhat higher incidences of hemorrhage (of uncertain significance) in small AVMs, AVMs of the temporal lobe, AVMs associated with neurologic deficits, and in females.

The natural risk of mortality and morbidity varies among individual hemorrhages, but Luessenhop and Rosa [32] consider 10% mortality and 30% morbidity to be good estimates, based on their own observations and a review of the literature.

In the Cooperative Study of Subarachnoid Hemorrhages and Intracranial Aneurysms, intracranial hemorrhage was the presenting complaint in 72% of infratentorial AVMs, as opposed to 66% of supratentorial lesions [38]. The incidence of intraventricular hemorrhage in angiomas of the posterior fossa reflects the common intraventricular extension or presentation of the majority of these malformations, except for the most peripherally located cerebellar AVMs [3].

Headaches are often migraine-like and are usually associated with AVMs in the posterior cerebral artery territory. Once started, they generally persist throughout the patient's lifetime [32]. Headaches can also be caused by hydrocephalus secondary to a subarachnoid or intraparenchymal hemorrhage.

The course of *seizures* is more difficult to predict, but they are rarely incapacitating if appropriate anticonvulsive therapy is initiated.

Progressive *neurologic deterioration* advances slowly and frequently stabilizes. In the absence of intervening hemorrhage, it rarely leads to severe deficits such as hemiplegia or aphasia [32]. Fluctuating or slowly progressing neurologic deficits are believed to result from chronic neuronal ischemia, which can also lead to seizures. Cerebral blood flow measurements in patients with angiomas indicate that large ischemic territories can exist in the vicinity of even small malformations [3].

Angiomas located on the medial aspect of the cerebral hemisphere and involving portions of the limbic system (15% of 164 AVMs in the series of Stein [47]) represent a special group of vascular malformations because of their obscure location and the difficulties encountered in their resection. They are prone to hemorrhage and evince complex venous drainage [47]. The arterial supply to these angiomas comes from deep and often obscure arteries, including trunks or branches of the anterior and posterior choroidal vessels and the posterior cerebral artery. Because of this, the malformations are often contiguous with the choroid plexus, which contains part of the feeding and draining vasculature.

Major draining veins extend to the sagittal sinus, via the cortex, and to the deep venous system, including the internal cerebral veins or vein of Galen and thence to the straight sinus. These features have important surgical implications [47, 48].

Luessenhop and Rosa [32] devised a *grading system for the natural risk and surgical risk of AVMs*, based on their observations of 450 cases over a period of 20 years. For the more common lateral hemispheric AVMs, they equated the risk to the maximum measured diameter in a lateral angiogram, which proved useful for predicting surgical outcome:

Grade I: lesions under 2 cm
Grade II: lesions of 2–4 cm
Grade III: lesions of 4–6 cm
Grade IV: lesions over 6 cm

Mortality and morbidity were low in grade I and grade II AVMs but reached the level of the natural risk in the higher-grade angiomas [31].

This classification by size does not take into account the hemodynamic and topographic aspects of the AVMs. An *anatomic grading system* has also been proposed in which the grades correspond to

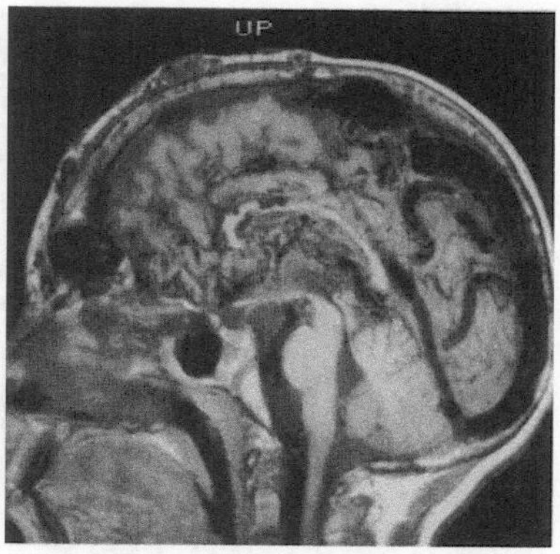

Fig. 14.1. Diffuse angiomatosis of the head in a 12-year-old boy with seizures. Bilateral involvement of external and internal carotid arteries. Sagittal scan, SE 0.6 s/15 ms (1.5 T)

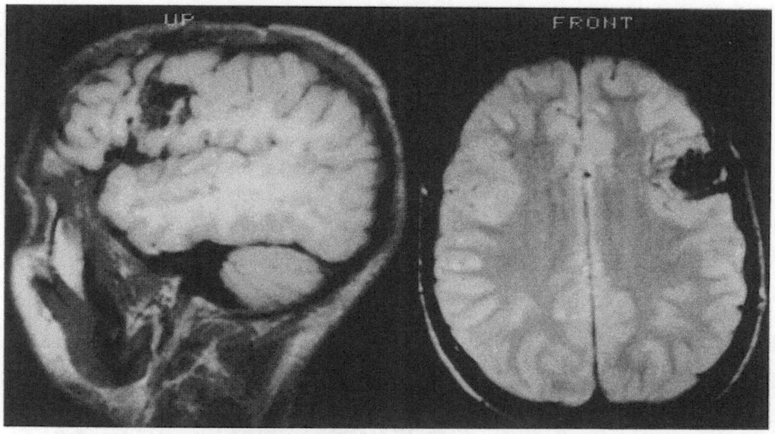

Fig. 14.2 a, b. AVM near Broca's center with superficial drainage in a 14-year-old boy with partial seizures. **a** Sagittal scan, SE 0.7 s/30 ms; **b** axial scan, SE 3.0 s/40 ms; (1.0 T)

the number of tertiary arteries directly supplying the malformation [31]. For deep AVMs, the grades correspond to the number of penetrating arteries participating. Other modifications are necessary for AVMs of the corpus callosum and choroid plexus. Spetzler and Martin [46] propose a grading system based on three of the most important variables: (1) the size of the AVM, (2) the pattern of venous drainage, and (3) the neurologic eloquence of the brain adjacent to the malformation. These variables embrace other critical factors related to the degree of surgical risk, such as the number of feeding arteries, the degree of vascular steal, and surgical accessibility. AVMs under 3 cm in diameter are rated as small, 3-6 cm as medium, and over 6 cm as large, corresponding to numerical scores of 1, 2, and 3 points respectively. Superficial drainage is scored 0 points, deep drainage 1 point. Likewise, a score of 1 is assigned to AVMs in eloquent brain regions, and of 0 in noneloquent regions. Areas considered eloquent include the sensorimotor, language, and visual cortex; the hypothalamus and thalamus; the internal capsule; the brainstem; the cerebellar peduncles; and the deep cerebellar nuclei. The grade (I-V) of an AVM is derived from the sum of the scores assigned for each of the three categories.

CT and MR Findings

Besides differences in blood flow velocity, other phenomena may be found in association with angiomas that are helpful in making a diagnosis: hemorrhages in various stages of liquefaction, perifocal edema, calcifications, or hemosiderin deposits as evidence of prior subclinical hemorrhage [12].

Arteriovenous malformations usually appear isodense on noncontrast CT scans, but they may also appear slightly hypodense or hyperdense, often with very high density calcifications. Contrast injec-

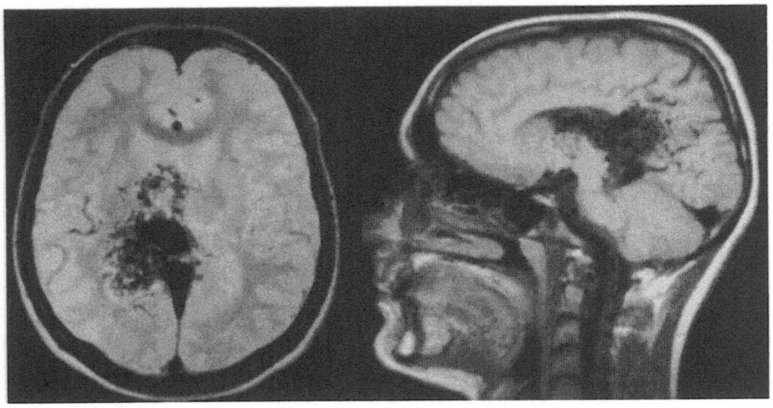

a b

Fig. 14.3 a, b. Large AVM of the region of the left basal ganglia in a 20-year-old woman with repeated episodes of headache after a normal pregnancy and delivery per vias naturales. Large AVM fed by all three major cerebral arteries including the lenticulostriate and choroidal arteries, and draining to an enlarged vein of Galen. **a** Axial scan, SE 3.0 s/45 ms, **b** sagittal scan, SE 0.4 s/17 ms (1.0 T)

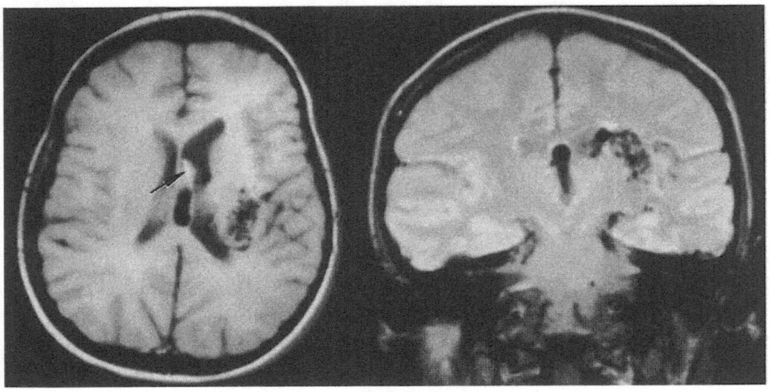

a b

Fig. 14.4 a, b. AVM of the right basal ganglia in a 23-year-old woman with spontaneous intraventricular hemorrhage. Small AVM involving parts of the putamen, the internal capsule, the external capsule, and the corona radiata, fed mainly by the posterior choroidal arteries and draining to the dilated internal veins. A small recent hemorrhage is seen near the foramen of Monro *(arrow)*. **a** Axial scan, SE 0.7 s/30 ms; **b** coronal scan, SE 2.5 s/35 ms (1.0 T)

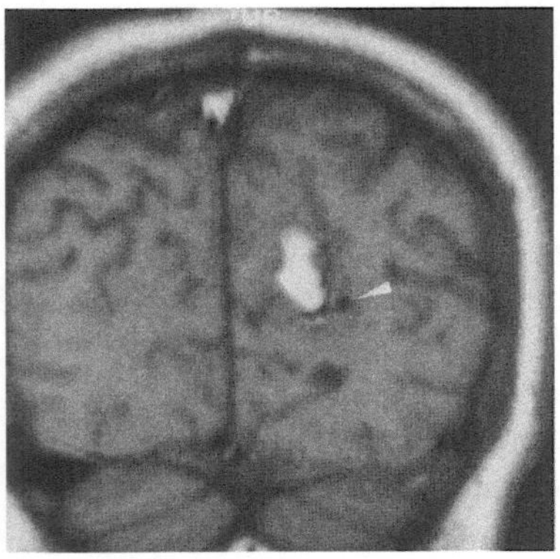

Fig. 14.5. Small AVM of occipital lobe in a 43-year-old man with sudden headache. Small subcortical hemorrhage of left occipital lobe. The dilated vessel lateral to the hematoma *(arrowhead)* arouses suspicion of an AVM, which was proven by surgery. Coronal scan, SE 0.5 s/30 ms (1.0 T)

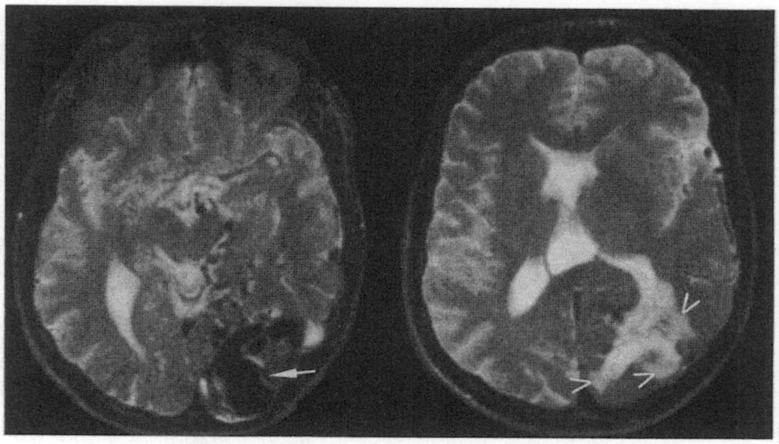

Fig. 14.6 a, b. AVM of the occipital lobe in a 30-year-old man with headache and visual disturbances. The nidus of this medium-size AVM is located in the occipital lobe, with feeding arteries from the middle and posterior cerebral arteries and extensively dilated draining veins *(arrow)*. Increased signal intensity of surrounding brain tissue may be related to edema or hypoxic damage *(arrow-heads)*. **a, b** Axial scans, SE 3.0 s/120 ms (1.0 T)

tion results in a marked, confluent pattern of enhancement of the vascular malformation. Feeding and draining vessels appear as serpiginous structures but cannot be distinguished within the nidus. While fresh hemorrhages can be identified by their high density, the differentiation from tumor in later stages of hematoma absorption, in which the blood appears isodense or hypodense, is uncertain. Calcifications are readily identified when they are large enough to escape the partial volume effect and their density values are well above those of a fresh hemorrhage. With less dense lesions, it may not be possible to distinguish between acute hemorrhages and light calcifications.

As mentioned previously (Sect. 5.3), MR is able to demonstrate blood flow without the use of contrast material. It can differentiate between the high-flow and low-flow compartments of AVMs, and between slow flow and thrombosis (see Sect. 5.3).

Angiomas appear on T1-weighted and T2-weighted images as a dark mass of blood vessels contrasting sharply with the surrounding brain. Within the mass, contours of individual vessels can be discerned with adequate window selection. Portions of the angioma may show a signal increase in the even-numbered echoes of a multiecho SE sequence owing to the phenomenon of even-echo rephasing in regions of venous or slow flow [6, 55] (see Sect. 5.3).

Moreover, the multiplanar images of MR are better than CT scans for evaluating the characteristics of angiomas that are essential in assessing the surgical risk (seen above). The main concerns in this regard are the size and location of the malformation and its relation to central and functionally vital regions. MR can demonstrate the extension of superficial angiomas to motor and sensory projection areas, and it can disclose involvement of the basal ganglia, internal capsule, and ventricular system by more deeply situated lesions (Figs. 14.1-14.6). It can show the relation of infratentorial malformations to the brainstem, pons, and medulla oblongata, and can confirm that a lesion is confined to the cerebellar hemispheres, vermis, tonsils, or cerebellopontine angle (Figs. 14.7, 14.8, 14.11). MR is more effective than CT and angiography in determining whether a given AVM is extrapial, lying on the surface of the central cerebral structures (hypothalamus, thalamus, corpus callosum, midbrain, brainstem, medulla oblongata) or whether it involves the parenchyma of the adjacent brain region.

Various pathologic processes such as tumors and infarctions can be mistaken for a vascular malformation on precontrast and postcontrast CT scans. On MR images, however, the only lesions apt to be confused with vascular malformations are calcifications.

CT is superior to conventional SE sequences in its ability to detect a fresh hemorrhage in the first 1-3 days following the acute episode. This type of hemorrhage appears dark on T2-weighted images (susceptibility effect, see Sect. 5.2).

Subacute and older hemorrhages are consistently displayed as high-intensity lesions (Figs. 14.4, 14.5), which is particularly advantageous in the CT-isodense phase of the hemorrhage. Hemosiderin deposits appear dark on T2-weighted images (see Sect. 5.2).

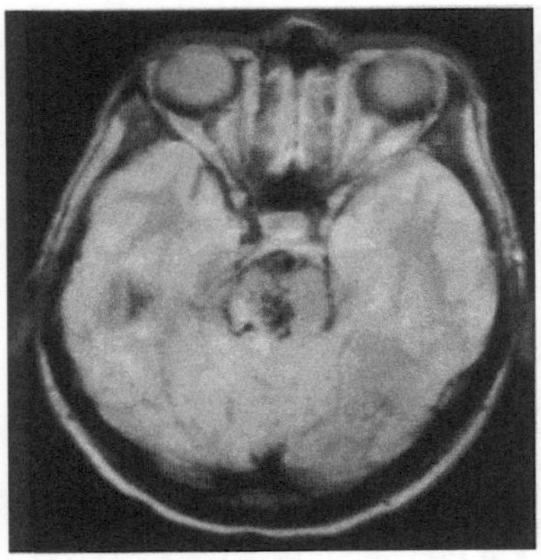

14.7

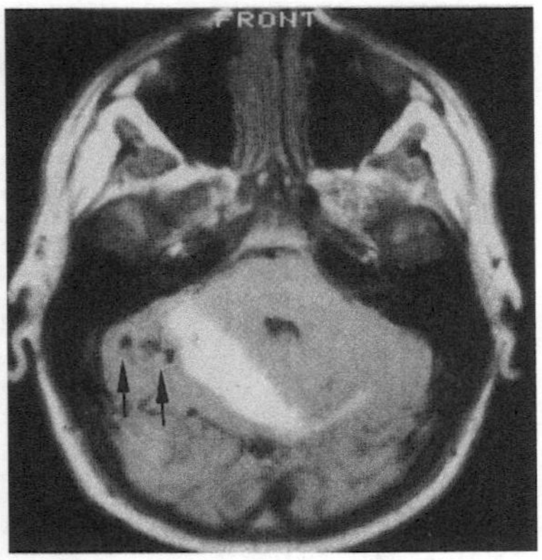

14.8

Fig. 14.7. AVM of the brainstem in a 37-year-old woman after a second episode of acute hemiparesis of her left side, cranial nerve palsy, and loss of consciousness. AVM of the midbrain and upper pons. Axial scan, SE 3.0 s/ 45 ms (1.0 T)

Fig. 14.8. AVM of the cerebellum with spontaneous hemorrhage in a 27-year-old man with sudden headache, dizziness, and nuchal rigidity. A small AVM *(arrows)* is seen in the lateral portion of the right cerebellar hemisphere, causing a major intracerebellar hematoma. Axial scan, SE 0.6 s/17 ms (1.0 T)

Calcifications may give very low signals on MR sequences. Small calcifications that have a tortuous, vessel-like shape can be difficult to distinguish from blood vessels, which likewise appear dark.

Perifocal edema, seen occasionally in association with angiomas but more frequently in hemorrhages, appears on T2-weighted images as a peripheral ring of increased signal intensity.

Varix or Aneurysm of the Vein of Galen

Varix or aneurysm of the vein of Galen is a rare vascular malformation in which direct communications exist between the circle of Willis arteries and the vein of Galen, which shows aneurysmal dilatation [21, 28]. The entire venous system may be dilated, and there may be a coexisting angioma [33].

Clinical symptoms appear when the volume of the shunted blood is sufficiently large (e.g., congestive heart failure; [45]), when CSF stasis develops (hydrocephalus), or when hemorrhages (usually subarachnoid; [33]) or seizures occur. In addition, the large malformation can lead to anoxic brain injury, which is most common and most severe in newborn infants [33]. The possibility of an intracranial AVM should always be considered in a newborn showing the clinical signs of congestive heart failure, even if a cranial bruit is not present.

CT and MR Findings

With an aneurysm of the vein of Galen, CT typically shows marked aneurysmal dilatation, accompanied clinically by a large head and pronounced internal hydrocephalus. Contrast injection produces marked enhancement of the aneurysm and its feeding and draining vessels. CT also gives information on the contents of the aneurysmal sac, any anoxic damage caused by the arteriovenous steal, calcifications, and hemorrhages [33, 9].

Roosen et al. [40] observed a region of high signal intensity within a large aneurysmal sac on T2-weighted images without ECG triggering, while the contents of the aneurysm appeared dark and featureless on proton-density images. The authors explain this finding by turbulent flow within the aneurysm and/or flow made up of different velocities.

Thrombus formation in the aneurysmal sac, which might result from regressive wall changes or fissuration, can initiate a process that culminates in the spontaneous disappearance of the aneurysm [9].

Venous Angiomas/-Anomalies

The true prevalence of venous angiomas has been appreciated only within the last few years. Sarwar and McCormick [43] and McCormick [34] showed in large autopsy series that venous angiomas are the most common vascular malformations detected at autopsy, with an incidence of about 3%. Venous angiomas have also been mentioned with increasing frequency since the advent of CT [41].

Microscopically, the lesions contain hypertrophied veins with walls made of a single layer of fibromuscular tissue lined by endothelium, with intervening normal brain parenchyma [16].

A venous angioma may consist of either a single large vein with many small venous tributaries or a compact tangle of such veins [42].

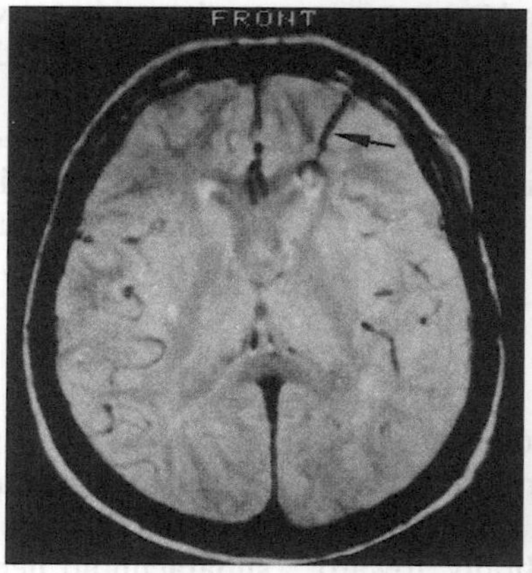

14.9

Fig. 14.9. Venous anomaly (incidental finding) in a 76-year-old woman complaining of headache. Transcortical vein *(arrow)* in the right frontal lobe. Axial scan, SE 3.0 s/40 ms (1.0 T)

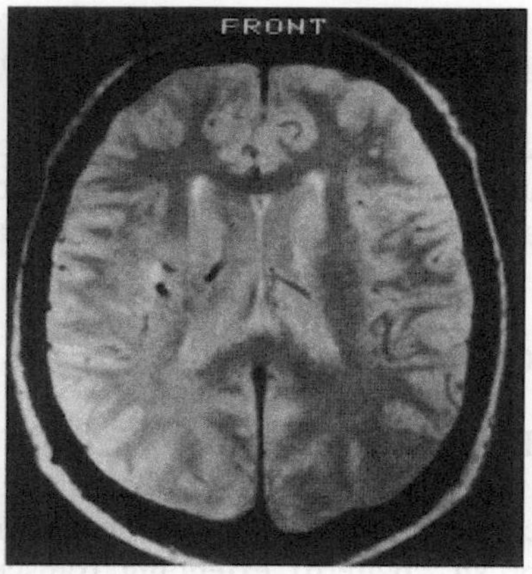

14.10

Fig. 14.10. Venous angioma in a 48-year-old man with a long history of headache after a new attack. Dilated vessels are seen lateral to the right ventricle. Angiography revealed a venous anomaly draining to the internal cerebral veins. Axial scan, SE 3.0 s/45 ms (1.0 T)

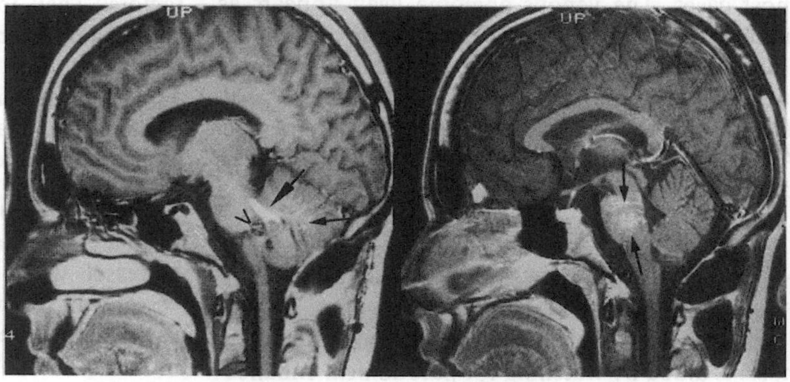

Fig. 14.11 a, b. Venous anomaly in a 20-year-old man. Control scans after hemorrhage from the associated cryptic AVM *(arrowhead)*. The involvement of the pons and cerebellum *(small arrows)* becomes obvious only after i.v. gadolinium-DTPA (**a, b**), which also enhances the large draining vein *(large arrow)*. Sagittal scans, SE 0.5 s/15 ms (1.5 T) **a** **b**

Two different groups of veins (superficial and deep) may be involved in the *drainage* of these lesions. The superficial medullary veins are short, begin juxtacortically, and run through the cortex to join the pial veins. The deep veins are longer; they begin subcortically and converge toward the subependymal veins of the lateral ventricles. There also exist anastomotic or transcerebral veins, which run from the pial to the subependymal veins (Fig. 14.9). Depending on the type of veins involved, the angioma may be drained superficially, deeply, or in both directions [54]. Valavanis et al. [54] classified cerebral venous angiomas into three groups based on their drainage pattern: (1) juxtacortical, (2) subcortical, and (3) paraventricular (Fig. 14.10).

The *clinical picture* is highly variable. Valavanis et al. [54] found on reviewing the literature that 29.3% of cerebral venous angiomas caused epileptic seizures (grand mal type), and that 17.2% produced headaches. The lesions were asymptomatic in 29.3% of cases, and in 13.7% they presented with an intracranial hemorrhage, more often subarachnoid than intracerebral. In the same study the majority of the angiomas occurred in the frontal lobes and cerebellum (Figs. 14.9, 14.11). Less common sites were the parietal lobe, temporal lobe, basal ganglia, and thalamus.

It is relevant to the assessment of *natural risk* that venous angiomas in the cerebellum are more prone to hemorrhage than those in other locations [36, 41]. The course of the hemorrhage may be acute and gradually progressive over a period of days, recurring, or acute and catastrophic [41]. Most of these hemorrhages occur in the cerebellar hemispheres close to the cerebellopontine angle. Because of this, a venous angioma should be suspected whenever a spontaneous cerebellar hemorrhage occurs, especially in younger patients.

Since the collecting vein of cerebral venous angiomas can also provide for the normal drainage of large areas of the brain, restraint should be exercised in the selection of patients for operation, unless, of course, urgent intervention is required for a hemorrhage with a significant mass effect.

CT and MR Findings

The classic angiographic picture of venous angioma is of a local network of small medullary veins which converge toward a large collecting vein ("paintbrush" pattern) extending transcerebrally toward the superficial veins or, less commonly, toward the deep veins [41].

Noncontrast CT scans are unremarkable in most cases. The venous angioma itself appears as an area of diffuse enhancement from which the transcerebral vein arises with an arcuate enhancement that can be followed on serial slices [30, 54]. The CT findings are characteristic but not specific. Angiography is indicated when it is necessary to distinguish a venous angioma from an AVM or a tumor.

On MR images, the collecting vein of the angioma appears dark when the flow velocity of the draining blood is sufficiently high (Figs. 14.9–14.11). If the blood is slow-moving, diagnosis is aided by watching for paradoxical enhancement and applying even-echo rephasing. No flow phenomena have been observed in the angioma itself [44]. Scott et al. [44] describe a high signal intensity of the venous angioma body due to a prolonged T2 and increased spin density, which they attribute to the large blood pool within the angioma. According to Augustyn et al. [1], a presumed increase in the T1 time of this blood pool could also account for the signal decrease on T1-weighted images.

For high-contrast definition of the collecting vein(s), these authors recommend T2-weighted sequences that accentuate the signal from the brain parenchyma, so as to provide better contrast with the low (flow-void) signal of the transcerebral vein [1, 5]. Intravenous contrast medium (e.g., gadolinium-DTPA) has proved to be very helpful for the visualization of the true extent of a venous malformation, as shown in Fig. 14.11. With the use of contrast agents, MR will be superior to CT in the evaluation of these lesions.

The venous angioma body was visualized in 57% of cases on T2-weighted images, matching the results achieved with contrast CT [1]. It is unlikely, however, that either modality can prove the presence of a venous angioma, and so angiography will continue to be necessary for differential diagnosis.

The differentiation of a true venous malformation and a venous anomaly remains difficult, even with angiography.

Aneurysms

Aneurysms are saccular or serpentine dilatations of arteries. They are the leading cause of spontaneous subarachnoid hemorrhages and are responsible for 20%–25% of all intracranial hemorrhages [23].

Aneurysms may be due to congenital defects in the vessel wall (medial gap) as well as to acquired factors. They may be classified etiologically into congenital, arteriosclerotic, mycotic, and syphilitic forms.

When assessing the operability of aneurysms, it is helpful to classify the lesions according to the morphologic scheme proposed by Krauland [26]:

Saccular (berry) aneurysms are believed to result from a congenital defect at the origin or bifurcation of vessels which leads to a local outpouching of the vessel wall, frequently aided by the presence of elevated blood pressure. Details on the potential significance of acquired factors in the pathogenesis of these lesions are beyond the scope of this text. Saccular aneurysms account for 66%–90% of all aneurysms. They most commonly involve the internal carotid artery and the anterior part of the circle of Willis, and occur at bifurcations of the major arteries or at the origins of small vessels branching from these arteries [23]. Major sites of occurrence include the terminal segment of the internal carotid artery, the origin of the anterior and posterior communicating artery, the trifurcation of the middle cerebral artery, and the basilar artery (Figs. 14.12, 14.13, 14.15). In 4%–5% of cases [23] multiple aneurysms can be found.

Fusiform aneurysms generally result from arteriosclerosis or other acquired causes. Such aneurysms of the cerebral vessels are very rare. The spindle-shaped dilatation involves a relatively long segment of vessel and thus cannot be clipped like a saccular aneurysm; it can be eliminated only by ligating the parent vessel (Fig. 14.14).

Clinical symptoms and complications of aneurysms include the following:

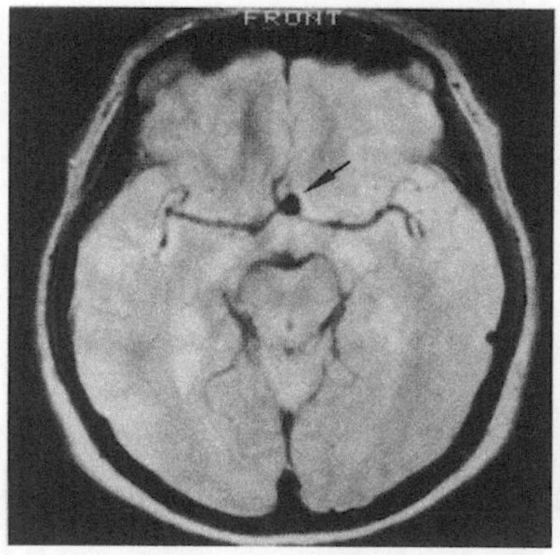

14.12

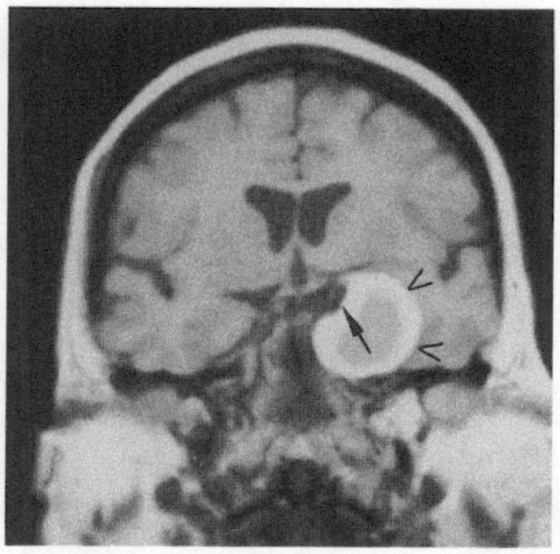

14.13

Fig. 14.12. Saccular aneurysm *(arrow)* of the anterior communicating artery (incidental finding) in a 65-year-old woman with repeated headache. Axial scan, SE 3.0 s/45 ms (1.0 T)

Fig. 14.13. Giant aneurysm of the internal carotid artery in a 55-year-old woman with headache and double vision. The sac of the aneurysm *(arrowheads)* is filled with a thrombus, which has a bright rim due to paramagnetic methemoglobin. Only a small medial part of the aneurysm *(arrow)*, which shows flow void on MR, is visible on angiography. Coronal section, SE 0.7 s/30 ms (1.0 T)

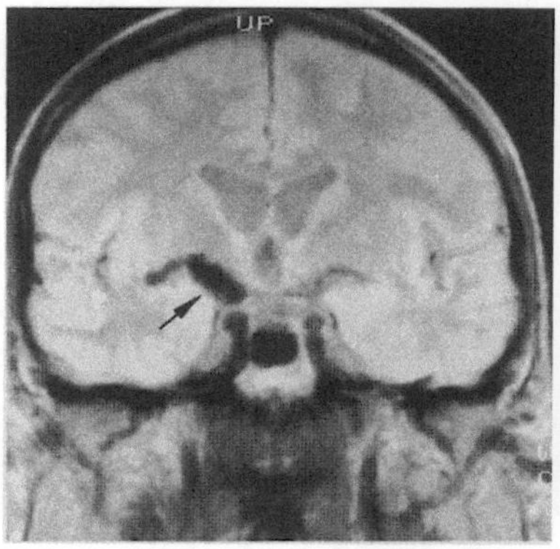

14.14

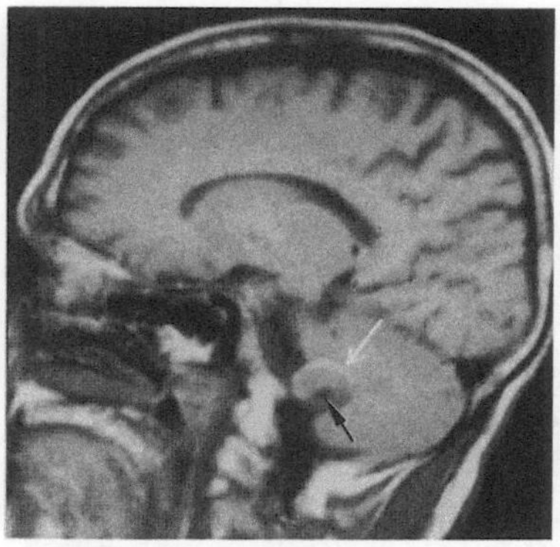

14.15

Fig. 14.14. Fusiform aneurysm *(arrow)* of the middle cerebral artery in a 55-year-old man with transient ischemic attack. Coronal scan, SE 0.5 s/35 ms (1.0 T)

Fig. 14.15. Incomplete thrombosis of aneurysm of the posterior inferior cerebellar artery in a 46-year-old man with recent subarachnoid hemorrhage. Round, isointense mass *(white arrow)* in the cerebellomedullary fossa adjacent to the vertebral artery. Only the lower portion of the aneurysm is dark due to flow void *(black arrow)*. Sagittal scan, SE 0.5 s/30 ms (1.0 T)

- Subarachnoid and/or intracerebral hemorrhage as an acute, dramatic episode
- Cranial nerve palsy (e.g., of nerves 3, 4, 6) caused by pressure from a large space-occupying aneurysm
- Cerebral infarction due to vasospasm secondary to a subarachnoid hemorrhage or spontaneous thrombosis of a large aneurysm (e.g., of the basilar artery)
- Hydrocephalus secondary to an acute hemorrhage obstructing the aqueduct or the foramina of the fourth ventricle (obstructive hydrocephalus) or due to the impaired absorption of CSF (malabsorptive hydrocephalus)
- Bone erosion caused by giant aneurysms of the internal carotid artery

CT and MR Findings

The goal of diagnostic imaging in aneurysms is not only detection of the lesion but also analysis of its morphologic features, which are important in explaining the clinical symptoms, assessing surgical risk, and planning the operation. The features of primary interest are the size and shape of the aneurysm, the width of its neck, and its relation to nearby blood vessels and nervous structures (e.g., the cranial nerves).

Angiography continues to be the method of choice for resolving these questions, especially when it is necessary to exclude an aneurysm. Nevertheless, angiography is an invasive procedure with risks which are not negligible, and it is proper to determine whether and to what extent it can be replaced by the noninvasive procedures of CT and MR imaging.

In CT, virtually any rounded structure whose size exceeds the caliber of the adjacent vessel and whose contrast dynamics match that of the parent vessel may represent an aneurysm. Even small aneurysms can be detected using modern CT equipment. In larger aneurysms, CT can show evidence of partial thrombosis and thus can demonstrate the

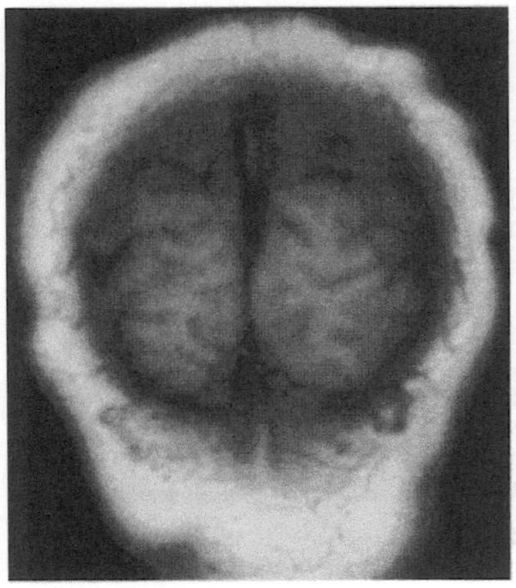

14.16

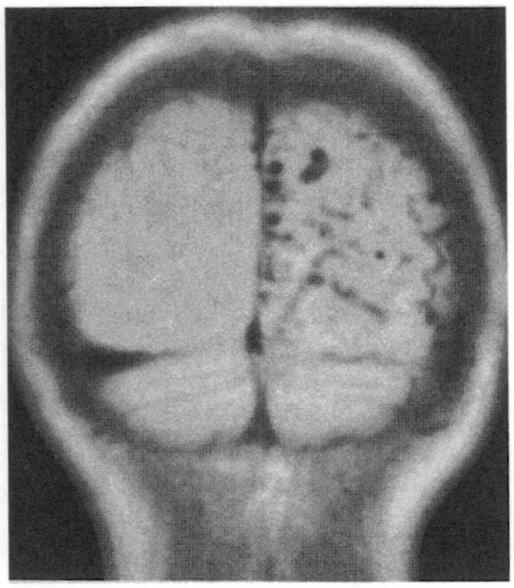

14.17

Fig. 14.16. Bilateral dural arteriovenous fistula in a 55-year-old man with headache and bilateral papilledema. Angiography revealed extensive bilateral dural arteriovenous fistula to the transverse sinus. The many dilated and tortuous scalp vessels are an indirect sign of the high flow. Coronal scan, SE 0.4 s/17 ms (1.0 T)

Fig. 14.17. Dural arteriovenous fistula in a 66-year-old woman with headache and pulsating tinnitus. Angiography showed varicosis of parieto-occipital cerebral veins due to retrograde flow from the fistula via the transverse sinus to the sagittal sinus and internal veins; the sigmoid sinus was occluded, and there was no connection of the transverse sinus to the torcular. Coronal scan, SE 3.0 s/28 ms (1.0 T)

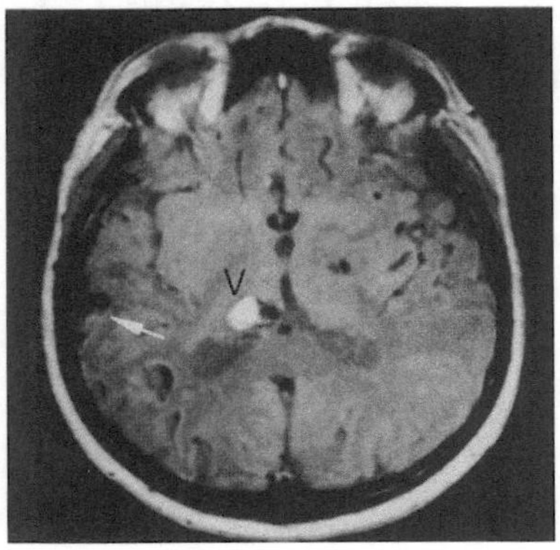

14.18

Fig. 14.18. Bilateral dural arteriovenous fistula in a 57-year-old woman with repeated dizziness, papilledema, and pulsating tinnitus. Varicose cerebral veins with aneurysmal dilatation *(arrow)* and small hemorrhage *(arrowhead)* due to the large shunt volume with venous congestion. Axial scan, SE 3.0 s/15 ms (1.5 T)

true size of the aneurysmal sac, whereas angiography would give the erroneous impression of a smaller lesion. However, the exact location of the aneurysm cannot be established with CT, and the neck of the lesion cannot be scrutinized. Neither can CT positively exclude an aneurysm or differentiate it from nodular masses of other etiology (e.g., a tumor).

Applying the same criteria, we find that MR imaging is quite useful in the detection and analysis of aneurysms. The multiplanar capabilities of MR are an advantage over CT, as is its ability to differentiate between moving and stationary protons (flowing blood vs thrombus, aneurysmal sac vs small nodular tumor). Flow-related artifacts create a new source of potential misdiagnosis, but they can be eliminated by changing the projection or image sequence or by the use of ECG triggering (see Sect. 5.3).

At present MR is incapable of excluding an aneurysm, and it is not an acceptable replacement for preoperative angiography.

Dural Arteriovenous Fistulas

Dural arteriovenous fistulas are relatively rare vascular lesions that cause shunting of blood between extracranial and meningeal vessels of the external carotid artery and the venous sinuses. Less commonly the meningeal and pial veins are involved. The etiology is still controversial. While a congenital etiology was once assumed, recently there has been convincing evidence that acquired injuries are causative in a number of cases [50]. Usually a unilateral thrombosis of the sigmoid sinus can be demonstrated, in which case the shunted blood drains extracranially through the sigmoid sinus of the opposite side. In the rare cases where the sigmoid sinus thrombosis is bilateral, or if there is a coexisting sinus anomaly in which the affected side does not communicate with the confluence of the sinuses, a damming back of the shunted blood into the cerebral veins will result (Figs. 14.17; 14.18). The clinical symptoms are determined by the volume, direction, and route of this retrograde flow. The disease is often progressive and can lead to increasing neurologic deficits, a rise of intracranial pressure, hydrocephalus (malabsorptive type), seizures, and extravasation from the stretched cerebral veins (Fig. 14.18) [29]. The lesions predominantly affect women over 40 years of age and occur mostly in the region of the transverse sinuses, although all the sinuses, including the cavernous, may be involved. A tinnitus synchronous with the pulse is frequently reported.

CT and MR Findings

For the diagnosis of dural arteriovenous fistulas, angiography is the method of choice.

In severe cases with thickened cerebral veins, CT may show hyperdense structures whose contrast dynamics and tortuous shape are consistent with dilated blood vessels.

MR images of fistulas with transcerebral drainage of the shunted blood show numerous hypointense (flow void), dilated veins on the cerebral surface or within the brain parenchyma (Figs. 14.17, 14.18). If drainage occurs to the contralateral transverse sinus or if the fistula is not very pronounced, there may be no appreciable dilatation of the cranial veins.

The similar signal intensities of bone and high-flow vessels explain why dural arteriovenous fistulas cannot be identified on conventional SE sequences. It is conceivable, however, that these fistulas occurring in or near bone can one day be diagnosed using flow-sensitive sequences (see Sect. 5.3). A marked proliferation and thickening of the scalp vessels may provide indirect evidence for the presence of such a fistula (Fig. 14.16).

14.1.2 Angiographically Occult Vascular Anomalies

The category of angiographically occult vascular anomalies includes *cavernous hemangiomas* and *capillary teleangiectases*. Certain small, thrombosed AVMs and venous angiomas also may be invisible on angiograms, but these lesions are classified among the angiographically demonstrable anomalies and are discussed under that heading.

The CT and MR features of cavernous hemangiomas and capillary teleangiectases will be discussed together, since both lesions have very similar appearances.

Cavernous Hemangiomas

Cavernous hemangiomas consist microscopically of large, closely clustered vessels, with or without intervening normal brain. Hemosiderin-containing macrophages and gliosis may be abundant in the surrounding nerve tissue.

Differentiation from capillary teleangiectases can be difficult [16]. Cavernous hemangiomas, however, have larger vessels that lack an elastic or muscular layer [52] and have relatively thick fibrous walls, in contrast with the one-layer, capillary-like vessels of the teleangiectases (see below).

Cavernous hemangiomas vary greatly in size from pinhead areas to sharply circumscribed nodules. They may form cysts and calcify. Transient enlargement during pregnancy has been reported by Yamasaki et al. [56].

The majority (about 75%) of these congenital vascular malformations are supratentorial, and about 25% are infratentorial [52, 56]. In the cerebrum many are cortical or subcortical and involve the region of the central sulcus or basal ganglia (Figs. 14.19, 14.21, 14.22). Favored sites in the posterior fossa are the pons and cerebellar hemispheres (Figs. 14.20, 14.22). Cavernous hemangiomas are multiple in 16%–33% of patients (Fig. 14.22).

In the subarachnoid cisterns cavernous hemangiomas can resemble an extra-axial mass lesion (Fig. 14.22d, e), and hemangiomas in the cerebellopontine angle can impinge upon the adjacent cranial nerves [24].

The major clinical symptoms are seizures (focal, generalized, or both), which are reported in about 55% of cases, intracerebral hemorrhages, in about 30%, and focal neurologic signs, in about 15% [52].

Capillary Teleangiectases

Capillary teleangiectases are composed of minute vessels (3 micrometers in diameter) lined by only one endothelial cell layer and separated from one another by normal brain parenchyma [35]. They are commonly found in the pontine base but also occur

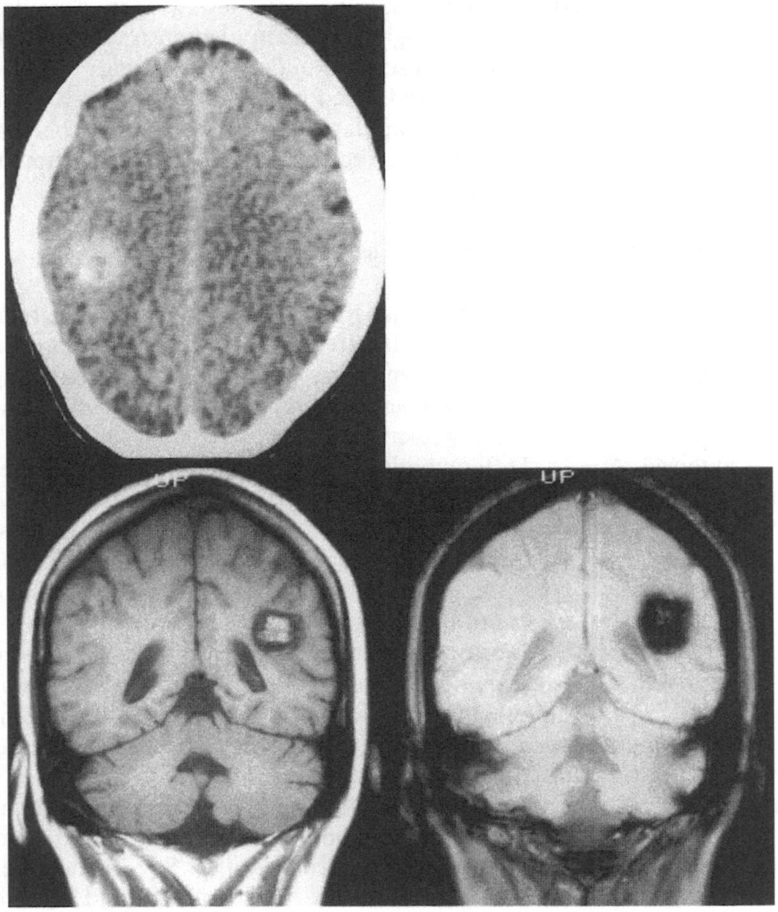

a b c

Fig. 14.19a–c. Occult vascular malformation in a 17-year-old girl with partial seizures. The ill-defined parietal lesion on CT (**a**) corresponds to the hypointense area in **c**, which in its center has higher signal corresponding to the recent hemorrhage shown in **b**. Coronal scans: **b** SE 0.6 s/15 ms, **c** FLASH 30°/0.1 s/15 ms (1.5 T)

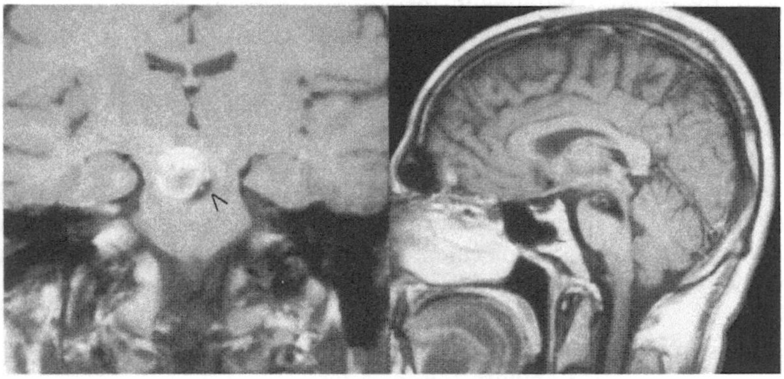

a b

Fig. 14.20a, b. Cryptic AVM in a 25-year-old man with acute tetraparesis and respiratory disturbances. Hyperintense subacute hemorrhage of midbrain and pons, hemosiderin deposits *(arrowhead)* of previous hemorrhages. On a T1-weighted control scan (**b**) after complete resorption 5 months later, a large area of hemosiderin is seen, which in the native CT scan appeared hyperdense. **a** Coronal and **b** sagittal scans, SE 0.3 s/30 ms (1.0 T)

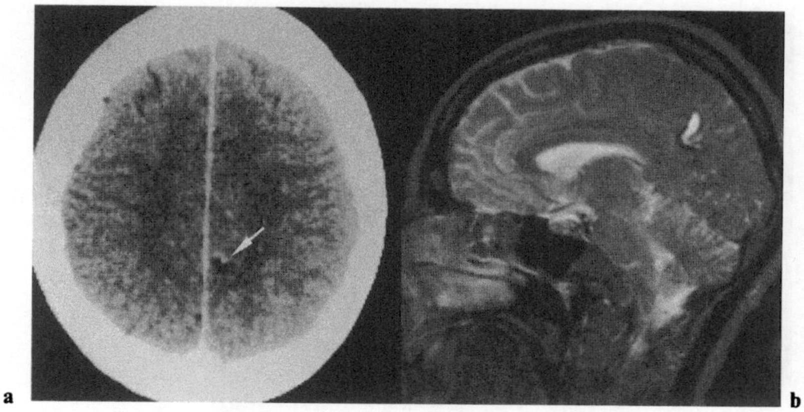

Fig. 14.21 a, b. Cavernous hemangioma in a 50-year-old woman with a first cerebral seizure. **a** CT shows a minute unspecific hypodense area *(arrow)*. **b** MR reveals subacute hemorrhage with a small rim of hemosiderin deposits caused by a cavernous hemangioma (proved by surgery). **b** Sagittal scan, SE 2.5 s/120 ms (1.0 T)

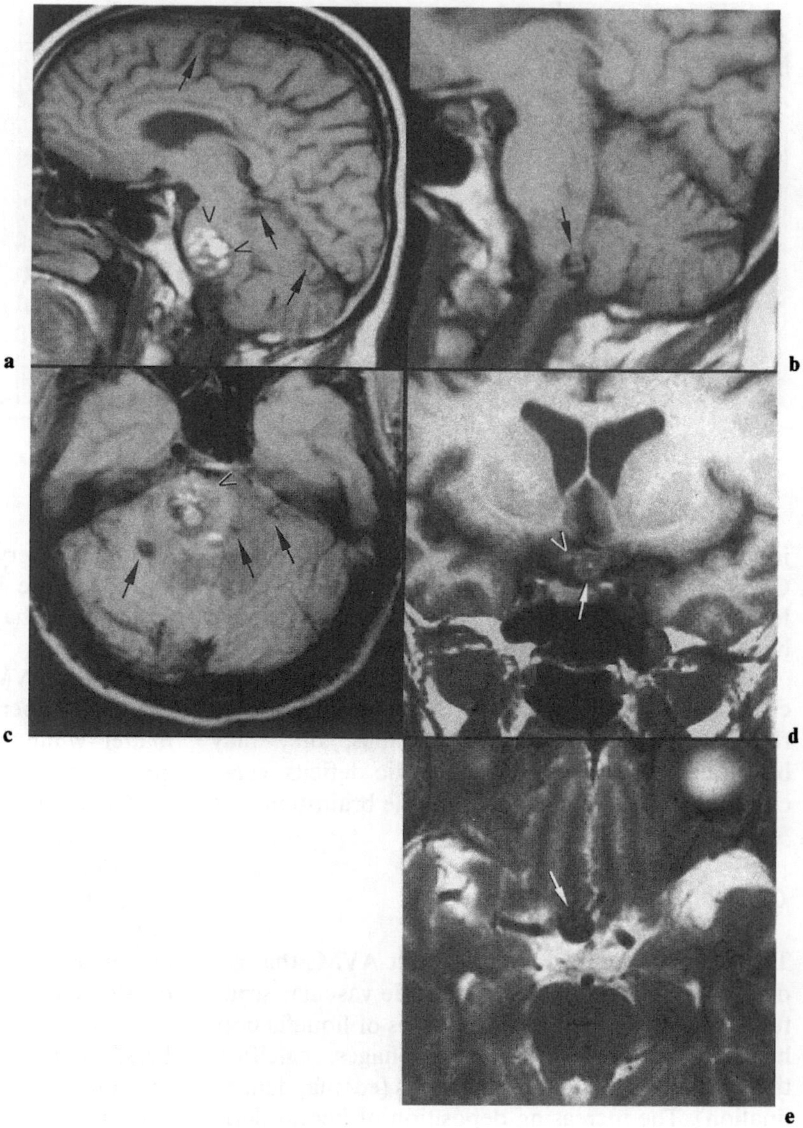

Fig. 14.22. a–c Multiple cavernous hemangiomas in a 49-year-old man with sudden hemiparesis. Multiple vascular malformations *(arrows)* of different size with recent hemorrhage in the lower pons *(arrowhead)*. **a, b** Sagittal scans, SE 0.7 s/30 ms; **c** axial scan SE 3.0 s/45 ms (1.0 T). **d, e** Cavernous hemangioma *(arrow)* attached to the chiasm *(arrowhead)* on the left in a 53-year-old woman with visual defects in the left eye. **d** Coronal scan, SE 0.6 s/15 ms; **e** axial scan, SE 3.0 s/90 ms (1.5 T)

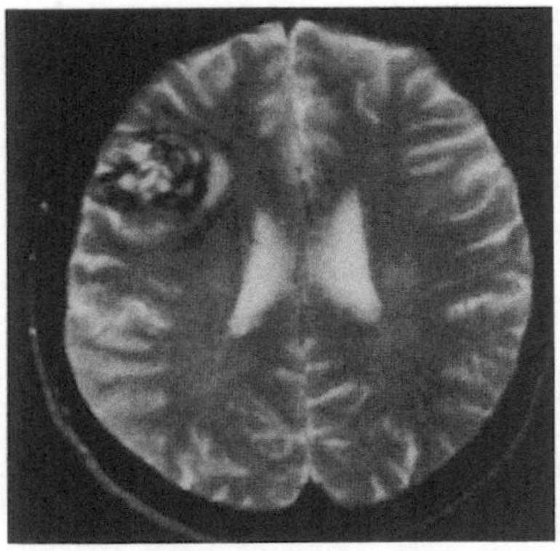

Fig. 14.23. Cryptic (cavernous) hemangioma in a 29-year-old man with focal seizure secondary to intracerebral hemorrhage. MR shows hemosiderin deposits, recent hemorrhage, and perifocal edema similar to the case illustrated in Fig. 14.24. The diagnosis was confirmed by surgery. Axial scan, SE 3.0 s/120 ms (1.0 T)

a 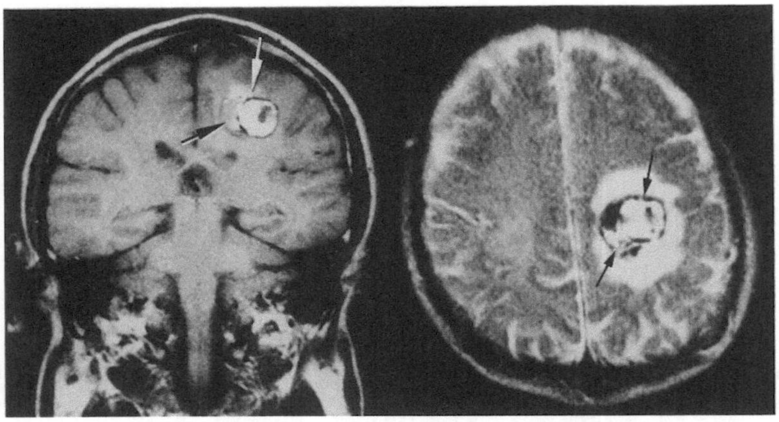 b

Fig. 14.24 a, b. Hemorrhage into an oligodendroglioma of the parietal lobe in a 47-year-old man, mimicking cryptic AVM. **a** Medium signal intensity of solid tumor *(arrows)* and high signal of the hemorrhage. **b** Rim of hemosiderin *(thin arrows)* and perifocal edema. **a** Coronal scan, SE 0.35 s/30 ms; **b** axial scan, SE 0.65 s/150 ms (1.5 T)

in the white matter of the cerebral hemispheres. Capillary teleangiectases in the lower brainstem can lead to slowly progressing neurologic deficits, perhaps due to small recurring hemorrhages [15].

Most capillary teleangiectases are discovered incidentally at autopsy. Though less prone to hemorrhage than cavernous hemangiomas, they may bleed and produce acute neurologic deficits, especially when bleeding occurs into the brainstem.

CT and MR Findings

The morphologic features of occult AVMs that are detectable with CT and MR include vascular structures, hemorrhages in various stages of liquefaction, hemosiderin deposits in macrophages, calcifications, and perifocal tissue reactions (edema, demyelination). The increasing deposition of hemosiderin at the periphery of hemorrhages is based on the inability of the brain tissue to remove the macrophages that have engulfed the extravasated blood [17].

Occult AVMs typically are found in the brainstem, in the periventricular white matter, at the gray matter–white matter junction, and in the basal ganglia (Figs. 14.19–14.23).

On plain CT scans the lesions appear as isodense or slightly hyperdense foci (maximum diameter 2–3 cm), many of which contain small calcifications (Figs. 14.19, 14.21). These minute calcifications may provide the only evidence of an occult angioma, and without them the lesion might be overlooked. A slight to moderate density increase is seen after the administration of contrast material. Fresh hemorrhages appear markedly hyperdense, but small hemorrhages may become isodense or hypodense within a few days, so that they can no

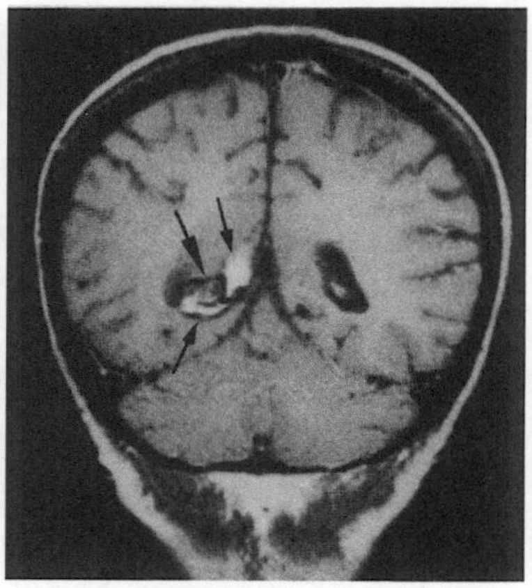

Fig. 14.25. Hemorrhage *(thin arrows)* from a small plexus papilloma *(arrow)* simulating cryptic AVM in a 63-year-old man. Coronal scan, SE 0.5 s/30 ms (1.5 T)

longer be identified as hemorrhages and are indistinguishable from a tumorous mass. Perifocal swelling is often present in the acute stage of a hemorrhage. Thus, the CT findings are nonspecific.

Small tangles of blood vessels are recognized on MR images by their serpentine, dark (flow void) structures. Usually, however, the images show rounded lesions whose hyperintense center is rimmed on T1-weighted and T2-weighted scans by an irregular, sharply contoured, more or less complete dark border [27, 37, 52]. The light and dark areas may also present an irregular, patchy appearance. Both the light areas and the dark border are believed to result from hemorrhage. These effects are seen so commonly in occult AVMs that they may be considered a characteristic sign of these vascular malformations.

Acute hemorrhages (where deoxyhemoglobin is present in intact blood cells) and hemosiderin (present as hemosiderin granules in macrophages) show a marked reduction of signal intensity on T2-weighted images, i.e., they appear dark. The cause is the susceptibility effect of these deposits. The complex signal characteristics of hemorrhages and their effects on MR images are discussed separately in Sect. 5.2.

These hemorrhagic effects require differentiation from dense calcifications and flow voids in vessels, which likewise appear hypointense on T1-weighted and T2-weighted images. Gomori et al. [18] state that this differentiation can be accomplished with high-field MR imagers with the help of certain criteria which are described in Sect. 5.2.

Even-echo rephasing, a property of slow flow, was not observed by Kucharzcyk et al. [27] and New et al. [37] in occult AVMs. This may be due to multidirectional flow or to a lack of net flow within the bed of small vessels of such lesions [2].

The areas of high signal intensity on proton-density and T2-weighted sequences may represent an organized thrombus within the vascular malformation. They may also be interpreted as evidence of an increased water content and decreased myelin content, as can be seen in the vicinity of these lesions after disruption of the blood-brain barrier and/or hemorrhage.

The "characteristic" MR findings of cryptic AVMs are related to the signal of hemosiderin deposits and of blood in various stages of evolution. Since the same mechanisms have to be considered in other cerebral lesions associated with hemorrhage, differential diagnosis should always include a neoplasm (glioma, metastasis, melanoma, etc.). For the differentiation of cryptic vascular malformations from hemorrhagic neoplasms no reliable criteria are available (Figs. 14.23–14.25) [51]. In some cases helpful information can be derived from CT, where cryptic vascular malformations are depicted as isodense or hyperdense areas with or without calcifications compared to hypodense or cystlike metastases. In still doubtful cases, careful follow-up will reveal an increase in size of a neoplasm but not of a vascular malformation.

14.2 Vascular Malformations Involving the Vertebral Canal

Reports on the incidence of spinal vascular malformations range between 3%–4% and 30%–40%, de-

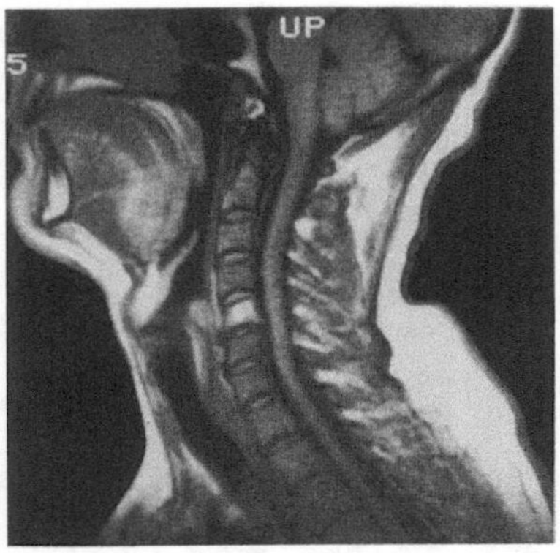

14.26

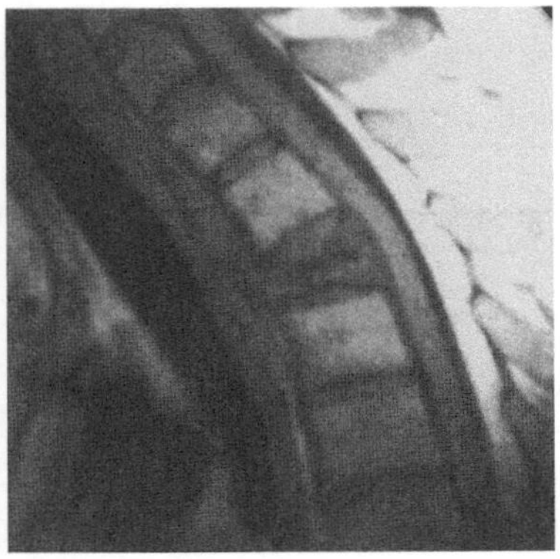

14.27

Fig. 14.26. Spinal angioma of C5 in a 56-year-old man with radicular symptoms of his upper extremities. The signal intensity was high in all three imaging sequences probably due to slow flow and increased proton density. Sagittal scan, SE 0.6 s/35 ms (0.5 T). (Courtesy of Drs. Kuhn, Steen, and Terwey, Oldenburg, FRG)

Fig. 14.27. Spinal angioma of T2 in a 25-year-old man with slowly progressive spasticity of his lower extremities. Pathologic fracture of T2 due to hemangioma leading to ventral compression of the cord. Sagittal scan, SE 0.4 s/17 ms (1.0 T)

pending on whether figures are based on autopsy series or on less selected neurosurgical populations.

14.2.1 Localization

The localization of spinal vascular malformations [22] varies according to the different layers involved (vertebral extradural, intradural, subpial arachnoidal, intramedullary), the site within the vertebral canal, and the spinal level.

Localization According to the Layers Involved

Isolated *spinal angiomas* are most commonly found in the middle and lower thirds of the thoracic spine. Lesions that expand into the extradural space can compress the spinal cord (Figs. 14.26, 14.27).

Extradural angiomas are relatively common, accounting for 15%-20% of all spinal vascular malformations. Their feeding vessels generally do not communicate with the spinal cord arteries and thus do not alter the blood supply to the cord. The differentiation of these mostly extradural angiomas from subdural or intramedullary angiomas is thus an important diagnostic concern.

Intradural angiomas are frequently found in isolation. They often penetrate the spinal cord but seldom extend into the epidural space (Figs. 14.28-14.31) [11].

Subpial angiomas are the classic and most common intradural vascular malformations. They may have one or more feeding vessels. Most subpial angiomas occur on the dorsal aspect of the spinal cord and do not communicate with the intramedullary vessels. In other cases a collateral system may exist which supplies the spinal cord to varying degrees. A "steal" effect by the angioma can cause cord ischemia.

Localization Within the Vertebral Canal

Almost all (93%) of the angiomas supplied by the anterior spinal artery (60% of all angiomas sited within the vertebral canal) have an intramedullary component, while the 40% of such angiomas supplied by the posterior spinal arteries are extramedullary or retromedullary in location. The posterior angiomas are therefore regarded as curable anomalies [10].

Localization According to the Spinal Level

Cervicothoracic and thoracic angiomas are found in about one-third of cases. Most are quite large and span three or more segments. Their two or three feeders usually arise unilaterally from the aortic intercostal vessels, and they are drained by the extradural veins to the sinuses and to the azygos vein and caval system.

Thoracolumbar, lumbar, and lumbosacral angiomas comprise about two-thirds of all spinal vascular malformations. They are usually smaller and are supplied by one large feeding artery from the caudal intercostal branches, the iliolumbar and internal iliac arteries, the artery of Adamkiewicz, or the posterolateral or posterior spinal arteries. They drain into the azygos vein and the caval system.

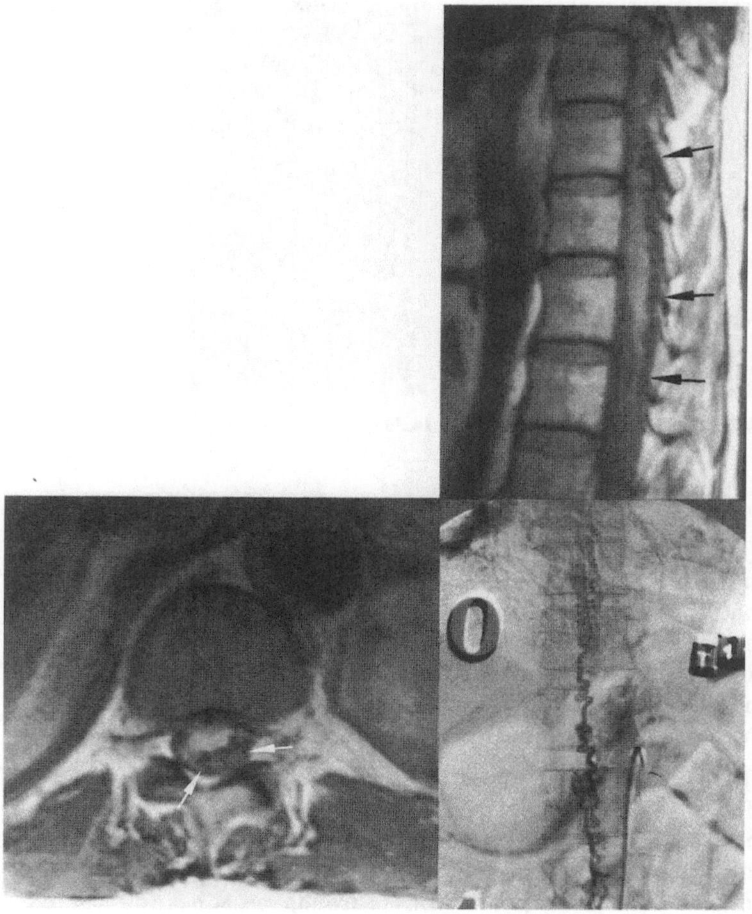

a b c

Fig. 14.28 a–c. Intradural arteriovenous fistula in a 72-year-old man with pain in his legs and progressive paraparesis. **a, b** Hypointense dilated and tortuous vessels at the dorsal aspect of the lower cord *(arrows)*. **a** Sagittal scan, SE 0.7 s/30 ms; **b** axial scan, SE 2.0 s/35 ms (1.0 T). **c** The fistula was confirmed by angiography (Courtesy of Profs. Picard and Moret, Nancy, France)

14.2.2 Classification

The following types of spinal vascular malformations and tumors are recognized in the classification of Rubinstein [42]:

1. Vascular malformations
   a) Arteriovenous malformation
   b) Capillary teleangiectasis
   c) Cavernous angioma
   d) Venous anomalies
2. Vascular tumors
   a) Capillary hemangioblastoma
3. Vascular tumors of the meninges ("angioblastic meningiomas")
   a) Hemangioblastoma
   b) Hemangiopericytoma

Vascular Malformations

Arteriovenous malformations are the most common type of spinal vascular anomaly and constitute 3%–11% of all spinal space-occupying lesions. They form a tortuous vascular mass of abnormal arteries and veins, which usually is found on the dorsal surface of the cord. AVMs located at higher levels are more likely than those occurring at more caudal levels to have several feeding vessels [20]. The leptomeninges are opaque due to fibrous thickening and to iron pigmentation resulting from prior spontaneous hemorrhage [22]. The draining vein may travel a considerable distance from the arteriovenous shunt cranially or caudally. Thrombosis of most of these lesions can cause AVMs to appear smaller on angiograms than they prove to be at operation [22].

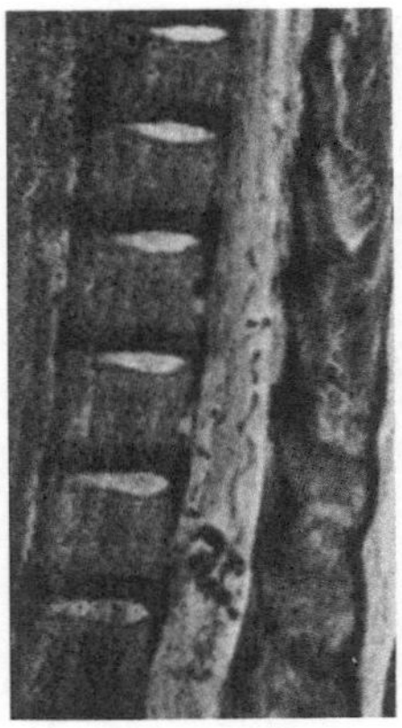

14.29

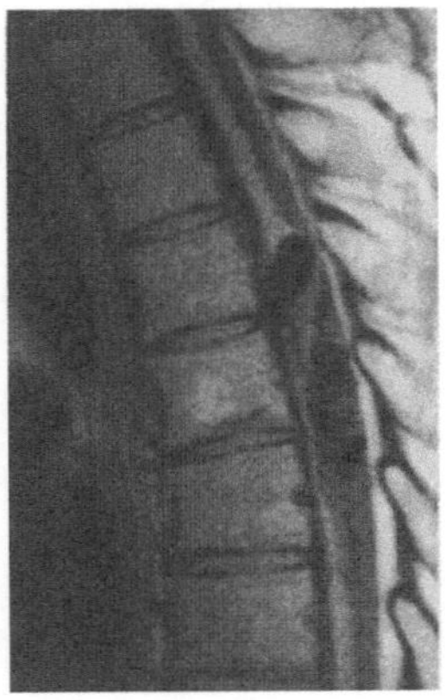

14.30

Fig. 14.29. Extramedullary AVM in a 21-year-old woman with slowly progressive gait disturbances for many years. A convolution of vessels is seen in the subarachnoid space, with tortuous hypointense structures extending cranially within the hyperintense CSF. Midsagittal scan, SE 1.8 s/100 ms (1.5 T)

Fig. 14.30. Intradural AVM in a 26-year-old man with repeated episodes of paraparesis leading to progressive neurologic deficit. At surgery an intradural AVM at T5-7 was found dorsal and lateral of the distorted cord. Sagittal scan, SE 0.6 s/30 ms (1.0 T)

Three patterns of AVMs are recognized [8]:

Type I: single coiled vessel or "adult" type. Most of these lesions are arteriovenous *fistulas* (Fig. 14.28) that consist of one or two tortuous vessels. This most common form of spinal AVM probably accounts for the majority of vascular anomalies formerly called "spinal varicosis" [22]. The flow in these lesions is slow [20].

Type II: or "glomus" type. These angiomas consist of a small vascular plexus confined to a short segment of the cord with one or more feeding arteries and draining veins (Figs. 14.29, 14.30). They occur only in adults [20, 22]. The flow is slow [8].

Type III: or "juvenile" type. Multiple large feeders supply an extensive mass of vessels that appears to fill the vertebral canal. Dilated veins extend up and down the spinal cord. This kind of AVM is seen mostly in children. The flow is rapid [8].

Capillary teleangiectases: Approximately 20% of spinal vascular malformations are teleangiectases (capillary angiomas), composed of abnormally dilated capillaries separated by interstitial or nervous tissue. Subpial teleangiectases can lead to subarachnoid hemorrhage, and intramedullary lesions to hematomyelia, myelomalacia, or diffuse progressive myelopathy [22].

Cavernous angiomas: The incidence of these malformations is 5%-16% in published series [22]. They consist of closely clustered, sinusoidal, thin-walled channels lined by a single endothelial layer, with little or no intervening parenchymal tissue. They are solitary, well-circumscribed lesions that occur mostly in the vertebral bodies and less commonly in the extradural or intradural space. Like capillary teleangiectases, they can lead to subarachnoid and intradural hemorrhage or progressive myelopathy (Fig. 14.31) [22].

Venous anomalies, known also as cirsoid or racemose varices, consist of a single, thickened, tortuous vein or a compact group of dilated veins. Histologically, these venous masses often show marked hyaline or collagenous thickening, thrombosis, or secondary inflammation. A severe structural abnormality of the vessel walls can make it difficult to distinguish veins from arteries [22].

Clinical Symptoms

In contrast to cerebral angiomas, which usually produce seizures and hemorrhages but no major neurologic deficits, the majority of spinal angiomas lead to paraplegia after a course of variable length.

The clinical course is marked by hemorrhages, pressure injury, ischemic changes (transient attacks or chronic disease), and chronic progressive radiculomyelopathy (Foix-Alajouanine disease). Major determinants of clinical symptoms are the presence of an intramedullary component and the level of the affected segments: The spinal cord is particularly sensitive to ischemic injury in the thoracic region, whereas the cervical cord is relatively protected owing to its rich blood supply.

Clinical deterioration may be slowly progressive (30%, similar to a tumor), intermittent (69%, with initially complete and later partial remissions), or paroxysmal (1%); the same neurologic segment is always affected [10].

The hemorrhagic tendency of all forms of spinal angioma is estimated to be high: 50% of all sub-

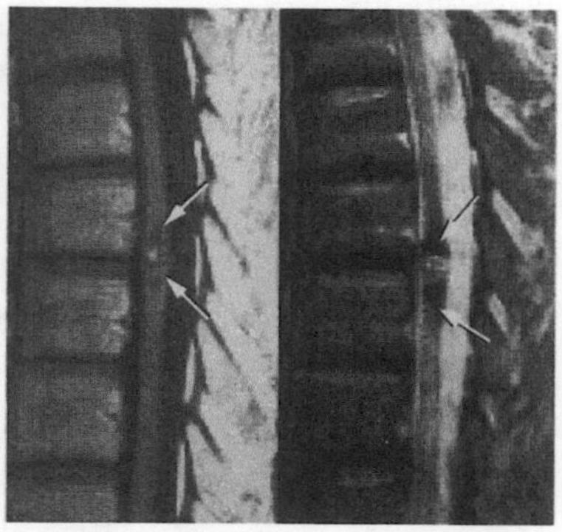

Fig. 14.31 a, b. Cavernous hemangioma of the spinal cord at T6 in a 50-year-old man with repeated paraparesis. At surgery a pea-sized hemangioma was found to be surrounded by hemosiderin deposits *(arrows)* which are most prominent on the T2-weighted scan (**b**). Sagittal scans: **a** SE 0.45 s/15 ms, **b** SE 2.5 s/70 ms (1.5 T)

arachnoid angiomas, one-third of subpial capillary angiomas, and about half of angiomatous tumors are accompanied by hemorrhages, which may be either subarachnoid or intramedullary (hematomyelia). The possibility of a spinal vascular malformation should always be considered in cases of spontaneous subarachnoid hemorrhage, especially in children [10].

Late sequelae of subarachnoid hemorrhages include adhesive arachnoiditis and the less common cystic arachnoiditis, which may form extensive, thick, calcified scars with a mass effect [39].

The subjective complaints associated with spinal angiomas are extremely diverse, making clinical diagnosis difficult and posing a significant danger of misinterpretation [39].

Various *dysplasias* are associated with spinal angiomas [22]:

- Cutaneous lesions: hemangiomas, nevi, angiolipomas
- Vertebral anomalies: scoliosis, kyphoscoliosis, vertebral angiomas
- Vascular dysplasias: soft tissue hemangiomas, angiomas, and arteriovenous fistulae of extremities, vascular deformities (variectases), disseminated hemangiomas, Klippel-Trenaunay-Weber syndrome, hemangiomas in viscera, Osler-Weber-Rendu disease, lymphatic dysplasias (angioelephantiasis)
- Vascular anomalies of the CNS: intracranial angioma, cerebrospinal angiomatosis, saccular aneurysms
- Vascular tumors: hemangioblastoma, retinocerebellar angiomatosis, von Hippel-Lindau disease, etc.
- CNS dysplasias: syringomyelia, spina bifida, etc.

The *differential diagnosis* of a spinal vascular malformation should include the following two conditions [20]: (1) "hypertrophied spinal artery syndrome," which may be found in congenital aortic obstructive conditions (coarctation), and paravertebral arteriovenous fistulas or vascular tumors; (2) hemangioblastomas of the spinal cord (see next subsection).

In rare cases, elongated, enlarged, and tortuous arteries (e.g. megadolichobasilar artery) may cause damage to the adjacent cord and brainstem by slowly increasing pressure and ischemia (Fig. 14.32 see also Fig. 5.15).

Vascular Tumors

Hemangioblastomas (capillary hemangioblastomas, hemangioendotheliomas), which probably arise from vasoformative elements, are relatively rare, comprising only 4%-5% of the tumors of the spinal cord and cauda equina. They are well circumscribed and may be either solid or cystic, containing yellow areas and dilated blood spaces. Histologically there is a tangle of closely packed, thin-walled blood vessels accompanied by large, polygonal interstitial cells with a foamy cytoplasm often showing considerable lipid storage [22].

Vascular Tumors of the Meninges (Angioblastic Meningiomas)

Spinal angioblastomas constitute 10%-20% of all spinal vascular malformations. They occur at all levels of the spinal cord but tend to favor the cervical or thoracic region. Most often they are single

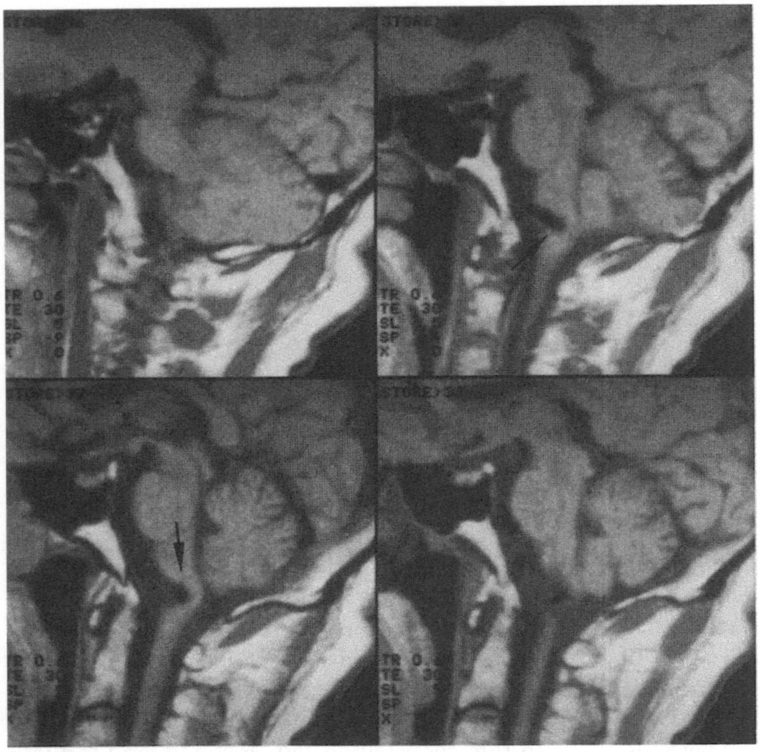

Fig. 14.32. Vasogenic myelopathy in a 60-year-old man with spastic tetraparesis. Compression and deformity of the upper cervical cord at the level of the foramen magnum by an elongated and tortuous vertebral artery *(arrow)*. Contiguous sagittal slices, SE 0.6 s/30 ms (0.5 T). (Courtesy Drs. Kuhn, Steen, Terwey, Oldenburg, FRG)

and intramedullary, and are associated with cysts in about 50% of cases. Syringomyelia is seen in 67% of intramedullary cases, and meningeal varicosity or AVM in 48% of all cases. Thirty-three percent of spinal cord angioblastomas exhibit other symptoms of von Hippel-Lindau disease (see Fig. 17.13) [22].

Hemangiopericytomas, which form about 1%-3% of intracranial "meningiomas," are extremely rare in the vertebral canal. These tumors arise from the pericytes, are attached to the meninges, and are encapsulated, occasionally lobulated, and solid. Histologically they show a vascular network of numerous vessels surrounded by densely packed, mostly spindle-shaped cells and frequent mitotic figures [22] (see Fig. 11.27).

MR and CT Findings

The goal of diagnostic imaging in spinal vascular malformations is similar to that in intracranial vascular anomalies, i.e., to establish the origin of the lesion, to determine the number of feeding vessels and distinguish them from the draining veins, and to establish the exact location of the vascular malformations with respect to the spinal cord. For hemodynamic evaluation, selective spinal cord angiography remains the procedure of choice.

CT can provide only axial scans of the vertebral canal, which often are obscured by bone artifact, and cannot furnish a direct longitudinal view of the canal displaying the course of the anomalous vessels along the long axis of the spine. After the injection of contrast material, an enhancing lesion whose time-density curve on dynamic CT resembles that of normal vessels may represent an angiomatous mass.

MR is able to utilize the special signal characteristics of moving protons to create a high-contrast image of blood flow. Because the signal intensity depends on the flow velocity, it is possible to distinguish between rapid and slow flow. Rapidly flowing blood in arteries (and large veins) appears dark on all image sequences, while the slow-moving blood in veins (or angiomatous masses) produces a more or less intense signal, depending on the nature and velocity of the flow. A certain range of slow velocities can enhance the MR signal compared with stationary protons (paradoxical enhancement; see

Sect. 1.3 and 1.4 and Fig. 5.14 for explanation of flow phenomena). If flow within the lesion is slowed as a result of surgery or embolization, its signal intensity may be increased. This gives MR imaging a potential role in the evaluation of response to treatment. Differentiation from other hyperintense structures with stationary protons, such as neoplasms and thrombi, can be accomplished by means of even-echo rephasing, phase imaging, the subtraction of images in time-shifted slice series, or cine studies with fast (gradient echo) sequences.

The rhythmic movements of the pulsating CSF can cause artifactual decreases in signal intensity that can mimic an angioma. On the other hand, CSF trapped in arachnoiditic pockets can produce a more intense signal than the "free" CSF in the rest of the vertebral canal. The phenomena that result from CSF flow effects are described in Sect. 5.3.

Sudden changes of contrast may lead to limited precision of object contrast in images reconstructed with the Fourier transformation. This phenomenon results from an alternating overshoot/undershoot approximation of the true signal and tends to accentuate or blur high-contrast interfaces. In anatomical regions with high-contrast boundaries, this edge effect (so-called Gibbs phenomenon) can be mistaken for a true signal abnormality, chemical shift, or flow phenomenon [4, 25].

References

1. Augustyn GT, Scott JA, Olson E, Gilmor RL, Edwards MK (1985) Cerebral venous angiomas: MR imaging. Radiology 156: 391-395
2. Axel L (1984) Blood flow effects in magnetic resonance imaging. AJR 143: 1157-1166
3. Batjer H, Samson D (1986) Arteriovenous malformations of the posterior fossa. J Neurosurg 64: 849-856
4. Bracewell RN (1978) Fourier transformation and its applications. McGraw Hill, New York (cited by Kelly 1987)
5. Cammarata C, Han JS, Haaga JR, Alfidi RJ, Kaufman B (1985) Cerebral venous angiomas imaged by MR. Radiology 155: 639-643
6. DeLaPaz RL, New PF, Buonanno FS, Kistler JP, Oot RF, Rosen BR, Taveras JM, Brady TJ (1984) NMR imaging of intracranial hemorrhage. J Comput Assist Tomogr 8: 599-607
7. Delitala A, Delfini R, Vagnozzi R, Esposito S (1982) Increase in size of cerebral angiomas. J Neurosurg 57: 556-558
8. DiChiro G, Doppman JL, Ommaya AK (1971) Radiology of spinal cord arteriovenous malformations. Prog Neurol Surg 4: 329-354
9. Diebler C, Dulac O, Renier D, Ernest C, Lalande G (1981) Aneurysms of the vein of Galen in infants aged 2 to 15 months. Diagnosis and natural evolution. Neuroradiology 21: 185-197
10. Djindjian R (1978) Clinical symptomatology and natural history of arteriovenous malformations of the spinal cord. In: Pia HW, Djindjian R (eds) Spinal angiomas. Springer, Berlin Heidelberg New York, pp 75-83
11. Djindjian R, Hurth M, Houdart R (1969) Les angiomes medullaires. Sandoz, Paris
12. Drake CG (1979) Cerebral arteriovenous malformations: considerations for and experience with surgical treatment in 166 cases. Clin Neurosurg 26: 145-208
13. Drayer BP (1984) Diseases of the cerebral vascular system. In: Rosenberg RN (ed) The clinical neurosciences. Neuroradiology. Livingstone, New York, pp 247-360
14. Erenberg G, Rubin R, Shulman K (1972) Cerebellar hematomas caused by angiomas in children. J Neurol Neurosurg Psychiatry 35: 304-310
15. Farrell DF, Forno LS (1970) Symptomatic capillary teleangiectasis of the brainstem without hemorrhage. Neurology 20: 341-346
16. Garcia JH (1985) Circulatory disorders and their effects on the brain. In: Davis RL, Robertson DM (eds) Textbook of neuropathology. Williams and Wilkins, Baltimore, pp 548-631
17. Gomori JM, Grossman RI, Goldberg HI, Zimmerman RA, Bilaniuk LT (1985) Intracranial hematomas: imaging by high-field MR. Radiology 157: 87-93
18. Gomori JM, Grossman RI, Goldberg HI, Hackney DB, Zimmerman RA, Bilaniuk LT (1986) Occult cerebrovascular malformations: high-field MR imaging. Radiology 158: 707-713
19. Graf CJ, Perret GE, Torner JC (1983) Bleeding from cerebral arteriovenous malformations as part of their natural history. J Neurosurg 58: 331-337
20. Heinz ER (1984) Arteriovenous malformations of the spinal cord. In: Rosenberg RN, Heinz ER (eds) The clinical neurosciences. Neuroradiology. Livingstone, New York, pp 943-947
21. Hirano A, Solomon S (1960) Arteriovenous aneurysm of the vein of Galen. Arch Neurol 3: 589-593
22. Jellinger K (1978) Pathology of spinal vascular malformations and vascular tumors. In: Pia HW, Djindjian R (eds) Spinal angiomas. Advances in diagnosis and therapy. Springer, Berlin Heidelberg New York, pp 18-44
23. Jellinger K (1979) Pathology and etiology of intracranial aneurysms. In: Pia HW, Langmaid C, Zierski J (eds) Cerebral aneurysms. Advances in diagnosis and therapy. Springer, Berlin Heidelberg New York, pp 5-19
24. Kawai K, Fukui M, Tanaka A et al. (1978) Extracerebral cavernous hemangiomas of the middle fossa. Surg Neurol 9: 19-25
25. Kelly WM (1987) Image artifacts and technical limitations. In: Brant-Zawadzki M, Norman D (eds) Magnetic resonance imaging of the central nervous system. Raven, New York, pp 43-83
26. Krauland W (1957) Die Aneurysmen der Schlagadern am Hirn und Schädelgrund und der großen Rückenmarksadern. In: Scholz W (ed) Nervensystem. Springer, Berlin Göttingen Heidelberg (Handbuch der speziellen pathologischen Anatomie und Histologie, vol 13/IB)
27. Kucharczyk W, Lemme-Plaghos L, Uske A, Brant-Zawadzki M, Dooms G, Norman D (1985) Intracranial vascular malformations: MR and CT imaging. Radiology 156: 383-389

28. Lagos JC (1977) Congenital aneurysms and arteriovenous malformations. In: Vinken PJ, Bruyn GN (eds) Handbook of clinical neurology, vol 31. North-Holland, Amsterdam, pp 137-209
29. Lasjaunias P, Chiu M, Ter Brugge K, Tolia A, Hurth M, Bernstein M (1986) Neurological manifestations of intracranial dural arteriovenous malformations. J Neurosurg 64: 724-730
30. Lotz PR, Quisling RG (1983) CT of venous angiomas of the brain. AJNR 4: 1124-1126
31. Luessenhop AJ, Gennarelli TA (1977) Anatomical grading of supratentorial arteriovenous malformations for determining operability. J Neurosurg 1: 30-77
32. Luessenhop AJ, Rosa L (1984) Cerebral arteriovenous malformations. Indications for and results of surgery, and the role of intravascular techniques. J Neurosurg 60: 14-22
33. Martelli A, Scotti G, Harwood-Nash DC, Fitz CR, Chuang SH (1980) Aneurysms of the vein of Galen in children: CT and angiographic correlation. Neuroradiology 20: 123-133
34. McCormick WF (1983) Selected topics in cerebrovascular disease. Presented at the Armed Forces Institute of Pathology Neuropathology annual short course, Jan 1983, Washington DC
35. McCormick WF, Notzinger JD (1966) "Cryptic" vascular malformations of the central nervous system. J Neurosurg 24: 865-875
36. McCormick WF, Hardman JM, Boulter TR (1968) Vascular malformations ("angiomas") of the brain, with special reference to those occurring in the posterior fossa. J Neurosurg 28: 241-251
37. New PF, Ojeman RG, Davis KR, Rosen BR, Heros R, Kjellberg RN, Adams RD, Richardson EP (1986) MR and CT of occult vascular malformations of the brain. AJNR 7: 771-779
38. Perret G, Nishioka H (1966) Report on the cooperative study of intracranial aneurysms and subarachnoid hemorrhage, section VI. Arteriovenous malformations. An analysis of 545 cases of cranio-cerebral arteriovenous malformations and fistulae reported to the cooperative study. J Neurosurg 25: 467-490
39. Pia HW (1978) Symptomatology of spinal cord angiomas. In: Pia HW, Djindjian R (eds) Spinal angiomas: Advances in diagnosis and therapy. Springer, Berlin Heidelberg New York, pp 48-74
40. Roosen N, Schirmer M, Lins E, Bock WJ, Stork W, Gahlen D (1986) MRI of an aneurysm of the vein of Galen. AJNR 7: 733-735
41. Rothfus WE, Albright AL, Casey KF, Latchaw RE, Roppolo HWN (1984) Cerebellar venous angioma: a "benign" entity? AJNR 5: 61-66
42. Rubinstein LJ (1972) Tumors of the central nervous system. In: Armed Forces Institute of Pathology. Atlas of tumor pathology, 2d series, fasc 6. Armed Forces Institute of Pathology, Washington DC, p 254
43. Sarwar M, McCormick WF (1978) Intracerebral venous angioma: case report and review. Arch Neurol 35: 323-325
44. Scott JA, Augustyn GT, Gilmor RL, Mealey JJr, Olson EW (1985) Magnetic resonance imaging of a venous angioma. AJNR 6: 284-286
45. Silverman BK, Brechx T, Craig J, Nadas A (1955) Congestive failure of the newborn, caused by cerebral arteriovenous fistula. Am J Dis Child 89: 539-543
46. Spetzler RF, Martin NA (1986) A proposed grading system for arteriovenous malformations. J Neurosurg 65: 476-483
47. Stein BM (1984) Arteriovenous malformations of the medial cerebral hemisphere and the limbic system. J Neurosurg 60: 23-31
48. Stein BM, Wolpert SM (1980) Arteriovenous malformations of the brain. I. Current concepts and treatment. Arch Neurol 37: 1-5
49. Stein BM, Wolpert SM (1980) Arteriovenous malformations of the brain. II. Current concepts and treatment. Arch Neurol 37: 69-75
50. Sundt TM Jr, Piepgras DG (1983) The surgical approach to arteriovenous malformations of the lateral and sigmoid dural sinuses. J Neurosurg 59: 32-39
51. Sze G, Krol G, Olsen WL, Harper PS, Galicich JH, Heier LA, Zimmerman RD, Deck MDF (1987) Hemorrhagic neoplasms: MR mimics of occult vascular malformations. AJNR 8: 795-802
52. Tagle P, Huete I, Mendez J, Del Villar S (1986) Intracranial cavernous angioma: presentation and management. J Neurosurg 64: 720-723
53. Tönnis W, Schiefer W (1955) Zur Frage des Wachstums arteriovenöser Angiome. Zentralbl Neurochir 15: 145-150
54. Valavanis A, Wellauer J, Yasargil MG (1983) The radiological diagnosis of cerebral venous angioma: cerebral angiography and computed tomography. Neuroradiology 24: 193-199
55. Waluch V, Bradley WG (1984) NMR even echo rephasing in slow laminar flow. J Comput Assist Tomogr 8 (4): 594-595
56. Yamasaki T, Handa H, Yamashita J, Paine JT, Tashiro Y, Uno A, Ishikawa M, Asato R (1986) Intracranial and orbital cavernous angiomas. J Neurosurg 64: 197-208

15 Inflammatory Diseases of the Central Nervous System

W. J. HUK, J. W. LOTZ, and R. H. HEWLETT

To date, little has been published on the MR imaging of inflammatory disorders of the CNS, and our own experience in this area is still very limited. To assist the reader to understand the mechanisms involved in producing an MR signal, it will be helpful to present a general discussion of the inflammatory process, paying particular attention to associated pathologic changes that can influence the signal characteristics on MR images. Experience with CT is included.

The general discussion will be followed by an examination of the specific features of various inflammatory diseases of the CNS.

15.1 General Aspects of the Inflammatory Process

Like other organs, the CNS and its coverings show relatively nonspecific patterns of response to physicochemical irritants and microbiologic agents.

General pathology recognizes two types of inflammation based on the outstanding feature of the inflammatory process:

1. Exudative inflammation, which may be classified as serous, fibrinous, purulent, or hemorrhagic according to the nature of the exudate
2. Proliferative or granulating inflammation

Generally the exudative inflammation takes an acute course, while the proliferative inflammation takes a more chronic course.

The neuroectodermal structures (nerve cells, glia) and mesodermal structures (vessels, connective tissue) of the CNS are closely interwoven. Inflammation-provoking irritants elicit a predominantly mesenchymal response of the vascular connective tissue and the meninges, which is most pronounced around the capillaries. A dense permeation of the tissue with leukocytes, lymphocytes, or plasma cells like that ordinarily occurring in inflamed tissue is rare in the brain. The capsule of the brain abscess consists of absorptive granulation tissue that originates from the mesenchymal tissue of the vessels and not from the glia.

The injury that provokes the inflammation also initiates profound physicochemical changes [59] which can affect the MR signal of the protons. These include changes in the ratio of sodium, potassium, and calcium (the normal ratio being 25:1:1), a rise of osmotic and oncotic pressure, a rise of temperature, and an increasing tissue acidosis (pH) resulting from an increase in the metabolic rate [59].

15.1.1 Exudative Inflammation

Exudative inflammation takes place at the capillary level. Local circulatory changes accompanying the inflammatory process raise the capillary permeability, leading to the outpouring of an exudate that may contain acellular blood plasma (serous) as well as formed blood constituents. The exudate has a higher protein content than transudate, and it may contain globulins and fibrinogen from the plasma. As proteins leave the bloodstream, they carry with them salts, protein degradation products, and enzymes. The latter can produce hemolysis and can split off iron in an ionized form.

The exudate collects mostly at the center of the inflammatory focus, while a vasogenic edema or transudate occurs in more peripheral areas, where there is less irritation of the vessel walls. This collateral edema can spread rapidly in loose tissue and in the brain. Accompanying changes in ion and salt contents and an increase in the protein content due to the rising osmotic and oncotic pressure contribute further to the fluid collection.

The inflammation is said to be *fibrinous* when the exudate contains significant amounts of fibrinogen, which congeals after leaving the capillaries to form flakes or threads of fibrin.

The exudate of *purulent* inflammation is rich in granulocytes. A purulent inflammation that spreads rapidly without becoming localized is known as cellulitis (also referred to as a phlegmon). Loose connective tissue and prior inflammatory edema create conditions favoring the development of cellulitis. Cellulitis can spread through the white matter, for example, as a result of encephalitis with abscess formation.

In abscess, the inflammation is confined to a localized area that is necrotic at its center. As leukocytes infiltrate the area and the necrosis becomes liquefied, pus is produced. Finally the leukocytes disintegrate, releasing absorbable proteins and poorly absorbable fats and lipoids. The purulent focus becomes walled off by a membrane of absorptive granulation tissue that contains fat and numerous foam cells. The absorption tissue increasingly forms collagenous fibers with the passage of time, and the membrane becomes divided into three zones: the absorption zone, the zone of connective tissue formation, and the finished connective tissue capsule.

A *hemorrhagic* inflammation is one in which erythrocytes are present in the inflammatory exudate. Red cell diapedesis in inflammation occurs just before the point of stasis when, due to permeability changes, virtually only erythrocytes are left in the capillaries. Hemorrhagic inflammations are rare, but their exudate can contain such a high proportion of blood that it is scarcely distinguishable from a true hemorrhage. The usual fate of the extravasated blood is hemolysis and absorption. Hemosiderin deposition is unknown.

The nature of the inflammatory exudate is determined not only by the particular nature of the tissue reaction but also by the site of the inflammation, its cause (or pathogenic agent), and the intensity of the injury. This is apparent in the pia mater, which reacts to pneumococci and meningococci with a purulent inflammation, to anthrax bacteria with a hemorrhagic inflammation, and to tubercle bacilli with a fibrinous inflammation.

15.1.2 Proliferative or Granulating Inflammation

Proliferative or granulating inflammation is a chronic form of inflammation that takes a protracted course.

If the proliferation of local connective tissue cells is accompanied or followed by the formation of new collagenous fibers and blood vessels, a granulation tissue is formed. In contrast to absorptive and reparative granulation tissue, the inflammatory granulation tissue exhibits features of exudation and cellular emigration. The inflammatory granulation tissue can also grow destructively with respect to surrounding tissues.

As the process advances, the granulation tissue becomes increasingly fibrous and less cellular and vascular, until only scar tissue remains.

15.2 Classification

In classifying inflammatory diseases of the CNS by their gross morphologic features, it is useful to subdivide the diseases according to whether they involve the meninges or the brain tissue itself (Table 15.1).

Table 15.1. Classification of inflammatory diseases of the CNS

Infections of the meninges	
Pyogenic infections	Leptomeningitis Tuberculous meningitis Subdural empyema Epidural abscess Infectious cerebral venous/sinus thrombosis (see Sects. 5.3, 13.2)
Viral infections	Aseptic meningitis
Infections of the brain tissue	
Bacterial (pyogenic) infections	Cerebritis/encephalitis Brain abscess Neurotuberculosis Sarcoidosis Syphilis Nonsyphilitic spirochaetosis
Viral infections	Aseptic meningitis Encephalomyelitis Acute postinfectious (perivenous) encephalitis Acute infective encephalitis - Herpes simplex virus - Rhabdovirus - Arthropod-borne virus Subacute sclerosing panencephalitis Cytomegaly (congenital cytomegalic inclusion disease)
Parasitic infections	Protozoal infections - Amebiasis - Malaria - Toxoplasmosis Metazoal infections - Cysticercosis - Echinococcosis or hydatid disease
Fungal infections	Candidiasis Aspergillosis Cryptococcosis Other fungal infections with worldwide distribution - Mucormycosis or zygomycosis - Actinomycosis and nocardiosis

Table 15.1. (continued)

Other, regional fungal infections - Cladosporiasis - Coccidioidomycosis - Histoplasmosis - Blastomycosis
Acquired immune deficiency syndrome (AIDS)

15.3 Infections of the Meninges

15.3.1 Pyogenic Infections

Infections of the pia and arachnoid can be caused by a variety of bacteria, viruses, fungi, and protozoans.

Leptomeningitis

In leptomeningitis the spread of exudate may be confined to the base of the brain or the convexities of the hemispheres, or it may cover the entire surface of the brain and spinal cord. In basilar meningitis, involvement of the internal CSF spaces is a consistent finding.

The initial stage of meningitis is characterized by congested pial vessels [44] and a serous exudate. Later, depending on the causative organism, the exudation becomes more purulent (staphylococci, meningococci, influenza bacteria) or more fibrinous (pneumococci, streptococci), and the meninges become thickened.

CT and MR Findings

CT and MR findings are normal in the early stage of meningitis and after its successful treatment. Less frequently, CT scans in early leptomeningitis may demonstrate the following changes [44]:

- Enlargement of CSF spaces
- Poor visualization of basal cisterns
- Decreased parenchymal attenuation
- Focal parenchymal enhancement
- General cerebral swelling
- Diffuse meningeal enhancement
- Communicating hydrocephalus
- Subdural effusion

A few days after the onset of the disease, enhancement of the meninges may be seen on postcontrast CT scans. A similar mechanism should produce enhancement with gadolinium chelate on MR images. Presumably this meningeal enhancement would be even more pronounced than on CT scans owing to the absence of bone artifact.

A number of *complications* can arise during the course of meningitis. Spread of the purulent inflammation with thickening of the arachnoid at the base of the brain can obstruct the circulation of CSF, leading to obstructive hydrocephalus. Venous thrombosis and arterial occlusion associated with vasculitis can cause foci of cerebral necrosis to appear [46, 73]. A variable pattern of infarction can develop, depending on the nature and localization of the vascular changes. Infarcts in the stage of edematous swelling have prolonged relaxation times, which are seen particularly well on T2-weighted MR sequences. Some authors consider this edema to be evidence of cerebritis [9]. Subdural effusion is seen in 10%–20% of small children with meningitis [73], and even ventriculitis may be seen, with inflammation of the ependyma and choroid plexus leading to obstruction of the sylvian aqueduct. The inflamed ependyma shows contrast enhancement on CT scans, and analogous enhancement would be expected with MR. The periventricular white matter shows edematous changes.

Tuberculous Meningitis

Tuberculous meningitis is discussed under the heading of neurotuberculosis (Sect. 15.4.1).

Subdural Empyema

Subdural empyema is a rapidly progressive infection of the subdural space that may follow infection of the paranasal sinuses, trauma, infection of a subdural hematoma, or meningitis. It can also result from hematogenous spread. The circumscribed collections of a more or less fluid, purulent exudate may be solitary or multiple and can occur over the convexities, in the interhemispheric fissure, or on the tentorium. Edema of the adjacent brain tissue may signify an incipient local encephalitis.

CT and MR Findings

CT usually shows an elliptical or sickle-shaped, hypodense or possibly isodense zone that is enclosed by an enhancing membrane [48]. The inflammatory edema of an encephalitis of the adjacent brain tissue appears hypodense.

On MR images the pus may appear dark on T1-weighted sequences due to its long relaxation times, as Davidson and Steiner [23] demonstrated in one case. By analogy with CT, enhancement of the membrane with gadolinium chelate would be expected.

Epidural Abscess

Epidural abscesses are rare. They usually arise by extension of infection from the paranasal sinuses, near the portal of entry of the infectious organism. Syphilis is one of the few causes of a primary epidural abscess (external pachymeningitis) [40, 85].

CT and MR Findings

Unlike subdural empyema, epidural abscesses can cross the midline. In other respects they are similar in appearance to subdural empyema. On CT there is contrast enhancement of the displaced, inflamed dura, which forms a thick membrane on the inner aspect of the abscess cavity [44]. Analogous MR findings would be expected after the administration of gadolinium chelate.

15.3.2 Viral Infections: Aseptic Meningitis

Viral diseases can give rise to an aseptic meningitis with a predominantly lymphocytic exudate and little protein elevation [15]. The major causative organisms of aseptic meningitis are enteroviruses [58], mumps virus, the virus of lymphocytic choriomeningitis (arenaviruses; [57]), and herpes simplex virus. Other viral infections (measles, influenza, hepatitis, atypical pneumonias) may also be accompanied by aseptic meningitis.

Aseptic meningitis does not produce any specific changes in brain tissue. Histologically the meninges are infiltrated by mononuclear inflammatory cells; these show perivascular cuffing that extends into the superficial layer of the cortex [15].

CT and MR Findings

The CT findings depend on the severity of the illness and the presence or absence of complications. Purulent forms cannot be confidently distinguished from viral forms by imaging procedures without supportive clinical data. Experience with MR imaging is not yet adequate to make a definitive assessment of its value.

15.4 Infections of the Brain Tissue

15.4.1 Bacterial (Pyogenic) Infections

Cerebritis/Encephalitis

Cerebritis represents the initial stage of a purulent inflammation of the brain tissue [3].

A suppurative encephalitis is incited by the passage of leukocytes from the capillaries. Astrocytes swell and proliferate, microglia are mobilized, and the tissue becomes edematous, hemorrhagic, and necrotic.

CT and MR Findings

Initially the inflammatory focus may produce no abnormalities on CT scans, or there may be a poorly marginated area of decreased density representing edema [62]. A diffuse, patchy enhancement is seen on postcontrast scans. The lesion may regress completely with antibiotic treatment, or it may evolve into an abscess.

MR is more sensitive to edematous changes in brain tissue and thus can demonstrate initial changes earlier than CT. As the perifocal edema of abscesses demonstrates, inflammatory edema is indistinguishable from edemas of other etiology. The edema is displayed best on T2-weighted sequences.

Brain Abscess

With the progression of an untreated or inadequately treated encephalitis (cerebritis), the area becomes walled off by the perifocal tissue reaction, and an abscess is formed. The center of the inflammatory focus becomes necrotic under the action of leukocytes, and it becomes surrounded by an inner wall composed of mesenchymal elements of the blood vessels. This is enclosed by a dense outer capsule formed by astroglia. The tissue at the center of the lesion liquefies and is replaced by pus. (Fig. 15.1, 15.2, 15.3, 15.4) Hemorrhages can occur within the capsule (see Section 5.4).

Fig. 15.1. Otogenic brain abscess in a 49-year-old man with a fracture of the petrous bone who was developing fever, headache and aphasia. The abscess shows an inhomogenous structure of moderately prolonged T2 probably indicating the area of cerebritis. There is pus in the underlying air cells of the pyramid *(arrow)* and edema of the adjacent brain tissue *(arrowheads)* and the extracranial soft tissue *(open arrow)*. Coronal scan, SE 2.5 s/120 ms (1.0 T)

Fig. 15.2. Brain abscess in a 45-year-old man with slight hemiparesis. The center of the abscess has prolonged relaxation times, appears inhomogenous, and is surrounded by a relatively thick rim, which is almost isointense to white matter. At biopsy during antibiotic therapy there was no firm capsule; the causative organisms could not be identified. Axial scan, SE 3.0 s/120 ms (1.0 T)

Fig. 15.3. Brain abscess in a 46-year-old man with sensorimotor hemiparesis. Large abscess in the right thalamus. After penetrating a firm abscess wall, pus containing streptococcus viridans and bacteroides chorodens could be removed from the abscess cavity by stereotaxic biopsy. The abscess is hyperintense to white matter, similar to CSF, suggesting long T2. There is a slight intensity gradient from the wall to the center, probably related to the stage of liquefaction of the necrotic tissue. The abscess is separated from the perifocal edema by a distinct, narrow hypointense border. Coronal scan, SE 2.5 s/120 ms (1.0 T)

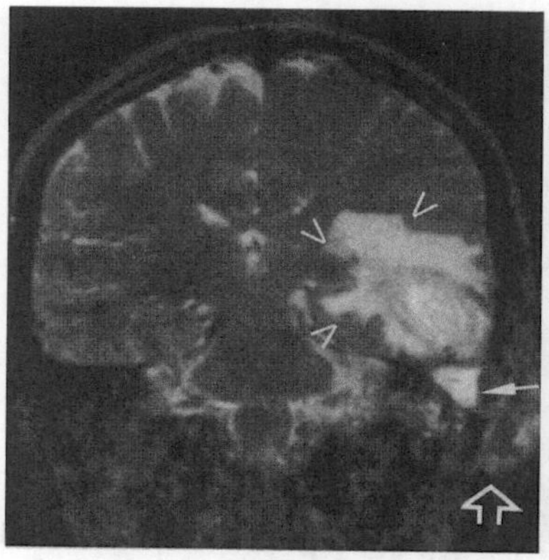

15.1

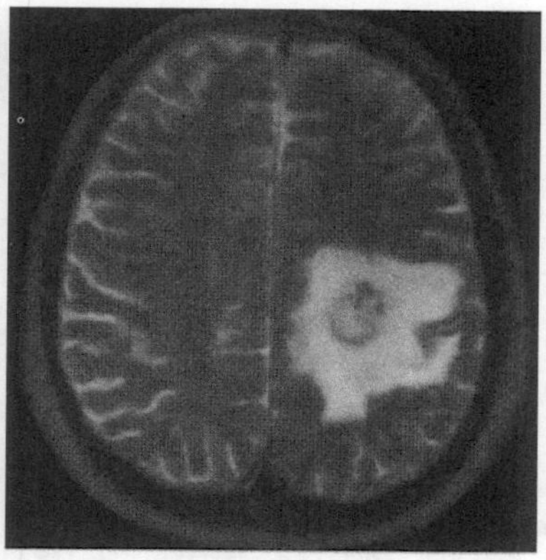

15.2

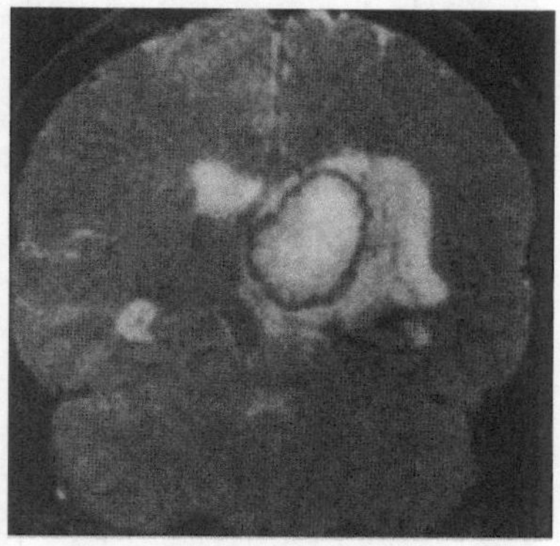

15.3

Abscesses can result from the direct extension of infection (e.g., from the paranasal sinuses), from penetrating wounds of the skull, or from the hematogenous spread of infection. The most common organisms found are staphylococci, streptococci, and pneumococci.

Any number of transitional states can exist, from a focal encephalitis, which responds satisfactorily to antibiotic drug therapy, to a pus-filled cavity walled off by dense collagenous tissue, which is curable only by surgical means [32]. Enzmann et al. [32] recognize four main stages in the evolution of an abscess based on their studies in experimental animals: (1) early cerebritis, (2) late cerebritis, (3) early capsule formation, and (4) late capsule formation.

CT and MR Findings

CT scans in early cerebritis show ill-defined patches of contrast enhancement in the area of the inflammatory edema. Late cerebritis presents a faint ring-like structure that shows delayed enhancement at its center. Thus, the appearance of a ring structure does not necessarily signify encapsulation. Ring enhancement in the stage of cerebritis can be distinguished from an abscess capsule by means of time-density analysis [13]:

In the case of formation of a collagenous capsule, maximum ring enhancement is seen earlier (5–10 min after contrast injection) than in late cerebritis, and the enhancement persists for a shorter time. The enhancement corresponds to the area of

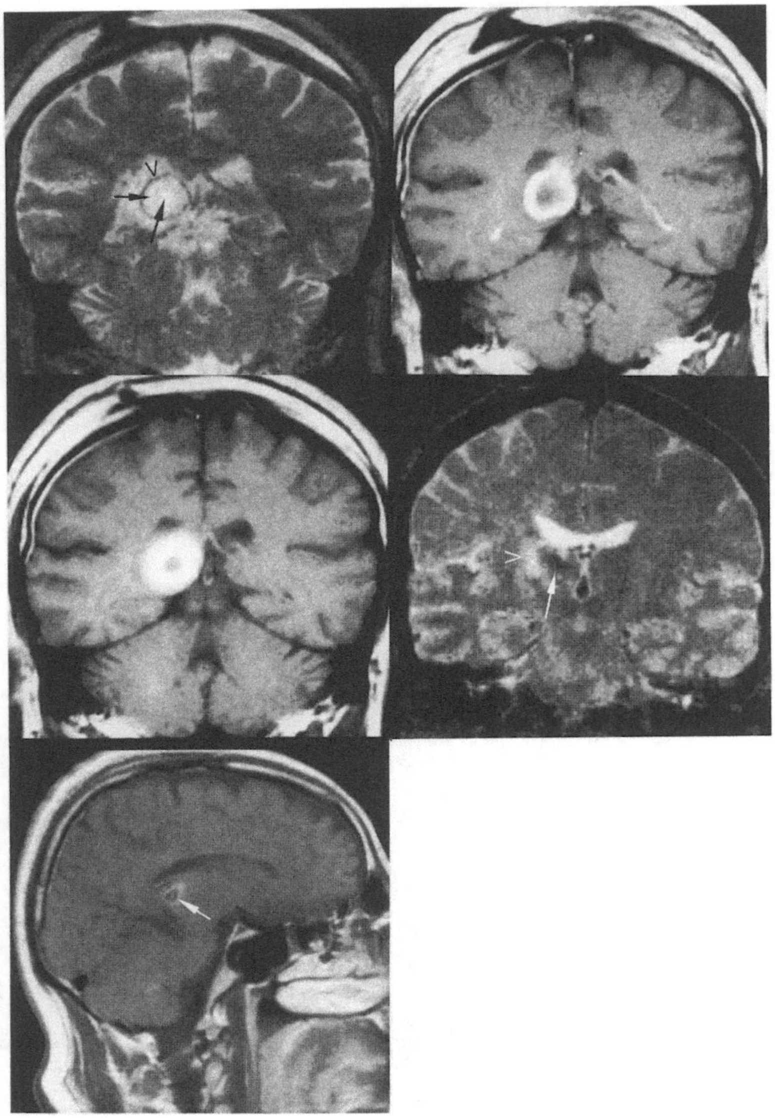

a b c d e

Fig. 15.4a–e. Abscess of the thalamus in a 45-year-old man with acute weakness of right leg and hemihypesthesia. Causative agent unknown. Within the abscess three layers can be distinguished, which are best seen in **a**: a dark, narrow rim of low signal intensity *(arrowhead)* indicating the abscess wall; an inner broader margin, probably corresponding to the area of cerebritis *(short arrow)* during the process of liquefaction, and, in the center, liquefied plus with prolonged relaxation times *(long arrow)*. **b** After i.v. injection of gadolinium-DTPA immediate enhancement of the dark rim and the adjacent inner and outer tissue is seen. **c** After 2 h the entire inner margin is enhanced, sparing only the pus in the center. The outer border is less well defined than in **b**. **d, e** Two weeks after stereotaxic puncture of the abscess and antibiotic therapy, only a small area of low signal intensity is recognized, probably corresponding to the shrinking capsule *(long arrow)* which still shows slight peripheral enhancement *(short arrow)* and perifocal edema *(arrowhead)*. Coronal scans (**a, d**) SE 2.5 s/120 ms, (**b, c**) SE 0.5 s/30 ms; parasagittal scan (**e**) 0.5 s/30 ms (1.0 T)

cerebritis. There eventually comes a point when central enhancement is no longer observed.

Rosenblum et al. [81] correlated the results of the medical treatment of brain abscesses with CT findings. Antibiotic therapy was successful when the medication was started before the abscess had developed a definite capsule and was no larger than 3 cm. A decrease in ring enhancement is a recognized criterion of successful drug therapy [12]. No comparable clinical studies utilizing MR have yet been performed.

The MR images in Figs. 15.3 and 15.4 show brain abscesses in the region of the thalamus. The signal intensity of the abscess in Fig. 15.3 is approximately equal to or slightly less than that of the surrounding brain on the proton-density image, and a faint, incomplete ring demarcates the abscess from the slightly higher intensity edema. With heavier T2 weighting of the sequence (SE TR 2.5 s/TE 120 ms), the contents of the abscess give a bright signal like that of CSF. It will be noted that the intensity of the signal gradually diminishes from the border of the lesion toward its center. The border, scarcely identifiable on the proton-density image, now stands out as a sharp, dark line (Figs. 15.3, 15.4a) and separates the abscess from the perifocal edema, which is less intense than the abscess contents or CSF. Following drainage and 2 weeks' antibiotic treatment (Fig. 15.4), both sequences display only a small, patchy, irregular paraventricular structure of low signal intensity with a minimal hyperintense rim of perifocal edema.

At present there is no accepted explanation for the hypointense ring, which at first sight might be interpreted as a collagenous capsule. This kind of ring structure is not specific for abscess capsule, however, and is also seen in association with brain tumors and hemorrhages. It may indicate hemorrhagic diapedesis in the abscess wall. Similar low signals can be produced by connective tissue structures, blood flow, calcifications, and hemosiderin deposits. Significant amounts of iron compounds have been suggested as a possible explanation, but no such compounds have been found in pathologic studies [100].

Neurotuberculosis

Tuberculosis of the brain tissue results from the hematogenous spread of *Mycobacterium tuberculosis* from a primary focus elsewhere in the body (lung, abdomen, genitourinary tract).

The complex and diverse nature of neurotuberculosis has been described by Dastur and Lalitha [21] and is generally acknowledged to be determined by individual variations of the host response. The pathologic processes fall into two main forms, in which either meningitis or tuberculoma predominates, with many instances of overlap.

Tuberculous meningitis begins with a leukocytic inflammation of the leptomeninges lasting several days, followed by a caseation of the exudate, especially around the vessels, with the formation of granulomatous nodules, mostly on the pial surface of the brain or within the superficial parenchyma. A heavy, fibrin-rich edema permeates the pia mater at the base of the brain. The brain tissue is invariably involved and may show edematous changes itself, or the inflammation may spread along the vessels of the pia mater to the cerebral cortex (meningoencephalitis).

Arteritis is invariably present, with widespread proliferative changes in the adventitia and intima, focal necrosis of the vessel wall, thrombosis, and (later) luminal obliteration (Heubner's specific endarteritis). This component of the disease is responsible for the frequent occurrence of ischemic parenchymal necrosis, especially of the deep gray matter and the brainstem (Figs. 15.5, 15.6).

Cranial nerve deficits occur secondarily in association with basilar meningoneuritis.

Involvement of the choroid plexus is common and leads to an increased production of CSF. This, together with obstruction of the foramina of Magendie and Luschka and the presence of purulent and fibrinous coagula in the CSF, can produce an obstructive or communicating hydrocephalus. The CSF typically shows lymphocytosis, a low glucose content, and a moderately to markedly elevated protein content, which congeals into a "fine cobweb" structure when allowed to settle in a test tube.

Tuberculoma formation characterizes many cases of neurotuberculosis and in childhood is frequently combined with frank meningitis. A capsule composed of dense granulomatous inflammatory infiltrate, fibroblasts, and granulation tissue surrounds a core of necrotic material which is usually solid (i.e., caseous). The caseous material does not become organized or absorbed, but calcifies; it undergoes fibrous tissue encapsulation in the event that "healing" occurs (Fig. 15.7). Less commonly the contents are liquefied, thereby conforming pathologically and radiologically to a true abscess. Not infrequently, these lesions are partly caseous and partly liquefied, or may undergo cystic degeneration. Macroscopic tuberculomas vary from 2 mm to several centimeters in size, may be single or multiple, and can occur anywhere within the cranium. In the subdural and subarachnoid spaces, tuberculomas tend to be elongated and lobulated, whereas parenchymal lesions are more rounded. Most cerebellar tuberculomas, though subarachnoid, take on the appearance of intraparenchymal masses due to the complexity of the folia. The process of exudate necrosis in meningitis is identical to that occurring in the tuberculoma, and in some cases mixed lesions occur, particularly at certain anatomic sites, e.g., over the insular cortex. This form of localized, caseating meningitis has been termed "tuberculomatosis" [22] and is particularly associated with superficial cortical vasculitis and ischemic necrosis, revealing itself radiologically as a dense, meningeal-parenchymal CT enhancement abnormality. Tuberculous encephalopathy is a diffuse disturbance of the hemispheric parenchyma that complicates some cases of tuberculous meningitis and is characterized by features of encephalitis, with lymphocytic perivascular cuffing, granulomatous arteriolitis, neuronal loss, demyelination, and gliosis.

Proliferative encasing granulomatous arachnoiditis can lead to tuberculous myelopathy through compression of the spinal cord and vasculitic

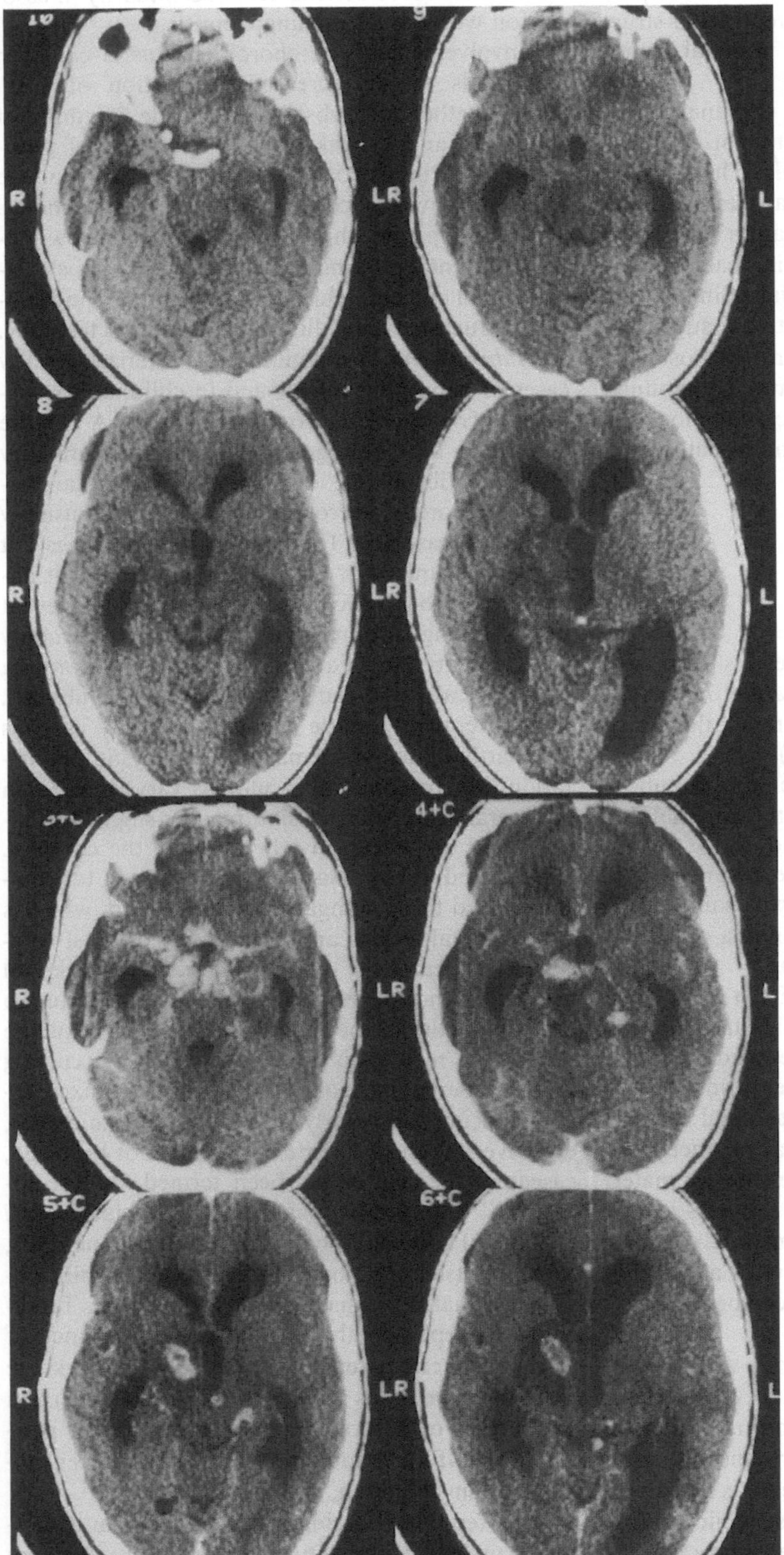

a

b

Fig. 15.5 a, b. Tuberculous meningitis in a 25-year-old woman with fever and severe organic psychosyndrome without focal neurologic deficits. **a** CT before administration of contrast medium. The basal cisterns are isodense, and there are ill-defined hypodense lesions in the basal ganglia and brainstem with some mass effect. **b** After administration of contrast medium. The cisterns are enhanced, and within the hypodense areas there is nodular enhancement suggesting caseous necrosis. (Courtesy of Dr. Backmund, Max Planck Institute of Psychiatry, Munich)

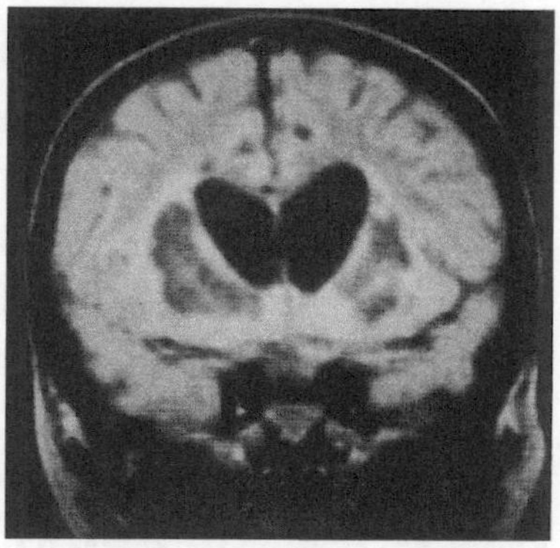

Fig. 15.6. Tuberculous meningitis. Bilateral, symmetrical basal infarcts are well demarcated from edema on the proton density image. An obliterative endarteritis is inferred. Internal hydrocephalus. Coronal scan, SE 2.0 s/27 ms

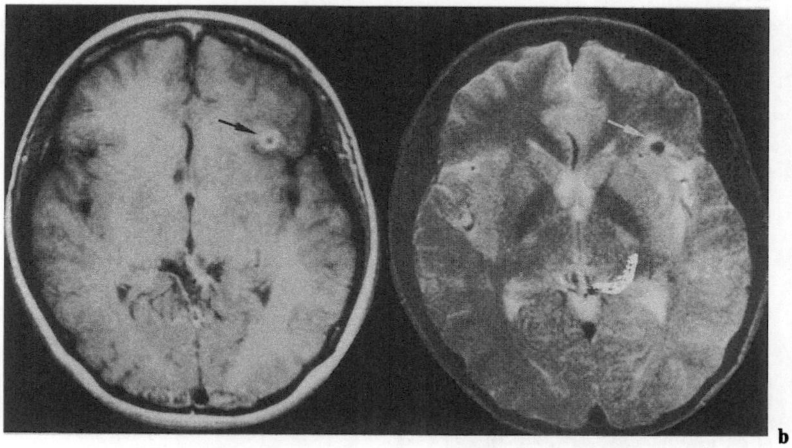

Fig. 15.7 a, b. Tuberculoma in a 23-year-old woman with known tuberculosis. The small tuberculoma *(arrow)* displays the characteristic target sign. Axial scans: **a** SE 0.5 s/30 ms, with i.v. gadolinium-DTPA; **b** SE 1.5 s/100 ms (1.5 T)

thrombosis of its vessels [91]. In rare cases this form may be unaccompanied by tuberculous vertebral caries (Pott's disease) [16, 51, 92] and encase the spinal cord within a thick, hard fibrinous-granulomatous layer that is fused to the cord.

Besides this more diffuse spread of granulomatous tissue in the subdural space, some authors have reported the occurrence of hard, tumorlike lesions several centimeters in diameter with relatively thin membranes, often containing granular calcified material [20, 86].

CT and MR Findings

Enhanced CT images in cases of tuberculous meningitis consistently show hyperdense basal cisterns and M1 segments of the middle cerebral arteries, very often associated with ventricular dilatation (Fig. 15.5).

Focal, hypodense, nonenhancing areas in the deep gray matter and the diencephalon indicative of ischemic necrosis also are commonly present [73, 90]. In patients with diffuse cerebritis, CT shows nondiscrete areas of enhancement scattered throughout the brain [5]. Focal mass lesions are round or lobulated, depending on the anatomic location, with rather thick, irregular rim enhancement. The centers of these lesions are isodense in caseous necrosis and hypodense in abscesses; surrounding edema is almost invariably present in the latter. Less frequently a nonenhancing, hyperdense nodule or a large, irregularly enhancing mass will be apparent [75]. The latter may be caused by conglomeration of multiple granulomas [27]. Densely enhancing lesions distributed en plaque along the tentorium have also been described [93] (cf. Fig. 15.5).

The presence of a central nidus of calcification or a central contrast enhancement within a ring-

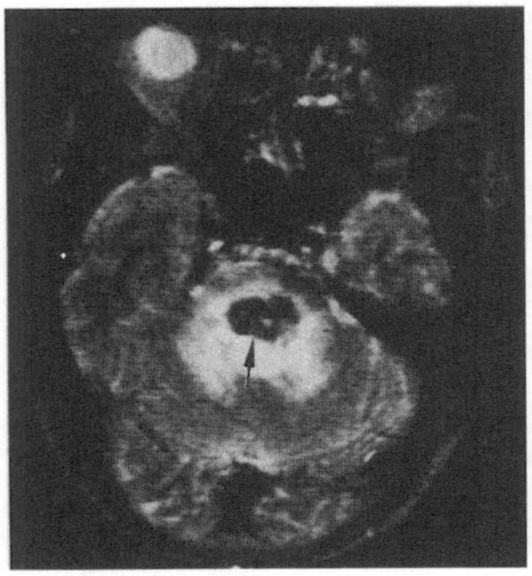

15.8

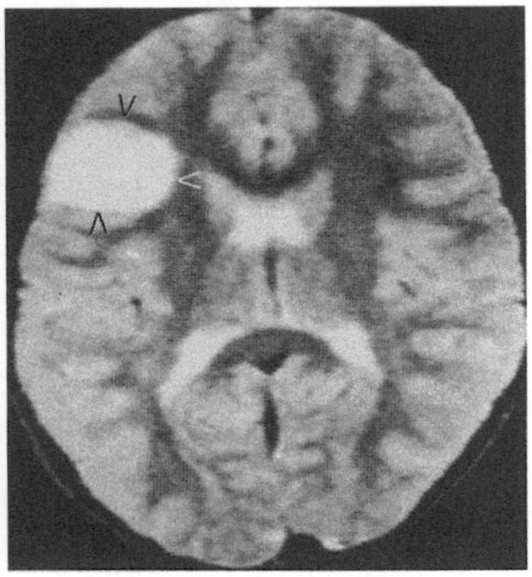

15.9

Fig. 15.8. Tuberculous granuloma. Well-demarcated low-intensity lesion (short T2) situated in the brainstem, probably corresponding to a caseating granuloma *(arrow)*. Axial scan, SE 2.0 s/120 ms (0.5 T). On CT, rim enhancement around an isodense center was seen

Fig. 15.9. Tuberculous abscess. The entire lesion has a high intensity on the T2-weighted image (SE 2.0 s/70 ms) and probably represents tuberculous abscess formation *(arrowheads)*. On CT, rim enhancement around a hypodense center was seen

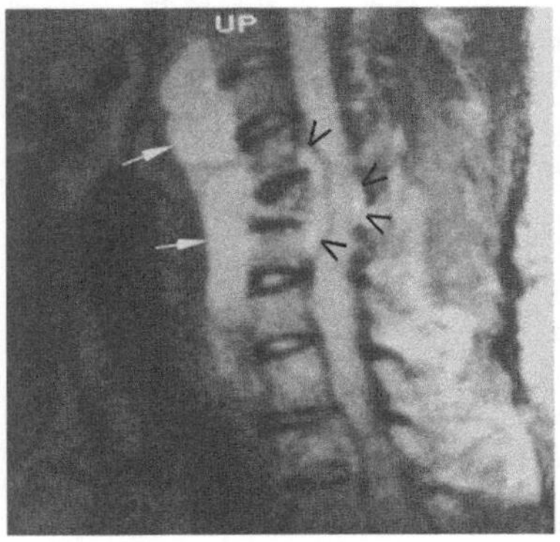

15.10

Fig. 15.10. Tuberculous abscess in a patient with known tuberculosis. There is destruction of the fifth vertebra with displacement of its dorsal border into the vertebral canal. The cord is also displaced and compressed by hyperintensive abscess material which surrounds it *(arrowheads)* and which extends as a large mass anterior to the vertebral column *(arrows)*. Sagittal scan, SE 2.0 s/70 ms (1.0 T). (Courtesy of T. Beydoun, MD, Dr. Erfan-Bagedo Hospitals, Jedda)

shaped lesion (target sign) is considered highly specific for tuberculosis by Welchman [93] (Fig. 15.7). The micro-ring appearance was not seen in sarcoidosis [94]. On the whole, however, the CT findings cannot be viewed as pathognomonic, and the diagnosis should be based on all supportive clinical data [90].

The basal, meningovascular enhancement abnormality demonstrated with CT has not been corroborated on MR, although the cisterns on T2-weighted images may be seen to contain loculi of fluid, which presumably consists mostly of CSF. This picture is accompanied by ventricular dilatation and periventricular edema. MR is superior to CT in the evaluation of focal parenchymal infarcts, which are clearly seen on T1 and proton density images as hypointense areas well demarcated from the surrounding edema (Fig. 15.6). As TR and TE are lengthened, these lesions become hyperintense, resulting in loss of differentiation. Focal tuberculous lesions are readily identified on MR images but are not specific in appearance and cannot be differentiated from other focal inflammatory masses.

The spectrum of signal intensity changes seen on T2-weighted images corresponds well with the forms of necrosis described above, as well as with the enhanced images on CT. Thus, a focal lesion with a high-intensity rim and low-intensity center (shorter T2) probably represents a caseating tuberculoma (Figs. 15.7, 15.8), whereas a lesion giving a homogeneous high signal (longer T2) would be consistent with a tuberculous abscess (Figs. 15.9, 15.10). Histologic proof of these assumptions is still needed, however.

The injection of MR-specific contrast material (gadolinium chelate) would be expected to produce a pattern of enhancement similar to that seen on CT, since the mechanism of contrast enhancement

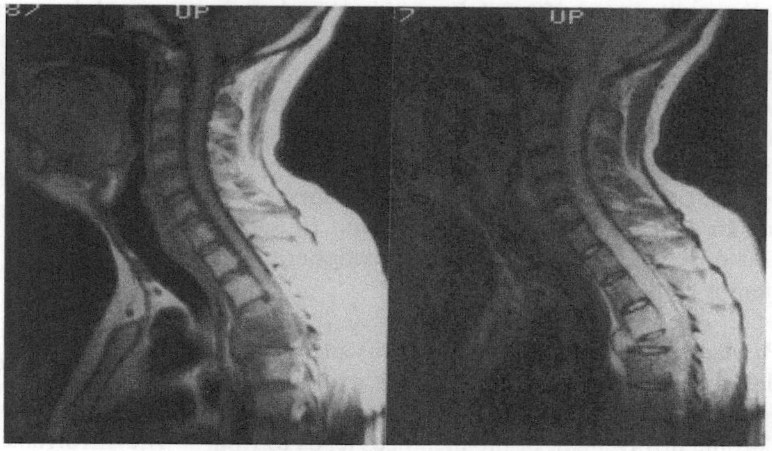

Fig. 15.11 a, b. Tuberculous spondylitis in a 31-year-old man with progressive paraparesis. The diagnosis was confirmed by biopsy. Note the preservation of the intervertebral disc (**b**). Midsagittal scans: **a** SE 0.4 s/17 ms, **b** SE 1.6 s/80 ms (1.0 T)

in both modalities is based on a disruption of the blood-brain barrier.

Granulomatous arachnoiditis of the vertebral canal can appear on CT images as a densely calcified intraspinal mass. The signal characteristics on MR images would presumably be analogous to those of intracranial granulomatous lesions. Compression of the cord may also be caused by tuberculous spondylitis (Fig. 15.11). In addition, the ischemic and pressure-related lesions of tuberculous myelopathy, which increase the relaxation times of the spinal cord through edema and demyelination, would be expected to produce high-signal areas on MR images. To reduce the chance of error, allowance should be made for the effects of CSF pulsations and arachnoiditic fluid pockets (see Sect. 5.3).

Sarcoidosis

Sarcoidosis resembles, clinically and pathologically, tuberculosis and other granulomatous infections. Its causative agent has not yet been identified, and its etiology is still not completely understood. The typical lesion consists of a focus of epithelial cells surrounded by lymphocytes and giant cells, but no caseation is seen.

In the CNS the tubercels of sarcoidosis, which are found in all regions of the body, induce granulomatous infiltration of the meninges and underlying parenchyma, particularly at the base of the brain [42].

Lesions of the chiasm and hypothalamus cause visual disturbances and signs of hypothalamic and pituitary dysfunction. Other manifestations include aseptic meningitis, hydrocephalus, cranial neuropathies, seizures, and adhesive arachnoiditis. Parenchymatous disease can lead to nodular mass lesions.

CT and MR Findings

Besides hydrocephalus, granulomatous nodules are frequently found. On CT, the latter are well-defined, slightly hyperdense masses with more or less extensive perifocal edema on noncontrast scan, and show homogeneous enhancement after i.v. contrast injection. En plaque enhancement of the basal cisterns is seen with infiltration of the meninges [14, 47, 54, 87].

On MR, the granulomatous masses may appear hyperintense, less frequently isotense or hypointense, on T2-weighted scans. MR has been found to be more sensitive than CT in evaluating hypothalamic and periventricular involvement and in detecting mass lesions of the brainstem [47].

Syphilis

Syphilis, caused by infection with *Treponema pallidum,* is divided into primary, secondary, and tertiary stages. CNS involvement can occur in any of these stages, from weeks to decades after infection. Neurosyphilis develops in about 5% of untreated patients [18].

The major symptomatic types of neurosyphilis are acute leptomeningitis in secondary syphilis and parenchymatous and meningovascular neurosyphilis in tertiary cases [50, 70]. Syphilitic vascular disease, tabes dorsalis, and gumma of the brain also may occur in neurosyphilis.

The parenchymatous type of neurosyphilis is encountered more frequently, causing widespread parenchymal damage and demyelination of the posterior column, dorsal roots, and dorsal root ganglia [50]. The meningovascular type causes infarction resulting from progressive endarteritis obliterans [73].

Pathologic findings in the meningovascular type include widespread thickening of the meninges and perivascular spaces with lymphocytic infiltration. Chronic involvement of the meninges leads to frontal lobe atrophy, ependymitis, and ventricular dilatation. In the parenchymatous type, diffuse proliferative inflammatory changes are seen within the cerebral cortex in general paralysis, occasionally associated with either miliary small or larger gummas. Gummas, on the rare occasions when they occur, vary from 1 mm to 4 cm in size. A central caseous or gummatous necrosis is surrounded by multiple dense epitheloid cells, spindle fibroblasts, and scattered multinuclear giant cells [50].

CT and MR Findings

CT can detect infarctions, (enhancing) gummas, and atrophy [42]. The CT findings can closely resemble a demyelinating or dysmyelinating disease of the white matter or a cerebrovascular insult.

MR imaging with proton-density and T2-weighted sequences has proved to be more sensitive than CT to abnormalities in the water content of tissues following multifocal infarction [50].

At the time of writing we are unaware of any published reports on the appearance of gummas on MR images. It is reasonable to assume that those lesions would behave similarly to other chronic inflammatory granulomas.

The CT and MR features of neurosyphilis that have been described to date indicate that a multicentric pattern of lesions is indicative of vasculitis, although the changes are not specific for neurosyphilis.

Nonsyphilitic Spirochaetosis of the CNS

Nonsyphilitic spirochaetosis of the CNS (erythema chronicum migrans, Borreliosis, Lyme disease) is caused by a tick-borne *(Ixodes ricinus)* infection with a nonsyphilitic spirochaete *(Borrelia burgdorferi)*. The spectrum of clinical reactions to this infection varies with the stage of the disease. It includes [2, 9]:

- In the early stage: erythema migrans and lymphadenoma benigna cutis,
- In the late stage: meningopolyneuritis Garin-Bujadoux-Bannwarth, oligoarthritis and myocarditis, and
- In the chronic form of the disease: acrodermatitis chronica atrophicans, progressive *Borrelia* encephalitis, and chronic polyarthritis.

The involvement of the CNS during the various stages shares common basic features; in the individual case, however, clinical manifestations may differ [49].

The peripheral nervous system is predominantly affected in European countries, whereas the North American form of the disease (Lyme disease) more often involves the CNS [77].

The symptoms of encephalomyelitis caused by *Borrelia* infection include tetra- or paraspastic paresis, disturbances of sensation and bladder function, cranial nerve palsy affecting also the optic nerve, cerebral seizures, and personality changes. In the CSF, pleocytosis, disruption of the blood-CSF barrier, and an increase of protein content are found.

Nonsyphilitic spirochaetosis of the CNS must be differentiated from cerebrospinal syphilis, progressive paralysis, and multiple sclerosis.

MR Findings

At the time of writing no reports on the MR features of CNS lesions of nonsyphilitic spirochaetosis were available to us. Figure 15.12a, b shows CNS lesions in patients with *Borrelia* encephalomyelitis which was confirmed by clinical and laboratory findings.

15.4.2 Viral Infections

Viral infections of the nervous system can be grouped into five categories: (1) aseptic meningitis, (2) encephalomyelitis, (3) postinfectious encephalitis, (4) acute infective encephalitis, and (5) subacute encephalitis [15]. With few exceptions, the reactions of the CNS to different viral infections are similar. They vary, however, in the prominence of certain modes of response and in their distribution.

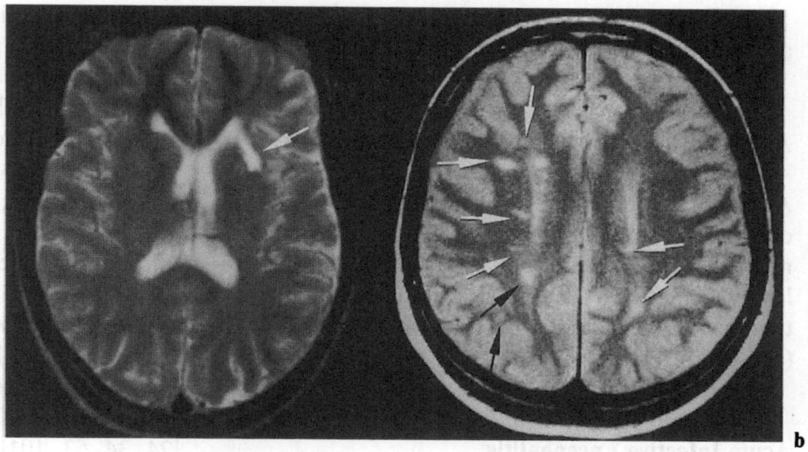

Fig. 15.12. Borreliosis (Lyme disease) in a (**a**) 29-year-old man with progressive spastic paraparesis. Antibodies against *Borrelia burgdorferi* in serum and CSF. Well-defined hyperintense lesion extending from the anterior horn of the lateral ventricle to the external capsule *(arrow)*. The pattern of this lesion resembles a small infarction in the territory of the lenticulostriate arteries. To explain the spinal symptoms an additional cord lesion has to be asumed. Axial scan, SE 3.0 s/112 ms (1.0 T). (**b**) 27-year-old woman with visual disturbances and slight weaknes on the right. Multiple, unspecific, white matter lesions *(arrows)*. Axial scan, SE 3.0 s/22 ms (1.5 T)

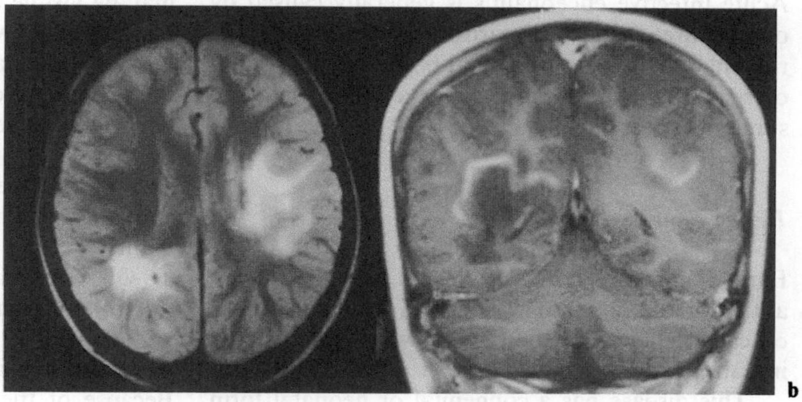

Fig. 15.13 a, b. Virus encephalitis in a 10-year-old girl presenting with rapidly progressing brachiofacial hemiparesis. Large, irregular, confluent lesions with prolonged relaxation times involving the white matter of both hemispheres without significant mass effect. With intravenous gadolinium-DTPA (**b**), incomplete rim enhancement is seen. Biopsy revealed virus encephalitis without identifying the virus. **a** Axial scan SE 3.0 s/45 ms, **b** coronal scan, SE 0.4 s/17 ms (1.0 T)

Macroscopic changes may not be apparent at autopsy, or there may be a circumscribed or general swelling of the brain and spinal cord with a prominent vascular pattern and a more or less pronounced softening of the nerve tissue (Fig. 15.13). Exceptions are changes in the brain associated with herpes simplex encephalitis and spinal cord changes related to poliomyelitis [15].

Microscopic features include:

- Inflammatory cell infiltration (polymorphonuclear leukocytes, lymphocytes)
- Hyperplasia and proliferation of microglial cells
- Astrocytosis (in response to tissue necrosis)
- Changes in neurons
- Inclusion bodies (in neurons, astrocytes, and oligodendroglial cells)
- Necrosis (of varying distribution)
- Demyelination
- Status spongiosus

Aseptic Meningitis

See Sect. 15.3.2.

Encephalomyelitis

The main representative of the encephalomyelitis group is encephalomyelitis caused by polio viruses.

The CNS may appear grossly normal in the acute stage of *poliomyelitis*, but in severe acute cases there will be vascular congestion, hemorrhages, or areas of necrosis involving the anterior horns of the spinal cord or the dorsal medulla. In these cases multiple foci of glial proliferation and neuronal necrosis may be found in the deep gray nuclei of the cerebrum, midbrain, pons, and cerebellum. In bulbar poliomyelitis, dense cellular infiltration is found in the nuclei of the motor cranial nerves. Similar areas of infiltration and neuronal necrosis are present in the cortex of the precentral gyrus [15].

No reports on the MR features of poliomyelitis are available at the moment.

Acute Postinfectious (Perivenous) Encephalitis

Acute postinfectious (perivenous) encephalitis occurs as a complication of viral infections such as measles, mumps, smallpox, and rubella, or may follow vaccinations. The most striking histologic feature is perivascular demyelination (Fig. 15.14) [15] (see Chap. 8).

Acute Infective Encephalitis

Acute infective encephalitis is generally caused by one of three (groups of) viruses: herpes simplex virus, rhabdovirus, or arthropod-borne viruses. Adenoviruses and enteroviruses also may be causative in some instances.

Herpes Simplex Encephalitis

Early diagnosis is critical in herpes simplex encephalitis, for today a drug therapy is available whose efficacy depends on the time at which treatment is initiated.

This disease has a congenital or neonatal form (type 2, HSV 2) and an adult form (type 1, HSV 1).

Type 1: Adult Form

The gross pathologic features of type 1 herpes simplex encephalitis are very characteristic but not pathognomonic: extensive, usually asymmetric areas of necrosis in the temporal lobes and frontobasal region accompanied by marked edema, which may expand to produce a general softening with zones of hemorrhage (Figs. 15.15). There is also a generalized brain swelling that is often more pronounced on one side than the other, and this may be associated with a shift of midline structures and tentorial herniation. The necrotic areas may involve the cortex as well as the white matter, hippocampus, amygdaloid nucleus and putamen, the parahippocampus and temporomedial regions, the insula, and the cingulate gyrus [15].

The microscopic features vary with the stage of the disease. The acute stage is marked by a diffuse meningoencephalitis, which is most pronounced around the necrotic areas. This is followed later by a cellular reaction around the necrotic foci in the form of glial hyperplasia. Finally, a great many lipid phagocytes appear together with lymphocytes and plasma cells in the meninges and around the vessels [15]. The necrotic areas lead to multifocal substance loss with cavitation mainly affecting the temporal lobes, whose borders show fibrosis and gliosis with an ongoing proliferation of microglia and lymphocyte infiltration [36].

CT and MR Findings. CT demonstrates ill-defined mass lesions of low density in one or both temporal lobes which extend in the white matter as far as the insula (island of Reil), sparing the lentiform nucleus [24, 34, 53, 101]. CT scans may appear normal before the 5th day. In other cases areas of hemorrhage may be visible after only 2 days [101]. Postcontrast scans may show streaklike changes after only three days. Occasionally the hyperdensities may precede the hypodense changes. Ringlike or garlandlike enhancement is seen at the borders of lesions and in the cortex [24, 34]. The hypodense areas may extend into the adjacent portions of the cerebral hemispheres [24]. Later, sharply marginated defects remain.

On MR scans the prolonged T1 and T2 times of the inflammatory edema produce areas of high signal intensity on proton-density and T2-weighted images, and low-signal areas on T1-weighted images. Because of the greater sensitivity of MR, inflammatory edema is visible earlier than on CT scans, and it manifests a greater extent (Fig. 15.15) [100].

Schroth and Kretzschmar [84] describe the demonstration of preferential lesions of the limbic system by MR before any CT changes appear. This observation supports the assertion that MR is the diagnostic procedure of choice for suspected viral encephalitis and should be performed even in uncooperative patients so that antiviral therapy can be initiated as soon as possible.

After injection of the MR-specific contrast agent gadolinium chelate, the lesions show enhancement similar to that in CT once the blood-brain barrier has become disrupted (see also Fig. 15.13) [100]. In the final stage of defect formation, the necrotic cavities are filled with CSF, whose relaxation times are the same as those of the intraventricular CSF. The signal from the periphery of the lesions will depend on the content of cellular and fibrous material and the presence of fat granule cells and foci of demyelination. Additional clinical observations are needed to characterize these findings more precisely.

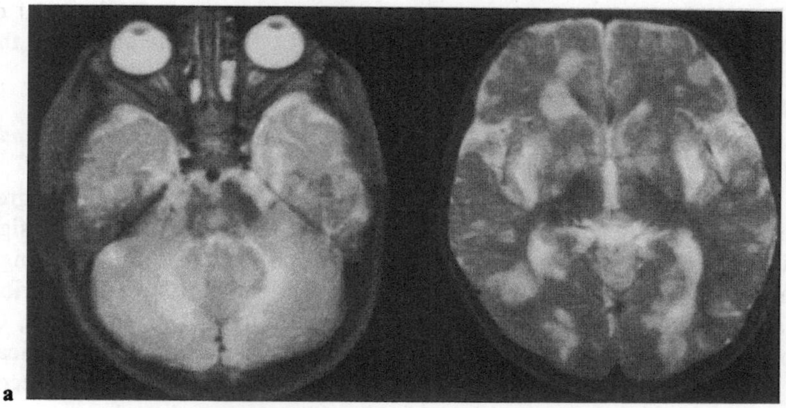

Fig. 15.14a, b. Postinfectious encephalitis in a 2-year-old boy with statomotor retardation, repeated episodes of fever and vomiting, and seizures. Multiple scattered lesions of varying size with prolonged relaxation times in both hemispheres and in the posterior fossa, involving both white and gray matter. Axial scans: **a, b** SE 3.0 s/120 ms (1.0 T)

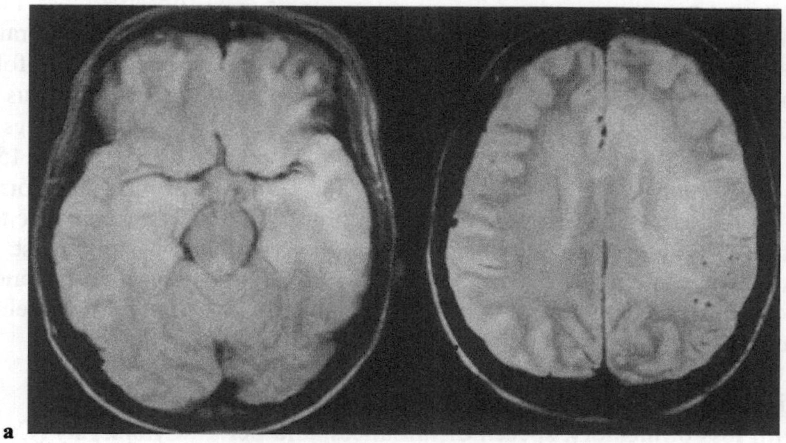

Fig. 15.15a, b. Herpes simplex encephalitis in a 32-year-old woman with organic psychosyndrome, cerebral seizures. Extensive, ill-defined area of prolonged relaxation times in both temporal lobes, predominantly on the right, extending to the parietal region. Axial scans: **a, b** SE 3.0 s/45 ms (1.0 T)

Type 2: Congenital or Neonatal Form

In type 2 herpes simplex encephalitis there may be extensive necrosis of the cerebrum, which is considered one cause of multiple cystic encephalomalacia [29, 71].

CT Findings. The earliest CT features of type 2 herpes simplex encephalitis can be very subtle, consisting of patchy areas of low density in both hemispheres that tend to spare the basal ganglia, thalami, and posterior fossa structures. As the disease progresses, areas of hemorrhage and calcification may occur in the thalami, the insular cortex, the periventricular white matter, and at the gray matter-white matter junction. The assessment of abnormal absorption coefficients is made difficult, however, by the immature white matter of the newborn, which is rich in water and poor in lipids and proteins compared with the brain at 9-12 months of age (see Chap. 6).

The finding of patchy low-density areas in both hemispheres of the neonatal brain should always raise suspicion of herpes simplex encephalitis [7]. Similar hypodense areas can be caused by a number of other processes, such as bacterial infections, hypoxia, and metabolic abnormalities [7].

At present we are unaware of any published reports on the MR features of type 2 herpes simplex encephalitis.

Rhabdovirus and Arthropod-borne Virus Infection

Encephalitis caused by these viruses consists in diffuse degeneration of nerve cells and scattered foci of varying size of inflammatory necrosis of the white matter and cortex. The brainstem usually is spared.

CT and MR Findings

The inflammatory foci appear hypodense in CT; after the injection of contrast medium patchy enhancement is seen. There is only very little mass effect.

On MR the irregular lesions have prolonged relaxation times. Fig. 15.13 shows two large foci of virus encephalitis, which was verified by biopsy; the causative virus could not, however, be identified. Rim enhancement of the lesions is seen after intravenous application of gadolinium-DTPA.

Subacute Sclerosing Panencephalitis

Subacute sclerosing panencephalitis (SSPE) is caused by infection with a measles virus (paramyxovirus). With Creutzfeld-Jakob syndrome, kuru, and progressive multifocal leukencephalopathy, it forms the group of slow virus infections in man (see also Sect. 9).

Symptoms appear, with few exceptions, from about 5-15 years of age, preferentially in boys, with an average latency of 4-5 years following an innocuous measles infection, which in most patients occurred before the age of 2 years [57].

The clinical picture varies with the stage of the disease. Insidious failure of intellectual function, with loss of memory, speech disturbances, and personality and behavioral deterioration, is followed by rigidity, hyperkinesia and dyskinesia, ataxia, spasticity, generalized seizures, and ultimately death in a vegetative state. The triad of dementia, extrapyramidal hyperkinesia, and muscle rigidity is most relevant for the diagnosis [72]. The disease may progress rapidly or more slowly.

Macroscopic changes in the brain are discreet, with induration and spotty gray discoloration of mainly the occipital and temporal white matter suggesting demyelination in chronic cases (Fig. 15.16). Some mild cortical atrophy, softening of the cortex, and symmetrical enlargement of the ventricles also may be seen.

Histologic findings of this form of encephalitis include patchy demyelination in the subcortical white matter, perivascular and leptomeningeal infiltrations of lymphocytes and plasma cells, proliferation and hypertrophy of astroglia in affected areas of gray and white matter, and intranuclear inclusion bodies [15]. Due to severe neuronal loss the cortex may appear ulegyric, and major loss of white matter may cause hydrocephalus ex vacuo.

Differential diagnoses include other slow virus infections and the leukodystrophies.

CT and MR Findings

When the progression of disease is rapid, CT scans may show no significant changes, although a general brain swelling with compression of the ventricles has been described [71]. In cases taking a more protracted course, CT shows patchy hypodense areas in the subcortical and periventricular white matter, which may account for the extrapyramidal motor disturbances seen with involvement of the caudate nucleus [30]. Contrast enhancement has not been observed [44]. Finally the disease leads to an extensive loss of brain substance. The changes are not specific, but follow the pattern characteristic of other slow virus infections.

MR findings in a patient with SSPE are demonstrated in Fig. 15.16. The areas of prolonged relaxation times correspond well with the site of predilection in the temporo-occipital lobe described by the pathologist. The greater sensitivity of MR enables earlier and more complete detection of diffuse brain swelling and focal white matter abnormalities.

Cytomegaly (Congenital Cytomegalic Inclusion Disease)

Prenatal infection with cytomegalovirus leads to the destruction of extensive brain areas, often accompanied by small foci of intracranial calcification.

CT and MR Findings

CT usually demonstrates a hydrocephalus ex vacuo and porencephalic defects due to tissue destruction, as well as periventricular calcifications. There may be inflammatory obstruction of the foramina of Monro (ependymitis), leading to CSF stasis and ventricular dilatation that is more prominent on one side than the other.

The defects are recognized on MR images by their CSF-like signal intensity. The small calcifications are displayed less clearly than with CT. Scarred brain tissue has signal characteristics that distinguish it from normal brain, although further clinical experience in this area is needed.

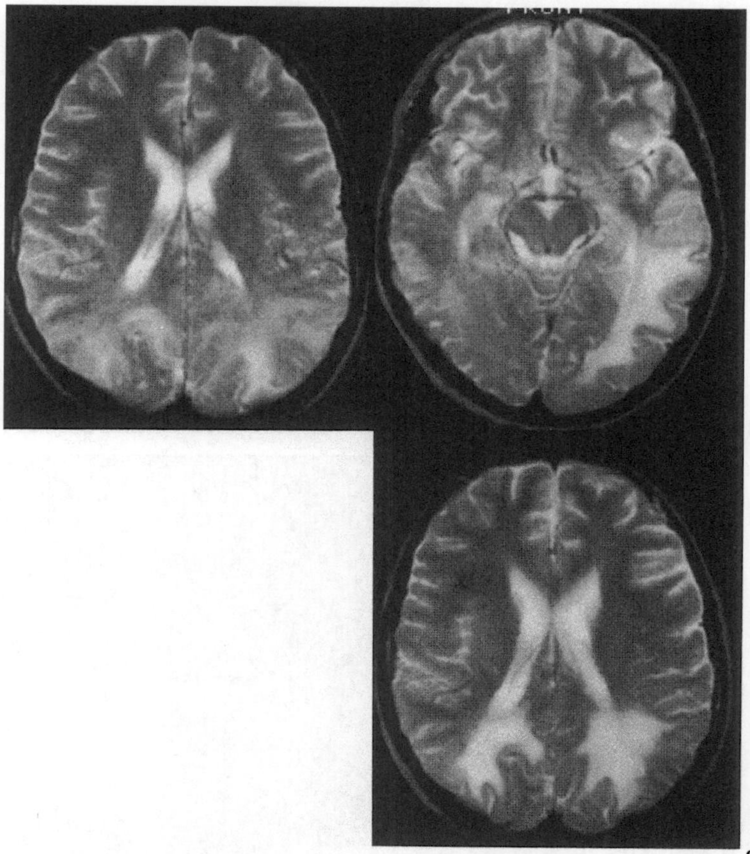

a b c

Fig. 15.16a–c. Subacute sclerosing panencephalitis in a 13-year-old boy with gradual onset 3–4 months previously of progressive symptoms including mental deterioration, disorientation, and ataxia. History of measles 12 years ago. **a** Large ill-defined areas of prolonged relaxation times of the dorsal portions of both hemispheres involving white matter and cortex. **b, c** Control scans 6 weeks later show greater changes of the relaxation times of the lesions, which now are better delineated and less extensive, and slight dilatation of the ventricles, indicating atrophy of white matter. The condition of the patient has worsened significantly. Axial scans, SE 3.0 s/120 ms (1.0 T)

15.4.3 Parasitic Infections

Protozoal Infections

The major protozoal infections that can involve the CNS are amebiasis, malaria, and toxoplasmosis.

Amebiasis

Infection by *Entamoeba histolytica* can lead in severe cases to meningoencephalitis and amebic abscess of the brain.

Malaria

Infection by the parasite *Plasmodium falciparum* can lead to cerebral involvement with brain edema, vascular congestion, and petechial hemorrhages. Hemorrhage into the white matter in the form of a disseminated vasculomyelopathy is especially common [89].

Toxoplasmosis

Cerebral toxoplasmosis is caused by the obligate intracellular organism *Toxoplasma gondii*. Two different patterns of disease, the adult and the neonate, are recognized according to whether the infection is acquired in an immunologically mature individual or prior to the development of immune competence [83].

Adult Type

In adults the organism causes a meningoencephalitis with lymphocytic infiltration of the leptomeninges, a metastatic focal encephalitis (Fig. 15.17), gliomatous nodules within the parenchyma (toxoplasmic granulomas) [64], and occasional parasitic cysts from 20 to 100 micrometers in size. An inflammatory reaction occurs only in the presence of cellular necrosis, as intracellular organisms do not incite this response [83].

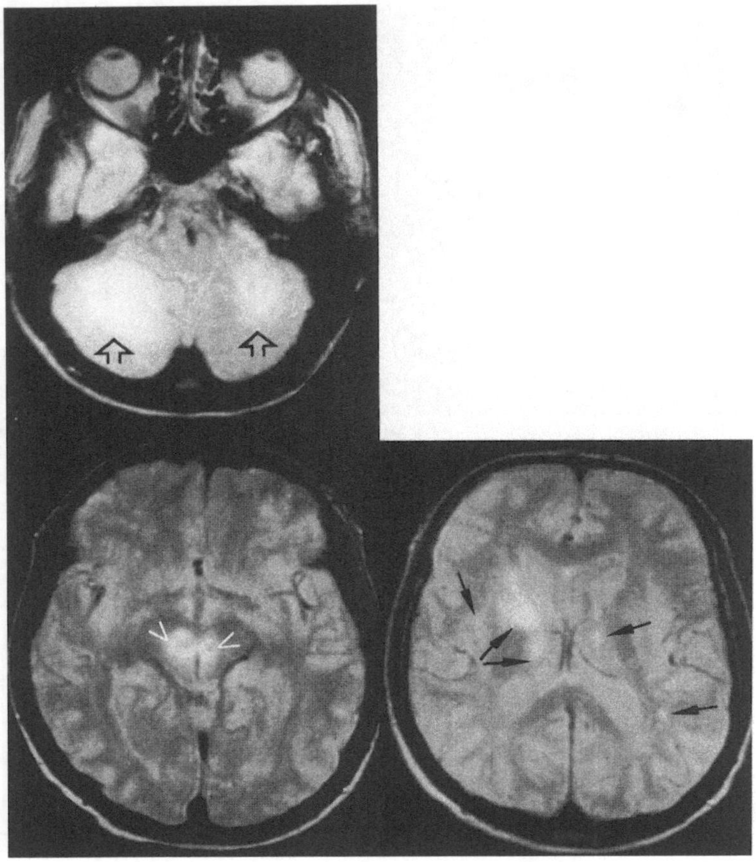

a

b

c

Fig. 15.17 a–c. Toxoplasmosis (confirmed by stereotaxic biopsy) in a 39-year-old man with known Boeck's disease presenting with cerebellar symptoms. **a** Hyperintense lesions within both cerebellar hemispheres *(open arrows)*. **b, c** Control scans 5 months later show new lesions in the midbrain *(arrowheads)*, in the basal ganglia, and in the white matter *(arrows)*; the cerebellar lesions have disappeared. Axial scans: **a–c** SE 3.0 s/45 ms (1.0 T)

CT and MR Findings. CT shows multiple, hypodense, densely enhancing nodules up to 4 cm in size at the gray matter–white matter junction and around the ventricles. Ring-enhancing lesions with thick or thin walls also may appear and can simulate a brain abscess [63]. The CT features of toxoplasmosis are nonspecific, and diagnosis relies on demonstrating the causative organism [64]. Exacerbation can occur in patients receiving cytostatic or immunosuppressive drugs [56] or suffering from some other immune weakness (e.g., AIDS; see Sect. 15.4.5) [74, 98], and multiple hypodense areas with small hemorrhagic foci may be seen in these patients [31]. The course in immune-deficient patients resembles that in neonates [8].

MR findings in toxoplasmosis are variable. Multiple high-signal zones of varying size generally are seen on T2-weighted images and may have no counterpart even on high-resolution CT scans. Fritze et al. [38] describe the lesions on T1-weighted SE images as rounded areas of decreased signal intensity rimmed by a hyperintense border that is indistinguishable from the main lesion on T2-weighted images. Concurrent shortening of T1 may be present as evidence of hemorrhage. The MR findings correlate better than CT findings with the results of postmortem examinations [64, 74]. Since effective therapy is available (sulfadiazine, pyrimethamine), it is proper to consider MR imaging a first-line study in patients suspected of having toxoplasmosis. MR is better than CT for establishing the optimum site for tissue biopsy, which is frequently indicated (Fig. 15.17).

Congenital Type

The congenital form of cerebral toxoplasmosis occurs only when the infection is acquired during pregnancy. The timing of the infection determines the severity of the fetal brain damage. The organisms proliferate in the ependyma and subependymal tissue and spread freely due to lack of antibodies, resulting in extensive tissue destruction [10].

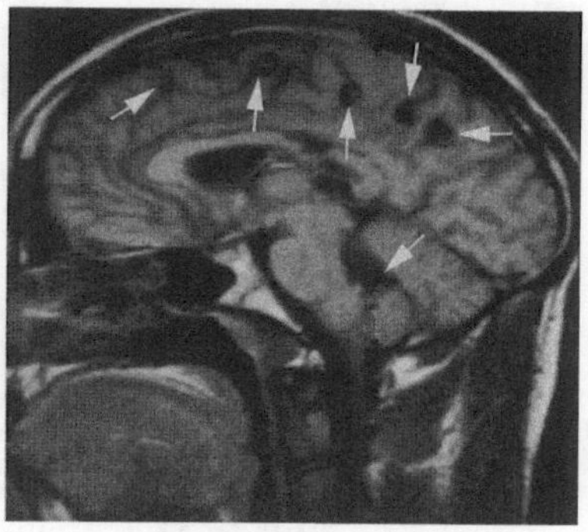

Fig. 15.18. Cysticercosis. Multiple cysts *(arrows)* related to the sulci, the corpus callosum, posterior to the thalamus and in the inferior part of the fourth ventricle. Sagittal section, SE 2.0 s/27 ms (0.5 T)

Toxoplasmic granulomas are scattered throughout the cerebral hemispheres, especially in the subcortical regions of the parietal and frontal lobes, the basal ganglia, the ventricular walls, and the choroid plexus [19]. Focal calcifications also develop in these regions. The aqueduct may become obstructed, leading to hydrocephalus, though the latter results more commonly from atrophic changes (hydrocephalus ex vacuo). When the damage is early and severe, microcephaly can result [83].

CT and MR Findings. The parenchymal substance losses in congenital toxoplasmosis are visible on both CT and MR and show densities or signal intensities similar to those of the dilated ventricles. T1-weighted sequences should be used owing to the good contrast that is obtained between CSF and brain.

The calcifications are clearly recognized as such on CT scans and are not displayed as well by MR.

Metazoal Infections

The metazoal infections include a number of parasitic infections, most of which occur in the tropics. The clinically important cestode larvae are cysticercus, echinococcus, and coenurus *(Taenia multiceps* or *Multiceps multiceps).* By far the majority of cases affecting the nervous system involve cysticercus, man serving both as an intermediate and as the only definitive host.

Cysticercosis

Cysticercosis occurs when man ingests the ova (oncospheres) of the tapeworm *Taenia solium,* and the larvae *(Cysticercus cellulosae)* penetrate the wall of the intestine to be dispersed by the circulation. Various forms of cysticercosis are recognized according to the anatomic or systemic location of the parasite in the human body:

- Disseminated cysticercosis (parasites in viscera, skin, and muscles)
- Ophthalmocysticercosis (parasites affecting the eyes and orbits)
- Neurocysticercosis (larvae lodged in the CNS)
- Mixed cysticercosis (involvement of more than one of the above locations) [99]

Neurocysticercosis

Infestation of the CNS by the encysted larvae can be further subdivided into cases with predominantly cerebral or spinal involvement. In the cranial cavity, the disease can assume three forms:

a *parenchymal* form, where the lesions are within the brain tissue proper; a *meningeal* form, where lesions are situated within the subarachnoid space; and a *ventricular* form. These different types may be present individually or in any combination in the same patient.

Cysticerci within the subarachnoid space tend to aggregate in the basal cisterns and usually are rather widely dispersed elsewhere. For reasons still unexplained, these meningeal parasites show a marked tendency toward cystic distention and may form structures up to several centimeters in diameter. This is in sharp contrast to the parenchymal organisms, which remain small (10 mm) throughout their viable existence. In many instances cysticerci are lodged deep within the sulci; inflammation and fibrosis lead to adhesions of the lips of the sulcus with sequestration of the parasites, which then be-

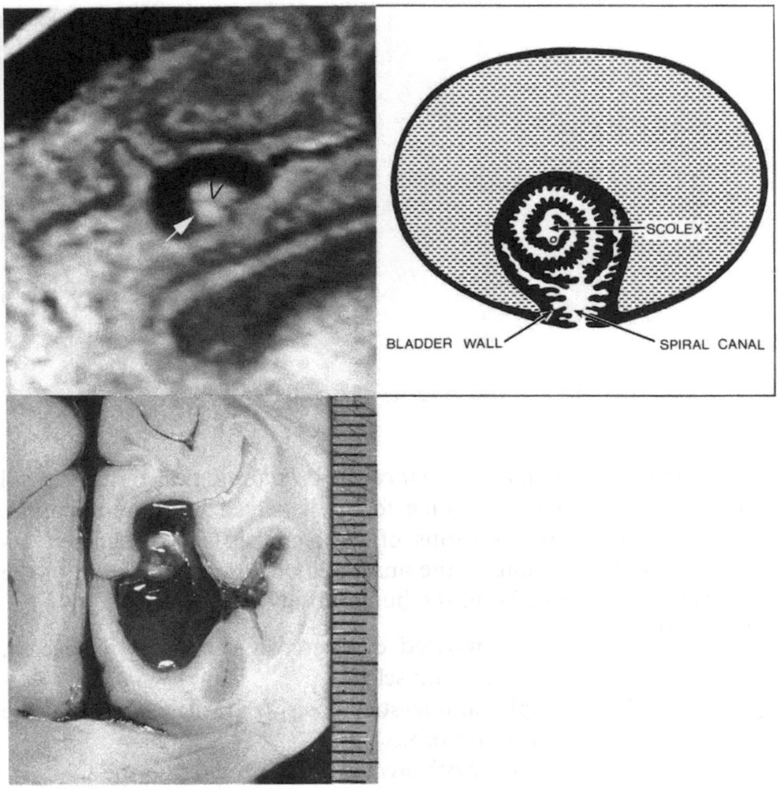

a b c

Fig. 15.19 a–c. Cysticercus cyst. **a** A typical lesion with fluid-filled cavity and mural nodule lies above the anterior corpus callosum. (**a**) Enlarged sagittal section, SE 0.5 s/27 ms (0.5 T). The cyst is located within the sulcal subarachnoid space. The cystic cavity surrounds an eccentric high-intensity nodule *(arrow)*, and the spiral canal *(arrowhead)* appears as a low-intensity tract traversing the nodule obliquely. **b** Schematic drawing of the cysticercus. The inverted protoscolex forms the spiral canal, surrounded by germinal tissue, contained within the bladder. **c** Section of the fixed brain, showing a parasitic cyst sequestrated within a sulcus and surrounded by gray matter. The opaque nodule represents degenerating germinal tissue of the dead protoscolex

come surrounded by gray matter and meninges. The literature contains conflicting reports on the incidence of parenchymal versus meningeal location of cysticerci [17, 76, 78, 79, 82, 88]. No doubt this has been partly due to the difficulty in localizing these deep sulcal parasites.

CT and MR Findings. A variety of "parenchymal" lesions have been described on scans, and patterns considered specific have been grouped as follows [65]: (1) Diffuse low densities with little or no enhancement; (2) focal low densities with well-defined, rounded, central enhancement; (3) round, cystic lesions with well-defined regular or irregular borders, exhibiting ring enhancement.

The CT features of cysticercosis vary with the stage of the disease. The acute encephalitic response is marked by the presence of nodular or localized lesions that appear on postcontrast scans as hyperdense nodules or ring structures. The encephalitis persists for 2–6 months, with the edema outlasting the enhancement. Calcifications can be demonstrated by about 8 months. Enhancing or nonenhancing hypodense cysts may also appear at this time [80].

With the advent of MR imaging, it has become evident that many, perhaps even most, cysticercus lesions are in fact situated in the sulcal subarachnoid space, where, on axial CT scanning, their sequestration gives the impression of a parenchymal location.

Because of its multiplanar capacity and high resolution, MR imaging is well suited to the investigation of neurocysticercosis. The anatomy of the parasite is well portrayed on three planes, and a characteristic lesion can often be defined. In particular, changes may be identified in the structure of the protoscolex which indicate death of the parasite. MR also demonstrates edema better than CT. Significant disadvantages of MR include its inability to show mineralization or the effects of presumed changes in the structure or function of the blood-brain barrier. The latter will require the injection of MR-specific contrast agents (gadolinium chelate).

The appearance of the typical lesion on T1-weighted images is that of a fluid-filled cyst with an eccentric, high-intensity mural nodule (Fig. 15.18, 15.19). The cyst fluid usually has a slightly higher intensity than CSF, indicating a shorter T1 (Fig. 15.20). The high signal from the

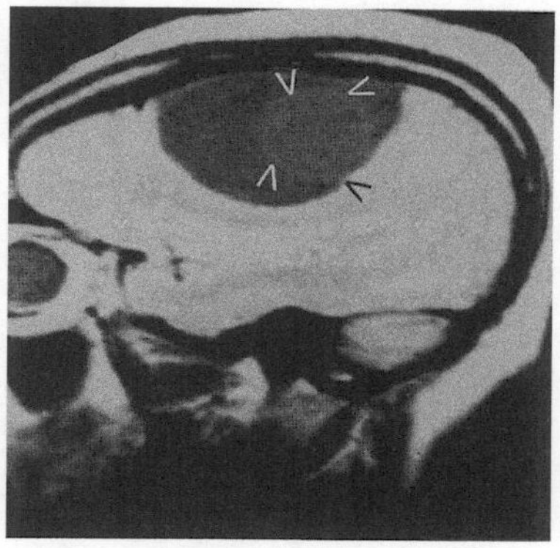

Fig. 15.20. Cysticercosis in a 46-year-old woman with focal seizures for 5 months, weakness of left arm for 2 months. Large cystic lesion in the parietal region with a smaller cyst of slightly higher intensity within the main cavity. The larger cyst was arachnoid in nature, the smaller cyst *(arrowheads)* was the parasitic bladder. Sagittal section, SE 2.0 s/27 ms (0.5 T)

mural nodule is a consistent feature, with T1 values longer than those of fat (Fig. 15.19 a). With lengthening of TR and TE, a narrow surrounding rim of high signal intensity can be consistently identified, which in most cases represents normal gray matter.

Localized cerebral edema is readily identifiable on T2-weighted images. It presents as a focal area of high signal intensity within the cerebral parenchyma and is presumably associated with the intraparenchymal variety of the disease. Heavier T2 weighting elicits a high signal from the entire cystic contents, and differentiation of structures is lost. Comparative morphologic studies have been performed to define the MR features of the typical parasitic lesion. Macroscopic brain sections demonstrate the bladder wall and cavity surrounding an eccentric, opaque nodule, which is typically elongated and measures 6×3 mm (Fig. 15.19). Microscopically the nodule consists of the invaginated protoscolex embedded in germinal tissue and surrounded by the bladder wall. In viable cysticerci, the protoscolex, bladder wall, and surrounding brain are practically in contact with one another (Fig. 15.19); with death of the parasite, the protoscolex becomes distended, the germinal tissue exhibits vacuolar swelling, and the bladder enlarges. In these circumstances the mural nodule enlarges and acquires a rounded shape. External to the bladder wall, meningeal compression obliterates the subarachnoid space, and there is variable inflammation and fibrosis. The sequestration of the parasite within the depths of a major sulcus (e.g., over the insula), combined with focal granulomatous meningitis, explains the genesis of larger cystic lesions. These are in fact arachnoid cysts, usually containing multiple bladders and bladder remnants, of the racemose type. Figure 15.20 demonstrates a well-demarcated cystic lesion of the parietal region. A second cystic structure is present in the posterior aspect of the larger cyst, whose contents show a high-intensity signal indicating a slightly shorter T1. Pathologic examination of these lesions revealed that the larger cavity represented an arachnoid cyst, while the smaller lesion was the cysticercus bladder.

Gray matter-white matter differentiation, and the demonstration of superficial cerebral anatomy in axial, coronal, and sagittal sections enable precise localization of the lesions on MR images. Neurocysticercosis is overwhelmingly a disease of the subarachnoid space and not of the cerebral parenchyma [76]. This finding is supported by autopsy studies, where lesions were found in the subarachnoid space in 79% and in the parenchyma in 35% of cases.

In Fig. 15.18 the subarachnoid location of the cyst can be readily appreciated: Cysts are directly related to the sulci and indent the cerebral cortex. A cyst is also present in the fourth ventricle. Microscopically, the bladder wall, compressed meninges, and brain are seen to be in contact with one another (Fig. 15.19 c).

MR is considered invaluable in the evaluation of intraventricular and cisternal cysticercosis cysts, which may be difficult to identify as such on standard CT studies [97]. Because the cysts can migrate, their location should be rechecked immediately before surgery is performed. The identification of intraventricular cysts in this situation can be lifesaving [97].

Echinococcosis or Hydatid Disease

Man and sheep are two of the many intermediate hosts for the organisms *Echinococcus granulosus* and *Echinococcus multilocularis,* and the incidence

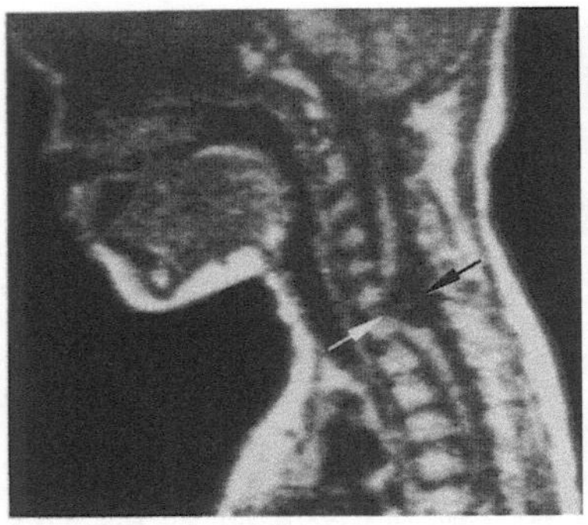

15.21

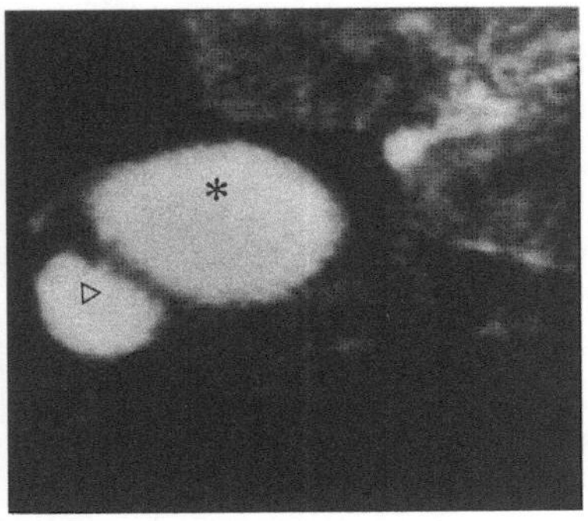

15.22

Fig. 15.21. Echinococcosis in a young child with progressive paraplegia. Compression and displacement of spinal cord by an intradural hydatid cyst *(arrows)* in the lower cervical region. Sagittal section, SE 0.5 s/30 ms (0.5 T)

Fig. 15.22. Hydatid cyst *(asterisk)* in the orbit displacing the eye *(triangle)*. Sagittal section, SE 2.0 s/100 ms (0.5 T)

of echinococcosis is highest in sheep-raising countries, where humans acquire the infection from their pet dogs. Larvae settle in the liver preferentially, with involvement of the lungs, bone, and brain in decreasing order of frequency. Most larvae are destroyed, but some survive to become encysted, enlarging slowly over a period of many years. The bladder or cyst wall has a distinctive, laminated external layer and an internal germinal layer from which innumerable daughter cysts or "brood capsules" develop, imparting a granular appearance to the interior of the cyst.

A unique and unexplained aspect of this infestation is the lack of an inflammatory response to the cyst in bone or brain. This accounts for the total absence of enhancement of the cerebral lesions on CT scans. Parasites in the liver or orbit, by contrast, incite a surrounding eosinophilic and granulomatous inflammatory response, with associated fibrosis.

The hydatid cysts can reach up to 10 cm in size. Escobar and Nieto [35] note that sites of predilection in the cerebral hemispheres are the region supplied by the middle cerebral artery (especially the retrorolandic artery) and the ventricles. Cysts may also form within vertebral bodies, leading to spinal cord damage as a result of pressure from the cyst or pathologic fracture [83] (Fig. 15.21).

CT and MR Findings

CT demonstrates hydatid cysts as hypodense, nonenhancing areas unaccompanied by perifocal edema.

In MR, the lesions in two cases of hydatid disease displayed the same basic features on both T1- and T2-weighted images, being purely cystic with contents exhibiting low intensity on T1-weighted images owing to long T1 values. No significant difference between CSF and cystic intensity was observed. On T2-weighted images the fluid content within the parasite showed typical long T2 values with high-level signals indistinguishable from CSF or ocular fluid.

Figure 15.21 shows a sagittal scan of the cervical spinal cord of a child from whom a temporal lobe hydatid cyst had been removed 2 years previously. The MR image clearly shows a cystic lesion with prolonged T1 and T2 values, together with displacement and compression of the spinal cord. In view of the patient's history, a tentative diagnosis of hydatid disease was made, and an intradural hydatid cyst was subsequently removed.

In Fig. 15.22, a sagittal section of the orbit demonstrates marked anterior displacement of the globe by a large cystic mass showing long T2 values on T2 weighting, with no significant difference in intensity between the contents of the lesion and the ocular contents. The anatomic relationships of the normal ocular structures and the lesion are readily appreciated. Surgical removal of this hydatid cyst was performed, and histology showed a prominent inflammatory-fibrous capsule.

In one patient with alveolar echinococcosis who had been treated with mebendazole for several years, Bauer et al. [6] saw a subcortical mass lesion with clumplike calcifications and perifocal edema in the parietal region. On MR images (SE TR 2.0, TE not specified) the lesion appeared hyperintense and irregular, but with sharply defined margins. Central zones of low signal intensity represented calcifications. Microscopic examination disclosed an alveolar echinococcosis with a chronic inflammatory reaction of the brain tissue accompanied by calcifications.

15.4.4 Fungal Infections

Fungal infections of the CNS are of two basic types:

- Infections caused by organisms of low pathogenicity (including *Candida, Mucor,* and *Aspergillus*) in patients whose resistance to infection is impaired (e.g., by diabetes mellitus, leukemia, lymphomas and other malignancies, AIDS, or long-term treatment with corticosteroids, antibiotics, cytostatics, or immunosuppressive drugs).
- Infections caused by more virulent organisms such as *Cryptococcus* and *Actinomyces/Nocardia,* which can induce primary disease. These mycoses also occur more commonly in the immune-compromised state.

Infection of the CNS is always secondary to a systemic primary focus. No single tissue alteration characterizes fungal infection: acute polymorphonuclear exudation, granulomatous inflammation, caseous necrosis, fibrosis, and calcification all vary from one infecting organism to another, depending as well on the host response and the site of the lesion. In general, the chronic granulomatous inflammatory response is more often associated with liquefactive necrosis than with caseation, qualifying it as an indolent abscess. Although most focal lesions are granulomatous, in a strict sense they should be further defined as abscesses or mycetomas, the latter containing enormous numbers of organisms embedded in a stroma of inflammatory cells and collagen. This pathologic concept has important clinical and radiologic implications.

Candidiasis

Infection with the organism *Candida albicans* is the most common fungal infection of the CNS [69]. Brain involvement by *Candida albicans* occurs by hematogenous spread late in the course of the generalized disease. Parker et al. [69] describe foci in all brain regions resembling hemorrhagic infarcts in the early stage and later appearing as abscesses and granulomas without central necrosis. Meningitis and pachymeningitis can also develop [43].

CT and MR Findings

The diverse pathologic changes in candidiasis produce a variety of CT findings: hydrocephalus secondary to leptomeningeal involvement; enhancing nodules with perifocal edema (granuloma with thick wall); calcified granuloma; signs of infarction and abscesses, which also can be simulated by thin-walled, enhancing granulomas [73]; irregular enhancing soft tissue masses; focal and diffuse low-density areas with ill-defined enhancement; hemorrhages; and enhancement of the basal cisterns and other CSF spaces [31, 68].

The formation of granulomas or abscesslike ring structures signifies a defensive reaction directed toward encapsulating the infectious focus. If the immune system is weakened and unable to contain the infection, the latter will spread freely and produce focal or diffuse, ill-defined hypodense areas on CT scans that show little or no peripheral enhancement with contrast material. This type of finding implies a poor prognosis. Differential diagnosis of the various types of fungal disease cannot be made on the basis of CT findings [31]. Enzman et al. [31] believe that the extent of lesions in patients with extensive disease tends to be underestimated from their appearance on CT.

Based on experience reported to date, MR appears to be more reliable than CT in demonstrating the pathologic changes associated with candidal infections. As with CT, however, the similarity of the CNS responses to different fungal species poses a major obstacle to differential diagnosis.

Aspergillosis

Aspergillus is a ubiquitous fungus with 350 known species, only a few of which are pathogenic to man [83].

The infection can enter the cranial cavity through the paranasal sinuses, ears, orbits, or hematogenously from the lungs, and the resulting intracranial changes may be unilateral or more widely distributed [83]. The fulminating form of aspergillosis can cause meningitis and meningoencephalitis with hemorrhagic infarcts caused by the thrombosis of vessels involved by the infection. More chronic forms lead to the formation of granulomas and abscesses [44].

CT and MR Findings

CT changes in the fulminating form of aspergillosis may be minor, contrasting markedly with the consumptive nature of the disease. There may be slight

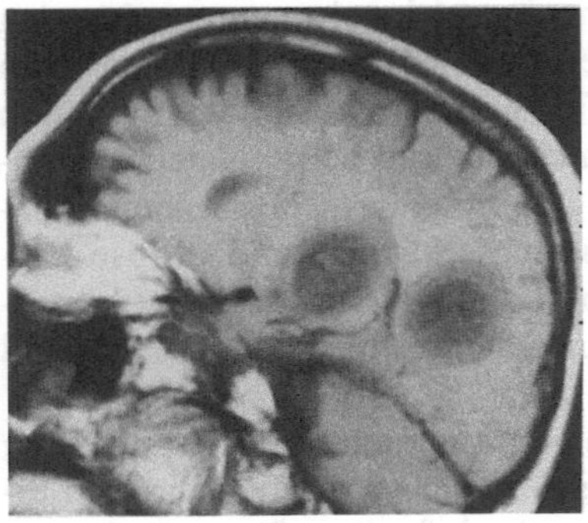

Fig. 15.23. Aspergillosis in a 67-year-old man with a long history of therapy with cortisone for endophthalmitis, presenting with hemiparesis, seizures, and drowsiness. Ring-shaped masses with a smooth outer hypointense ring and a darker, inhomogeneous center. The diagnosis was confirmed by biopsy and autopsy. Sagittal scan SE 0.7 s/30 ms (1.0 T)

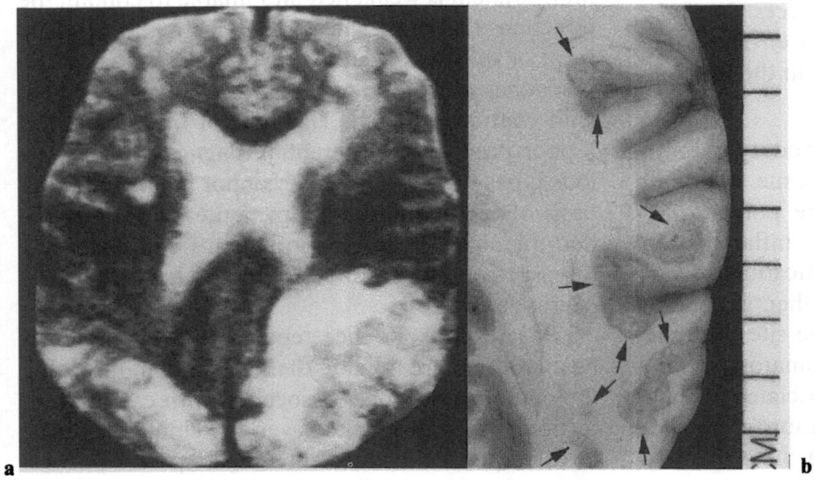

Fig. 15.24 a, b. Cryptococcosis. Multiple discrete low intensity lesions following the line of the cortical ribbon are surrounded by prominent perifocal edema (**a**). These correspond to the multiple cryptococcomas *(arrows)* seen in the fixed brain section (**b**). Axial section, SE 2.0 s/100 ms (0.5 T)

evidence of hypodense mass lesions with minimal enhancement and no ring structure, implying a poor prognosis. The demonstration of solid nodules or ring enhancement similar to abscesses (Fig. 15.23) signifies a more benign course of the infection [44, 45]. An obstructive hydrocephalus can result from involvement of the meninges.

In patients with a rhinocerebral form of aspergillosis (or mucormycosis; see below) soft tissue masses, usually unilateral, are seen in the paranasal air sinuses. Examination of the orbit may disclose thickening and displacement of both muscles and the optic nerve, infiltration of the orbital fat, and bone destruction.

Jinkins et al. [52] describe five cases with varying radiological findings, including large tumorlike enhancing granulomatous masses within the brain tissue, nodular meningeal granulomas, peripontine enhancement compatible with meningitis, paranasal sinus and orbital masses with bone destruction, infarctions due to vasculitis, and aneurysm.

In one case MR revealed a well-delineated inhomogeneous mass with low signal intensity compared to the surrounding edema and also the normal brain tissue on the proton-density scan. Mikhael et al. [67] mention an intermediate signal intensity of a granulomatous lesion with similar imaging parameters, surrounded by perifocal edema.

Cryptococcosis (Torulosis)

Cryptococcosis (infection by *Cryptococcus neoformans*) is unique among the mycoses in that it can involve the nervous system predominantly, without overt disease elsewhere. Its occurrence in chronically sick individuals raises the possibility of endemic disease.

Spread is usually hematogenous from a focus in the lung. The lesions are described as gelatinous (paucireactive) or granulomatous, although these forms may coexist in the CNS. In most cases organisms invade the subarachnoid space and are confined there, inciting a chronic inflammatory cell response (meningitis, meningoencephalitis). In the case of severe or progressive infection, there is widespread penetration of the Virchow-Robin spaces with formation of cryptococcal granulomas or "cryptococcomas" in the superficial parenchyma. These gradually coalesce, becoming grossly visible as sago-like structures (Fig. 15.24b) whose gelatinous appearance has also been termed cystoid. It is probably on account of the relative size of the organisms and the cerebral arterioles that cryptococcosis is limited to the gray matter (of the cerebral hemispheres, basal ganglia, and cerebellum). Intraparenchymal and intraventricular masses are rare [61], are poorly displayed on noncontrast CT scans, and enhance poorly after contrast injection [96].

CT and MR Findings

CT scans show contrast enhancement of the meninges (due to fungal invasion) and ventricular dilatation. These are frequently accompanied by focal ischemic changes and cortical atrophy. Hyperdense nodular granulomas with perifocal edema show additional enhancement [44]. They also may calcify.

MR images of CNS cryptococcosis are shown in Fig. 15.24. In this case multiple, discrete lesions are seen following the line of the cortical ribbon. They have a low signal intensity on T2-weighted images, contrasting with the surrounding cerebral edema, and were found pathologically (Fig. 15.24b) to consist of cryptococcomas about 5 mm in diameter. The hypointense signal presumably reflects their glycogen- and mucin-rich composition.

Other Fungal Infections with Worldwide Distribution

Mucormycosis or Zygomycosis

Zygomycetes are ubiquitous fungi and mucormycosis is the most acutely fatal mycosis in man [66]. The disease typically affects immune-compromised patients (e.g., diabetics) and is initially manifested in the region of the nasopharynx and orbits, from which the fungi invade the meninges and frontal lobes through penetrating vessels [66]. Mucormycosis also occurs in a disseminated form that does not involve the orbits and may produce solitary or multiple brain lesions without prior involvement of the lungs or paranasal sinuses [66].

CT and MR Findings

Paranasal sinus changes have been described with CT that resemble benign thickenings of the mucosa. At this time we are aware of no reports on MR findings.

Involvement of the orbits and the deep paranasal structures is a sign of impending intracranial invasion. Short-term follow-up investigations of the skull base region are indicated because of the rapid progression of the disease, with particular attention to any obliteration of normal fat density in the infratemporal and pterygopalatine fossa and to bone destruction. In the orbital region the fungus may infiltrate the retrobulbar fat and muscles, posing a danger of spread to the cavernous sinus.

Involvement of the cerebral vessels (by direct endothelial injury or the endovascular growth of hyphae) can lead to thrombosis as well as mycotic emboli, resulting in distal noncontiguous brain infarctions or abscess formation.

Usually, however, CT demonstrates low-density masses with variable peripheral enhancement and minimal perifocal vasogenic edema at the base of the anterior and middle cranial fossae. Bland infection may be difficult to distinguish from abscess with CT [41].

Because intracranial involvement signifies a grave prognosis – according to Gamba et al. [41] mortality is 80% – early detection of the organisms is of extreme importance.

Actinomycosis and Nocardiosis

The *Actinomyces* and *Nocardia steroides* organisms cause chronic suppurative lesions, of which craniofacial actinomycosis is the most common, with local contiguous spread to the meninges and brain.

The tissues are indurated to a woody texture, a change explained by the presence of intense fibrosis in which are interspersed granules of fungi surrounded by inflammatory cells. This is a proliferative-destructive process that involves a diffuse, sieve-like erosion of the bone, including skull and vertebrae. Although the cranial meninges are not a barrier to the infection, inflammatory tissue spreads in the spinal extradural spaces, where it produces cord compression. Because of the unreliability of reporting, particularly with regard to accurate laboratory diagnosis, the incidence of actinomycosis and nocardiosis is difficult to determine. Hematogenous brain abscess can occur in both infections but is much commoner in nocardiosis (together with pulmonary involvement), while the finding of a craniofacial mass distinctly favors actinomycosis.

CT and MR Findings

The usual forms of the rare CNS involvement by actinomycosis are brain abscess and meningitis. The abscesses may be unifocal or multifocal. In a review of the literature, Khosla et al. [55] describe epidural abscesses, subdural empyemas, cranial vault osteomyelitis, granulomas of the gasserian ganglion, and primary actinomycosis of the third ventricle. The same authors describe a case of actinomycosis associated with a marked "hyperostosis" of the frontal and parietal bones with some osteolysis and a large enhancing mass in the frontal parafalcine region with marked edema, similar to a meningioma, on the contrast CT scan. This bone expansion is interpreted as a marked periostitis secondary to an intraosseous granuloma [55].

The MR features of a case of craniocervical mycetoma are well illustrated in Fig. 15.25. These axial and sagittal images give more information on the pathologic process and demonstrate the direct involvement of cerebral parenchyma to better advantage than CT. An axial image of the brain in Fig. 15.28b shows bone involvement, marked meningeal thickening, and infiltration of the underlying temporo-occipital lobes. There is a prominent soft tissue mass together with signs of infiltration of the temporal bone in that region. The cerebral lesions appear as poorly demarcated areas of low signal intensity due to their short T2 values, an appearance consistent with the chronic sclerosing granulomatous process observed histologically.

A sagittal image of the head and neck of the same patient demonstrates the extent of the disease process in the upper cervical and craniocervical junction regions. Figure 15.28a shows a large soft tissue mass occupying the back of the neck, destroying the spinous processes and posterior elements of the upper cervical vertebrae, including the dens, and extending anteriorly to expand the tissues of the oropharynx and nasopharynx. The process, shown pathologically to be a sclerosing granulomatosis typical of actinomycosis, has also spread to surround the cervical cord. Rostrally it has displaced the medulla, eroded the clivus and posterior clinoids, and is infiltrating the pituitary fossa. Dilatation of all four ventricles, presumably secondary to meningeal involvement in the basal cisterns, is also apparent on this image.

Figure 15.26c shows increased parenchymal water and "invasion" of the posterior aspects of the occipital lobes and cerebellum. A relatively nondestructive process was inferred from the fact that vision was preserved. This patient had presented with quadriplegia and respiratory failure. MR yielded much of the diagnostic information, including evidence of brainstem compression. Laboratory studies subsequently identified the organism as *Nocardia brasiliensis*.

Other, Regional Fungal Infections

Fungal infections restricted to certain geographic locations include cladosporiosis, coccidioidomycosis, histoplasmosis, and blastomycosis.

Cladosporiosis

Cladosporiosis caused by *Cladosporium bantianum*, occurs in temperate regions throughout the world.

Coccidioidomycosis

Infections with *Coccidioides immitis* are reported in North and South America. They are characterized by the formation of multiple granulomas in the basal cisterns, which account for the communicating hydrocephalus that is a very frequent complication of cerebral coccidioidomycosis [28]. On CT, contrast enhancement of the basal cisterns and other cisternal spaces probably relates to formation of new vessels in granulation tissue and to the extravasation of contrast medium through the vessels with weak endothelial junctions [33]. However, CT scans may be normal early in the course of the disease [100]. At present we are unaware of any published MR findings on this condition.

Histoplasmosis and Blastomycosis

Infections by *Histoplasma capsulatum* occur in North and South America, Africa, and Australia. Infection with *Blastomyces dermatitidis* is restricted to North America. Both diseases are of the yeast form, producing granulomatous lesions within the brain substance. *Blastomyces* granulomas are visible on noncontrast CT scans and show significant enhancement after the injection of contrast material.

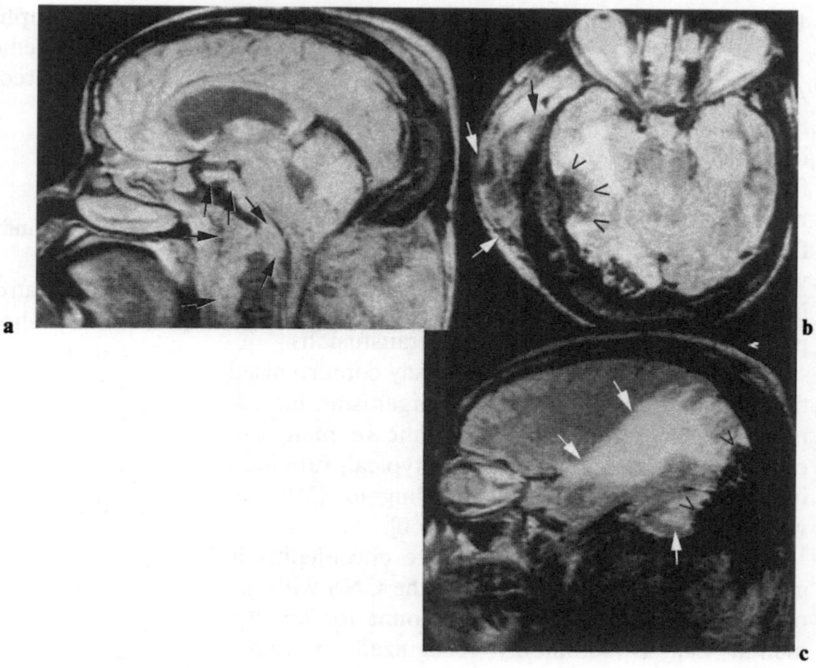

Fig. 15.25 a–c. Nocardiosis *(Nocardia braziliensis).* **a** Large soft tissue mass in the posterior cervical region with destruction of the posterior neural elements of the upper cervical vertebra and the dens; the process extends into the extradural space, up the clivus and the pituitary fossa *(arrows).* **b** In the left temporal region the soft tissue swelling overlies an area of meningeal thickening and direct cerebral involvement *(arrows).* **c** Extensive cerebral edema *(arrows).* The low intensity of the cerebral lesions *(arrowheads* in **b***)* due to short T2 is consistent with the chronic sclerosing granulomatous process shown on histology. **a** Midsagittal scan, SE 2.0 s/27 ms; **b** axial, and **c** parasagittal scans, SE 2.0 s/70 ms (0.5 T)

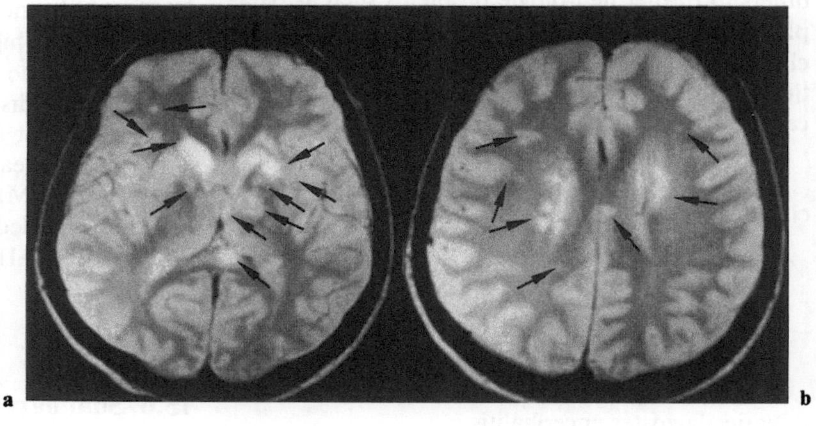

Fig. 15.26 a, b. Cerebral lesions in a 33-year-old man with AIDS, gait disturbances. Multiple patchy, partly confluent, lesions with prolonged relaxation times in the periventricular white matter, but also involving the basal ganglia *(arrows).* The causative agent was not identified. Axial scans: **a, b** SE 3.0 s/45 ms (1.0 T)

Manifestations in the CNS may be found in less than 25% of cases of acute or chronic pulmonary histoplasmosis in infants, elderly, or immunocompromised patients. Isolated CNS involvement has also been described [26, 96]. It includes miliary granulomas, basal leptomeningitis, and solitary granulomas (histoplasmomas).

CT and MR findings are described as nonspecific. In cases of solitary granulomas the lesions may be mistaken for neoplasms; they are well defined in noncontrast scans with early ring enhancement and perifocal edema. On MR, a nodular mass has been described with a hypointense rim separating it from perifocal edema, the center being isointense to gray matter on the proton-density image and hyperintense on the T2-weighted scan [26].

15.5 Acquired Immune Deficiency Syndrome

AIDS, known since 1981, is caused by a human retrovirus (human immuno-deficiency virus, HIV), identified in 1983/1984. The virus damages the function of the cellular immune apparatus. Transmission occurs by direct contact with infected body fluids of AIDS patients, accounting for the prevalence of the syndrome in homosexuals, users of intravenous drugs sharing syringes and needles, and patients requiring frequent blood transfusions.

The immune system is so severely compromised that a great many environmental organisms, including those not ordinarily pathogenic in man, can produce diseases which take an atypical, fulminating, and generalized course leading to CNS involvement in about 40% of cases [60].

It is suggested that a subacute encephalitis is caused by a primary infection of the CNS with the neurotropic HIV. This could account for the dementia that is commonly recognized in young AIDS patient and has thus been referred to as AIDS-related dementia complex [11, 37]. These patients have been found to be more susceptible than others to further neurologic problems such as paraplegia and incontinence. Pathologic findings include atrophy of white matter, perivascular infiltrations, and the presence of macrophages and giant cells.

The opportunistic infections of the CNS associated with AIDS include the following [11]:

Viral infections:
- Atypical aseptic encephalitis
- Herpes simplex encephalitis
- Cytomegaly
- Progressive multifocal leukoencephalopathy
- Varicella-zoster encephalitis

Nonviral infections
- Toxoplasmosis
- Cryptococcosis
- Candidiasis
- Coccidioidomycosis
- Cerebrospinal syphilis
- Tuberculous meningitis
- Aspergillosis
- Histoplasmosis
- Bacterial meningitis

Malignant neoplasms found with increased frequency in AIDS patients include:
- primary lymphomas of the CNS,
- CNS involvement by systemic lymphomas, and
- Kaposi's sarcoma (seldom found intracranially) [39]

CT and MR Findings

Besides the atrophy mentioned above, imaging studies may show solitary, multiple, or diffusely scattered lesions of varying size and shape that appear hypodense on CT scans and show prolonged T1 and T2 values on MR images. The findings are not specific for AIDS with either modality (Figs. 15.26; see Fig. 15.17). Some authors have emphasized the greater sensitivity of MR, stating that it allows more reliable confirmation or exclusion of CNS lesions than is possible with CT and an optimum choice of the site for surgical biopsy. The latter is an important consideration, since the nonspecific nature of imaging features often compels reliance on (stereotaxic) biopsy to establish a diagnosis. Thus, MR appears to be the imaging modality of choice for the detection and follow-up of the CNS complications of AIDS [25].

In areas of high signal intensity on T2-weighted images, with no differentiation apparent between the lesion and its perifocal edema, the use of intravenous contrast material (e.g., gadolinium chelate) can help to reveal the true size and shape of the lesion. Contrast MR should, in fact, be the only imaging study needed in the majority of cases for the evaluation of AIDS patients with neurologic symptoms [25].

15.6 Summary

Experience with MR in inflammatory diseases of the CNS is still quite limited. Cerebritis and brain abscess are recognized more easily from their secondary edema than from the primary process. Meningitis may cause edema and thickening of the meninges with increasing intensity on T2-weighted images. In the evaluation of various granulomatous processes, MR without the use of contrast material is not as useful as CT in staging the disease. Whereas CT demonstrates enhancement during the acute inflammatory stage, MR may not show a significant change in appearance from the initial edematous through the late gliotic stage unless contrast material (gadolinium chelate) is used. Moreover, the calcifications that form in the chronic stage of many of these diseases may not be identifiable on MR images with the same reliability as on CT scans.

In summary, we may say that MR, by virtue of its high sensitivity, is the imaging modality of choice in the acute stage of inflammatory diseases of the CNS. When contrast injection is used, the multiplanar capabilities of MR make it superior to CT even in the chronic stage for the detection of granulomatous changes. CT continues to have an important role, however, in the detection of calcifications.

References

1. Ackermann R (1986) Erythema-migrans-Borreliose und Frühsommer-Meningoenzephalitis. Dtsch Ärztebl 83 (24): 1765-1774
2. Ackermann R, Gollmer E, Rehse-Küpper B (1985) Progressive Borrelien-Enzephalomyelitis. Dtsch Med Wochenschr 110: 1039-1042
3. Alvord EC Jr, Shaw CM (1977) Infections, allergic, and demyelinating diseases of the nervous system. In: Newton TH, Potts DG (eds) Radiology of the skull and brain: anatomy and pathology, vol 3. Mosby, St Louis, pp 3088-3172
4. Adams RA, Victor M (1985) Principles of neurology, 3rd edn. McGraw-Hill Book, New York
5. Bachman DS (1980) Computed tomography in a verified case of tuberculous meningitis. Neurology 30: 347
6. Bauer WM, Obermüller H, Vogl T, Lissner J (1984) MR bei zerebraler alveolärer Echinikokkose. Digitale Bilddiagn 4: 129-131
7. Benator RM, Magill HL, Gerald B, Igarashi M, Fitch SJ (1985) Herpes simplex encephalitis: CT findings in the neonate and young infant. AJNR 6: 539-543
8. Best T, Finlayson M (1979) Two forms of encephalitis in opportunistic toxoplasmosis. Arch Pathol Lab Med 103: 693-696
9. Bilaniuk LT, Zimmerman RA, Brown L, Yoo HJ, Goldberg HI (1978) Computed tomography in meningitis. Neuroradiology 16: 13-14
10. Binford CH, Connor DH (eds) (1976) Pathology of tropical and extraordinary diseases. Armed Forces Institute of Pathology, Washington DC
11. Biniek R, Brockmeyer N, Balzer K, Gesemann M, Scheiermann N, Gerhard L, Lehmann HJ (1987) Neurologische Erkrankungen bei HIV-Infektion. Dtsch Ärztebl 84 (27): 1297-1302
12. Brant-Zawadzki M, Enzmann DR, Placone RC Jr, Sheldon P, Britt RH, Brasch RC, Crooks LA (1983) NMR imaging of experimental brain abscess: comparison with CT. AJNR 4 (3): 250-253
13. Britt RH, Enzmann DR, Yeager AS (1981) Neuropathological and computerized tomographic findings in experimental brain abscess. J Neurosurg 55: 590-603
14. Brooks BS, El Gammal T, Hungerford GD (1982) Radiological manifestations of neurosarcomatosis: role of computed tomography. AJNR 3: 513-521
15. Brownell B, Tomlinson AH (1984) Viral diseases of the central nervous system. In: Adams JH, Corsellis JAN, Duchen LW (eds) Greenfield's neuropathology. Wiley, New York, pp 260-303
16. Bucy PC, Oberhill HR (1950) Intradural spinal granulomas. J Neurosurg 7: 1-12
17. Byrd SE, Locke GE, Biggers S, Perey AK (1982) The computed tomographic appearance of cerebral cysticercosis in adults and children. Radiology 144: 819-823
18. Clark EG, Danbolt N (1964) The Oslo study of the natural course of untreated syphilis. Med Clin North Am 48: 613-623
19. Collins AT, Cromwell LD (1980) Tomography in the evaluation of congenital cerebral toxoplasmosis. J Comput Assist Tomogr 4 (3): 326-329
20. Compton JS, Dorsch NW (1984) Intradural extramedullary tuberculoma of the cervical spine. Case report. J Neurosurg 60: 200-203
21. Dastur DK, Lalitha MD (1973) The many facets of neurotuberculosis. In: Zimmerman HM (ed) Progress in neuropathology, vol 11. Grund and Stratton, New York, pp 351-408
22. Dastur DK, Lalitha VS, Udani PM, Parekh U (1970) The brain and meninges in tuberculous meningitis: gross pathology and pathogenesis in 100 cases. Neurol India: 86-100
23. Davidson HD, Steiner RE (1985) Magnetic resonance imaging in infections of the central nervous system. AJNR 6: 499-504
24. Davis JM, Davis KR, Kleinman GM, Kirchner HS, Taveras JM (1978) Computed tomography of herpes simplex encephalitis, with clinicopathological correlation. Radiology 129: 409-417
25. DeLaPaz R, Floris R, Brant-Zawadzki M, Norman D, Newton TH (1986) MRI of CNS complications of acquired immune deficiency syndrome (AIDS). Presented at the 24th Annual Meeting of the American Society of Neuroradiology, Jan 18-23, San Diego
26. Dion FM, Venger BH, Landon G, Handel SF (1987) Thalamic histoplasmoma: CT and MR imaging. J Comput Assist Tomogr 11 (1): 193-194
27. Draouat S, Abdenabi B, Ghanem M, Bourjat P (1987) Computed tomography of cerebral tuberculoma. J Comput Assist Tomogr 11 (4): 594-597
28. Dublin AB, Phillips HE (1980) Computed tomography of disseminated cerebral coccidioidomycosis. Radiology 135: 361-368
29. Dubois PJ, Heinz ER, Wessel HB, Zaias BW (1979) Multiple cystic encephalomalacia of infancy: computed tomographic findings in two cases with associated intracerebral calcification. J Comput Assist Tomogr 3: 97-101
30. Duda EE, Huttenlocker PR, Patronas NJ (1980) CT of subacute sclerosing panencephalitis. AJNR 1: 35-38
31. Enzmann DR, Brant-Zawadzki M, Britt RH (1980) CT of central nervous system infections in immuno-compromised patients. AJNR 1: 239-243
32. Enzmann DR, Britt RH, Yeager AS (1979) Experimental brain abscess evolution: computed tomographic and neuropathologic correlation. Radiology 133: 113-122
33. Enzmann DR, Norman D, Mani J, Newton TH (1976) Computed tomography of granulomatous basal arachnitis. Radiology 120: 341-344
34. Enzmann DR, Ranson B, Norman P, Talberth E (1978) Computed tomography of herpes simplex encephalitis. Radiology 129: 419-425

35. Escobar A, Nieto D (1972) Parasitic diseases. In: Minckler J (ed) Pathology of the nervous system. McGraw-Hill, New York, pp 2503-2521
36. Esiri MM (1982) Herpes simplex encephalitis: an immunohistological study of the distribution of viral antigen within the brain. J Neurol Sci 54: 209-226
37. Farthing CF, Brown SE, Staughton RCD, Cream JJ, Mühlemann M (1986) AIDS. Schwer, Stuttgart
38. Fritze J, Beyer HK, Schlichting P, Spittler JF (1986) Toxoplasmen-Enzephalitis - multiple Sklerose: Differentialdiagnose durch Kernspintomographie. Nervenarzt 57: 56-60
39. Gärtner HV (1987) AIDS-Pathomorphologie: lichtmikroskopische, immunhistologische und elektronenoptische Befunde. In: Klietmann W (ed) AIDS. Schattauer, Stuttgart, pp 77-103
40. Galbraith JG, Barr VW (1974) Epidural abscess and subdural empyema. Adv Neurol 6: 257-267
41. Gamba JL, Woodruff WW, Djang WT, Yeates AE (1986) Craniofacial mucormycosis: assessment with CT. Radiology 160: 207-212
42. Godt P, Stoeppler L, Wischer U, Schroeder H (1979) The value of computed tomography in cerebral syphilis. Neuroradiology 18: 197-200
43. Gorell JM, Palutkas WA, Chason JL (1979) Candida pachymeningitis with multiple cranial nerve pareses. Arch Neurol 36: 719-720
44. Grossmann RI, Zimmermann RA (1985) Infectious diseases of the brain. In: Latchaw (ed) Computed tomography of the head, neck and spine. Year Book, Chicago, pp 119-151
45. Grossmann RI, Davis KR, Taveras JM, Beal MF, O'Carroll CP (1981) Computed tomography of intracranial aspergillosis. J Comput Assist Tomogr 5: 646-650
46. Grossmann RI, Wolf G, Biery D, McGrath J, Kundel H, Aronchick J, Zimmerman RA, Goldberg HI, Bilaniuk LT (1984) Gadolinium enhanced nuclear magnetic resonance images of experimental brain abscess. J Comput Assist Tomogr 8: 204-207
47. Hayes WS, Sherman JL, Stern BJ, Citrin CM, Pulaski PD (1987) MR and CT evaluation of intracranial sarcoidosis. AJNR 8: 841-847
48. Heiss E, Huk W (1981) Computer tomographic findings in subdural empyemas. In: Schiefer W, Klinger M, Brock M (eds) Advances in neurosurgery, vol 9. Springer, Berlin Heidelberg New York, pp 134-137
49. Hörstrup P, Ackermann R (1973) Durch Zecken übertragene Meningopolyneuritis (Garin-Bujadoux, Bannwarth). Fortschr Neurol Psychiatr 41: 583-606
50. Holland BA, Perrett LV, Mills CM (1986) Meningovascular syphilis: CT and MR findings. Radiology 158 (2): 439-442
51. Jenkins RB (1963) Intradural spinal tuberculoma with genitourinary symptoms. Arch Neurol 8: 539-543
52. Jinkins JR, Siqueira E, Al-Kawi MZ (1987) Cranial manifestations of aspergillosis. Neuroradiology 29: 181-185
53. Kaufmann DM, Zimmermann RD, Leeds NE (1979) Computed tomography in herpes simplex encephalitis. Neurology 29: 1392-1396
54. Kendall BE, Tatler GLV (1978) Radiological findings in neurosarcoidosis. Br J Radiol 51: 81-92
55. Khosla VK, Banerjee AK, Chopra JS (1984) Intracranial actinomycoma with osteomyelitis simulating meningioma. J Neurosurg 60: 204-207
56. Krick JA, Remington JS (1978) Current concepts in parasitology. Toxoplasmosis in the adult. An overview. N Engl J Med 298: 550-553
57. Leestma JE (1985) Viral infections of the nervous system. In: Davis RL, Robertson DM (eds) Textbook of neuropathology. Williams and Wilkins, Baltimore, pp 704-787
58. Lennette EH, Magoffin RL, Knouf EG (1962) Viral central nervous system disease. An etiologic study conducted at the Los Angeles County General Hospital. JAMA 179: 687
59. Letterer E (1959) Allgemeine Pathologie. Grundlagen und Probleme. Thieme, Stuttgart
60. Levy RM, Rosenbloom S, Perrett LV (1986) Neuroradiologic findings in AIDS: a review of 200 cases. AJNR 7: 833-839
61. Long IA Jr, Herdt IR, DiChiro G, Cramer HR (1980) Cerebral mass lesions in torulosis demonstrated by computed tomography. J Comput Assist Tomogr 4: 766-769
62. Marcu H, Hacker H, Vonofakos D (1979) Bilateral reversible thalamic lesions on computed tomography. Neuroradiology 18: 201-204
63. McLeod R, Berry PF, Marshall WH Jr et al. (1979) Toxoplasmosis presenting as brain abscess: diagnosis by computerized tomography and cytology of aspirated purulent material. Am J Med 67: 711-714
64. Menges HW, Fischer E, Valavanis A, Schubiger O (1979) Cerebral toxoplasmosis in the adult. J Comput Assist Tomogr 3: 413-416
65. Mervis B, Lotz J (1980) Computed tomography (CT) in parenchymatous cerebral cysticercosis. Clin Radiol 31: 521-528
66. Mikhael MA (1979) Cerebral phycomycosis. J Comput Assist Tomogr 3: 417-420
67. Mikhael MA, Rushovich AM, Ciric I (1985) Magnetic resonance imaging of cerebral aspergillosis. Comput Radiol 9 (2): 85-89
68. Newton TH, Norman D, Alvord EC et al. (1977) The CT scan in infectious diseases of the CNS. In: Norman D, Korabkin M, Newton TH (eds) Computed tomography. University of California Press, San Francisco, pp 719-740
69. Parker JC Jr, McCloskey JJ, Lee RS (1981) Human cerebral candidiasis. A postmortem evaluation of 19 patients. Hum Pathol 12: 23-28
70. Parker JC, Dyer ML (1985) Neurologic infections due to bacteria, fungi and parasites. In: Davis RL, Robertson DM (eds) Textbook of neuropathology. Williams and Wilkins, Baltimore, pp 632-703
71. Pedersen H, Wulff CH (1982) Computed tomographic findings of early subacute sclerosing panencephalitis. Neuroradiology 23: 31-32
72. Poeck K (1987) Neurologie. Springer, Berlin Heidelberg New York
73. Post MJD, Hoffman TA (1984) Cerebral inflammatory disease. In: Rosenberg RN, Heinz ER (eds) The clinical neurosciences. Neuroradiology. Churchill Livingstone, New York, pp 525-594
74. Post MJD, Chan JC, Hensley GT, Hoffman TA, Moskowitz LB, Lippmann S (1983) Toxoplasma encephalitis in Haitian adults with acquired immunodeficiency syndrome: a clinicopathologic-CT correlation. AJNR 4: 155-162
75. Price H, Danziger A (1978) Computed tomography in cranial tuberculosis. AJR 130: 769-771

76. Rabiela-Cervantes MT, Rivos-Hernandes A, Rodriguez-Ibarra J, Castillo-Medina S, Cancino F de M (1982) Anatomopathological aspects of human brain cysticercosis. In: Flisser A, Wilms K, Ladette JP, Lerrolde C, Ridaura C, Beltran F (eds) Cysticercosis: present state of knowledge and perspective. Academic, New York, pp 139-162
77. Reik L, Steere AC, Bartenhagen H, Shope RE, Malawista StE (1979) Neurologic abnormalities in Lyme disease. Medicine (Baltimore) 58: 281-294
78. Rodriguez-Carbajal J, Boleaga-Duran B (1982) Neuroradiology of human cysticercosis. In: Cysticercosis: present state of knowledge and perspectives. Academic, New York, pp 139-162
79. Rodriguez-Carbajal J, Palacios E, Zee C-S (1983) Neuroradiology of cysticercosis of the central nervous system. In: Palacios E, Rodriguez-Carbajal J, Taveros M (eds) Cysticercosis of the central nervous system. Thomas, Springfield, pp 101-143
80. Rodriguez-Carbajal J, Salgado P, Gutierrez-Olvarado R, Escobar-Izquierdo A, Aruffo C, Palacios E (1983) The acute encephalitic phase of neurocysticercosis: computed tomographic manifestations. AJNR 4: 51-55
81. Rosenblum ML, Hoff JT, Norman D, Weinstein PR, Pitts L (1978) Decreased mortality from brain abscess since advent of computerized tomography. J Neurosurg 49: 658-668
82. Santin G, Vorgos J (1966) Roentgen study of cysticercosis of the central nervous system. Radiology 86: 520-528
83. Scaravilli F (1984) Parasitic and fungal infections of the nervous system. In: Adams JH, Corsellis JAN, Duchen LW (eds) Greenfield's neuropathology. J Wiley and Sons, New York, pp 304-337
84. Schroth G, Kretzschmar K (1986) MRI of cerebral infections. Presented at the XIII. Symposium Neuroradiologicum, June 23-26, Stockholm
85. Segall HD, Rumbaugh CL, Bergeron RT, Teal JS, Gwinn JL (1973) Brain and meningeal infections in children: radiological considerations. Neuroradiology 6: 8-16
86. Slade HW, Glazer N (1955) Extramedullary spinal tuberculoma. J Pediatr 46: 288-295
87. Stern BJ, Krumholz A, Johns C, Scott P, Nissim J (1985) Sarcoidosis and its neurological manifestations. Arch Neurol 42: 909-917
88. Suss RA, Maravilla KR, Thompson J (1986) MR imaging of intracranial cysticercosis: comparison of CT and anatomopathologic features. AJNR 7 (2): 235-242
89. Toro G, Roman G (1978) Cerebral malaria. A disseminated vasculomyelopathy. Archives of Neurology 35: 271-275
90. Vengsarkar US, Pisipaty RP, Parekh B, Panchal VG, Shetty MN (1986) Intracranial tuberculoma and the CT scan. J Neurosurg 64: 568-574
91. Vlcek B, Burchiel KJ, Gordon T (1984) Tuberculous meningitis presenting as an obstructive myelopathy. Case report. J Neurosurg 60: 196-199
92. Wadia NH, Dastur DK (1969) Spinal meningitides with radiculo-myelopathy. Part 2. Pathology and pathogenesis. J Neurol Sci 8: 261-297
93. Welchman JM (1979) Computerized tomography of intracranial tuberculomata. Clin Radiol 30: 567-573
94. Whelan MA, Stern J (1981) Intracranial tuberculoma. Radiology 138: 75-81
95. Whelan MA, Stern J, de Napoli RA (1981) The computed tomographic spectrum of intracranial mycosis: correlation with histopathology. Radiology 141: 703-707
96. Young RF, Gade G, Grinnell V (1985) Surgical treatment for fungal infections in the central nervous system. J Neurosurg 63: 371-381
97. Zee CS, Segall H, Ahmadi J, Schultz D (1986) MRI of neurocysticercosis. Presented at the XIII. Symposium Neuroradiologicum, June 23-28, Stockholm
98. Zee CS, Segall HD, Rogers C, Ahmadi J, Apuzzo M, Rhodes R (1985) MR imaging of cerebral toxoplasmosis: correlation of computed tomography and pathology. J Comput Assist Tomogr 9 (4): 797-799
99. Zentenaro-Alaris GH (1982) A classification of human cysticercosis. In: Flisser A, Wilms K, Ladette JP, Lerrolde C, Ridaura C, Beltran F (eds) Cysticercosis: present state of knowledge and perspectives. Academic, New York, pp 139-162
100. Zimmerman RD, Becker RD, Devinsky O, Petito CK, Haimes AB, Deck MDF (1986) MRI features of cerebral abscesses and other intracranial inflammatory lesions (excluding Aids patients). Presented at the XIII. Symposium Neuroradiologicum, June 23-28, Stockholm
101. Zimmermann RD, Russell EJ, Leeds NE, Kaufman D (1980) CT in the early diagnosis of herpes simplex encephalitis. AJR 134: 61-66

16 Head Injury

W. J. Huk

In the acute phase of head injuries the imaging procedures have two tasks to perform:

- Immediate, reliable demonstration of space-occupying hemorrhages so that the necessary life-saving surgery can be carried out without delay
- Evaluation of inoperable brain lesions (choice of conservative therapy, prognosis) and
- assessment of persistent post-traumatic damage (e.g., legal proceedings)

This distinction can also be applied to the classification of head injuries (Table 16.1).

Because the majority of head injuries are associated with intracranial hemorrhage, it is helpful to review the general appearances of hemorrhages on MR images, which are described fully in Sect. 5.2.

Table 16.1. Classification of head injuries

I. Intracranial, extracerebral hemorrhage
1. Epidural hematoma
2. Subdural hematoma
- Acute and subacute
- Chronic
- Subdural hygroma
II. Blunt brain injuries
1. Focal injuries
- Cerebral concussion
- Cerebral contusion
- Lacerations
- Intracerebral hemorrhage
- Traumatic subarachnoid hemorrhage
2. Diffuse injury
- Diffuse axonal injury
- Diffuse brain swelling
- Hypoxic brain damage
- Brain edema
III. Open head injuries
1. Depressed injury
2. Penetrating injury
3. Perforating injury
4. CSF fistula
IV. Other sequelae of injuries
1. Fat embolism
2. Air embolism
V. Late sequelae of head injuries

16.1 Intracranial Extracerebral Hemorrhages

Life-threatening, space-occupying extracerebral hemorrhages are common even in relatively trivial head injuries that show little brain involvement. Prompt detection and evacuation of the hemorrhage are necessary to preserve life or avert serious brain damage. Trauma may cause hemorrhage into the epidural, subdural, or subarachnoid space, into the brain substance, or into the ventricles, and intracranial hemorrhages are classified accordingly.

16.1.1 Epidural Hematoma

Epidural hematoma (EDH), in which blood accumulates between the skull and the dura, results from the tearing of meningeal arteries and, less commonly, of veins or sinuses. The dura, which is less firmly adherent to the skull in younger patients, is progressively pushed away from the skull as the volume of blood increases, giving the hemorrhage its familiar biconvex (discoid) shape.

Most EDH occur in the temporoparietal region after tearing of the middle meningeal artery by a fracture of the thin temporal squama. About one-third occur frontally, parietally, or in the posterior fossa, and a few are bilateral. Hematomas from the fractured bone usually take a less fulminating course and attain a smaller size.

CT and MR Findings

The typical CT appearance of acute EDH is that of a markedly hyperdense, biconvex mass lesion separating the brain surface from the inner table of the skull, with or without accompanying edema of the adjacent brain. With heavier blood loss (e.g., in multiple trauma), or if clotting is impaired, the EDH may appear less dense or even isodense with the brain. Because the blood overlies the dura, it can cross the midline or sinuses.

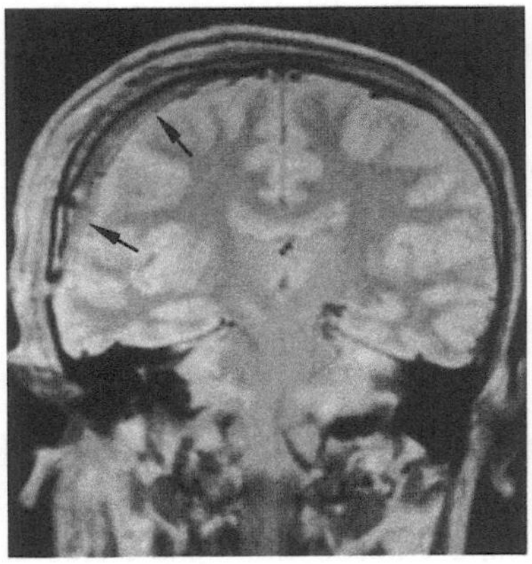

16.1

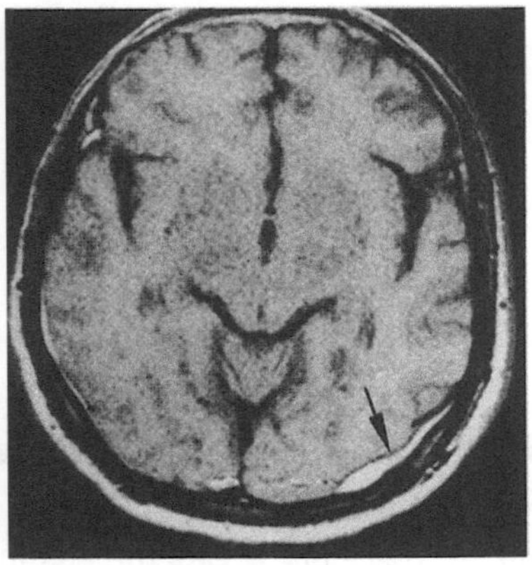

16.2

Fig. 16.1. Epidural hematoma in a 38-year-old man examined a few hours after craniotomy. The epidural blood *(arrows)* appears hypointense. Coronal scan, SE 3.2 s/30 ms (1.0 T)

Fig. 16.2. Subacute epidural hematoma in a 48-year-old man after head injury. The dura *(arrow)* is depicted as a dark line. Axial scan SE 0.65 s/50 ms (1.5 T)

The MR signal intensity of the blood changes over time. This process is described fully in Sect. 5.2. In the acute stage (less than 2 days), the blood has a short T2 because of the high magnetic susceptibility of the deoxyhemoglobin in intact red cells, and consequently it appears dark on T2-weighted images. The dura also gives a low signal and is difficult to separate from the hemorrhage. In the subacute stage, the paramagnetic effect (hydration effect) of the methemoglobin becomes operative, and the T1 of the hemorrhage decreases as its T2 becomes somewhat longer. At that point the hemorrhage appears hyperintense on T1-weighted and T2-weighted images and is clearly demarcated from the dura, which still gives a low signal (Figs. 16.1-16.2).

16.1.2 Subdural Hematoma

Acute and Subacute

Subdural hematoma (SDH) occupies the space between the dura and arachnoid, where it can spread freely over the surface of the brain. As a result, SDH are more extensive and are often less thick than epidural hemorrhages. Pure SDH are caused by the rupture of bridging veins and can produce a mass effect within periods ranging from minutes to hours. The extravasated blood remains clotted for 48 h to several days before starting to liquefy, and by about 3 weeks no further evidence of coagulation can be found [18].

Acute SDH from superficial cerebral vessels (mainly arteries) caused by a hemorrhagic contusion of the adjacent brain take a much more rapid course. Most of these "burst lobe" injuries are seen in the frontal and temporal areas [2, 4]. Arterial hemorrhage and contusional swelling lead rapidly to a life-threatening intracranial mass effect.

CT and MR Findings

On CT the acute SDH presents a crescent shape owing to its free spread between the dura and brain surface. If the hematoma is not absorbed spontaneously, its CT density decreases as liquefaction progresses. Fresh secondary bleeding can create a patchy appearance with hyperdense areas or a fluid level. With the formation of neomembranes in chronic SDH the hematoma finally assumes a more biconvex shape (see next subsection). It should be noted that an acute SDH may appear isodense or hypodense in patients who are anemic.

As with CT, the MR appearance of the extravascular blood changes over time (Figs. 16.3, 16.4). The sequence of changes corresponds basically to that described for EDH (see also Sect. 5.2). There is evidence that MR is more sensitive than CT in detecting a concomitant contusional swelling of the brain (see Sect. 16.2.1).

Chronic

Chronic SDH is a separate entity that can occur weeks or months after a seemingly minor head injury. Many patients are unable to report a history of head trauma; this is especially common in the elderly or alcoholic patient and in patients taking anticoagulant medication. The pathogenesis of

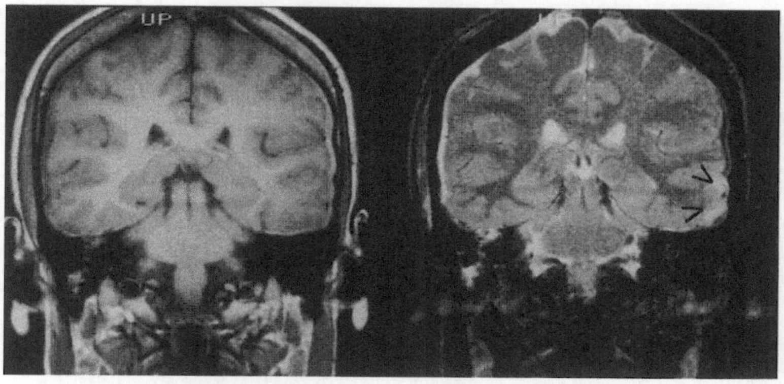

a b

Fig. 16.3 a, b. Subdural hemorrhage in a 15-year-old boy 2 days after head injury with transient unconsciousness and vomiting. CT 1 day after the accident was normal. Subdural fluid collections over both hemispheres. On the left the subdural hematoma is still hypointense on the T_2-weighted image (**b**); on the right the subdural effusion appears hyperintense. Small cortical contusions *(arrowheads)* of left temporal lobe which were not seen on the T_1-weighted image (**a**) and on CT. Coronal scans: **a** SE 0.6 s/15 ms, **b** SE 3.1 s/110 ms (1.5 T)

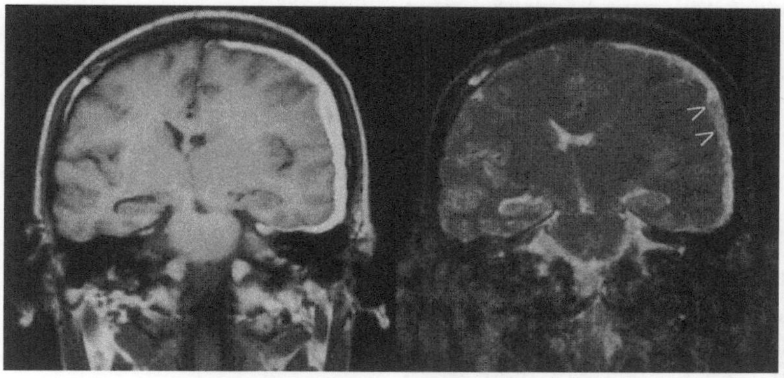

a b

Fig. 16.4 a, b. Subacute subdural hematoma in a 33-year-old man 5 days after head injury. The hematoma appears bright in **a** due to short relaxation times of methemoglobin, the darker portions *(arrowheads)* in **b** indicating still coagulated clots. Moderate mass effect. Shallow, probably epidural hematoma on the opposite side. Coronal scans: **a** SE 0.5 s/30 ms, **b** SE 2.5 s/120 ms (1.0 T)

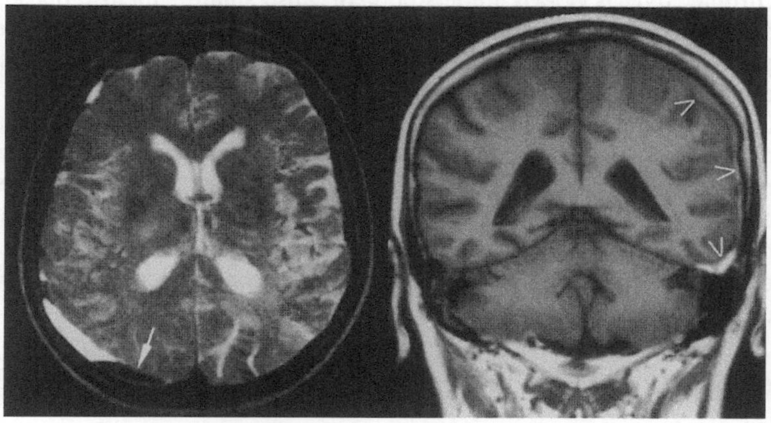

a b

Fig. 16.5 a, b. Chronic subdural hematoma in a 76-year-old woman 3 weeks after minor head injury, now presenting with increasing occipital headache. Sickle-shaped fluid collection over the left hemisphere *(arrowheads)* with different relaxation times. The hypointense part (*arrow* in **a**) with fluid level represents sedimentation of erythrocytes. **a** Axial scan, SE 3.0 s/100 ms; **b** coronal scan, SE 0.6 s/15 ms (1.5 T). The hematoma was isodense on CT

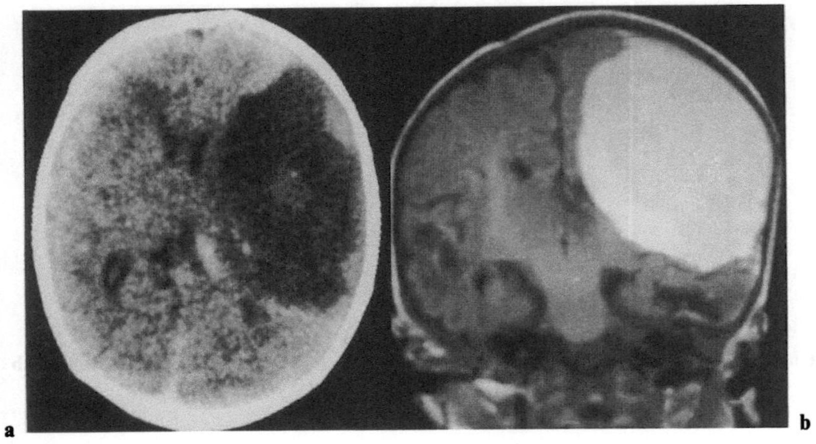

Fig. 16.6 a, b. Chronic subdural hematoma (perinatal) in a 7-days-old baby with large, assymmetric head. **a** The cyst is hypodense in CT. **b** The short and long relaxation times on MR performed 3 days after CT indicate old hemorrhage, which was proven by surgery. Coronal scan (**b**) SE 0.7 s/30 ms (1.0 T)

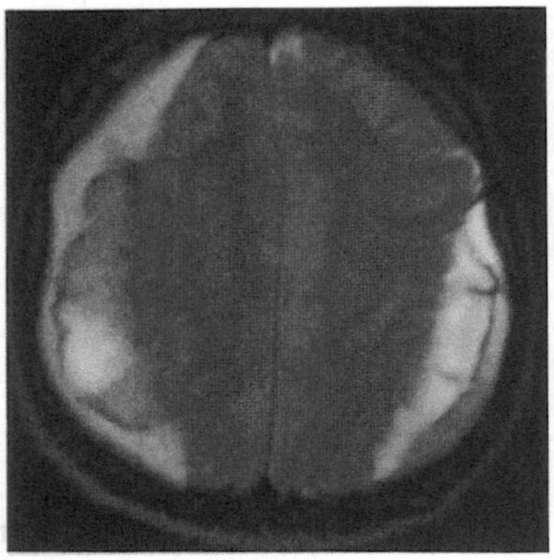

Fig. 16.7. Chronic subdural hematoma in a 35-year-old male after recent head injury. In addition the patient has a history of intracranial infection with syphilis, HIV for 1 year, herpes simplex, and toxoplasmosis. Multiple, bilateral subdural hematomas, with different signal intensities because they are at different stages of liquefaction, separated by thin membranes. Axial scan, SE 3.0 s/120 ms (1.0 T)

chronic SDH is poorly understood. Because small SDH normally are spontaneously reabsorbed, it appears that a pathologic change in the dura must exist in order for chronic SDH to develop. It is usual at operation to find an old, liquefied hematoma that is enclosed by membranes of varying thickness, may be loculated, and may contain fresher components that are still clotted. The clinical symptoms result from a local rise of intracranial pressure over the affected hemisphere, which later becomes more generalized.

CT and MR Findings

From 10% to 25% of chronic subdural hemorrhages are isodense on CT scans and so are not easily detected by that method. As in CT, the MR signal intensities of extravasated blood change as the collection undergoes hemolysis (see Sect. 5.2). The hyperintense phase of the hemorrhage on MR images is caused by methemoglobin and lasts considerably longer than the high-density phase in CT (Figs. 16.5–16.7). Therefore hematomas that are isodense on CT scans are easily recognized with MR. The capability of MR for direct coronal imaging is particularly useful for demonstrating very shallow hemorrhages over the hemispheres, basally, and on the tentorium, where evaluation by CT is complicated by bone artifacts or partial volume effects.

Subdural Hygroma

Subdural hygroma can develop in small children due to an arachnoid tear following a minor head injury [17]. The hygroma often consists of encapsulated xanthochromic fluid and can stimulate excessive cranial growth.

CT and MR Findings

The MR signal of subdural hygroma corresponds to that of CSF when the fluid collection results from an arachnoid tear [17]. While differentiation from a markedly hypodense SDH can be difficult on CT scans, the high protein content of a hematoma and its methemoglobin residues will shorten the relaxation times sufficiently to distinguish it from CSF on MR images (see Fig. 16.3).

16.2 Blunt Brain Injuries

16.2.1 Focal Injuries

Cerebral Concussion

By definition, cerebral concussion does not produce structural damage to the brain, although experimental studies have disclosed minimal, nonspecific neuronal changes [1, 13]. Generally the diagnosis of concussion is made clinically on the basis of mild, transient subjective complaints or objective neurologic deficits. CT in these cases may show no clear evidence of general or focal abnormalities. Recent studies with MR, however, have shown that this modality can demonstrate circumscribed signal changes, indicating contusional edema or a shallow effusion or hematoma, even when CT studies are negative. If these observations are confirmed, we will be compelled to formulate new guidelines for the diagnosis of cerebral concussion.

Cerebral Contusion

Cerebral contusion is defined as a bruise of the brain surface covered by intact dura [14]. By this definition, contusions are a focal type of brain damage in regions relatively unimportant to immediate survival, and they are followed by an uneventful recovery. Deeper lesions are considered to come under the heading of diffuse brain damage, which is of greater clinical significance [4].

Contusions can occur directly at the site where a blow is inflicted (coup contusion) or at a site diametrically opposed (contrecoup contusion). They may be found in the margins of brain hernias (herniation contusion), occurring mainly about the edges of the falx, tentorium, and foramen magnum. Other, very common sites of occurrence are the frontal poles, the orbital surface of the frontal lobes, the lateral and inferior surface of the temporal lobes, and the cortex above and below the sylvian fissures (sphenoid wing) [3].

Contusions may be limited to the crests of the gyri, or they may involve deeper layers of the cortex including portions of the white matter. Early cases are marked by punctate hemorrhages or streaks of hemorrhage that are essentially perivascular in location [4].

Later the hemorrhages spread in the cortex and infiltrate the digitate white matter. Ischemic cell changes signify necrosis of neurons in the adjacent cortex. The white matter response to the hemorrhage is manifested by a proliferation of capillaries, astrocytes, and microglia. Concurrent edematous swelling of the adjacent brain region is seen in the acute stage. Irreversibly damaged tissues are finally broken down, leaving behind a shrunken and gliosed, rather fenestrated scar containing macrophages filled with residual hemosiderin.

CT and MR Findings

The appearance of contusion on CT depends on the age of the injury and the extent of hemorrhagic infiltration. In the acute stage there is a patchy mass lesion with hyperdense zones of hemorrhage, hypodense zones of necrosis, and acute edema. Between day 3 and day 7 after the trauma there is a breakdown of the contused tissue, leading to the formation of additional edema with accentuation of the mass effect. At this stage smaller hemorrhages can no longer be identified because of the edematous influx. Between the 1st and 3rd weeks, vascular proliferation is seen at the periphery of the contused area, with an associated disruption of the blood-brain barrier. Contrast injection at this time produces edge enhancement of the contusion, similar to that seen around an intracerebral hematoma or infarction. Unless the history is known, differentiation from a tumor or infarct will be difficult. Between 3 and 6 months after the injury the damaged tissue is broken down, resulting in a substance loss with reactive expansion of the adjacent portions of the ventricles.

In comparative CT and MR studies of cerebral contusions in the subacute stage [15, 38], MR disclosed many sites of contusion that were not detected by CT (see Fig. 16.3). This was particularly true in the frontobasal, temporopolar, and temporobasal regions, which are difficult to evaluate with CT because of bone artifact. Shearing injuries of the

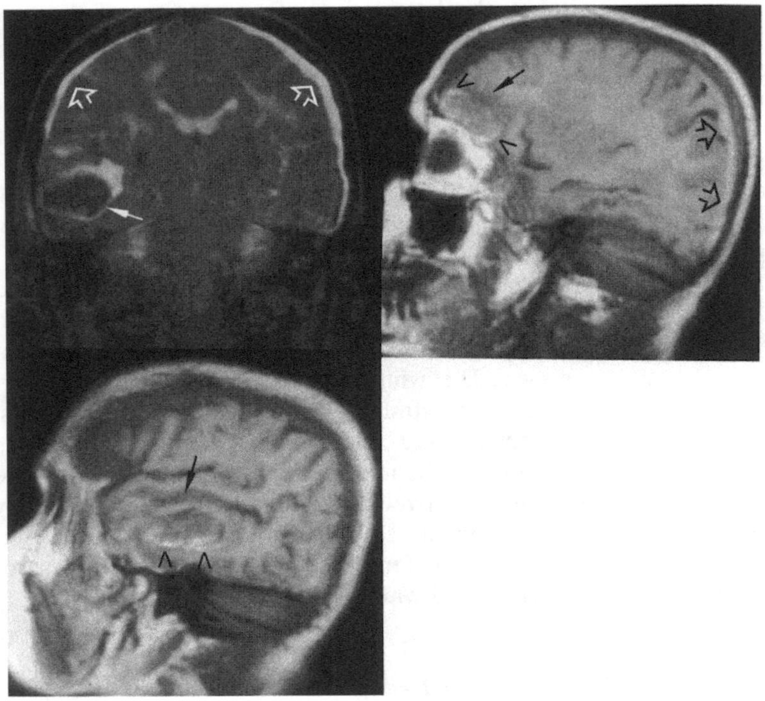

a b c

Fig. 16.8 a–c. Hemorrhagic contusions and bilateral subdural hemorrhage, in the subacute stage, in a 75-year-old woman 1 day after head injury. The patient was awake and able to communicate. Right temporal and left frontal hemorrhagic contusions *(arrows)* with perifocal edema. The hematomas appear isointense (**b, c**) or hypointense (**a**) with methemoglobin formation beginning on the periphery *(arrowheads)*. Hemorrhagic effusion covering both hemispheres *(open arrows)* is hyperintense on T1-weighted and T2-weighted images. Its relaxation times are shorter in the posterior regions of the head when the patient is supine, indicating a higher concentration of constituents of blood. **a** Axial scan, SE 2.5 s/120 ms; **b, c** sagittal scans, SE 0.4 s/17 ms (1.0 T)

white matter (see "Diffuse Axonal Injury" in Sect. 16.2.2) and brainstem also were more clearly visualized. Small hemorrhages in contusions, which appear isodense with the edema on CT scans, could be clearly identified as hemorrhages on T1-weighted images. Gentry et al. [12] state that the major advantage of MR over CT is its greater sensitivity in the detection of nonhemorrhagic cortical white matter lesions, and subcortical gray matter lesions (Figs. 16.8–16.10).

Lacerations

A laceration is a tear or rent in normal tissue that is produced by mechanical forces [14]. Lacerations show the same spatial distribution as contusions and are especially common along fracture lines and at sites of penetrating injury. Lacerations are consistently located in the corpus callosum and the rostral brainstem. Rents of the pontomedullary junction [27] and cerebral peduncles are presumably caused by sufficient hyperextension to stretch and snap the axons at these sites [14]. Hemorrhages extend rostrally from the pontomedullary junction into the tegmentum of the pons [24].

CT and MR Findings

MR imaging may well afford the first opportunity to demonstrate lacerations in the brainstem region clearly, without the problem of bone artifact that is so troublesome in CT. Frontal and sagittal images would be best for demonstrating these lesions, although we have no personal experience in this area.

Contusional edema gives an intense signal on proton-density and T2-weighted images. Hemorrhages in the initial acute phase appear dark on T2-weighted images and later appear bright on T1-weighted images.

Intracerebral Hemorrhage

Traumatic intracerebral hemorrhages (ICH) occur in contused brain tissue. They may coalesce into a larger mass within a few hours, or it may take several days for a delayed post-traumatic hematoma to form. "Shear hemorrhages" occur at the boundaries of tissues with different consistencies, such as the area of the corpus callosum and basal ganglia (see "Diffuse Axonal Injury" in Sect. 16.2.2).

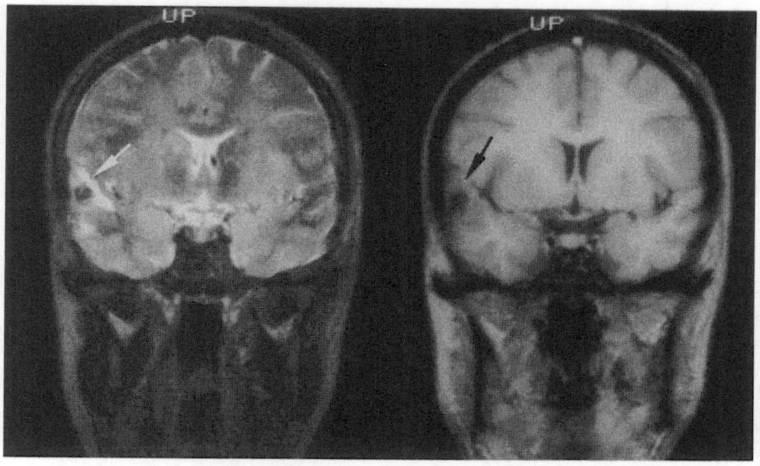

Fig. 16.9 a, b. Hemorrhagic contusion in a 13-year-old girl after head injury with unconsciousness of 20 min duration, 3½ days after the accident. The hemorrhagic infiltration *(arrows)* is more clearly demonstrated on MR images with heavier T2 weighting (**a**) or with FLASH (**b**). It was not seen on the T1-weighted SE image. Coronal scans **a** SE 2.8 s/110 ms, **b** FLASH 50 s/0.1 s/10 ms (1.5 T)

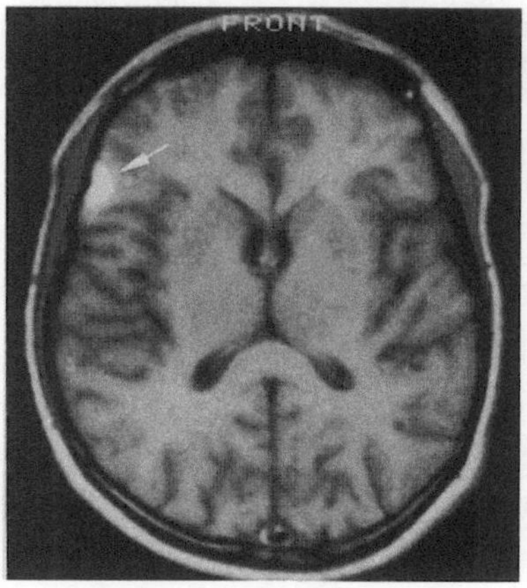

Fig. 16.10. Hemorrhagic cerebral contusion in a 24-year-old man 3 weeks after head injury presenting with headache. Small recent hemorrhage into a superficial frontotemporal contusion *(arrow)* which was not seen on CT. It was hyperintense also on the T2-weighted image. Axial scan SE 0.4 s/17 ms (1.0 T)

CT and MR Findings

Acute ICH presents a very high density on CT scans. It is often surrounded by a low-density border, thought to represent extravasated serum. As days go by the mass effect increases due to spreading perifocal edema. At the same time, the density of the hematoma decreases from its periphery, and its volume dwindles (see Sect. 5.3). However, the mass effect of the hematoma does not decrease at the same rate as its density. Absorption of the blood takes a considerably longer time than the decline of radiopacity, which basically corresponds to the degree of liquefaction. The absorption and resolution of large hemorrhages may take months to accomplish. The final parenchymal defect is usually quite a bit smaller than the original hematoma, unless the accompanying contusion was very extensive. A reactive expansion of adjacent ventricles and sulci is commonly observed.

The changes in MR signal intensity are influenced by the paramagnetic effect of the hemoglobin breakdown products (see Sect. 5.2). This denaturing process starts at the edge of the hematoma and proceeds toward its center, accounting for the initial rise of peripheral signal intensity that is seen on T1-weighted images (SE with short TR/TE). Whereas the liquefied, hypodense hematoma is scarcely distinguishable from perifocal edema on CT scans, the hyperintense hematoma contrasts sharply with the dark edema on T1-weighted MR images due to the long relaxation times of the edema (Figs. 16.8–16.10). In larger hematomas the hyperintense phase may persist for several months.

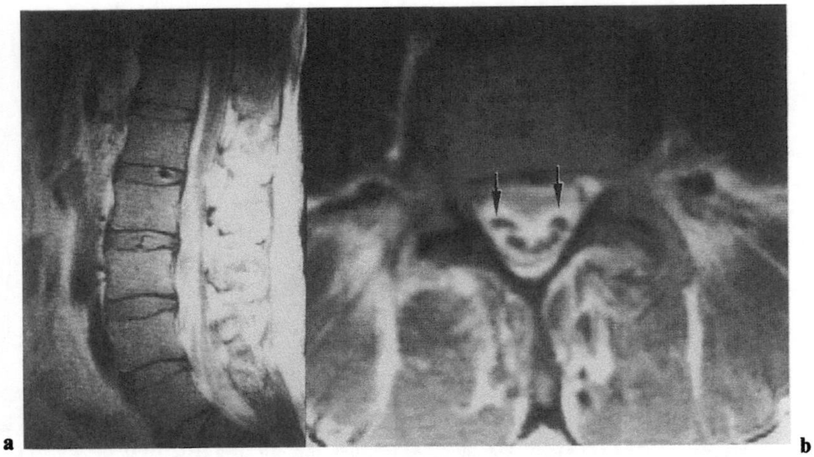

Fig. 16.11 a, b. Subarachnoid hemorrhage in a 32-year-old man a few days after lumbar puncture with intrathecal hemorrhage. The lumbar CSF appears bright due to methemoglobin and thus contrasts well with the dark nerve roots *(arrows)*. **a** Midsagittal scan, SE 0.4 s/30 ms; **b** axial scan, SE 0.6 s/30 ms (0.5 T). (Courtesy of Drs. Kuhn, Steen, and Terwey, Oldenburg, FRG)

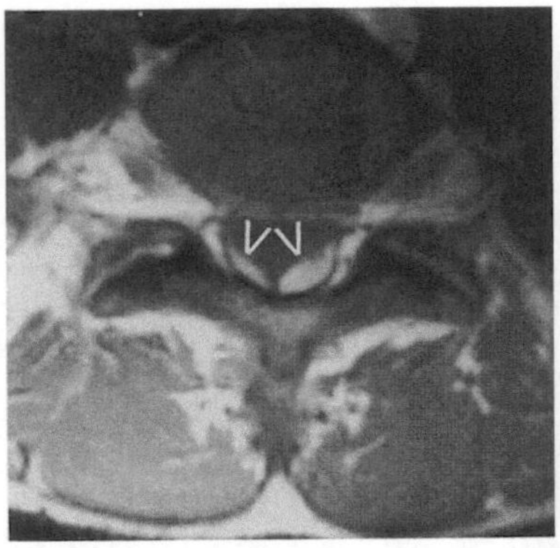

16.12

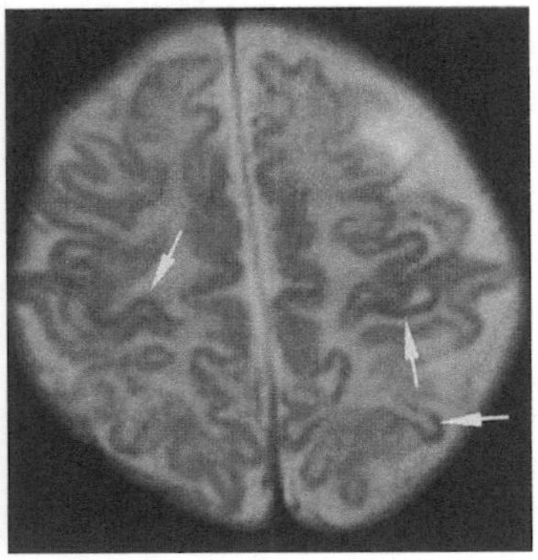

16.13

Fig. 16.12. Subacute subdural hematoma *(arrowheads)* of the lumbar spine in a 25-year-old boxer presenting with pain in the neck and back. Axial scan, SE 0.6 s/26 ms (1.5 T)

Fig. 16.13. Perinatal trauma in a 6-week-old boy with a history of perinatal subarachnoid hemorrhage. Hemosiderin deposits *(arrows)* in parts of the cortical gray matter. Axial scan, SE 3.0 s/120 ms (1.0 T)

After about 2 weeks, at the start of the chronic phase, iron from the hemoglobin is deposited in macrophages at the periphery of the hemorrhage, which then appears dark on T2-weighted images (see Sect. 5.2). Finally the hematoma cavity contains only nonparamagnetic hematoidin [5, 32].

Traumatic Subarachnoid Hemorrhage

Traumatic subarachnoid hemorrhages (SAH) usually occur in association with contusions and lacerations. Sometimes they are the only sign of such injuries on CT scans. Aseptic meningitis develops with polymorphonuclear leukocytes, lymphocytes, and macrophages. The latter consume the red blood cells in a matter of days or weeks. Malabsorptive hydrocephalus can result from massive or recurring SAH.

CT and MR Findings

Chakeres and Bryan [10] performed in vitro MR and CT measurements (T1 and T2, Hounsfield units) in mixtures of normal human CSF and normal heparinized blood ranging from 0% to 100% by volume. The MR measurements were made in a low-field scanner (6 MHz) using IR and SE pulse sequences for T1- and T2-calculated relaxation times. The authors found that MR distinguishes varying blood/CSF mixtures on the basis of relaxation times better than does CT on the basis of Hounsfield units. However, a more severe hemorrhage appears hyperdense on CT scans and so is easily distinguished from normal brain, whereas a concentrated acute SAH has relaxation times on MR images similar to those of brain, making it roughly isointense with the brain tissue [10].

Bradley and Schmidt [6] state that an acute SAH is difficult to identify on MR images because of the minimal shortening of the T1 value of the blood-tinged CSF. With the appearance of methemoglobin about a week later, the images become easier to interpret (Figs. 16.11, 16.12) [6]. After perinatal trauma, hemosiderin deposits in cortical gray matter may be secondary to subarachnoid hemorrhage (Fig. 16.13) (see also Sect. 6.3).

16.2.2 Diffuse Injury

Diffuse Axonal Injury

If a severe head injury is followed by immediate unconsciousness that progresses to a vegetative state or death after a protracted period, it is very likely that a diffuse axonal injury has occurred. In the past this condition was commonly diagnosed as brainstem contusion; it appears, however, that diffuse damage to the brain is always present [4]. Theoretical, experimental, and morphologic studies have shown that diffuse axonal injury of the cerebral white matter, brainstem, corpus callosum, fornix, internal capsule, deep gray matter, and cerebellar folia is produced by a sudden angular rotation of the head [14, 26]. This type of brain damage has been referred to as a shearing injury [29] or a diffuse white matter shearing injury [34, 35].

Distributed lesions containing reactive axonal swellings (reaction balls) are found in the affected regions. After a few weeks, clusters of microglial cells develop at these damaged sites and may replace the swollen axons. Long tract degeneration will evolve. According to Adams [1], this Wallerian-type degeneration can also be found in the white matter of the hemispheres, including the subcortical white matter and internal capsule. Reduced bulk and increased consistency of the white matter and thinning of the corpus callosum with resulting ventricular dilatation will follow [1]. Small foci of hemorrhage and necrosis may form in connection with the subsequent cellular reactions [14]. When such hemorrhagic and necrotic lesions occur in the periaqueductal tissue, they may be responsible for the prolonged coma and unfavorable outcome associated with these injuries.

CT and MR Findings

CT in the acute stage of diffuse axonal injury demonstrates small hemorrhages in the corpus callosum, at the corticomedullary junction, in the internal capsule, the basal ganglia, and the upper brainstem. The torn axons are not visible. At 2–3 weeks post injury, areas of decreased density can be seen in the white matter, accompanied by atrophic changes with dilatation of the ventricles and external CSF spaces [33].

As described in Sect. 5.2, the small hemorrhages of the acute injury are not easily identified on MR images. The best evidence for their presence is the edema that develops within a few hours following the injury. In the subacute stage, hemorrhages give a very intense MR signal and are readily distinguishable from edema (see above). Diffuse axonal injury also should be presumed in cases where the absence or mildness of CT changes is inconsistent with the poor clinical condition (coma) of the trauma patient. Zones of increased signal intensity on T2-weighted sequences have been described in the white matter (corpus callosum, basal ganglia, gray matter–white matter junction) [37]. It is anticipated that MR imaging can contribute to diagnostic evaluation in a significant number of cases.

Diffuse Brain Swelling

Diffuse brain swelling can result from a general brain edema or from cerebral hyperemia secondary to vasoparalysis. It leads to increased intracranial pressure. The brain swelling occurs following a heavy, blunt head injury and tends to be especially pronounced in children. The degree of the swelling is variable, and mild cases are difficult to diagnose. The swelling may subside with no sequelae, or it may progress within hours to an acute general edema (malignant edema) with a poor prognosis.

A negative prognostic factor in such cases is the acute venous congestion that results from acute cortical compression, and which in turn causes a secondary global ischemia by lowering the perfusion pressure to critical levels (see below), establishing a vicious cycle of edema formation.

Histologic criteria of cerebral edema include pallor of the myelin, distension of the perivascular and pericellular spaces, rarefaction of subpial spaces, a vacuolar appearance of the neuropil, and pools of protein-rich fluid in the spongy-appearing areas [14, 25]. Grossly there is symmetric narrowing of the ventricles and compression of the basal cisterns and sulci [9, 31, 36].

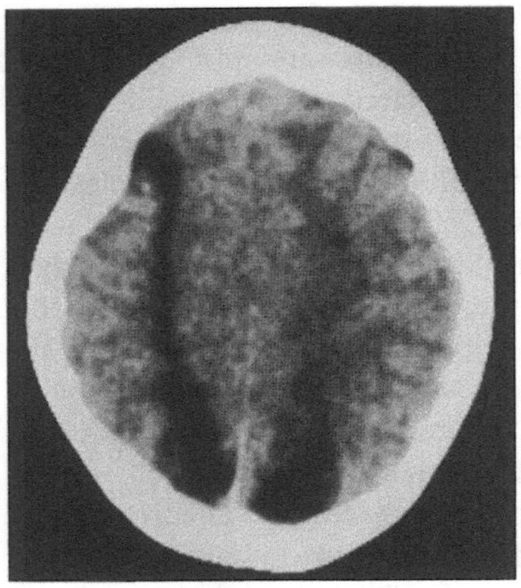

Fig. 16.14. Hypoxic brain damage affecting the boundary zones of major cerebral vessels, with bilateral infarctions of posterior cerebral artery, in an 11-year-old girl with Fallot's disease. CT scan

CT and MR Findings

The initial changes on CT scans in cases of diffuse brain swelling consist of narrowing and compression of the ventricles and perimesencephalic cisterns. Because the ventricles and cisterns usually are already narrow in children, the patient's clinical status must be known for proper evaluation of the scans. So far there are no reports on MR examinations of this acute swelling, nor do we have any personal experience. It is reasonable to assume that the progression to acute edema could be demonstrated earlier and more reliably with MR than with CT (see also Sect. 5.1).

Hypoxic Brain Damage

A decrease in the supply of oxygen to the brain is a potentially serious complication of head injuries. Posttraumatic cerebral hypoxia can have several causes:

- Circulatory insufficiency (shock)
- Obstructed airways and respiratory arrest
- Increased intracranial pressure with reduced perfusion pressure
- Intracranial arterial spasm

The hypoxic damage to the brain can have various localizations and patterns of distribution. The most common form of hypoxic damage affects the boundary zones between the territories of the major cerebral arteries (Fig. 16.14). The second most common form presents as diffuse damage to the cortex of both hemispheres, while the third and least common form involves the territories of the anterior and/or middle cerebral arteries. When circulation in the posterior cerebral arteries is compromised due to a rise of intracranial pressure, hypoxic damage can be seen in Ammon's horn and the basal ganglia [30] as well as in the medial occipital cortex.

The acute initial brain swelling (vasoparalysis), which can progress to diffuse edema, leads to venous congestion by lowering the perfusion pressure. The result of this is an ischemic edema which further raises the intracranial pressure. Contusional swelling and intracranial hemorrhage can also contribute to the pressure increase.

CT and MR Findings

On CT, the edema of hypoxic brain damage decreases the density of the swollen brain, with parenchymal structures appearing blurred and indistinct.

When local damage occurs to individual cerebral vessels (e.g., the posterior cerebral artery in tentorial herniation, post-traumatic vasospasm, extracranial vascular injury), a circumscribed ischemic edema develops in the affected area. This condition may be reversible when the cause of the vascular insufficiency (e.g., acute epidural hematoma causing increased intracranial pressure) is eliminated in time. The CT features of these ischemic changes correspond to those of cerebral infarction. A similar assumption is made for MR findings (see Sect. 13.1).

16.3 Open Head Injuries

Open head injuries occur when a sharp object penetrates the skin, skull, and dura, or when a basal

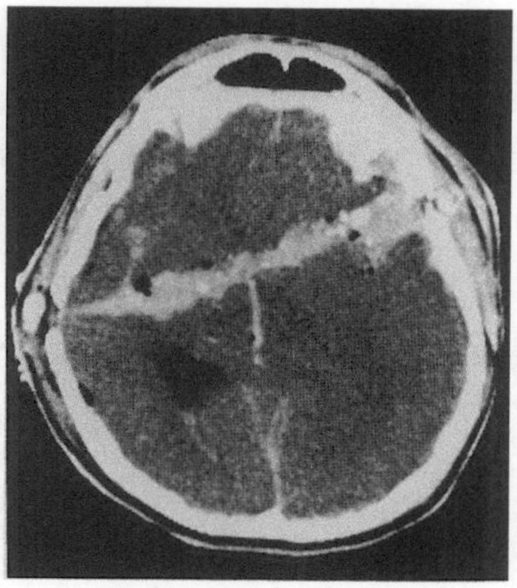

Fig. 16.15. Perforating shotgun injury in a 19-year-old man. Axial CT shows blood, pieces of bone, and air along the bullet track, swelling of right hemisphere, and subarachnoid and intraventricular hemorrhage

skull fracture communicates with the subarachnoid space. Several types of injury can occur, depending on the energy absorbed:

1. *Depressed injuries* with fracture contusion and dural laceration. The brain damage is usually circumscribed [22].

2. *Penetrating injuries* caused by an object (nail, pen, knife, bullet, etc.) that penetrates the skull without traversing it. The extent of the brain damage depends on the size of the object and its depth of penetration. These injuries carry a high risk of infection in the form of meningitis or brain abscess.

3. *Perforating injuries* in which the object (usually a bullet) enters and exits the skull. High-velocity projectiles typically produce a larger exit wound than entry wound, whereas low-velocity bullets inflict more damage upon entry. The missile can drive pieces of skin, bone, and clothing into the interior of the skull, resulting in severe laceration of the brain, hemorrhage, and necrosis (Fig. 16.15). The cross-section of the wound canal exhibits three zones: a central zone with brain tissue and blood, an intermediate zone of necrotic tissue, and a peripheral zone with slightly discolored tissue. Additional injuries are found distant from the bullet track. Typically these consist of herniation contusions at the tentorial margin and at the rim of the foramen magnum caused by an acute rise of pressure during passage of the bullet [20]. As in penetrating injuries, the risk of infection is high.

CT and MR Findings

With MRI, the diagnosis of skull fractures is less reliable than with CT. A fissure will only be visualized by the high signal of fluid or blood filling the cleft. This is also true in fractures of the petrous bone and paranasal air sinuses. Since air, cortical bone and dura are hypointense, the evaluation of the auditory ossicles and of intracranial air in open fractures of the skull base is limited with MRI.

Depressed fractures, indriven bone fragments, and other foreign bodies exhibit a high density on CT images, and their location and effect on the brain tissue can be readily assessed. Fresh hemorrhages along a puncture or bullet track and intracranial air contrast sharply with surrounding tissues. For these reasons CT continues to be the mainstay in the diagnostic evaluation of acute open head injuries.

Before MR imaging is performed, the absence of intracranial metal fragments must be confirmed by X-ray, unless the nature of the injury is such that the presence of metal fragments may be safely excluded. The appearance of small bone fragments and other nonmetallic foreign bodies is less characteristic than on CT, since cortical bone gives a very low signal that resembles air, CSF, blood vessels, and even edema, while fat-containing cancellous bone can mimic a subacute hemorrhage. The brain itself exhibits the features characteristic of hemorrhagic contusion and ischemic brain damage. If infection occurs, the appearance may be that of regional cerebritis, brain abscess, empyema, or meningitis. The MR features of these complications are described in Chap. 15.

16.3.1 Cerebrospinal Fluid Fistula

A CSF fistula cannot be detected on noncontrast MR images. DiChiro et al. [11] attempted to dem-

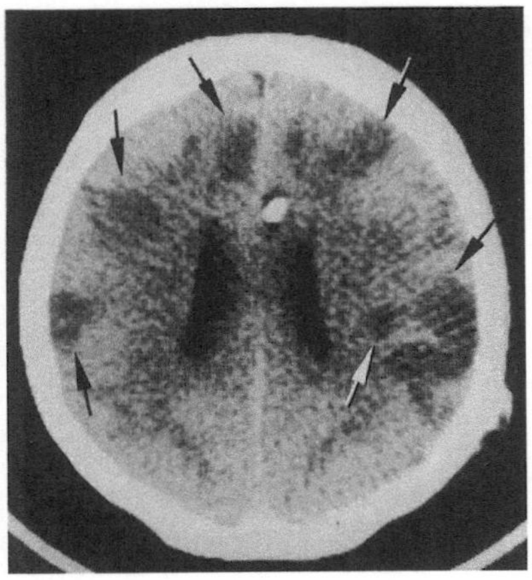

Fig. 16.16. Air embolism in a 66-year-old woman during craniotomy. CT scan 2 days after the acute event. Patchy, ill-defined areas of hypoxic edema

onstrate the path of spontaneous CSF rhinorrhea in beagle dogs following the intrathecal injection of gadolinium-DTPA (10 mM gadolinium-DTPA solution, 2 ml). Extracranial passage of the contrast agent was clearly seen in the images after 1 h and 2 h [11]. It is expected that this technique will be useful for investigating traumatic or spontaneous CSF fistulas in man, once gadolinium chelate has been approved for intrathecal use in human patients.

16.4 Other Sequelae of Injuries

16.4.1 Fat Embolism

Cerebral fat embolism can occur in multiply traumatized patients who have sustained skeletal injuries. The brain may appear normal, or there may be scattered pericapillary, ring and ball type petechial hemorrhages in the white matter [19]. Microscopic examination reveals fat globules in the smaller arterioles and capillaries, necrosis of capillary walls, foci of myelin pallor, or perivascular infarcts. In the gray matter, whose capillaries are short and anastomose more frequently than the vessels of the white matter, fat globules are as abundant as in the white matter, but hemorrhage and tissue damage are not observed [19].

MR Findings

At the time of writing, no reports were available concerning the MR features of fat embolism. It is reasonable to expect that any hemorrhages or ischemic changes in the white matter would be well displayed on T1-weighted and T2-weighted images.

16.4.2 Air Embolism

The neuropathologic effects of air embolism can be difficult to distinguish from those of decreased cerebral blood flow due to other causes. In some cases there is focal perivascular ischemic damage to the neurons, which often are outlined by a narrow zone of pallor of staining, creating the "geographical" outline that is typical of larger lesions [8, 7].

CT and MR Findings

On CT scans of air embolism, diffuse, ill-defined or, at a later stage, more circumscribed hypodense lesions indicative of hypoxic edema are seen (Fig. 16.16).

At present we are unable to relate personal or other experience with the MR features of air embolism. Grossly visible ischemic lesions should be apparent on T2-weighted and proton-density images. The shape and distribution of the foci, representing edema and demyelination, would presumably match the neuropathologic observations and the CT findings.

16.5 Late Sequelae of Head Injuries

In evaluating the late effects of head trauma, it is necessary to distinguish between focal postcontusional lesions and diffuse brain damage.

Fig. 16.17. **a** Tissue defects *(arrows)* after bilateral fronto-basal hemorrhagic contusion in a 49-year-old woman with anosmia. On T2-weighted scans hemosiderin deposits were depicted in the wall of the scar. Coronal scan, SE 0.6 s/15 ms. **b** Hemosiderin deposits *(arrowheads)* after hemorrhagic contusion of cerebellum and cerebral peduncle (along the tentorial notch) on the left in a 16-year-old girl. Additional tissue defect *(open arrow)* of the left temporal lobe near the sphenoid wing. Axial scan, SE 3.0 s/90 ms (1.5 T)

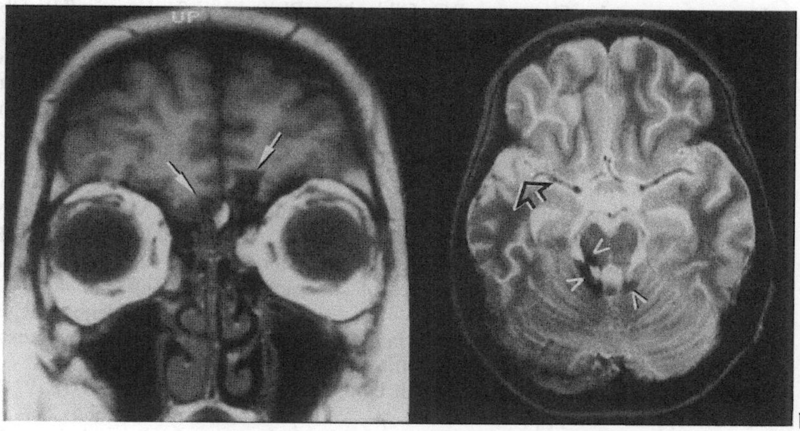

Diffuse axonal injury and hypoxic brain damage, which may be caused by brain swelling or prolonged pressure from a hematoma, lead to a reduction in brain volume with a compensatory dilatation of the ventricles and external CSF spaces. This usually results in persistent disability [28].

Focal brain damage leads to a circumscribed substance loss with formation of a glial scar. Even when the damage is relatively severe, recovery may be good. Focal brain damage may result from a contusion that causes vascular disruption beyond the area of mechanical tissue destruction, leading to areas of necrobiosis [23]. Post-traumatic vascular occlusions (arterial spasm, compression in tentorial herniation, etc.) result in encephalomalacia of the affected vascular territory. Traumatic intracerebral hemorrhage can develop in a parenchymal defect that is small in relation to the original volume of the hemorrhage.

CT and MR Findings

The late CT findings after head injuries are nonspecific. Dilatations of the internal and external CSF spaces indicate diffuse damage to the brain. Circumscribed expansions of portions of the ventricles or regional sulci and parenchymal defects are indicative of a focal substance loss.

Both diffuse and local substance losses in the brain appear on CT scans as CSF-filled spaces, with the scarred tissue at the periphery of the defects showing some degree of hypodensity. MR can demonstrate these changes more accurately on direct coronal and sagittal T1-weighted sequences, which are unhampered by bone artifact and partial volume effects (Fig. 16.17). According to Langfitt et al. [21], the extent of the encephalomalacic areas at the periphery of the defects is defined better by MR than by CT.

It is difficult to establish cause-and-effect relationships on the basis of a single examination. As morphologic methods, CT and MR can provide information on macroscopic changes in brain tissues but not on the functional status of the imaged structures. Only serial CT and/or MR studies which document the initial post-traumatic findings and then follow the subsequent course, including all complications - effusions, secondary hemorrhages, traumatic subarachnoid hemorrhages with CSF stasis (transient or requiring surgery), brain edema infections, etc. - can furnish useful information on the extent of the traumatic injury and any functional deficits that may exist. Nevertheless, there are cases in which brain function is significantly altered, yet CT is able to demonstrate only minor morphologic changes. Comparative studies are needed to determine whether MR has diagnostic capabilities surpassing those of CT in cases of this type. The detection and evaluation of the extent of a functional brain disturbance will continue to rely on appropriate function studies.

References

1. Adams JH (1975) The neuropathology of head injuries. In: Vinken PJ, Bruyn GW (eds) Handbook of clinical neurology, vol 23. Elsevier, New York, pp 35-65
2. Adams JH, Graham DI, Scott G, Parker LS, Doyle D (1980) Brain damage in fatal non-missile head injury. J Clin Pathol 33: 1132-1145
3. Adams JH, Graham DI, Gennarelli TA (1982) Neuropathology of acceleration-induced head injury in the sub-

human primate. In: Grossman RG, Gildenberg PL (eds) Head injury: basic and clinical aspects. Raven, New York, pp 141-150

4. Adams JH (1984) Head injury. In: Adams JH, Corsellis JAN, Duchen LW (eds) Greenfield's neuropathology. Wiley, New York, pp 85-124
5. Bradley WG Jr (1987) Pathophysiologic correlates of signal alterations. In: Brant-Zawadzki M, Norman D (eds) Magnetic resonance imaging of the central nervous system. Raven, New York, pp 23-42
6. Bradley WG, Schmidt PG (1985) Effect of methemoglobin formation on the MR appearance of subarachnoid hemorrhage. Radiology 156: 99-104
7. Brierley JB, Graham DI (1984) Hypoxia and vascular disorders of the central nervous system. In: Adams JH et al. (eds) Greenfield's neuropathology, 4th edn., John Wiley and sons', New York, pp 125-207
8. Brion S, Psimaras A, Gallissot MC (1974) Neuropathologie de l'embolie gazeuse humaine au cours de la chirurgie cardiaque. In: Arfel G, Naquet R (eds) L'embolie gazeuse du systeme carotidien. Doin, Paris, pp 194-198
9. Bruce DA, Alavi A, Bilaniuk LT, Kolinskas C, Obrist W, Uzzell B (1981) Diffuse cerebral swelling following head injuries in children; the syndrome of "malignant brain edema". J Neurosurg 54: 170-178
10. Chakeres DW, Bryan RN (1986) Acute subarachnoid hemorrhage: in vitro comparison of magnetic resonance and computed tomography. AJNR 7: 223-228
11. DiChiro G, Girton ME, Frank JA, Dietz MJ, Gansow OA, Wright DC, Dwywer AJ (1986) Cerebrospinal fluid rhinorrhea: depiction with MR cisternography in dogs. Radiology 160: 221-222
12. Gentry LR, Godersky JC, Thompson B, Dunn VD, Ehrhardt J (1986) Magnetic resonance of closed cranial trauma: prospective MR/CT comparative study. Presented at the 24th Annual Meeting of the American Society of Neuroradiology, Jan 18-23, San Diego
13. Groat RA, Windle WF, Magoun HW (1945) Functional and structural changes in the monkey's brain during and after concussion. J Neurosurg 2: 26-35
14. Hardman JM (1985) Cerebrospinal trauma. In: Davis RL, Robertson DM (eds) Textbook of neuropathology. Williams and Wilkins, Baltimore, pp 842-882
15. Hesselink JR, Dowd CF, Healy MF, Luerssen TG (1986) Magnetic resonance imaging of cerebral concussion. Presented at the 24th Annual Meeting of the American Society of Neuroradiology, Jan 18-23, San Diego
16. Horton JA (1985) Cranial trauma. In: Latchaw RE (ed) Computed tomography of the head, neck and spine. Year Book, Chicago, pp 55-69
17. Jaeckle KA, Allen JH (1979) Subdural hygroma: diagnosis with computed tomography. Comput Tomogr 3: 201-206
18. Jennett B, Teasdale G (1981) Management of head injury. Davis, Philadelphia
19. Kamenar E, Burger PC (1980) Cerebral fat embolism: a neuropathological study of a microembolic state. Stroke 11: 477-484
20. Kirkpatrick JB, Di Maio V (1978) Civilian gunshot wounds of the brain. J Neurosurg 49: 185-198
21. Langfitt TW, Obrist WD, Alavi A, Grossman RI, Zimmerman R, Jaggi J, Uzzell B, Reivich M, Patton DR (1986) Computerized tomography, magnetic resonance imaging, and positron emission tomography in the study of brain trauma. Preliminary observations. J Neurosurg 64: 760-767
22. Lindenberg R (1971) Trauma of meninges and brain. In: Minckler J (ed) Pathology of the nervous system, vol 2. McGraw-Hill, New York, pp 1705-1765
23. Lindenberg R, Freytag E (1960) The mechanism of cerebral contusion. A pathologic-anatomic study. Arch Pathol 69: 440-469
24. Lindenberg R, Freytag E (1970) Brainstem lesions of traumatic hyperextension of the head. Arch Pathol 90: 505-515
25. Manz HJ (1974) The pathology of cerebral edema. Hum Pathol 5: 291-313
26. Oppenheimer DR (1968) Microscopic lesions in the brain following head injury. J Neurol Neurosurg Psychiatry 31: 299-306
27. Patscheider H (1962) Zur Entstehung von Ringbrüchen des Schädelgrundes. Dtsch Z Gesamte Gerichtl Med 52: 13-21
28. Strich SJ (1956) Diffuse degeneration of the cerebral white matter in severe dementia following head injury. J Neurol Neurosurg Psychiatry 19: 163-185
29. Strich SJ (1961) Shearing of nerve fibres as a cause of brain damage due to head injury. Lancet II: 443-448
30. Strich SJ (1976) Cerebral trauma. In: Blackwood W, Corsellis JAN (eds) Greenfield's neuropathology, 3rd edn. Edward Arnold, London, pp 327-360
31. Teasdale E, Cardoso E, Galbraith S, Teasdale G (1984) CT scan in severe diffuse head injury: physiological and clinical correlations. J Neurol Neurosurg Psychiatry 47: 600-603
32. Whisnant JP, Sayer GP, Milikan GH (1963) Experimental intracerebral hematoma. Arch Neurol 3 (9): 586-592
33. Zimmerman RA, Bilaniuk LT (1984) Head trauma. In: Rosenberg RN, Heinz ER (eds) The clinical neurosciences. Neuroradiology. Livingstone, New York, pp 483-524
34. Zimmerman RA, Bilaniuk LT, Bruce D, Dolinskas C, Obrist W, Kuhl D (1978) Computed tomography of pediatric head trauma: acute general cerebral swelling. Radiology 126: 403-408
35. Zimmerman RA, Bilaniuk LT, Gennarelli TA (1978) Computed tomography of shearing injuries of the cerebral white matter. Radiology 127: 393-396
36. Zimmerman RA, Bilaniuk, LT, Gennarelli TA, Bruce D, Dolinskas C, Uzzell B (1978) Cranial computed tomography in diagnosis and management of acute head trauma. AJR 131: 27-34
37. Zimmerman RA, Bilaniuk LT, Hackney DB, Goldberg HI, Grossman RI (1986) Head injury: early results of comparing CT and high-field MR. AJNR 7: 757-764
38. Zimmerman RD, Snow RB, Heier LA, Lin DPC, Deck MDF (1986) MRI features of acute traumatic and spontaneous intracerebral hemorrhage. Presented at the 24th Annual Meeting of the American Society of Neuroradiology, Jan 18-23, San Diego

17 Diseases of the Vertebral Column and Spinal Cord

F. E. ZANELLA and G. FRIEDMANN

Magnetic resonance imaging is able to demonstrate the vertebral column and especially the structures of the vertebral canal without hazard to the patient, in many cases obviating the need for more invasive diagnostic procedures.

17.1 Examination Technique

The pulse sequence most commonly used for examinations of the axial skeleton is the spin-echo (SE) technique. Inversion recovery (IR) is of minor importance at the present time. T1- or T2 weighted images may by obtained by gradient-echo techniques also. Gradient-echo pulse sequences allow very short acquisition times, and therefore motion artifacts are reduced. With some refinements, this technique promises to replace spin-echo pulse sequences in certain cases. Because both T1-weighted and T2-weighted images are necessary for spinal evaluations, echo and repetition times of varying length must be employed [27, 28, 32, 33, 41, 49, 52, 60, 62, 67, 84, 91].

First a transaxial "fast" image of the spine is obtained to assist orientation, and then a series of sagittal T1-weighted images are initiated (TR 0.25-0.5 s/TE $\leqslant$ 30 ms). With these parameters the spinal cord gives an intense signal while the CSF appears dark, so the spinal cord contrasts sharply with the subarachnoid space and with extradural structures (Fig. 17.1 a).

Spinal nerve segments visualized at the level of the intervertebral foramina give less intense signals than the surrounding fatty tissue and so are easily distinguished from it (Fig. 17.1 b).

The medullary spaces of the vertebral bodies show a somewhat higher signal intensity because of their fat content, while the cortical bone and ligaments contain few protons and thus generate a lower signal. The intervertebral discs show a homogeneous signal intensity that is somewhat lower than the adjacent vertebral bodies.

Next a series of T2-weighted images are obtained, again on the sagittal plane. We recommend using the double-echo technique with a TR of 1.5-2.0 s and a TE of 50/100 ms. The CSF, with its long T1 and T2, appears brighter in this sequence than the adjacent extradural structures, and masses projecting into the subarachnoid space from the outside are displayed with exceptional clarity (Fig. 17.2 a). However, this increased signal intensity of the CSF makes it more difficult to distinguish from epidural fat, the nerve roots, the spinal cord, and the conus medullaris. Lengthening TR to more than 2.0 s increases the CSF signal intensity to such a degree that the spinal cord gives a less intense signal than the subarachnoid space (MR myelography). T2-weighted images of the spinal cord may be degraded by CSF pulsation artifacts, which can obscure small lesions (e.g., infarcts, multiple sclerosis plaques). ECG and respiratory gating can markedly improve image definition and make lesions visible that would otherwise go undetected [20]. This technique, as well as cine studies with fast (gradient echo) sequences, will help to unmask flow artifacts and thus avoid false-positive findings (see Chap. 5.3).

The intervertebral discs give an intense signal by virtue of their high proton content, with the bright portion representing the nucleus pulposus and the inner ring of the anulus fibrosus. Low signals are produced by the outer ring of the anulus fibrosus, which contains few protons, and by the adjacent cortical bone. After 30 years of age it is common to find a central cleft of lower signal intensity, which represents connective tissue ingrowth (Fig. 17.2 b). Axial images should additionally be obtained, especially in patients with intervertebral disc disease. The examiner may either return to T1 weighting for this series (TR 0.25-0.5 s/TE $\leqslant$ 30 ms) or employ a "mixed" sequence (TR 2 s/TE 30 ms). The T1-weighted sequence has the advantage of short imaging time with good visualization of the nerve roots within the hypointense CSF (dural sac) or hyperintense fat (intervertebral foramina) (Fig. 17.3 a). The mixed sequence yields very high contrast that

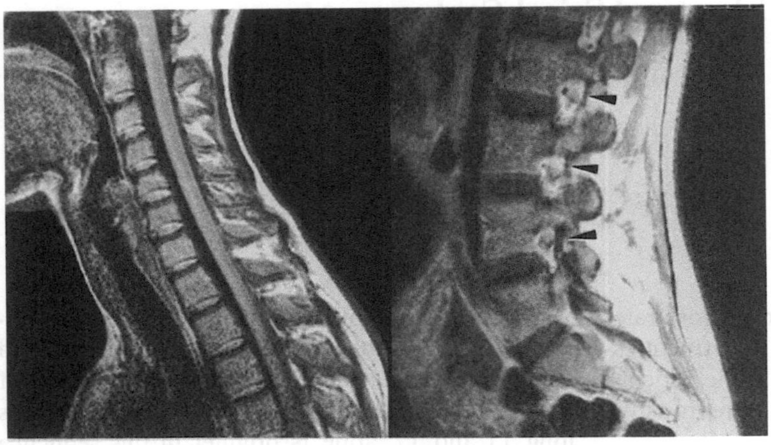

Fig. 17.1. **a** Normal cervical canal in a 28-year-old woman. The spinal cord is clearly depicted as a structure of medium intensity within the hypointense subarachnoid CSF space. Physiological signal intensity of vertebral bodies and intervertebral discs. Sagittal scan, SE 0.4 s/30 ms; surface coil. **b** Normal anatomy of the intervertebral foramina of the lumbar spine in a 30-year-old woman. The low signal intensity of the spinal nerve roots *(arrowheads)* contrasts well with the hyperintense fat of the foramina. Sagittal scan, SE 0.4 s/30 ms

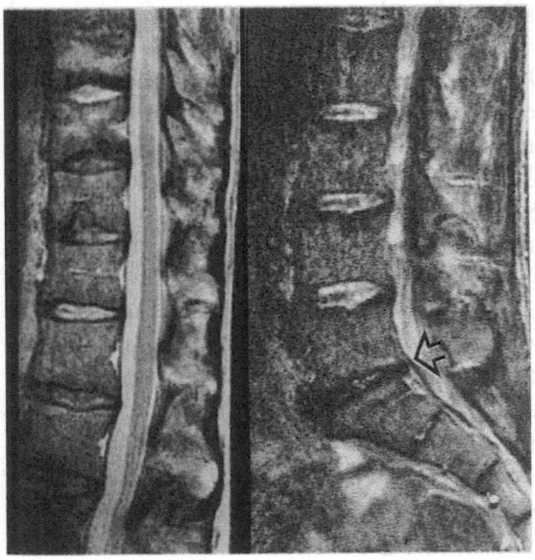

Fig. 17.2. **a** Thoracolumbar junction in a 47-year-old woman with metastasizing carcinoma of the breast presenting with progressive paraparesis of both legs. Normal intraspinal findings. Extradural tissue and hypointense cord contrast well with the hyperintense CSF (MR myelography). Multiple metastases of vertebral bodies are seen. Sagittal scan, SE 1.5 s/100 ms. **b** "Intranuclear cleft" in a 46-year-old man with sciatica. Tapelike hypointense structure in the center of the intervertebral discs of L1/2–L4/5. Degeneration of the discs with lowering of the intervertebral space and small prolapse *(open arrow)* at L5/S1. Sagittal scan, SE 2.0 s/100 ms

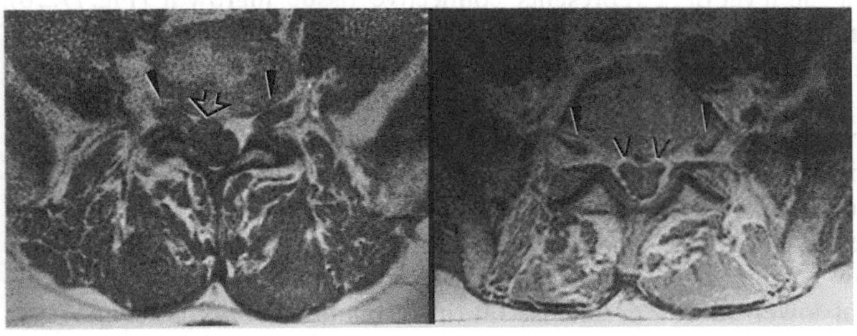

Fig. 17.3. **a** Mediolateral disc prolapse on the right at L5/S1 in a 51-year-old man with progressive flaccid paresis of the right leg. Within the intervertebral foramina the dural sack and nerve roots *(arrows)* are well delineated. The right lateral recessus is occupied by the prolapse *(open arrow)*. Axial scan, SE 0.35 s/30 ms. **b** Normal axial section of lumbar spine in a 65-year-old man. Good differentiation of anatomical details of dural sack, nerve roots *(arrows)*, and fat. SE 2.0 s/30 ms

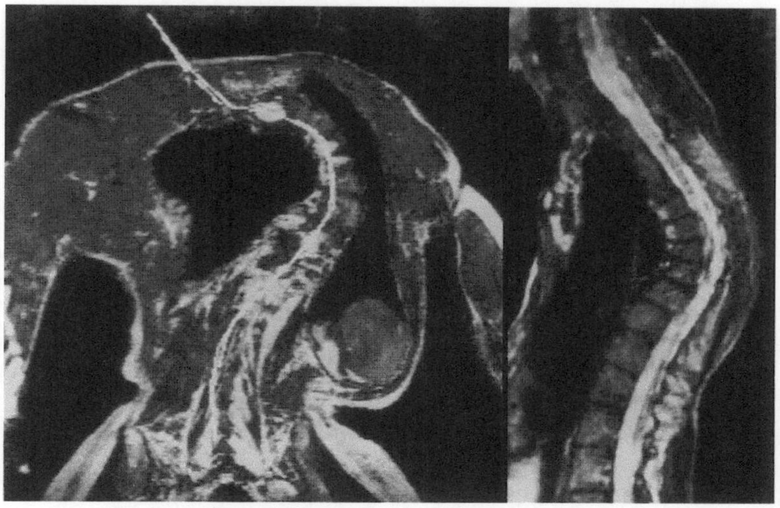

a b

Fig. 17.4 a, b. Extreme scoliosis of the spine in a 59-year-old woman. The sagittal scan in **b**, slice thickness 1.6 mm, was reconstructed along the white line marking the cord in **a**

provides good differentiation of the fat and nerve roots. These images are comparable in appearance to thin-section CT scans (Fig. 17.3 b). Disadvantages are a long acquisition time and the need to match the angulation of the scan to the individual disc spaces.

A slice thickness of 5 mm is generally recommended for sagittal and coronal images, and 8-10 mm for axial images of the spinal cord. For disc examinations, the slice thickness should not exceed 3 mm. The poorer signal-to-noise ratio of these sections makes it advantageous to use higher field strengths, although this makes the images more susceptible to artifacts.

The number of acquisitions greatly influences the signal-to-noise ratio. The lower the expected signal (e.g., axial image of cervical spine) and the thinner the slice (e.g., axial image to check for disc herniation), the more acquisitions are needed to achieve an acceptable image quality. This increases the imaging time by a factor equal to the number of acquisitions. Two acquisitions are sufficient for good image quality, and four are recommended for axial imaging of the cervical discs.

The spatial resolution depends in part on the matrix size, generally 256×256.

Surface coils are widely used for spinal examinations. The disadvantage of the reduced field of view is more than offset by the higher spatial resolution resulting from the improved signal-to-noise ratio. Because the signal intensity falls off with distance from the coil, structures situated anterior to the vertebral bodies are difficult to evaluate [3].

Paramagnetic contrast agents have expanded the capabilities of MR, especially in the diagnosis of intramedullary lesions. Many tumors show significant contrast enhancement on T1-weighted images and on that basis can be distinguished from surrounding edema.

The acquisition time can be shortened if the information provided by the T1-weighted images is sufficient to make a definitive evaluation. The disadvantage of omitting T2-weighted images is that it is then more difficult to evaluate extradural stenosing processes and demonstrate perifocal edema [11, 52, 62, 79].

In severe scoliosis, a continuous view of the spine and cord is not possible with routine two-dimensional imaging. This problem can be solved by means of three-dimensional data acquisition and subsequent reconstruction of images along a predefined line which connects points of interest in different planes. With this technique, coronal images of a scoliotic spine can be created in which the deformation of the spine in the sagittal plane is eliminated (Fig. 17.4 a, b). In the same way, sagittal scans can be obtained with correction of scoliosis in the coronal plane [35].

17.2 Intraspinal Processes

17.2.1 Intramedullary Processes

Only about 10%-15% of intraspinal tumors are intramedullary. Most of these are ependymomas; gli-

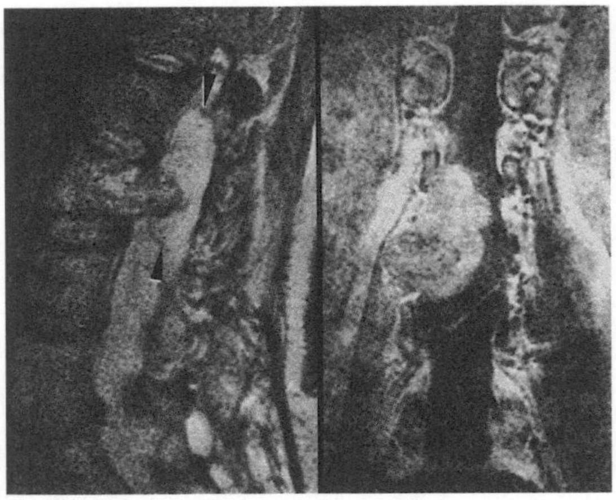

a b

Fig. 17.5 a, b. Ependymoma. Tumor recurrence in a 65-year-old man with renewed weakness of both legs 4 years after primary surgery. With T1-weighting the tumor and the adjacent portion of L1-vertebra were equally hypointense and of homogeneous structure. With T2-weighting (**a**) increased signal intensity of tumor mass *(arrowheads)* is seen. Less intense changes of adjacent dorsal portion of L2 vertebra. Reduced contrast between tumor and equally hyperintense CSF. Sagittal scan, SE 1.8 s/100 ms. **b** Coronal scan with i.v. gadolinium-DTPA: increased signal intensity of intraspinal tumor. No corresponding change of signal intensity of the suspected tumor portion within the vertebra; at surgery scar tissue instead of tumor was found. Sharp delineation of the borderline of the tumor. The coronal scan shows the tumor predominantly on the right side. SE 0.4 s/30 ms (0.5 T)

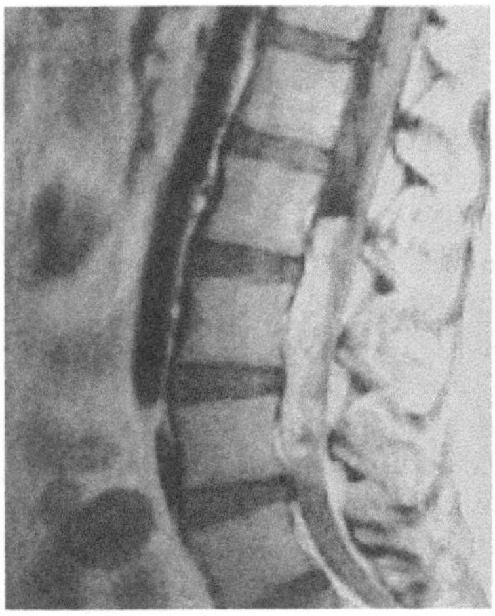

17.6

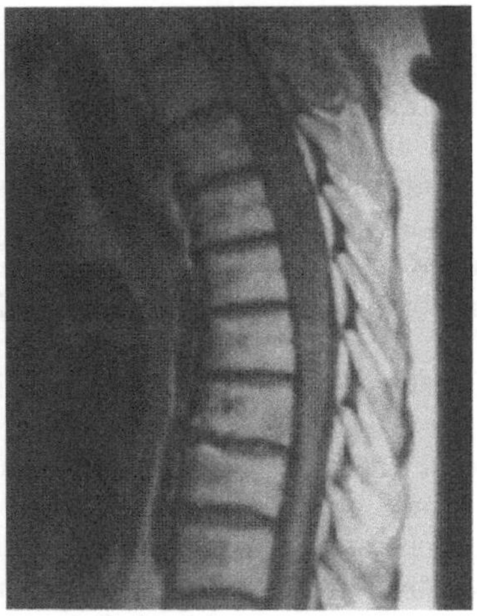

17.7

Fig. 17.6. Myxopapillary ependymoma of the lumbar region (WHO grade 1) in a 30-year-old woman with bilateral radicular pain. Sagittal scan, with i.v. gadolinium-DTPA, SE 0.4 s/17 ms (1.0 T)

Fig. 17.7. Ependymoma (WHO grade 1) in a 58-year-old woman with spasticity of both legs. Hypointense lesion of enlarged thoracic cord simulating "haustrated" syringomyelia. Midsagittal scan, SE 0.7 s/30 ms (1.0 T)

omas and other neoplasms are less common [5, 16, 19, 34, 38, 55, 74, 76, 80, 85].

Ependymoma

Ependymomas (see Sect. 10.2.4) form the majority of tumors arising from the spinal cord. They are most prevalent between the third and sixth decades of life and are somewhat more common in males. Ependymomas grow slowly, and many remain asymptomatic for a long period. Most cases prove histologically benign, although individual extraneural tumor deposits have been described.

The tumors most commonly involve the posterior part of the spinal cord over several lumbosacral segments. In that position they can be surgically enucleated after incision of the cord, and radiotherapy is indicated only in the event of incomplete removal or recurrence [5, 16, 34, 55, 74, 76].

MR Findings

Generally, by the time the ependymoma is diagnosed it already extends over multiple cord segments. It typically consists of solid and cystic components.

The *solid* tumor components and portions of the spinal cord infiltrated by tumor produce a high signal on T2-weighted images (Fig. 17.5 a, b). A marked, often nonhomogeneous enhancement is seen on T1-weighted images following paramagnetic contrast injection (Figs. 17.5 b; 17.6) [12].

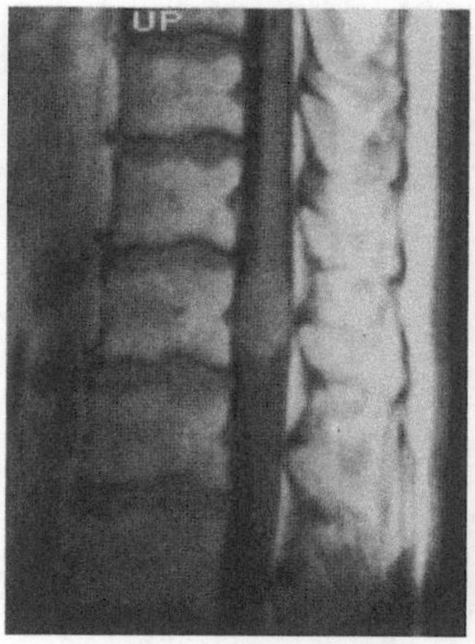

17.8

Fig. 17.8. Pilocytic astrocytoma (WHO grade 1) in a 42-year-old man with radicular symptoms mimicking lumbar disc disease. Isointense, club-like thickening of conus. Midsagittal scan, SE 0.4 s/17 ms (1.0 T)

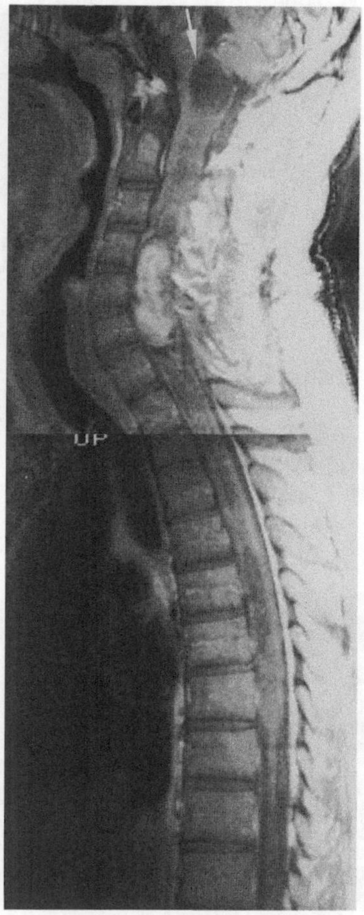

17.9

Fig. 17.9. Pilocytic astrocytoma (WHO grade 1) in a 21-year-old man with progressive clumsiness of arms and legs. Tumor of the cervical and thoracic cord with inhomogeneous structure and marked contrast enhancement. Adjacent syringomyelia with large cyst *(arrow)* in the medulla oblongata. Midsagittal scans (with gadolinium-DTPA), SE 0.4 s/17 ms (1.0 T)

The *cystic* portions of the tumor give a low signal on T1-weighted images (Fig. 17.7) and a high signal on T2-weighted images. Unlike a syrinx cavity, the cystic tumor components often do not present a spindle shape; they usually are less sharply marginated and situated eccentrically in the spinal cord. Also, expansion of the cord is usually less pronounced in syringomyelia [4, 15, 19, 25, 52, 62, 73, 84, 91].

A recurrence of ependymoma shows the same features as the original tumor, and its extent and direction of growth can be ascertained at an early stage (Fig. 17.5 a, b).

Sagittal images are excellent for demonstrating the expansion of the vertebral canal with posterior excavation of the vertebral bodies that so often accompanies the myxopapillary type of ependymoma.

Ependymomas are heavily vascularized, and so spontaneous subarachnoid hemorrhages are possible with these tumors.

Glioma

Spongioblastomas, known also as pilocytic astrocytomas, comprise the majority of intramedullary gliomas (Figs. 17.8; 17.9). Astrocytomas and glioblastomas are decidedly rare (Figs. 17.10–17.12).

Gliomas can present an elongated ("pencil") shape (see Fig. 17.12) similar to syringomyelia and ependymoma situated near the midline or between the posterior columns. Pilocytic astrocytomas comprise about 20%–25% of tumors arising from the spinal cord and generally are benign [5, 16, 34, 55,

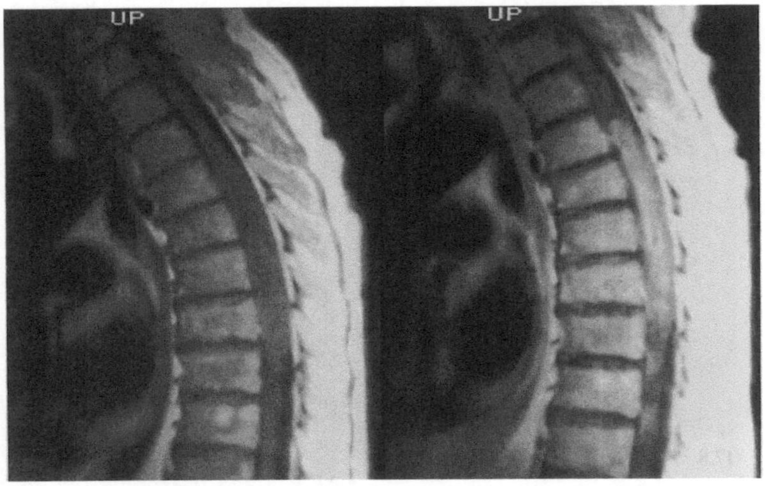

a b

Fig. 17.10 a, b. Fibrillary astrocytoma (WHO grade 2) in a 72-year-old woman with progressive spasticity of both legs. Fusiform thickening of the thoracic cord with prolonged relaxation times and slightly irregular enhancement after i.v. gadolinium-DTPA. Midsagittal scans: **a** without, **b** with gadolinium-DTPA, SE 0.4 s/17 ms (1.0 T)

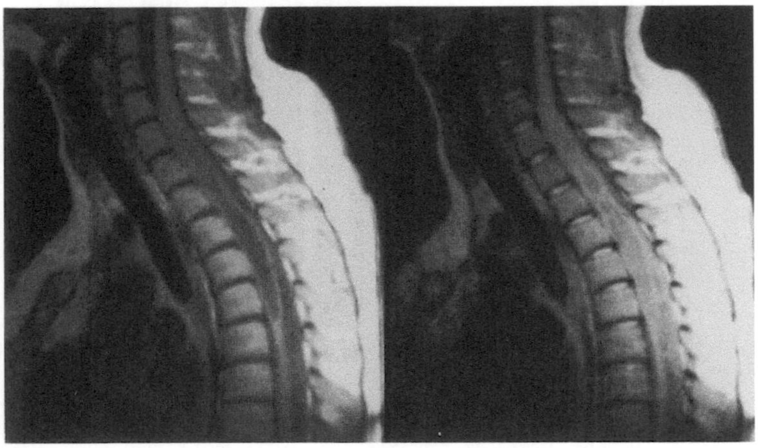

a b

Fig. 17.11 a, b. Astrocytoma (WHO grade 2) in a 26-year-old man with slowly progressive spasticity of arms and legs. Cyst like lesion in **a** without flow void sign in **b**. Midsagittal scans: **a** SE 0.7 s/30 ms, **b** SE 2.0 s/30 ms (1.0 T)

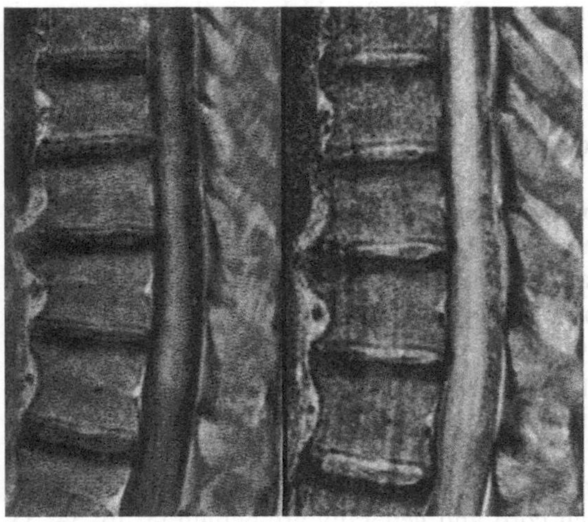

a b

Fig. 17.12 a, b. "Pencil" glioma of caudal thoracic cord in a 65-year-old man with progressive paraplegia of both legs. Circumscribed but ill-defined, hyperintense lesion predominantly in the anterior section of the cord. The area of increased signal intensity is larger in **b** than in **a**, indicating perifocal edema. Sagittal scans: **a** with i.v. gadolinium-DTPA, SE 0.4 s/30 ms; **b** SE 2.4 s/50 ms (1.5 T)

74, 76, 85]. Their incidence is maximal between the ages of 20 and 50 years and they most commonly involve the thoracic and cervical spine, in that order of frequency.

MR Findings

Gliomas usually cause a fusiform swelling of the spinal cord that is apparent on T1-weighted images. Like ependymomas, they may contain cystic elements, which appear as areas of relatively low signal on T1-weighted images (Fig. 17.9). Calcifications are rarely encountered and do not yield a signal [4, 11, 15, 25, 41, 49, 60, 73, 84, 91].

The response of the tumors to paramagnetic contrast injection is inconstant. The enhancement effect on T1-weighted scans is less pronounced than with ependymoma. The enhancement may be nonhomogeneous, and maximal enhancement may be somewhat delayed (Fig. 17.9). The use of contrast material is justified, however, because these tumors may induce an extensive perifocal edema, which contrasts poorly with the tumor on T2-weighted images because of its almost identical signal intensity (see Fig. 17.12b).

Hemangioblastoma

The overall incidence of hemangioblastomas of the vertebral canal is low. They are intramedullary in 60% of cases and comprise about 1%–3% of tumors arising from the spinal cord. They are multiple in one-fifth of cases, and 20%–40% are accompanied by cerebral hemangioblastoma (von Hippel-Lindau).

Intramedullary hemangioblastomas usually become clinically apparent between 20 and 30 years of age. About 40% involve the cervical cord and 50% the thoracic cord.

Tumors that are well demarcated can be completely removed at operation. Untreated, their blastomatous growth leads to progressive paralytic symptoms consistent with transverse cord damage [5, 16, 34, 55, 74, 76, 85].

MR Findings

The MR findings in hemangioblastoma vary with the size of the lesion. A richly vascularized but small tumor nodule that has not expanded the spinal cord may be missed, or merely presumed on the basis of a circumscribed zone of decreased signal intensity. But if the tumor is surrounded by cystic and fat-containing glial structures, a high-intensity ring will be visible around the hypointense center. The vertebral canal above the lesion may be expanded [4, 15, 52, 73].

After intravenous administration of paramagnetic agents, enhancement of solid tumor nodules may be seen (Fig. 17.13a, b).

Owing to the rich tumor blood supply, bleeding can occur into the spinal cord or subarachnoid space, depending on the tumor site (see Sect. 11.1.2).

Rare Intramedullary Tumors

The rare intramedullary tumors include lipomas, which often develop under the pia mater and, when extramedullary (see also p. 169), can mimic an intramedullary growth or subsequently spread to involve the spinal cord itself (Fig. 17.22).

Also included in this group are hemangiopericytoma, ganglioneuroma, intramedullary metastases from a cerebral tumor [5, 14, 34, 55, 74, 85]; and others (Fig. 17.14). Typical MR findings have not been reported.

Differential Diagnosis of Intramedullary Processes

Even non-neoplastic processes can produce swelling of the spinal cord. They include syringomyelia (see Sect. 7.3.4), acute hematomyelia, intramedullary vascular malformations, inflammatory spinal cord changes, and radiation effects.

MR Findings

As yet we have no information on MR findings within 48 h after the onset of *hematomyelia,* but analogy with fresh cerebral hemorrhages implies that a low signal intensity would be seen on T2-weighted images. After that period a high signal intensity is seen on both T1-weighted and T2-weighted images. It should be noted that fat-containing or cholesterol-containing tumors (lipomas, dermoids) also give high signal intensities on T1-weighted and T2-weighted images, but the history and clinical presentation should suffice for differentiation.

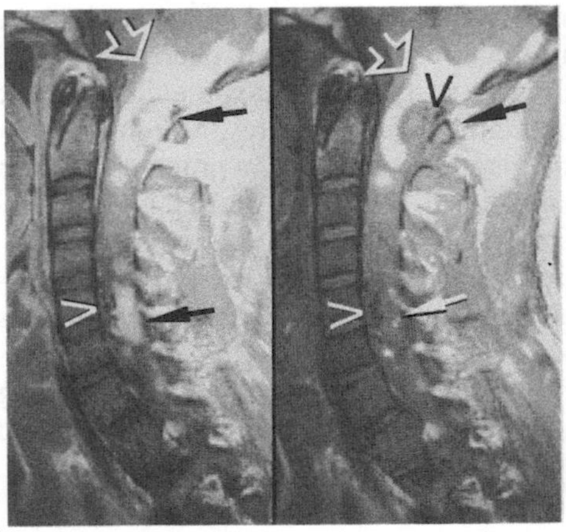

a b

17.13

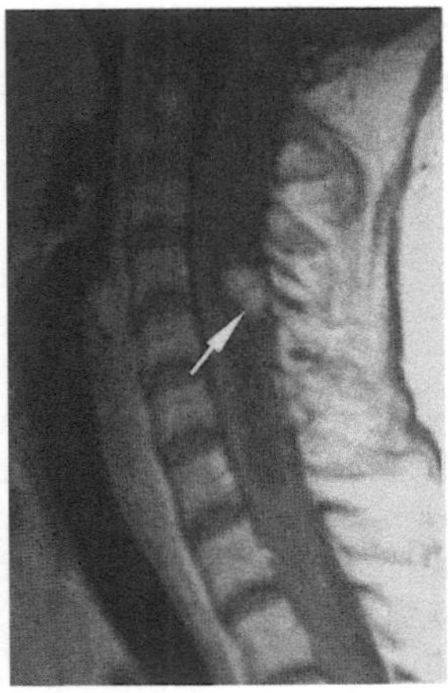

17.14

Fig. 17.13 a, b. Multiple hemangioblastomas in a 23-year-old man one week after acute hemorrhage *(open arrow)* into the medulla oblongata and subarachnoid space. With iv gadolinium-DTPA (**a**) enhancing tumor nodules *(arrows)* with pathological vasculatur *(arrowheads)* are seen. Sagittal scans, SE 0.45 s/15 ms (1.5 T)

Fig. 17.14. Angioglioma and astrocytoma (grade 2 WHO) in a 45-year-old woman with progressive spasticity. Fusiform thickening of cervical cord by the hypointense astrocytoma. After IV gd-DTPA only the nodular angioglioma *(arrow)* enhances. Sagittal scan, SE 0.6 s/15 ms (1.5 T)

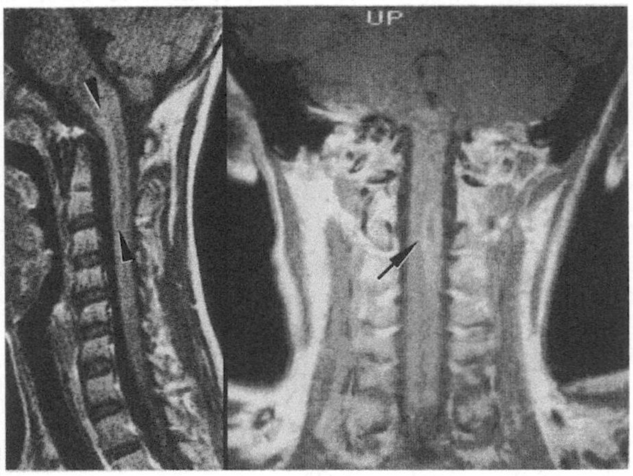

a b

Fig. 17.15 a, b. Myelitis (clinical diagnosis). **a** A 13-year-old boy with paraplegia. No pathological findings in the plain scan. With i. v. gadolinium-DTPA, slight enhancement of the anterior portion of the cervical cord is seen *(arrows)*. Sagittal scans, SE 0.4 s/50 ms (0.5 T). **b** A 23-year-old women with sensory deficit in the left arm; no CSF changes suggesting multiple sclerosis. With i. v. gadolinium-DTPA, enhancement of the posterior portion of the slightly thickened cervical cord on the left *(arrow)*. Coronal scan, SE 0.6 s/15 ms (1.5 T)

T1 weighting is necessary to detect *intramedullary vascular malformations,* for it can differentiate the low-intensity vascular structures from the higher-intensity spinal cord and from the surrounding CSF, which also gives a slow signal (Fig. 17.16 b; see Figs. 14.30, 14.31). On the other hand, T2 weighting is necessary for the much more common extramedullary vascular malformations to provide contrast with the high-intensity CSF [4, 15, 19, 52, 62] (see Figs. 14.28, 14.29).

As a general rule, images should be recorded in two planes so that the extent of the vascular malformation can be established.

The most important of the *inflammatory changes of the spinal cord* is involvement of the cord by disseminated encephalitis [43]. Spinal cord involvement without coexisting intracerebral foci is very rare. As in the cerebrum, the spinal lesions give a high signal on T2-weighted images, although their approximate isointensity with the CSF can make small lesions difficult to detect. The use of paramagnetic contrast agents can aid in this evaluation (see Sect. 8.22; Fig. 8.12).

In one case of diffuse myelitis involving the cervical cord and parts of the medulla oblongata, there was very little expansion of the spinal cord, far less than would be expected with a tumorous mass lesion of comparable extent (Fig. 17.15). The accompanying edema produced an increase of signal intensity on T2-weighted images. Injection of a paramagnetic agent produced only minimal enhancement on T1-weighted images (Fig. 17.15 a, b; see also Fig. 8.12).

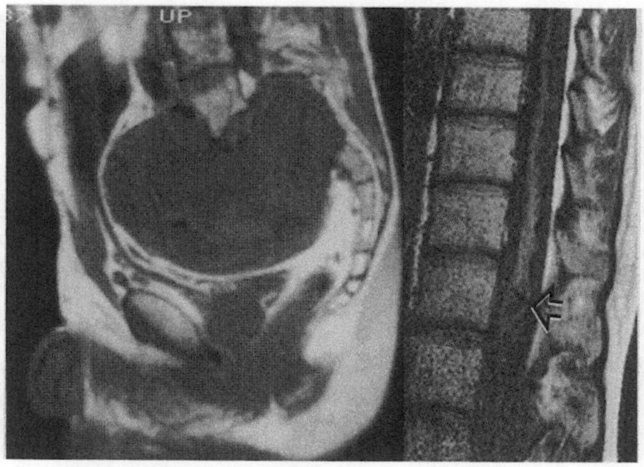

Fig. 17.16. **a** Neurinoma in a 50-year old man with disturbances of gait and rectovesical function. Tumor recurrence 10 years after primary surgery. Huge, well-delineated, nodular tumor in the pelvis with destruction of the sacrum and invasion of the sacral canal and adjacent soft tissue. Sagittal scan, SE 0.4 s/17 ms (1.0 T). **b** Intramedullary AVM of the conus in a 21-year-old woman with slowly progressive gait disturbances for several years. Hypointense notches in the area of the conus *(open arrow)* and irregular dorsal border of the cord. Sagittal scan, SE 0.3 s/ 30 ms (0.5 T)

17.2.2 Extramedullary Processes

Extramedullary processes usually begin with radicular or segmental pain, before enlargement of the lesion leads to progressive neurological deficits [34, 59, 76, 85]. They may be subdivided into intradural and extradural forms.

Extramedullary Intradural Processes

Neurinomas and meningiomas are the most common extramedullary intradural processes and are far more prevalent than angiomas, lipomas, metastases, and mass lesions of other etiology [5, 38, 47, 54, 55, 59, 74, 76, 85].

Neurinoma

Neurinomas, which are also called schwannomas and perineural fibroblastomas, are derived from the Schwann cells. Neurofibromas contain an additional fibrous tissue component consisting of proliferating perineural fibroblasts.

About 30% of all intraspinal tumors are neurinomas. They can occur at any level in the vertebral canal but show a predilection for the upper and middle cervical cord and the upper thoracic cord segments. Multiple foci should arouse suspicion of neurofibromatosis. Reports on sex ratio vary from 1:1 to a 2:1 predilection for females.

Because spinal neurinomas arise almost exclusively from the posterior nerve roots, more than 90% of them occur in the posterolateral quadrant of the vertebral canal. They are predominantly solid but may contain isolated cystic or hemorrhagic components; calcifications are rare. Grossly the tumor may be round, ovoid, or lobulated. Usually it is only a few centimeters in diameter, although lumbar neurinomas can attain a considerable size (Fig. 17.16 a). The tumors show no tendency to recur after complete removal [5, 34, 55, 59, 65, 74, 76, 80, 85].

MR Findings

Most neurinomas and neurofibromas have a signal intensity similar to that of adjacent neural structures, so they contrast well on T1-weighted images with the dark ambient CSF (Fig. 17.17 a, b). They present a slightly higher signal intensity on T2-weighted images, but then they contrast poorly with the equally bright CSF. Nevertheless, T2-weighted images are an essential part of the examination, because they can reflect the sometimes diverse histologic structures of the tumors. For example, mucinous neurinomas appear only slightly hyperintense to CSF on T1-weighted images and thus are more difficult to distinguish from CSF (Fig. 17.18) [4, 22, 23, 27, 28, 41, 79, 91].

If the adjacent intervertebral foramen is involved by an hourglass-shaped neurinoma, the expansion of the foramen can be detected on axial images (Fig. 17.19). The extent of paraspinal involvement is best appreciated on coronal sections (Fig. 17.20). Contrast images are useful only in ex-

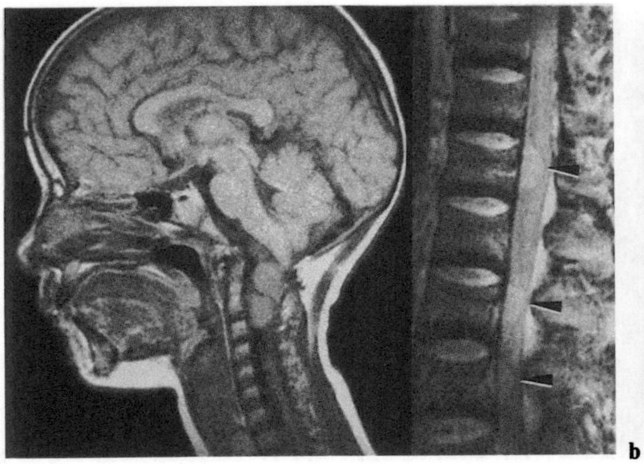

17.17

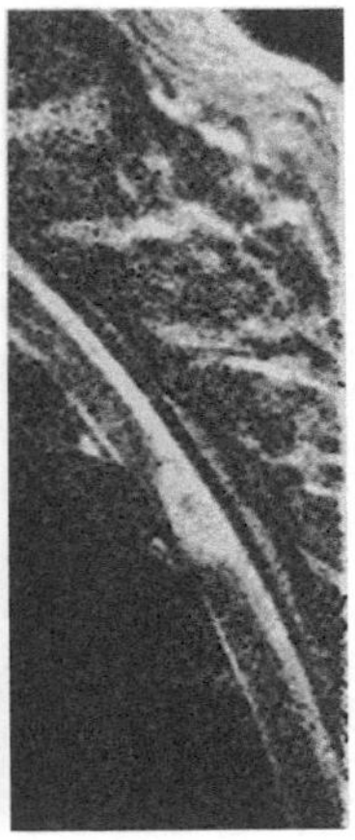

17.18

Fig. 17.17. **a** Neurofibromas in an 8-year-old boy with von Recklinghausen's disease. Three nodular lesions of varying signal intensity at the craniocervical junction with dorsal displacement of medulla and cord. They are well delineated by the dark CSF. **b** Multiple neurinomas in a 36-year-old man. Three clearly depicted hyperintense nodular tumors at the T12, L2, and L3 segments *(arrows)*. Sagittal scans: **a** SE 0.4 s/50 ms, **b** SE 1.5 s/50 ms (0.5 T)

Fig. 17.18. Neurinoma of the thoracic spine with mucoid degeneration in a 53-year-old man with progressive gait disturbances. Poor delineation of a hypointense mass at the level of T4 with T1-weighting. With heavy T2 weighting the extramedullary tumor mass can be differentiated from the cord more clearly due to its CSF-like signal intensity. Sagittal scan, SE 0.65 s/200 ms (0.5 T)

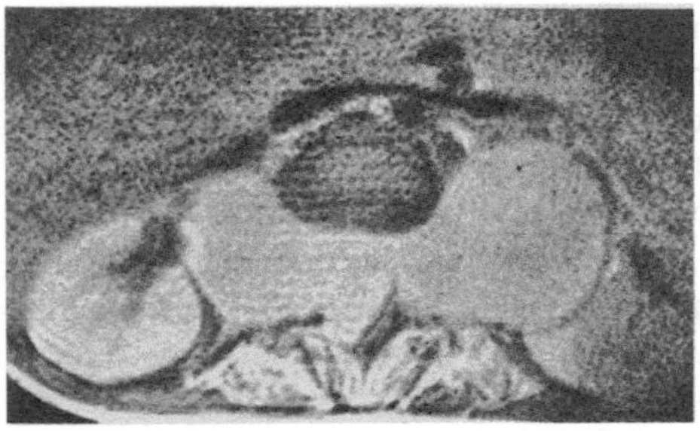

17.19

Fig. 17.19. Large hourglass neurinomas with bilateral dilatation of intervertebral foramina in a 12-year-old boy with slowly progressive gait disturbances for several years. The tumor extends bilaterally through the enlarged foramina into the paravertebral tissue. Axial scan with i.v. gadolinium-DTPA, SE 0.95 s/30 ms (0.5 T)

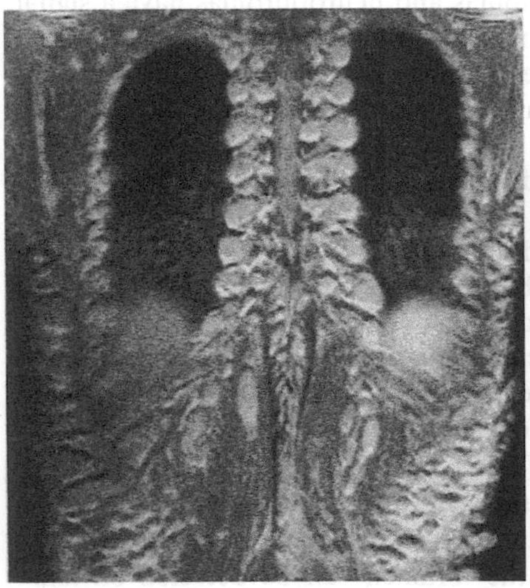

17.20

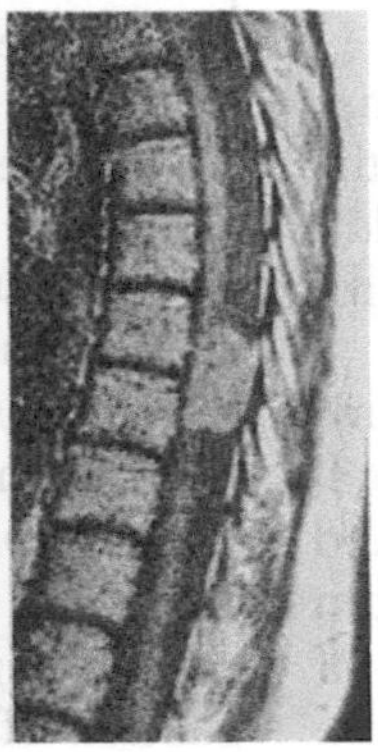

17.21

Fig. 17.20. Multiple neurinomas in a 29-year-old man with von Recklinghausen's disease. Tumor growth is seen in all intervertebral foramina of the thoracic spine. The paravertebral extension of the neurinomas is demonstrated clearly by this coronal section. SE 1.2 s/50 ms (0.5 T)

Fig. 17.21. Meningioma of the thoracic spine in a 51-year-old woman with progressive gait disturbances. Extramedullary, intradural, medium-intensity, nodular mass at T8/9 with anteriorly displaced spinal cord, which contrasts well with the dark CSF. Sagittal scan, SE 0.5 s/50 ms (0.5 T)

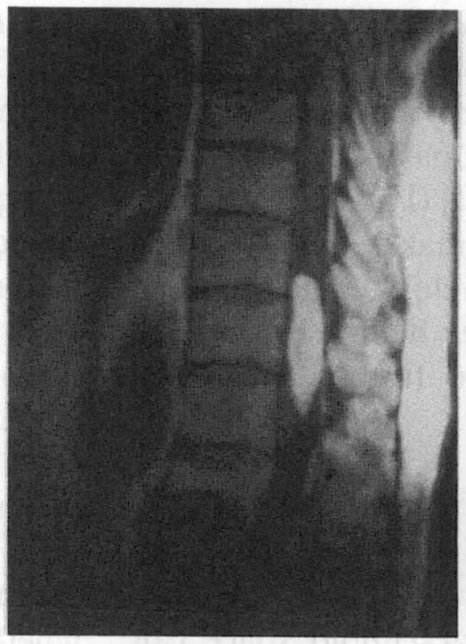

17.22

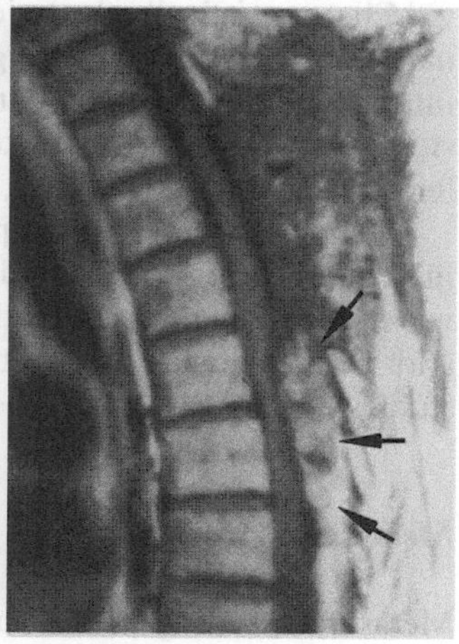

17.23

Fig. 17.22. Intradural lipoma in a 74-year-old man with progressive paraparesis, no additional dysraphic symptoms. The lipoma which seems attached to the cord was infiltrating the medullary conus. Sagittal scan, SE 0.5 s/30 ms (1.0 T)

Fig. 17.23. Hemangiolipoma in a 62-year-old woman with progressive paraplegia of lower extremities. Extradural dorsal mass of inhomogeneous structure, compressing the cord. Tumor recurrence caudal to the site of previous surgery. Sagittal scan, SE 0.3 s/17 ms; with i.v. gadolinium-DTPA rapid and marked enhancement of the tumor *(arrows)* was seen (1.0 T)

ceptional cases, because neurinomas generally stand out clearly in the low-intensity subarachnoid space, and the location and extent of the lesion are more important considerations for operative planning than tissue classification. Even with contrast injection, often it is not possible to make a pathologic diagnosis or differentiate the lesion from a meningioma.

Meningioma

Meningiomas develop mainly in the upper and middle thoracic region; they are extremely rare below L1. Females predominate by about 4:1. The tumors are most commonly detected between the fourth and seventh decades of life, substantially later than neurinomas and intramedullary tumors. Multiple meningiomas, especially when associated with neurinomas, are suspicious for neurofibromatosis.

Most meningiomas are globular in shape and, unlike neurinomas, may be situated anterior, lateral, or posterior to the spinal cord within the vertebral canal.

In contrast to the radicular symptoms of neurinomas, meningiomas tend to produce paraspastic signs and sensory disturbances [5, 34, 55, 59, 65, 74, 76, 80, 85].

MR Findings

The signal intensity of meningiomas corresponds to that of adjacent nerve tissues, so the lesions (like neurinomas) contrast well with the dark CSF on T1-weighted images (Fig. 17.21). Meningiomas usually appear isointense with the ambient CSF on T2-weighted scans [4, 30, 40, 79, 84, 91].

Hourglass-shaped growths are rare, but calcifications are often considered to be pathognomonic, especially in the psammomatous forms. On MR images these calcifications produce voids with little or no signal because of their low proton content.

The same considerations apply to the use of paramagnetic agents as for neurinomas. Nonspecific signal enhancement is seen only in uncalcified meningiomas.

Angioma

Arteriovenous malformations of the spine and spinal cord are described in detail in Chap. 14 (see Fig. 17.16 b).

Lipoma

Lipomas are most commonly found in the posterior part of the thoracic and lumbosacral vertebral canal. Extension over multiple segments is not unusual. These tumors are histologically benign; they may, however, infiltrate the spinal cord along the septa, so that complete removal is associated with a high risk of postoperative neurologic deficit (Fig. 17.22) [36, 57, 78, 87]. The origin of intradural spinal lipomas is unknown (see Sect. 7.3.4).

MR Findings

Lipomas are highly variable in size, shape, and extent.

Characteristically the lesions produce a high signal intensity on both T1-weighted and T2-weighted images, although the comparably high signal intensity of CSF on T2-weighted images creates problems of separation [4, 49, 60, 91] (Fig. 17.22).

It should be noted that lipomas frequently occur in conjunction with maldevelopmental tumors, vertebral anomalies, and other neoplastic lesions, and that this may necessitate further diagnostic studies (Fig. 17.23).

Metastases

Metastatic seeding in the subarachnoid space can occur in association with neuroepithelial tumors or cerebellar metastasis, but is relatively uncommon [76, 85].

MR Findings

Despite their typically small size, metastatic tumors give a relatively high signal on T1-weighted images isointense to the cord that contrasts well with the low-signal CSF. While most metastases appear as circumscribed foci, some may form a more plaque-like growth. With T2 weighting the lesions are easily missed because of their isointensity with the CSF.

Paramagnetic agents are indicated when non-contrast MR scans are negative or equivocal, because they produce enhancement of the metastases, similar to the effect of intravenous contrast medium in CT (Fig. 17.24).

Spinal Arachnoiditis

Spinal arachnoiditis produces circumscribed adhesions and thickenings of the meninges and presents both a cystic and a fibrous-adhesive form. It is most commonly seen in the upper thoracic cord or upper caudal region. Spinal arachnoiditis spanning several segments can result as a delayed complication of surgical procedures on the spinal cord, traumatic spinal injuries with bleeding into the meninges, and spinal meningitis. Less frequent causes are oily dye residues following myelography and a local reaction of the meninges to intraspinal tumors. Often the cause remains unknown [34, 76, 85].

MR Findings

In the portions of the subarachnoid space filled with foreign tissue of soft tissue density, the normally hypointense signal of the CSF space is not appreciated on T1-weighted images. The spinal cord may be displaced or distorted and may be poorly delineated. When changes are severe, differentiation from tumor or tumor recurrence can be difficult (Fig. 17.25; 17.26, see Fig. 17.44). Experience indicates that spinal arachnoiditis commonly does not produce hyperintensity on T2-weighted images, nor does it enhance on T1-weighted images after paramagnetic contrast injection. It remains unclear whether the age of the arachnoiditis can be established from its signal characteristics [49, 62, 91].

Spinal Subarachnoid Hemorrhage

After ruptured intracranial aneurysms, the most common causes of spinal subarachnoid hemorrhage are trauma (see Sect. 16.2) and vascular malformations. Other potential causes are anticoagulant drug therapy and bleeding from neoplasms [76, 85].

MR Findings

Very few reports on spinal subarachnoid hemorrhage are available, and its MR appearance is not well known. However, it is reasonable to expect that the MR features would correspond to those described for intramedullary hemorrhages (Fig. 17.27; see Figs. 5.5, 5.6, 16.11).

Extramedullary Extradural Processes

Extradural lesions arising from the vertebrae, the disc space, or the structures surrounding the vertebral canal can lead to intraspinal involvement that is best displayed on T1-weighted images; deformation of the subarachnoid space and displacement of the spinal cord can be appreciated very well on T2-weighted images [4, 22, 28, 34, 52, 81, 83, 91].

Lymphoma

When the spine becomes involved by a paravertebral lymphogranulomatosis or non-Hodgkin's lym-

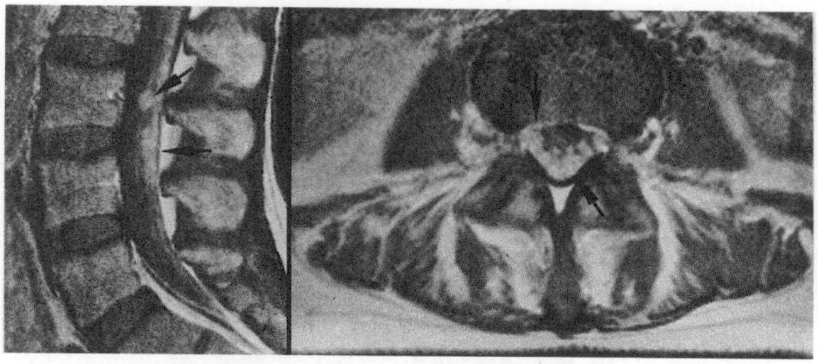

a b

Fig. 17.24 a, b. Intraspinal metastasis (meningiosis carcinomatosa) following radiotherapy of cerebellar metastasis of breast cancer in a 45-year-old woman with radiating pain in both legs. The nearly isointense metastases *(arrows)* enhance after i.v. gadolinium-DTPA. Midsagittal scan, **a** SE 0.4 s/30 ms; **b** axial scan, SE 0.4 s/30 ms (0.5 T)

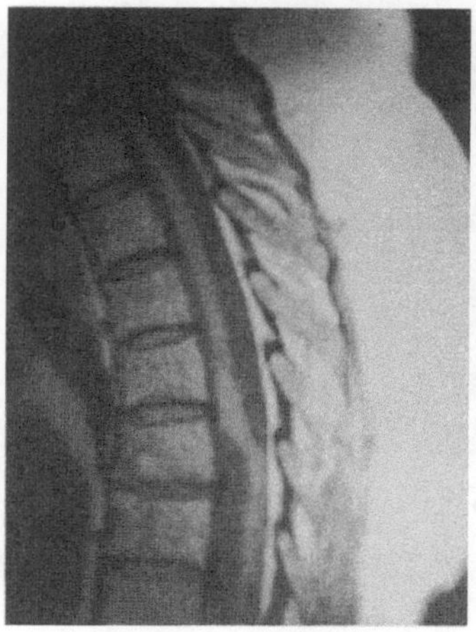

17.25

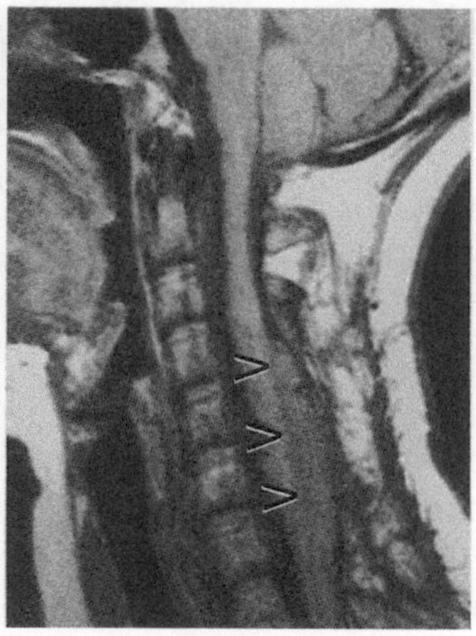

17.26

Fig. 17.25. Arachnopathy with adhesions and cysts (operative finding) in a 58-year-old woman with spastic paraparesis. Complete obstruction on myelography. Midsagittal scan, SE 0.4 s/35 ms (0.5 T). (Courtesy of Drs. Kuhn, Steen, and Terwey, Oldenburg, FRG)

Fig. 17.26. Spinal arachnopathy in a 41-year-old woman after removal of ependymoma of the cervical cord with progressive complaints in both arms. Dorsal mass lesion *(arrows)* of medium signal intensity separated from the spinal cord by a thin hypointense line. No displacement of the cord. Sagittal scan, SE 0.5 s/30 ms (0.5 T)

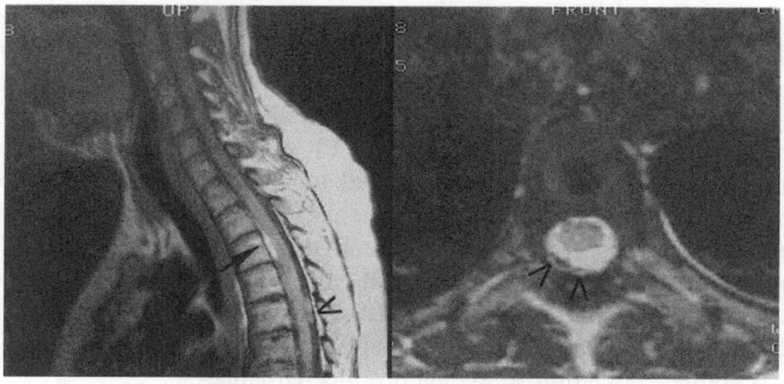

a b

Fig. 17.27 a, b. Spontaneous spinal subarachnoid hemorrhage from small dural-AV-fistula in a 36-year-old woman presenting with incomplete transient paraplegia, bloody lumbar tap, and complete stop in myelography. **a** One day after admission hyperdense (*arrow* at the level of T3) and isodense *(arrowhead at T5)* portions of the hematoma surrounding the cord were seen on T1-weighted images. Eight days later the clot at T3 is no longer seen, and in the axial scan **b** at the level of T5 hypointense clots *(arrowheads)* are attached to the wall of the subarachnoid space. **a** SE 0.45 s/15 ms; **b** SE 3.0 s/90 ms (1.5 T)

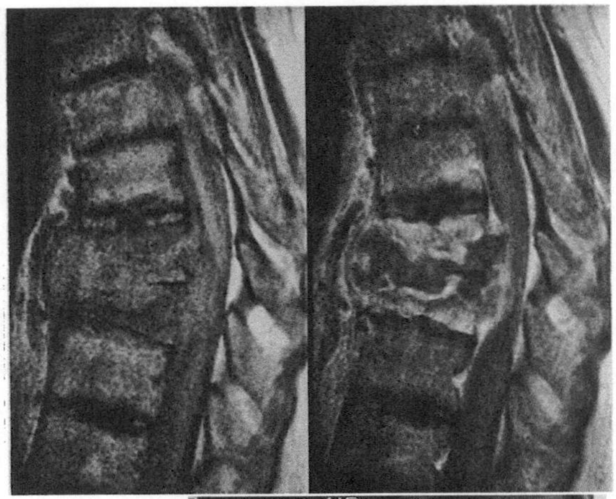

a b

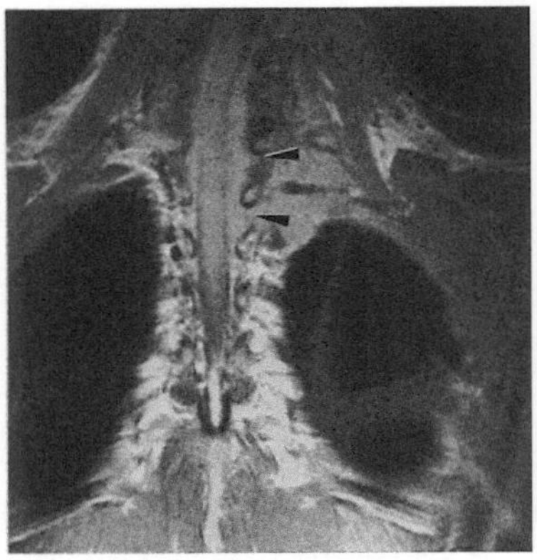

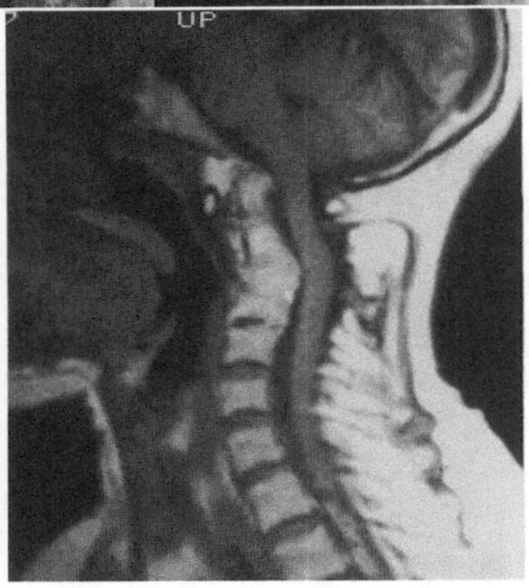

c

17.28 17.29

Fig. 17.28. Hodgkins lymphoma of the cervicothoracic junction in a 20-year-old woman with progressive weakness of arms and legs. Isointense, extradural mass lesion in the dorsal aspect of the spinal canal extending over five segments with ventral displacement of spinal cord. The tumor is well delineated by the hypointense dura mater. Infiltration of the intervertebral foramina on the left *(arrows)*. Coronal scan, SE 0.5 s/30 ms (1.5 T)

Fig. 17.29. a, b Epidural abscess (spondylodiscitis) at T8/9 in a 61-year-old woman with severe back pain and progressive paraparesis of both legs: **a** slightly hypointense mass lesion with paravertebral extension and compression of the spinal cord. The intervertebral disc cannot be differentiated; **b** with i.v. gadolinium-DTPA, enhancement of the affected vertebral bodies and part of the intervertebral disc, as well as better delineation of the paravertebral and intraspinal extension of the abscess. Sagittal scans: **a** SE 0.5 s/30 ms, **b** SE 0.4 s/30 ms (0.5 T). **c** Fused vertebrae (C2/3) after osteomyelitis in a 64-year-old woman with neck pain and slight difficulty in walking. Deformation of the vertebrae and anterior compression of the cord by the gibbus. Midsagittal scan, SE 0.4 s/17 ms (1.0 T)

phoma, the tumor tissue usually invades the vertebral canal through the intervertebral foramina and produces neurologic symptoms corresponding to the level of involvement.

MR Findings

Lymphomatous tissue overlying the spinal dura shows a moderate signal intensity on T1-weighted and T2-weighted images. The epidural location of the tumor is indicated by a dark boundary line, representing the displaced dura, between the tumor and the subarachnoid space or spinal cord. The total extent of the lesion can be established by the use of multiple image planes (Fig. 17.28) [9, 15, 31].

Paramagnetic contrast agents produce enhancement on T1 images only in tumor tissue that is still active.

Epidural Abscess

Spinal epidural abscess is usually hematogenous or postsurgical and is associated with severe pain, fever, inflammatory changes in the CSF, and tenderness to pressure and percussion over the affected area. The midthoracic and upper lumbar spinal segments are most commonly involved.

Compression of the vertebral canal by the abscess, combined with a disturbance of spinal blood flow, leads to rapidly progressive transverse cord symptoms [76, 85]. These symptoms may also be secondary to late sequelae of osteomyelitis.

MR Findings

The epidural abscess produces an elongated indentation of the subarachnoid space. It presents a moderate signal intensity on T1-weighted images, and heavier T2 weighting usually produces a marked rise of signal intensity.

Paramagnetic agents cause enhancement on T1-weighted images, clearly demarcating the abscess from the dark subarachnoid space (Fig. 17.29 a–c, see Fig. 17.55).

Rare Space-Occupying Lesions

Leukemic infiltration of the dura and sarcomas arising from the leptomeninges or vascular adventitia are not detectable with MR as long as the process is confined to the spinal meninges. Lesions that spread to the epidural space are visible on MR but are indistinguishable from other space-occupying lesions.

17.3 Spinal Tumors

17.3.1 Tumors Arising from Bone

Approximately 10% of primary bone tumors arise from the vertebral column. About 85% of these are benign and 15% malignant [21, 34, 36, 56, 58, 70, 85].

Previous experience with MR imaging of bone tumors indicates high sensitivity but low specificity, suggesting that the main value of MR is in defining the extent of a lesion in the medullary cavities and surrounding soft tissues. MR is a poor source of information on cortical bone changes or any pathologic calcifications that may be present [17, 52, 62, 68, 78].

As in other spinal disorders, the multislice SE technique is considered optimal for the evaluation of spinal tumors. T1-weighted images (TR 0.25–0.5 s/TE $\leqslant$ 30 ms) with a slice thickness of 5–10 mm are of particular value and can be effectively supplemented in some cases by an IR sequence. Surface coils can improve the signal-to-noise ratio for greater diagnostic accuracy and are especially useful for smaller lesions [3]. Further tissue characterization with MR (cystic component, hemorrhage) requires additional T2-weighted imaging. For a lesion that is already detected and unaccompanied by perifocal reaction, this can be satisfactorily accomplished by a multiecho single-slice acquisition (e.g., TR 0.9 s/TE 50/100/150/200 ms). If the tumor has infiltrated the surrounding soft tissue, a T2-weighted multislice series should be added (TR 1.3–2.0 s/TE 50/100 ms).

Most tumors of this group are hypointense on T1-weighted images and hyperintense on T2-weighted images. There is no clear explanation for this, although it may relate to an increased water content in the tissue [17, 68, 78].

Osteoid Osteoma

Osteoid osteomas predominantly affect males in the second and third decades of life. About 20% involve the vertebral column, showing a predilection for the neural arch and articular processes of the thoracolumbar vertebrae [21, 34, 56, 57, 70, 85].

MR Findings

Because the nidus may be hypervascularized and sclerotic, its signal characteristics are variable. There is some evidence that a predominantly high-signal nidus is a consistent feature on T2-weighted images and thus could be used for differential diagnosis, but this has not been proved. Also, we have little information on the degree of the bone density increase and sclerosis that are associated with this tumor [17, 78].

Osteoblastoma

Osteoblastomas comprise the largest proportion (40%) of benign spinal tumors. They mostly affect children and adolescents and, like osteoid osteomas, show a predilection for the neural arch [34, 70, 85].

MR Findings

Expansion of the bone by the tumor is apparent on T1-weighted sequences. The hypointense periphery of the lesion, visible on T1-weighted and T2-weighted images, represents the calcium-dense shell. Calcifications are usually present in the tumor and create signal voids. There are no signs of perifocal reaction. The increased signal intensity on T2 images reflects the hypervascularity of the lesion. The relation of the tumor to the intraspinal space is well appreciated on sagittal sections [17, 68, 78].

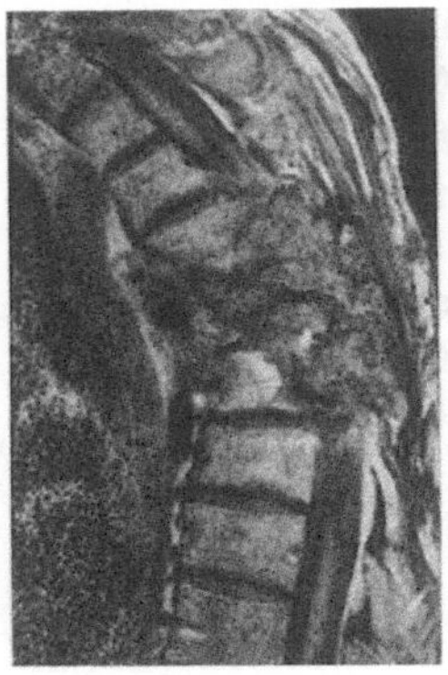

17.30

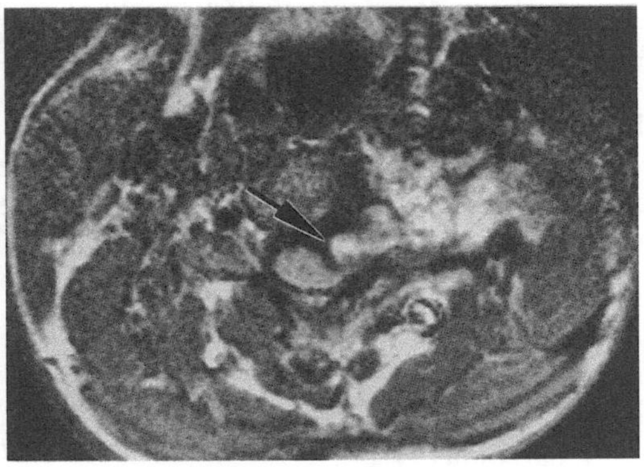

17.31

Fig. 17.30. Chondroblastoma in a 64-year-old man with unsteady gait. Nodular mass with inhomogeneous structure between T4 and T6, extending into the paravertebral and dorsal soft tissue. Midsagittal scan, SE 0.55 s/30 ms (0.5 T)

Fig. 17.31. Chondroma at C4–C6 in a 22-year-old man with multiple cartilaginous exostoses. Irregular, nodular, hyperintense mass involving the vertebrae C4–C6; compression of the cord by intraspinal extension of the tumor *(arrow)*. Axial scan, SE 0.4 s/30 ms (0.5 T)

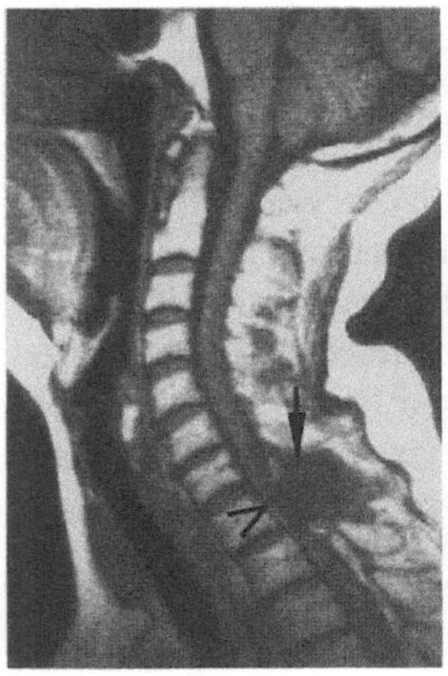

17.32

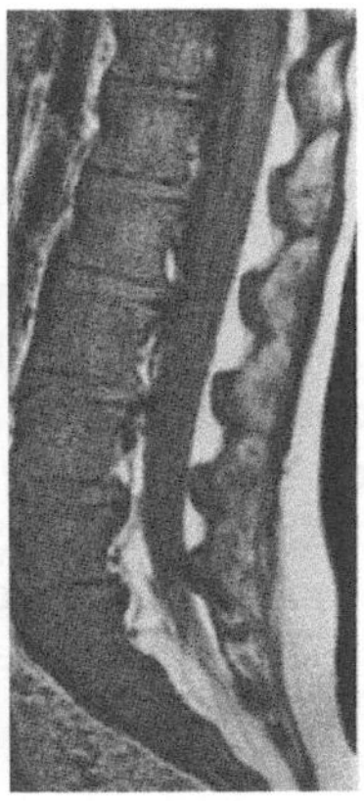

17.33

Fig. 17.32. Chondrosarcoma of first thoracic vertebra in a 55-year-old woman with paraplegia, accentuated on the right. Extradural tumor *(arrow)* with long T1 and T2 with destruction of the neural arch and spine compressing the cord *(arrowhead)*. Midsagittal scan, SE 0.4 s/35 ms (0.5 T). (Courtesy of Drs. Kuhn, Steen, and Terwey, Oldenburg, FRG.)

Fig. 17.33. Normal vertebrae in a 2-year-old child. Physiological, low signal intensity of infantile bone marrow compared to high signal intensity of adult bone marrow with fatty degeneration. Sagittal scan, SE 0.4 s/30 ms (1.5 T)

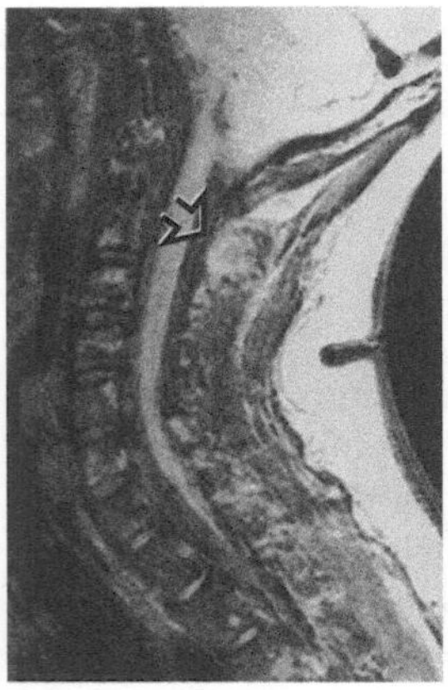

17.34

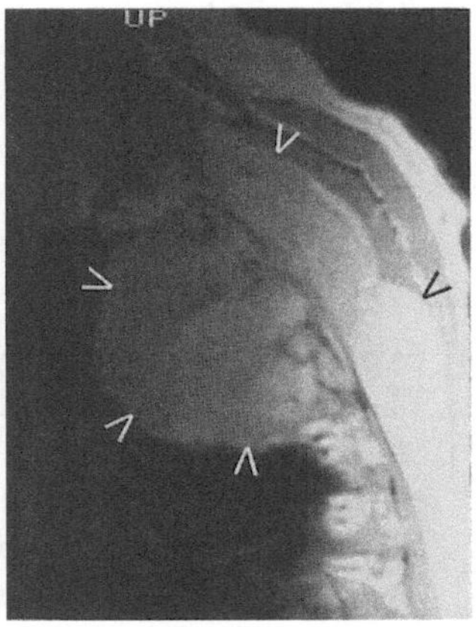

17.35

Fig. 17.34. Plasmocytoma in a 42-year-old man with neck pain and osteolysis of spinous process of C2 as seen on plain X-ray. Irregular distension of spinous process of C2 with low to medium signal intensity on the T1-weighted image. With heavier T2 weighting the signal of the osteolytic process increases *(open arrow)*. Multiple, patchy areas of increased signal intensity are seen also in other vertebrae of the cervical and thoracic spine without intraspinal tumor extension. Midsagittal scan, SE 2.4 s/50 ms (0.5 T)

Fig. 17.35. Known plasmocytoma in a 55-year-old man. Large paravertebral tumor mass *(arrowheads)* invading the vertebral canal, the paravertebral tissue and the thorax. Sagittal scan, SE 2.0 s/30 ms (1.0 T)

Chondroblastoma, Chondroma, Osteochondroma

Chondroblastoma, chondroma, and osteochondroma are rare in the vertebral column and are most prevalent in persons under 30 years of age. The MR findings correspond basically to those of osteoblastoma (Figs. 17.30; 17.31; 17.32).

Osteoclastoma

Given the rich vascularity of osteoclastoma (vertebral giant cell tumor) and its typical extension over multiple segments, it is reasonable to expect marked hyperintensity on T2-weighted images and marked enhancement on T1-weighted images after paramagnetic contrast injection [17, 68, 78].

Sarcoma

The various types of sarcoma are very rarely (0.8%–2%) seen in the axial skeleton. They are mostly found in the lumbar and sacral regions (Fig. 17.32). MR changes specific for sarcoma are unknown. Malignancy is evidenced by signs of infiltration and destruction of surrounding tissues, irregular margins, and extension over two or more segments [17, 68, 78].

17.3.2 Tumors Arising from the Bone Marrow and Blood Cells

Normal bone marrow in adults consists mostly of fat (yellow) marrow and therefore gives a signal like that of fatty tissue (nonpolar storage fat: short T1, long T2). The bone marrow in children, on the other hand, contains a larger proportion of hematopoietic (red) marrow, which yields a lower signal on T1-weighted images and can make it more difficult to detect infiltrations of the marrow (Fig. 17.33).

Even in older patients, the bone marrow of the vertebral bodies is richer in cellular elements than the femur or the flat bones, and thus has a generally lower MR signal intensity. Thus, primary or at least supplementary examination of the pelvis and femur is indicated if there is suspicion of diffusely infiltrating bone marrow disease [13, 17, 27, 52, 62, 78].

Bone marrow tumors primarily involve areas of high hematopoietic activity, like the pelvis and vertebral bodies. As the infiltration increases the cellularity and water content of the affected bone marrow, its T1 becomes longer, resulting in decreased signal intensity on T1-weighted images. The degree of signal decrease depends on the degree of infiltration.

The changes are portrayed best on sagittal SE multislice images with T1 weighting (TR 0.25–0.5 s/TE $\leq$ 30 ms). T2-weighted images generally are unnecessary. A multiecho single-slice image (TR 0.9 s/TE 50/100/150/200 ms) may be obtained for tissue characterization.

Plasmocytoma

Plasmocytomas account for about 10%–15% of primary tumors of the spinal column. They generally originate from the vertebral bodies, are usually multiple, and may spread to involve the paravertebral soft tissues [21, 34, 57, 58, 70, 85].

MR Findings

The plasmocytoma displaces the normal bone marrow, producing a focus of decreased signal intensity on T1-weighted images and a hyperintense focus on T2-weighted images (Figs. 17.34, 17.35; similar to Fig. 17.36).

The advantage of MR imaging is its ability to establish the number of involved vertebrae and confirm or exclude involvement of the spinal cord and paravertebral soft tissues in a single examination.

Leukemia

Vertebral involvement is generally present in granulocytic leukemia as well as in the lymphatic forms. There may be direct medullary infiltration as well as paraspinal or intraspinal extension.

MR Findings

Lesions cause a decrease in MR signal intensity on T1-weighted images commensurate with the degree of infiltration. For example, an acute exacerbation (e.g., a blast crisis in chronic granulocytic leukemia) leads to an almost total loss of signal, while a more patchy signal pattern is characteristic of the chronic forms. The potential value of MR for detecting changes and recurrences and for monitoring response to bone marrow transplantation is unclear at

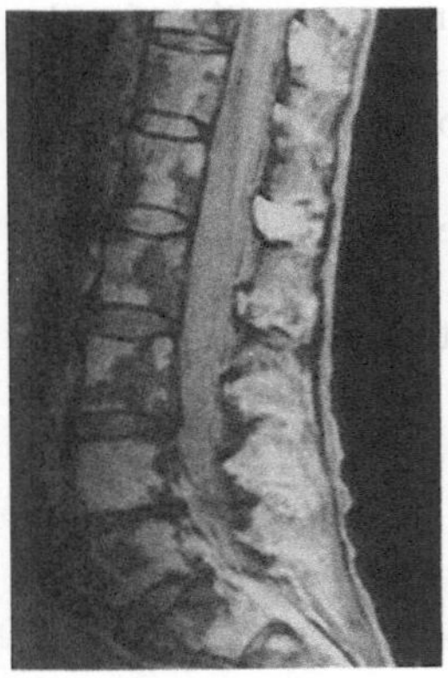

17.36

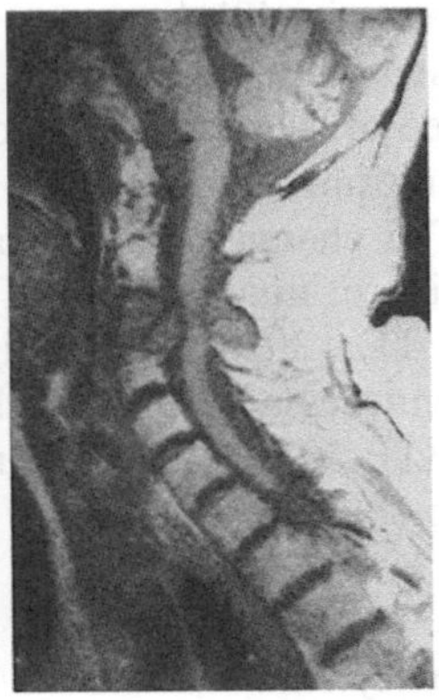

17.37

Fig. 17.36. Non-Hodgkin lymphoma with infiltration of bone in a 64-year-old man with symptoms of cauda and conus compression. Multiple patchy areas of decreased signal intensity are seen within several vertebrae of the lower spine; no intraspinal extension. Sagittal scan, SE 2.4 s/50 ms (1.5 T)

Fig. 17.37. Osteolytic metastasis of hypernephroma at C3 in a 66-year-old woman after radiotherapy of the cervical spine, presenting with transverse lesion of the cord. Destruction of vertebra C3 by a hypointense mass lesion, with ventral and dorsal compression of the cord. Increased signal intensity of vertebrae C1-C6 secondary to radiotherapy. Sagittal scan, SE 0.4 s/30 ms (1.5 T)

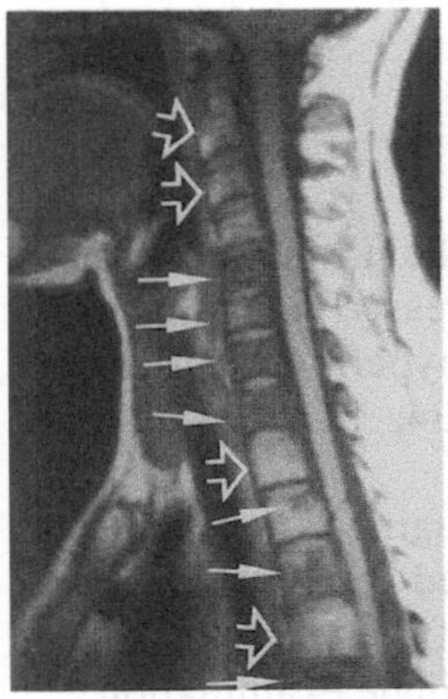

17.38

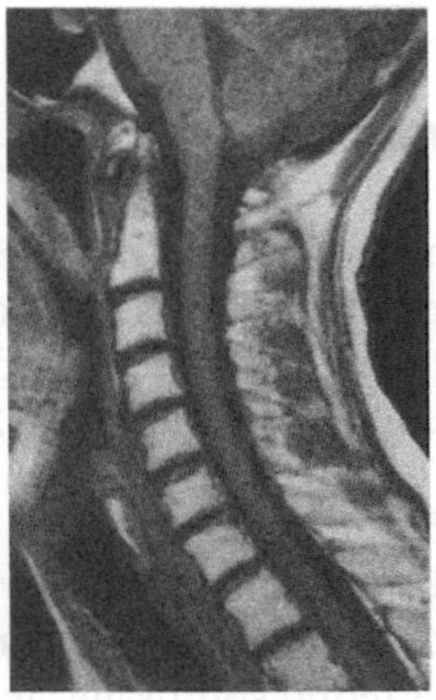

17.39

Fig. 17.38. Multiple metastases in a 45-year-old woman with carcinoma of the breast. Multiple lesions in the spine *(arrows)* which are hypointense compared to the normal vertebrae *(open arrow)*. Sagittal scans, SE 0.4 s/17 ms (1.0 T)

Fig. 17.39. Condition after radiotherapy of glomus (caroticum) tumor. Increased signal intensity of cervical vertebrae within the radiation field used to treat the glomus tumor. Sagittal scan, SE 0.25 s/30 ms (1.5 T)

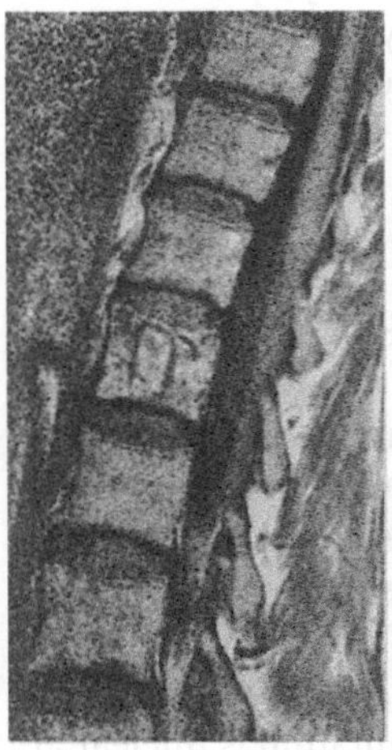

17.40

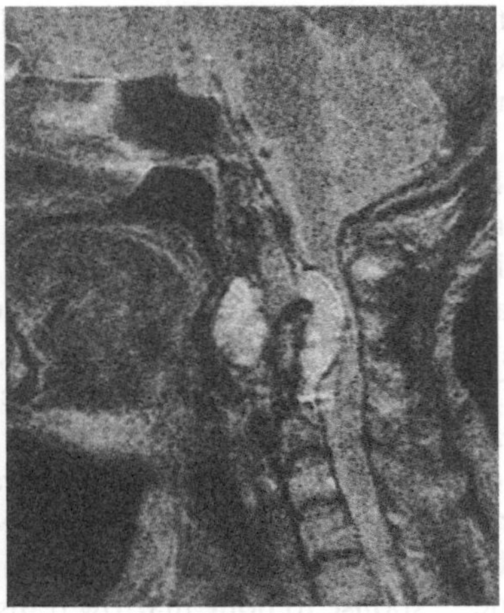

17.41

Fig. 17.40. Hamartoma of vertebra L1 in a 51-year-old woman with nonspecific back pain. Slight increase of signal intensity of the body of vertebra L1 with hypointense trabeculae. The lesion, which does not extend into the vertebral canal, cannot be distinguished from histiocytosis X (see Fig. 17.42). Midsagittal scan, SE 0.5 s/30 ms (0.5 T)

Fig. 17.41. Chordoma of the cervical spine: recurrent tumor in a 47-year-old woman. The extradural location is indicated by the sharp, hypointense convex borderline of the tumor. On the T2-weighted scan (SE 1.35 s/100 ms) the paravertebral and intraspinal portions of the hyperintense tumor and the dorsal displacement of the hypointense cord can be evaluated (0.5 T)

the present time. Normalization of the MR bone marrow signal has been observed, but occurs later than normalization of the biopsy findings and clinical course [13, 17, 52, 62, 78].

Lymphoma

Lymphomas, especially the non-Hodgkin's variety, can lead to primary osseous involvement as well as to paraspinal changes that spread secondarily to the bone.

MR Findings

Lymphomas tend to form focal lesions within the bone marrow of the vertebral bodies. These foci give relatively low signals on T1-weighted images and can be demonstrated earlier than with scintigraphy (Fig. 17.36). Similar signal changes are seen following infarctions and in association with inflammation, myelofibrosis, metastases, and sarcomas [17, 27, 37, 48, 52, 62, 68, 69, 75, 78, 82, 88].

Metastases

The primary tumors most commonly giving rise to vertebral metastases in adults are bronchial carcinoma, breast carcinoma, renal carcinoma, and prostatic carcinoma.

MR Findings

Osteolytic foci have a long T1 and are clearly demonstrated on T1-weighted images (Figs. 17.37, 17.38). If findings are questionable, metastases can be recognized as high-signal foci on T2-weighted images.

Osteoplastic metastases with new bone formation give a low signal on T1-weighted and T2-weighted images.

MR cannot replace scintigraphy or conventional roentgenography in the diagnosis of vertebral metastases, but it can supply useful information if the findings are equivocal (e.g., severe pain with a negative isotope scan) and can confirm or exclude spinal involvement [17, 52, 62, 78].

Radiation Effects

From about a month after radiotherapy, T1-weighted images may show an increase in signal intensity caused by the destruction of normal hematopoietic tissue and its replacement by fatty tissue (Figs. 17.37, 17.39). A recurrence causes the signal intensity to decrease; a similar picture can be seen in aplastic anemia [17, 52, 62, 66, 68, 78].

17.3.3 Tumors of Vascular Origin

Hamartoma

Most vertebral hamartomas occur in the lower thoracic or upper lumbar spine, and many are discovered fortuitously. The tumors generally involve the vertebral body, and about 90% are solitary [21, 34, 56, 57, 70, 85].

MR Findings

Hamartomas are exceptional among vertebral body tumors in that they appear hyperintense on both T1-weighted and T2-weighted images, owing to their short or moderate T1 and long T2. It is common to see rootlike voids within the hyperintense vertebral body which represent bony trabeculae (Fig. 17.40). The expansion of the vertebral body can be seen on sagittal images, while neural arch involvement is displayed better on axial sections [17, 39, 78].

MR permits the early detection of hamartoma, whereas conventional roentgenograms and X-ray tomograms do not show abnormalities until more than 25% of the vertebral body is involved.

17.3.4 Other Tumors and Tumor-Like Lesions

Chordoma

Approximately 15%–20% of malignant primary vertebral tumors are chordomas. These tumors, which grow by infiltration, usually develop in middle-aged patients at the craniocervical, lumbosacral, or sacrococcygeal junction and involve multiple segments. The prognosis is poor [21, 34, 58, 70, 85].

MR Findings

MR examination of these tumors reveals no signs typical of chordoma except the location. Infiltrative growth and extension into the vertebral canal with compression of intraspinal structures are best appreciated on sagittal images (Fig. 17.41) [17, 42, 71, 86].

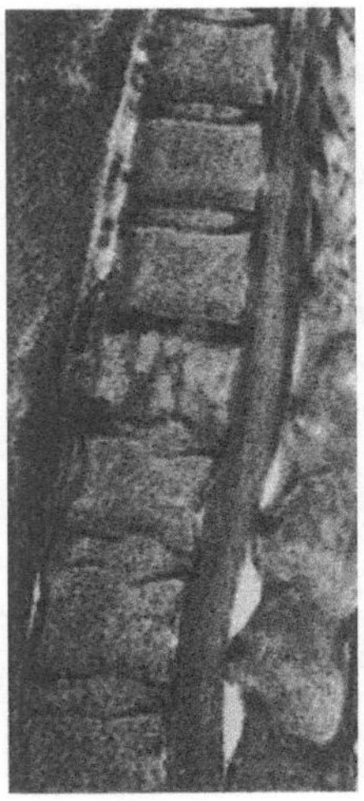

17.42

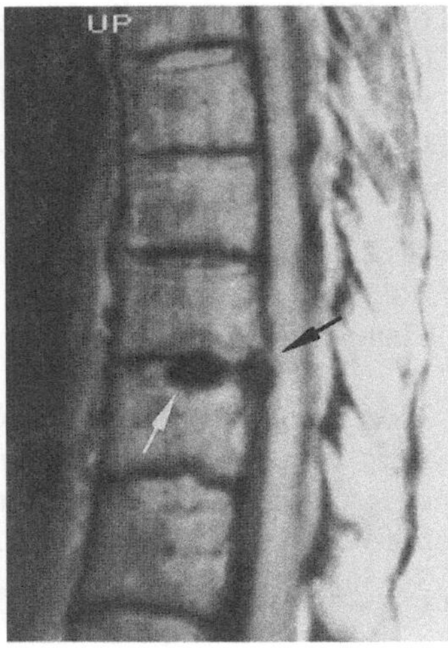

17.43

Fig. 17.42. Histiocytosis X at L1 in an 18-year-old man with back pain. Prolonged T1 and T2 of L1 with hypointense focal lesion within the body of the vertebra. The sagittal diameter of the body is slightly elongated with flattening of its anterior portion. Discreet dorsal dislocation of the cord. Decreased signal of the adjacent intervertebral disc. With i.v. gadolinium-DTPA, enhancement of L1 was seen, the streaky hypointensities remaining unchanged. Sagittal scan, SE 0.5 s/30 ms (1.5 T)

Fig. 17.43. Granulomatous calcinosis in a 54-year-old woman with severe back pain. Small, intraspinal mass lesion at the level of the intervertebral disc with dislocation and compression of the spinal cord *(arrows)*. The lesion is hypointense in all sequences due to the calcification. Midsagittal scans, SE 1.6 s/35 ms (1.5 T)

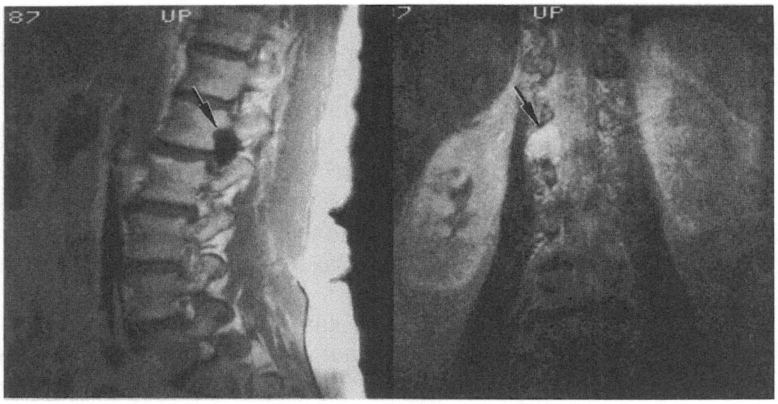

a b

Fig. 17.44 a, b. Chronic adhesive cystic arachnoiditis in a 66-year-old woman with radicular symptoms on the right. At surgery a cyst *(arrows)* was found, formed by scar tissue and containing clear fluid. **a** Sagittal scan, SE 0.4 s/17 ms; **b** coronal scan, SE 2.0 s/90 ms (1.0 T)

Aneurysmal Bone Cyst

Aneurysmal bone cysts usually originate from the vertebral bodies, are most common in younger patients, and mainly affect the cervical and thoracic vertebrae [21, 34, 70, 85].

MR Findings

The osteolytic defect of the aneurysmal bone cyst gives a low signal on T1-weighted images, is usually confined to one vertebra, and does not incite a perifocal reaction. With larger cysts, involvement of adjacent structures (e.g., ribs) may be seen. The calcium-dense border of the cyst forms a smooth, sharp wall devoid of signal. Low-signal areas within the cyst represent bony septa. Because of its rich vascularization, the lesion produces an intense signal on T2-weighted images. Enhancement on T1-weighted images would be expected to occur after paramagnetic contrast injection [7, 17, 78].

Histiocytosis X

A systemic disease, histiocytosis X is most prevalent in children and adolescents. If the vertebral column is involved, additional foci are present in more than 50% of cases, especially in the flat bones [34, 57, 78] (see also Sect. 10.5).

MR Findings

In the one case of histiocytosis X that we have examined thus far, we observed lacunar defects in the affected vertebra. The features seen on T1-weighted and T2-weighted images were identical to those described for vertebral hamartoma. Injection of paramagnetic contrast material produced marked enhancement of the lesion on T1-weighted scans (Fig. 17.42).

Granulomatous Calcinosis

The etiology of granulomatous calcinosis is obscure but the disease is believed to relate to a metabolic abnormality. The calcinosis may be composed of hyaline cartilage from the vertebral body end-plates. Noncontrast X-rays show calcifications in the disc space and often lead to the misdiagnosis of a calcified nucleus pulposus [70].

MR Findings

Sagittal T1-weighted and T2-weighted images at the level of the affected intervertebral space show a hypointense or signal-free mass projecting into the epidural space, resembling a ruptured and dehydrated disc (Fig. 17.43). For comparison, see the case of chronic adhesive cystic arachnoiditis depicted in Fig. 17.44. On T1-weighted images the lesion appears hypointense, as in granulomatous calcinosis. With T2 weighting, however, the cystic lesion has a high signal intensity while the signal of the calcification remains low.

17.4 Degenerative Diseases of the Spine

17.4.1 Intervertebral Disc Disease

MR imaging using surface coils and thin-section technique can provide results at least comparable to those attainable with CT, especially when a high-field system is used. Other advantages of MR are its high contrast resolution and its ability to depict individual spinal segments without superimposition by the use of variable image planes and acquisition sequences [3, 18, 44, 50, 51, 67, 89, 90].

The examination begins with a "fast" axial scan that provides orientation for the initial sagittal multislice series. The sagittal sections permit accurate evaluation of the structures of the intervertebral disc, including the nucleus pulposus and anulus fibrosus, and they enables the signal intensities of adjacent discs to be directly compared. They also demonstrate the relation of the disc to the posterior longitudinal ligament and dural sac.

If an abnormality is detected, supplementary axial images are taken at an angle matching the orientation of the disc space being examined.

It is standard practice to use SE multislice sequences for this examination, with TR 1.5-2.0 s and TE $\leqslant$ 20-100 ms. The recommended slice thickness is 5 mm for sagittal images and 3 mm for axial images. The signal-to-noise ratio is improved by the use of flexible surface coils [3, 18, 52, 64].

Normal Disc Anatomy on MR Images

The normal intervertebral disc appears on sagittal images as a transverse oval-shaped structure of high signal intensity situated between the thin, dark cortical end-plates of the adjacent vertebral bodies. The high signal intensity with long TR results from the high water content of the disc, which ranges from 70% to 85% depending on the age of the patient [38, 45, 55, 64, 67]. The nucleus pulposus and inner ring of the anulus fibrosus form the high-intensity core of the disc. The outer ring of the anulus fibrosus gives a less intense signal because of the lower water content of the collagenous fibrocartilage; the signal is especially low in the posterior part of the disc space. The dark line often seen at the center of the disc (Fig. 17.2b) has been identified histologically as connective tissue ingrowth [1, 18, 64]. The posterior longitudinal ligament running behind the intervertebral disc contrasts sharply with the high-intensity CSF (T2 weighting) because of its lack of signal. The ligament forms a dark boundary line that includes the dura, which also is devoid of signal.

The high signal intensity of epidural fat on both T1-weighted and T2-weighted sequences serves to demarcate it from the adjacent bony structures and ligaments. The fatty tissue may be seen posterior to the vertebral bodies, in the lateral recess, and in the intervertebral foramina; it is not visible at the level of the disc spaces. It varies greatly in conspicuousness among individuals.

Degenerative Disc Changes

Normal aging processes as well as premature degeneration of the disc tissue alter the consistency of the avascular nucleus pulposus. Its water content is decreased, and the associated reduction in proton

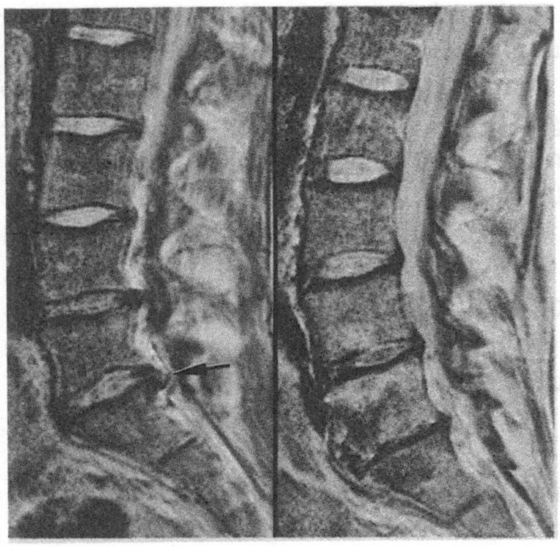
a b

Fig. 17.45. **a** Prolapse of degenerated discs of L4/5 and L5/S1 segments in a 21-year-old man. Moderate decrease of signal intensity of L4/5 and L5/S1 discs. At L5/S1 sequestration of part of nucleus pulposus behind S1 is seen *(arrow).* Sagittal scan, SE 2.0 s/50 ms. **b** Various grades of disc degeneration in a 56-year-old woman. The signal of L1/2 and L2/3 intervertebral spaces reflects normal hydration of the discs. At L3/4 slight decrease of water content is indicated by a reduced signal intensity. At T12/L1, L4/5, and even more so at L5/S1, severe degeneration of the discs is revealed by further decrease of the signal. At L5/S1 a signal of the disc is no longer seen. Osseous reaction predominantly at L5. Sagittal scan, SE 1.8 s/50 ms (1.5 T)

content lowers its signal intensity on proton-density and/or T2-weighted images until it becomes indistinguishable from the anulus fibrosus. All gradations exist between the healthy disc, which gives an intense MR signal, and the degenerated disc, which gives no signal (Fig. 17.45 a, b). Changes in signal intensity and narrowing of the disc space are most commonly seen in the lumbar region, whereas structural and morphologic irregularities tend to be seen in the cervical region [1, 44, 50, 53, 64, 67, 89].

It is relatively rare for degenerating discs to herniate. On the other hand, herniation is common in discs that are appropriately hydrated for age, especially when the disc is subjected to sudden compressive forces. Long-standing protrusions consistently produce a loss of signal intensity.

Intervertebral Disc Herniation

The neurologic symptoms of disc herniation depend on the level of the herniation, the volume of the herniated material, and the direction of the protrusion (posterior, posterolateral, lateral) as well as on the surrounding anatomic structures. Even a small protrusion will cause complaints in a narrow vertebral canal, while a larger protrusion may be well tolerated in the presence of a thick epidural fat layer [8, 10, 23, 24, 58, 76, 77, 80, 85, 87].

Pathoanatomically, a disc herniation involves the protrusion of a portion of the nucleus pulposus through a tear in the anulus fibrosus, with associated stretching of the posterior longitudinal ligament. A distinction is made between a disc protrusion, which is reversible, and a disc prolapse in which portions of the nucleus pulposus herniate through a complete rupture of the fibrous ring.

A progressive posterior or posterolateral herniation can even lead to rupture of the posterior longitudinal ligament and tearing of the dura mater [8, 12, 24, 38, 55, 58, 84]. Calcifications may form within the herniated disc material but are not easily identified with MR. The extruded portion of the nucleus pulposus may become detached, forming a sequestrum (see Fig. 17.3 a). The fragment may lie in front of or behind the posterior longitudinal ligament and may migrate some distance from the affected segment.

Herniated discs are displayed best on T2-weighted images because of the good contrast between the herniated material and CSF, and we recommend that T2-weighted images be obtained in these cases as a primary study.

T1-weighted images are useful for distinguishing the lower-signal nerve roots from the high-signal epidural fat in the region of the intervertebral foramina (Fig. 17.1 b).

If the nucleus pulposus and the inner ring of the anulus fibrosus still show a sufficient signal intensity, it may be possible to see the divergence of the lower-intensity outer ring of the anulus fibrosus on sagittal images when a prolapse exists (Fig. 17.46). However, this is not a reliable morphologic criterion for distinguishing between protrusion and prolapse, so that, as in CT, attention must be paid to the degree of the herniation, its effect on the dural sac, and the possible involvement of the spinal cord or cauda equina.

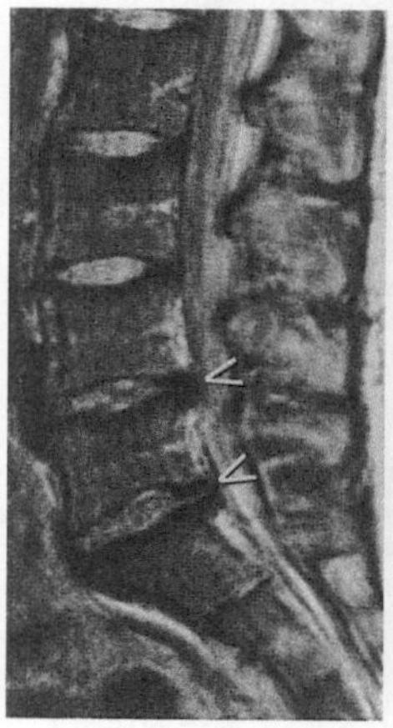

17.46

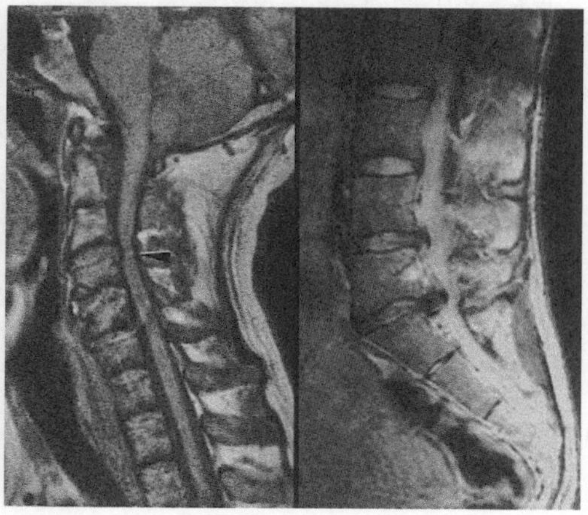

17.47 b

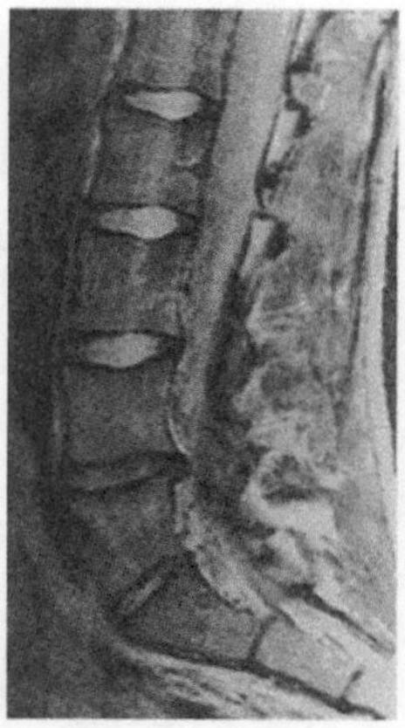

17.48

Fig. 17.46. Dissociation of anulus fibrosus in a 21-year-old man with sciatica. At L4/5 and L5/S1 the diverging anulus fibrosus *(arrows)* gives way to a tongue-shaped dorsal dislocation of the nucleus pulposus. Sagittal scan, SE 2.0 s/30 ms (1.5 T)

Fig. 17.47. **a** Cervical disc prolapse at C3/4 in a 38-year-old man with spastic tetraparesis. Collar-button-shaped prolapse of nucleus pulposus at C3/4 with cord compression *(arrow)* which is aggravated by a narrow canal. Note the anomaly of the dens axis. Sagittal scan, SE 0.3 s/30 ms. **b** Simultaneous prolapse of L4/5 and L5/S1 intervertebral discs in a 19-year-old man with back pain for 1 year radiating into the right leg, incipient paresis. The bulging disc material is tongue-shaped at L4/5, compared to the more dumbbell-shaped prolapse of L5/S1. Sagittal scan, SE 1.5 s/60 ms (1.5 T)

Fig. 17.48. Disc prolapse with intact posterior longitudinal ligament in a 20-year-old man with sciatica. Hypointense signal of L4/5 and L5/S1 intervertebral spaces due to dehydration. Disc prolapse at L4/5 lumbar segment. Hypointense borderline dorsal to the intervertebral discs of L2/3, L3/4, and L4/5 indicates an intact posterior longitudinal ligament. Sagittal scan, SE 2.4 s/50 ms (1.5 T)

A dumbbell-shaped or collar-button configuration of the hyperintense disc tissue is strongly suggestive of a prolapse (Fig. 17.47 a, b).

In cases where the disc still presents an adequate signal intensity, and the sagittal image shows the dark boundary line of the posterior longitudinal ligament bulging toward the vertebral canal but displaying no discontinuities, it is likely that a rupture does not exist (Fig. 17.48).

Differentiation between a posterior and a posterolateral herniation can usually be accomplished with multislice images on the sagittal plane. A posterolateral herniation is recognized by its tendency to obliterate, on lateral sections, the epidural fat in the vicinity of the intervertebral foramen on the side of the affected segment (Fig. 49 a–c) [12, 63, 67, 90].

However, axial images permit a more accurate appraisal of the situation because of the improved visualization of nervous structures (Fig. 49 b). Axial images are essential, in fact, for demonstrating a lateral herniation. In these cases the use of a mixed sequence with TR of 2.0 s and TE of 30 ms provides maximal contrast between the structures of interest [18, 50–53, 64, 67]. The long TR also permits the acquisition of numerous sections without prolonging the examination time, making it possible to image about three segments concurrently. It should be added, however, that perfect angulation is usually obtained for only one segment in the multislice series.

The herniation is recognized by lateral disparities in the epidural fat layer, the visible presence of foreign tissue, and edematous thickening of the altered nerve roots.

Dehydrated disc tissue is unfavorable for MR imaging, because the reduced signal intensity makes it difficult to distinguish such tissue from posterior osteophytes. Occasionally the spondylophytes undergo secondary spongiform changes, making them easier to identify (Fig. 17.49 c). On the

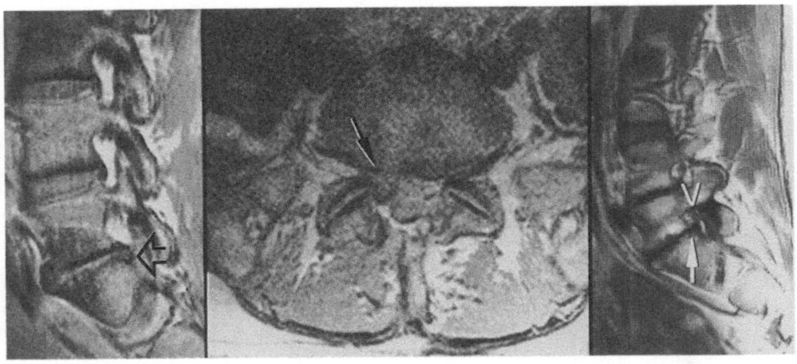

a b c

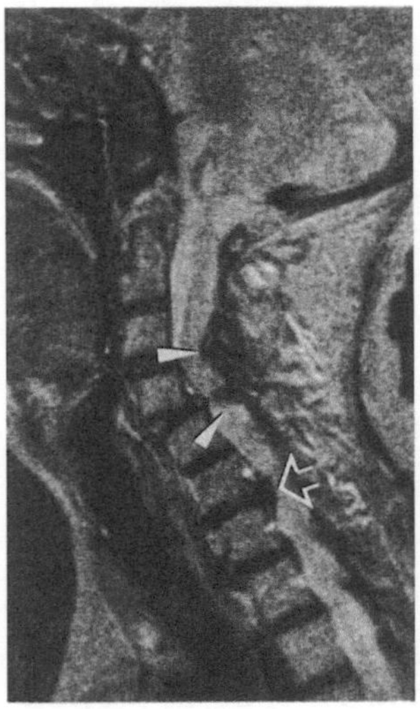

17.50

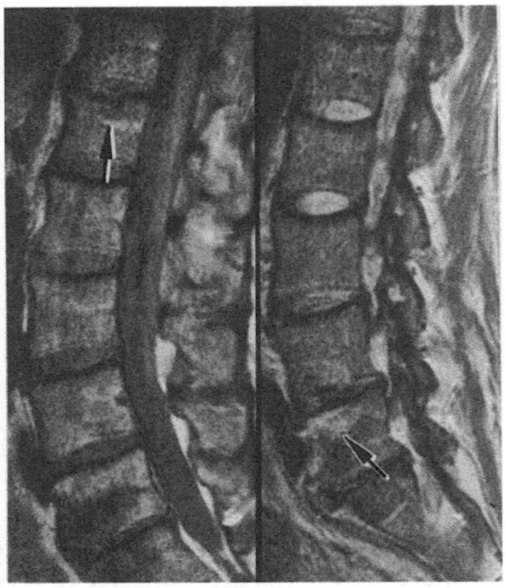

a b

17.51

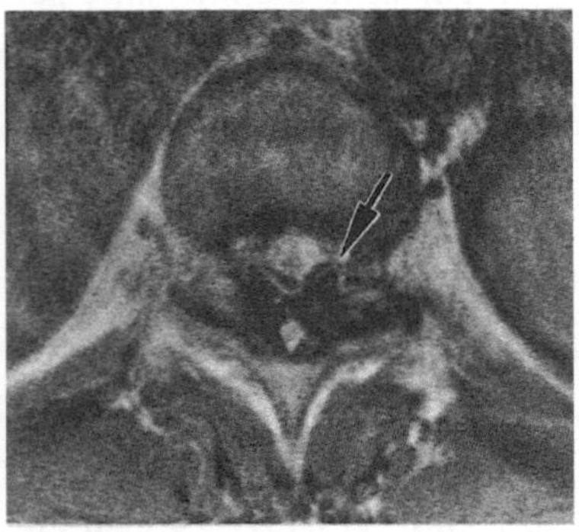

17.52

Fig. 17.49. a Mediolateral disc prolapse on the right in a 59-year-old man with pain and progressive paresis of the right leg. Parasagittal scan with disc prolapse at L5/S1, which is indicated by the missing fatty tissue and the deformation of the intervertebral foramen *(open arrow)*. Sagittal scan, SE 1.5 s/30 ms. **b** Mediolateral disc prolapse on the right in a 33-year-old man with radiating pain and paresis of right leg. In this axial scan the obliteration of the lateral recess and parts of the intervertebral foramen by disc material is shown *(arrow)*. Dislocation of dural sac to the opposite side, SE 2.0 s/30 ms (1.5 T) **c** Spondylophytes of L5/S1 segment in a 53-year-old woman with radicular symptoms (S1). Dorsolateral spondylophytes *(arrow)* associated with lowering of the intervertebral space cause narrowing of the intervertebral foramen with root *(arrowhead)* compression. Parasagittal scan, SE 0.45 s/15 ms (1.5 T)

Fig. 17.50. Hypointense cervical disc prolapse in a 62-year-old woman with progressive spastic tetraparesis. Hypointense impression of the dural sac at C6/7 *(open arrow)*. The lesion cannot be differentiated clearly from dorsal osteophytes. Stenosis of vertebral canal at the level of C3-C5 cervical segment secondary to hypertrophy of the ligamenta flava *(arrows)* and subluxation of C4/5. Sagittal scan, SE 2.0 s/100 ms

Fig. 17.51. a Osteochondrosis of L4/5 and L5/S1 lumbar segments in a 57-year-old woman with sciatica. The ventral portions of the lower end-plate of L5 and the upper end-plate of S1, as well as ankylosing osteophytes of the same level appear hypointense, also with T_2-weighting. Note a disc prolapse into the spongiosa of L1 *(arrow)*. Sagittal scan, **a** SE 0.4 s/30 ms. **b** Osteochondrosis of L4/5 and L5/S1 in a 57-year-old woman. Triangular zone of increased signal intensity at the anterolateral edge of L5 vertebra *(arrow)*. With heavier T2 weighting the signal intensity of the upper end-plate of L5 *(arrow)* increases; this is also true to a lesser degree for the lower end-plate of L4. Degeneration of the intervertebral discs of T12/L1, L3/4, L4/5, and L5/S1. Sagittal scan **b** SE 1.8 s/100 ms (1.5 T)

Fig. 17.52. Osseous stenosis of vertebral canal at T11/12 in a 51-year-old man with back pain radiating into both legs. Hypointense osseous structures attached to the left vertebral joint with cone-shaped protrusion into the vertebral canal *(arrow)*. Axial scan, SE 1.8 s/50 ms (1.5 T)

other hand, the use of surface coils and thin sections in high-field imagers is making it possible to distinguish dehydrated herniated tissue from bony structures, for even dehydrated discs still give a detectable signal and usually show a demonstrable relationship to the intervertebral space (Fig. 17.50) [1, 3, 18, 52, 64, 90].

17.4.2 Degenerative Changes in Bone

Degenerating discs incite degenerative changes in the adjacent vertebral bodies, altering their signal characteristics. In some cases a decrease in signal intensity is seen on both T1-weighted and T2-weighted images (Fig. 17.51 a). On the other hand, it is not unusual to see the signal intensity increase with T1 and T2 weighting (Fig. 17.51 b). The reason for this discrepancy is open to argument, although it has been suggested that the degenerative changes are age-dependent. In that case the increase in signal intensity would represent an increased incorporation of fat and thus a long-standing change, whereas a loss of signal intensity would reflect sclerosing processes of more recent onset [51, 52, 64, 67].

17.4.3 Spinal Stenosis

The term spinal stenosis is used to denote narrowing of the vertebral canal in which there is a disproportion between the width of the canal and the neural structures contained therein.

Acquired spinal stenosis usually develops gradually as a result of parallel changes in the intervertebral disc and intervertebral joints. Especially in the lumbar region, degenerative disc diseases lead to narrowing of the intervertebral space, placing excessive loads upon the intervertebral joints with consequent osteoarthritis and osteophytosis [10, 38, 44, 50, 51, 58, 76, 77, 80, 85, 87].

On MR, the dural sac may be displaced and the epidural fat decreased in volume. Sagittal images are best for portraying the extensive or segmental circumferential narrowing of the vertebral canal, especially from the posterior aspect (hypertrophied ligamenta flava; see Fig. 17.50). Images also show osteoarthritic changes with osteophytic deposits about the facet joints (Fig. 17.52). The hypertrophy of the ligamenta flava represents a fibrotic response to chronic traumatization, rather than a functional adaptation. The above structures cannot be differentiated on MR images because of their isointensity.

The degree of the stenosis is best appreciated on T2-weighted images, where the bright CSF contrasts sharply with the dark extradural structures. Axial images are also useful, mainly because they permit an accurate measurement of the width of the verterbral canal, the intervertebral foramina, and the lumen of the dural sac.

If there is need for more accurate differentiation of structures that give little or no MR signal (cortical bone, calcifications, hypertrophied ligaments, artifacts from particles of metallic debris), CT imaging should be performed as an adjunctive study.

17.4.4 Postoperative Changes

Postoperative complaints, whether acute, subacute, or chronic in nature, increasingly are a cause for referral for MR examination.

Following cervical disc surgery through the anterior approach, it is common to see loss of signal intensity in the adjacent vertebral bodies on T1-weighted images for a period of 6-12 months. Increased signal intensity usually becomes apparent as the images are weighted toward T2. This finding is not considered to be pathologic [50, 52, 67].

Cervical fusion operations that leave behind metallic debris produce significant image artifacts (overshoot phenomenon) that hinder or preclude evaluation of the operated area (Fig. 17.53) [29].

Changes following posterior operations on the lumbar spine mainly affect the dorsal soft tissues in the acute and subacute stage. Besides epidural hemorrhage, abnormal CSF collections can form as a result of dural injury (Fig. 17.54), and soft tissue hematomas (see Fig. 17.64) or abscesses may develop. Abnormal signal intensities in the back muscles may persists for several months, even with an uncomplicated postoperative course [50, 52, 67].

Several changes have been described following chemonucleolysis [32, 45, 52]:

- Narrowing of the disc space
- Loss of disc signal intensity on T2-weighted images as possible evidence of a change in the water-binding capacity of the nucleus pulposus
- Loss of signal intensity in the adjacent vertebral bodies on T2-weighted sequences [49], believed to indicate an inflammatory response similar to that seen in spondylodiscitis (Fig. 17.55).

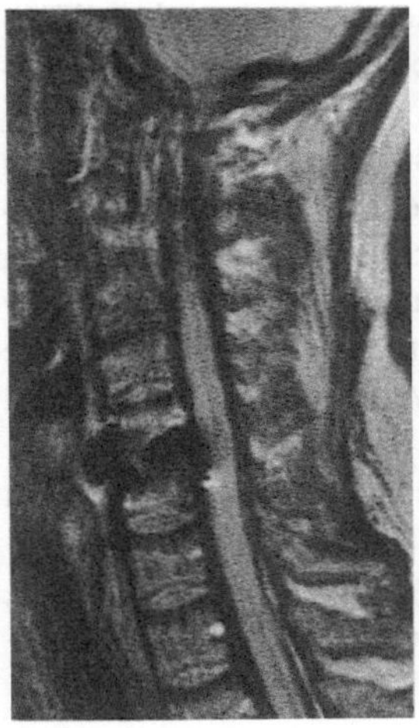

17.53

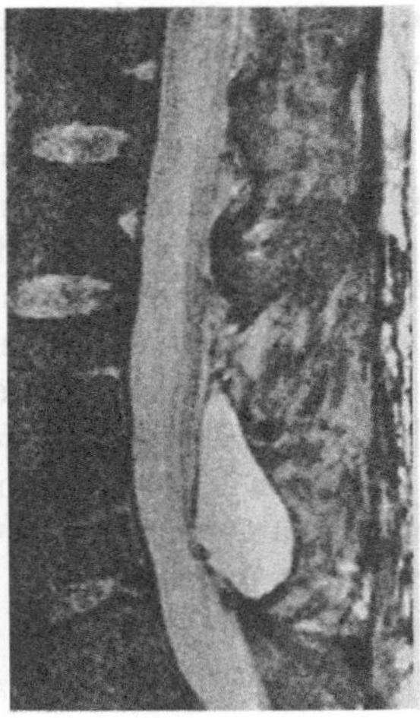

17.54

Fig. 17.53. Metal artifacts after Cloward's procedure at the C5/6 segment in a 51-year-old woman. Signal void in the operated C5/6 segment caused by metal particles originating from surgical instruments, rendering the diagnostic evaluation of this segment impossible. Sagittal scan, SE 1.8 s/50 ms (1.5 T)

Fig. 17.54. Postoperative pseudomeningocele in a 44-year-old man with persistent back pain after disc operation. Pear-shaped hyperintense structure dorsal to the dural sac at L3 and L4. The signal of the encysted fluid is more intense than that of pulsating CSF. The signal of the soft tissue of the back is inhomogeneous secondary to the operation. No signal is seen from the L3/4 intervertebral disc. Sagittal scan, SE 1.8 s/100 ms (1.5 T)

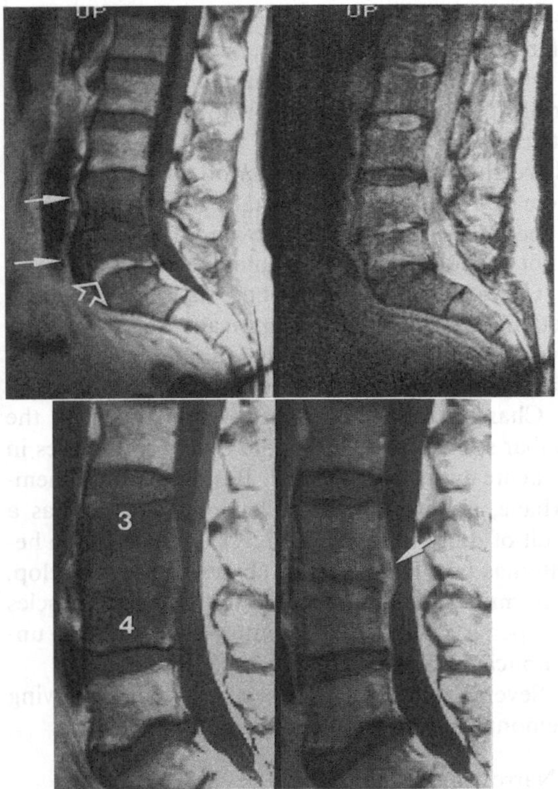

a b c d

Fig. 17.55. a, b Spondylodiscitis at the L4/5 segment in a 55-year-old man presenting with severe back pain and markedly increased blood sedimentation rate about 6 weeks after disc surgery; the pain decreased with bed rest. The inflammatory edema causes a prolongation of T1 and T2 of the bone marrow of the vertebrae involved *(arrows)*. The focus of fatty degeneration of L5 *(open arrow)* remains unchanged. Midsagittal scans: **a** SE 0.4 s/17 ms, **b** SE 1.6 s/80 ms (1.0 T). **c, d** Spontaneous spondylodiscitis in a 60-year-old man at L3/4; causative organism: streptococcus. With gadolinium-DTPA **(d)** enhancement of the affected vertebrae and the epidural inflammatory granulation tissue *(arrow)* is seen. On the T2-weighted scan the signal of L3 and L4 was only slightly increased compared to normal vertebrae. Midsagittal scans, SE 0.4 s/15 ms (1.5 T)

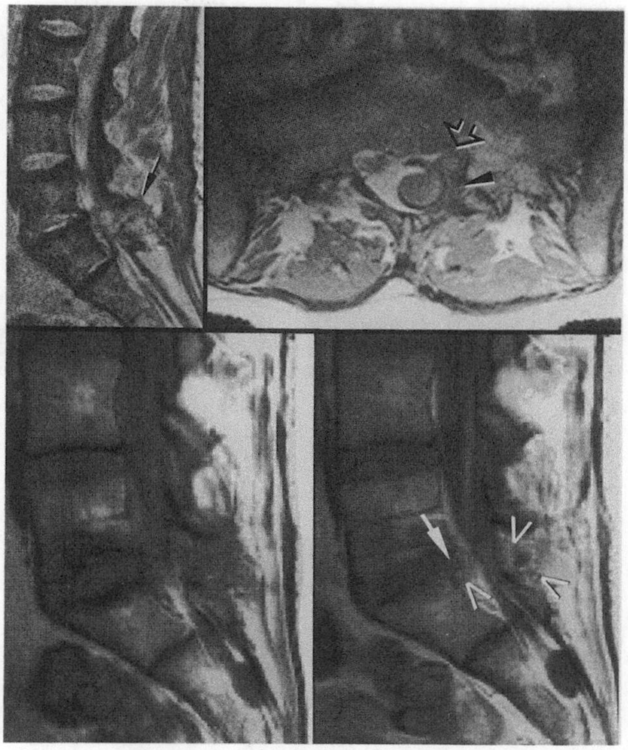

Fig. 17.56 a–d. Scar tissue. **a** In a 42-year-old woman 4-years after disc surgery. Inhomogeneous structure and varying signal intensity (from low to medium values) of dorsal soft tissue *(arrow)*. The foreign tissue invades the vertebral canal posteriorly. Sagittal scan, SE 1.8 s/100 ms. **b** In a 59-year-old man presenting with recurrent radicular pain on the left several years after disc surgery. Hypointense en plaque structure extending in the left dorsolateral part of the vertebral canal *(arrow)*. Ipsilateral distortion of the dural sac. Enlarged nerve root on the left *(open arrow)*. Axial scan, SE 1.2 s/30 ms (1.5 T). **c, d** Hyperintense scar tissue *(arrowheads)* surrounding a nonenhancing, small recurrent disc herniation *(arrow)* in a 45-year-old woman 4 months after disc surgery. Sagittal scans, SE 0.45 s/15 ms, **b** after i.v. gadolinium-DTPA (1.5 T)

With successful treatment, a regression of the disc protrusion can usually be observed [32].

Differentiation between recurrent disc herniation and scar is difficult both with CT and with MR. Previous experience suggests that an area of decreased signal intensity seen on both T1-weighted and T2-weighted images more than 3 months after surgery represents the proton-poor fibrotic tissue of a scar, rather than a recurrent disc herniation (Fig. 17.56 a, b). Also, scars usually show continuity with similar changes in the back muscles, whereas a herniation often is seen to communicate with the intervertebral disc space. Since early postoperative scar tissue shows significant enhancement, intravenous injection of contrast medium (e.g., gadolinium-DTPA) can be used as an auxiliary measure to differentiate recurrent disc herniation from scar tissue in the first 5–6 months following surgery (Fig. 17.56 c, d).

If the disc material is heavily dehydrated, it may be impossible to distinguish a recurrent herniation from a scar. The scar, in fact, may display higher signal intensities than the herniation.

Scar tissue or disc material obliterating the lateral recess is more easily differentiated form nerve roots by MR imaging than by CT owing to the higher contrast resolution and better tissue characterization of MR, made possible by the variety of pulse sequences that can be employed.

17.4.5 Relative Values of Imaging Procedures in the Diagnosis of Disc Disease

MR offers greater certainty than CT in the diagnosis of cervical spinal disorders, for it is free of the superimpositions, "hardening" artifacts, and partial volume effects that can degrade the results of CT.

The low signal of the small vertebrae is also a problem with MR, however, leading to a reduction of image detail. This signal loss is especially noticeable on axial images, where long repetition times or multiple acquisitions are needed to obtain optimal results.

In the lumbar region, high-resolution thin-section CT offers a diagnostic accuracy rate approaching 95%. CT remains the method of choice, therefore, in patients with advanced osteochondrosis or radicular symptoms referrable to lumbar disease.

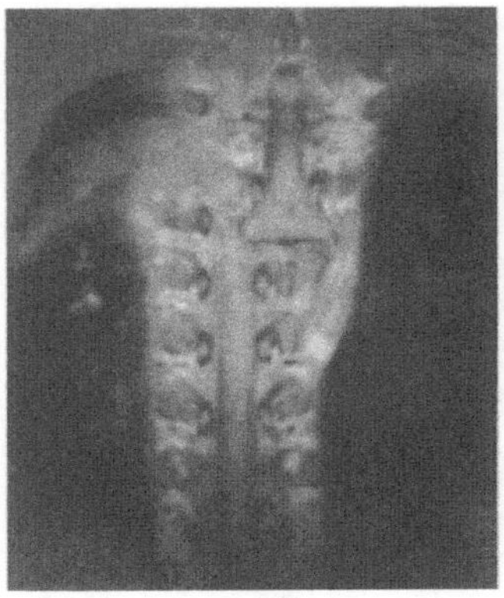

17.57

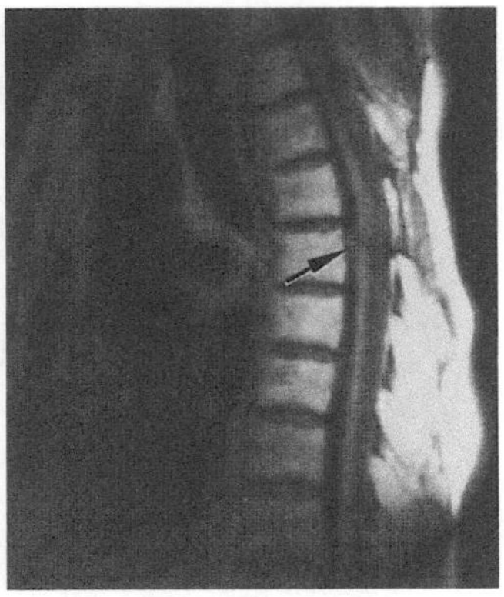

17.58

Fig. 17.57. Flexion-rotation trauma of the thoracic spine with lateral dislocation in a 27-year-old woman 3 months after a motorcycle accident. Complete disruption of the cord. Coronal scan, SE 0.7 s/30 ms (1.0 T)

Fig. 17.58. Stab wound *(arrow)* of the spinal cord in a 71-year-old woman presenting with spastic monoparesis of the right leg. Midsagittal scan, SE 0.4 s/35 ms (0.5 T). (Courtesy of Drs. Kuhn, Steen, and Terwey, Oldenburg, FRG.)

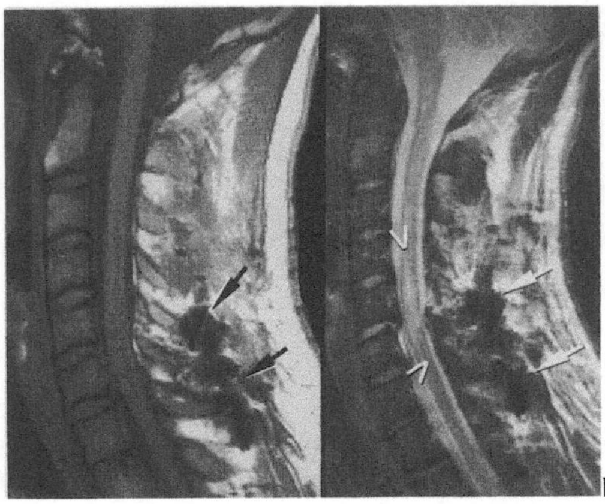

a b

Fig. 17.59 a, b. Persistent transverse lesions in a 32-year-old man 1 day after open reduction and internal fixation of bilateral facet dislocation of C5/6, due to edematous swelling of the adjacent cord segment *(arrowheads)*. Only minor metal artifacts (signal void) from the fixation wire *(arrows)*. Sagittal scans, **a** SE 0.4 s/15 ms; **b** SE 2.5 s/70 ms (1.5 T)

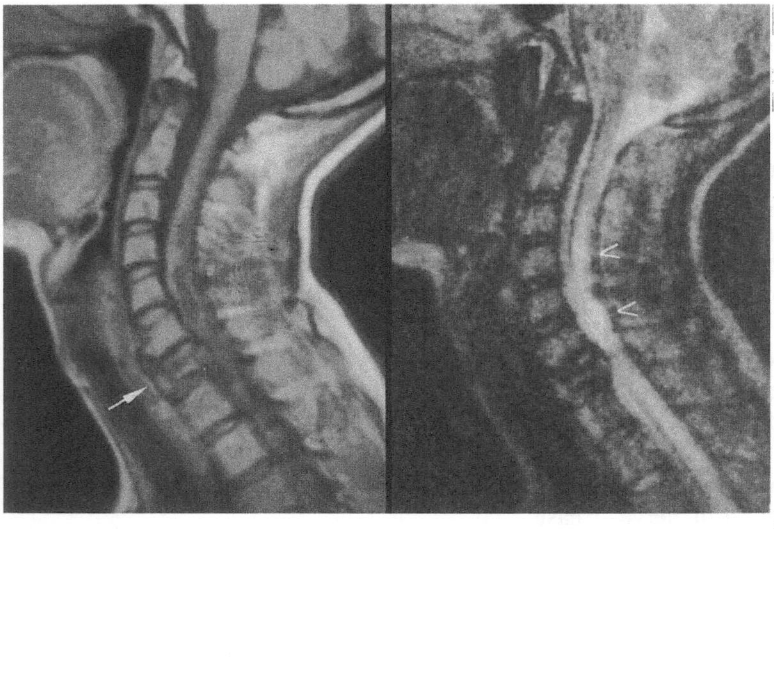

a b

Fig. 17.60 a, b. Post-traumatic syringomyelia in a 23-year-old woman with tetraplegia after fracture of the seventh cervical vertebra with compression of the cord *(arrow)*. The small syrinx and prolonged relaxation times in the cord segments cranial to the site of injury indicate the extent of the cord damage *(arrowheads)*. Midsagittal scans: **a** SE 0.4 s/35 ms, **b** SE 1.6 s/140 ms (0.5 T). (Courtesy of Drs. Kuhn, Steen, and Terwey, Oldenburg, FRG.)

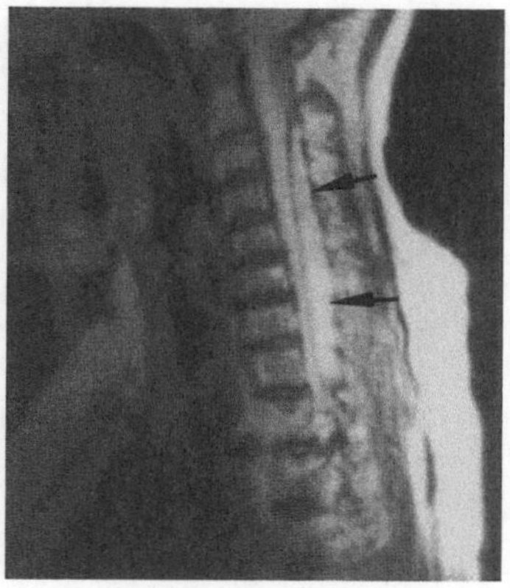

Fig. 17.61. Arachnoid cyst of the cervical spine in a 50-year-old woman with progressive, proximal spastic paraparesis and a history of detachment of right cervical plexus 4 years previously. The cyst is probably caused by a valve action at the site of the arachnoid tear leading to compression of the cord *(arrow)*. Midsagittal scan, SE 1.6 s/90 ms (1.0 T)

But MR is still considered the primary study (1) for localizing disease, owing to the excellent general view afforded by the sagittal projection; (2) for suspected spinal tumors, owing to the good contrast resolution obtainable with different pulse sequences and image planes; and (3) for postoperative complaints of unknown cause, especially in younger patients with adequately hydrated intervertebral discs that give an intense MR signal.

Owing to its capability for sagittal and axial views using variable pulse sequences, MR is able to demonstrate a narrow vertebral canal and a coexisting disc herniation with greater speed and reliability than CT, despite the scant epidural fatty tissue often seen in these cases.

For the reasons stated, it is likely that reliance on myelography will decline as the capabilities of MR become better known and applied.

17.5 Trauma

Injuries of the vertebral column show different features in the cervical, thoracic, and lumbar regions [6].

Injuries of the *cervical spine* may cause:

- Vertical compression or dispersion fractures of one or more vertebral bodies, which are stable
- Extension or retroflexion injury with rupture of the anterior longitudinal ligament
- Unilateral or bilateral facet dislocation with or without fracturing of the facets and with anterior displacement by about half the diameter of the vertebral body

Injuries of the *thoracic spine* lead mostly to vertical compression or flexion-rotation trauma, with or without displacement (Fig. 17.57). The thoracic vertebral canal is relatively narrow and provides little compensatory space for displaced bone fragments or disc protrusions.

Injuries of the *lumbar spine* are mainly associated with flexion-rotation injuries of varying severity (90%-92%), compression dispersion (8%-10%), and hyperextension injuries (1%).

The junction of the relatively rigid thoracic spine and the flexible lumbar spine is especially vulnerable to traumatic injury.

Penetrating injuries of the vertebral column and spinal cord are rare (Fig. 17.58).

Associated injuries involve the muscles and ligaments of the vertebral column and include strains and sprains, lacerations, and hemorrhages, which can eventually lead to cicatricial changes.

Injuries of the *spinal cord* may be classified by severity as spinal concussion, spinal contusion, or crushing or transection of the cord. These injuries result in edematous swelling, internal hemorrhage (hematomyelia), and necrosis in the affected segments, and these changes may spread proximally and distally from the traumatized site (Fig. 17.59). Space occupying epidural hemorrhages are rare (Fig. 17.64). Direct spinal cord injuries are produced by indriven bone fragments or by the gross displacement of a fractured vertebra.

Late sequelae of spinal cord trauma include glial scars with demyelination, atrophy, arachnitic adhesions, and post-traumatic syringomyelia (Fig. 17.60; 17.61). The latter is reported in up to 8% of patients with post-traumatic transverse cord symptoms [72] and is of special interest because of its operability [2].

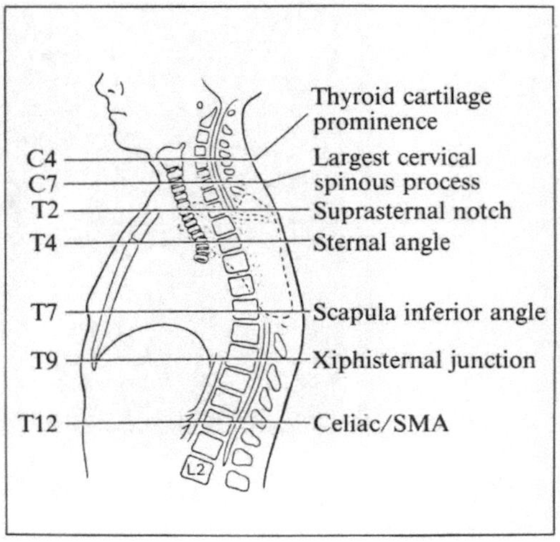

17.62

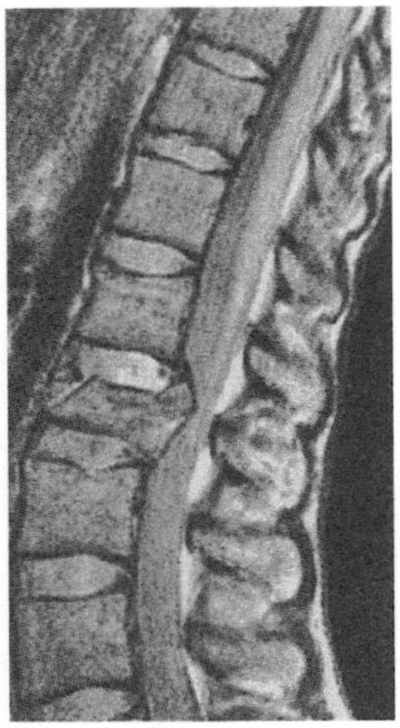

17.63

Fig. 17.62. Surface coil placement guide (from [61])

Fig. 17.63. Compression fracture of L2 in a 44-year-old woman with persisting back pain. Deformation of vertebral body L2 with a small fragment projecting into the dark subarachnoid space. Slight dorsal dislocation of nervous structures. Sagittal scan, SE 0.5 s/50 ms (1.5 T)

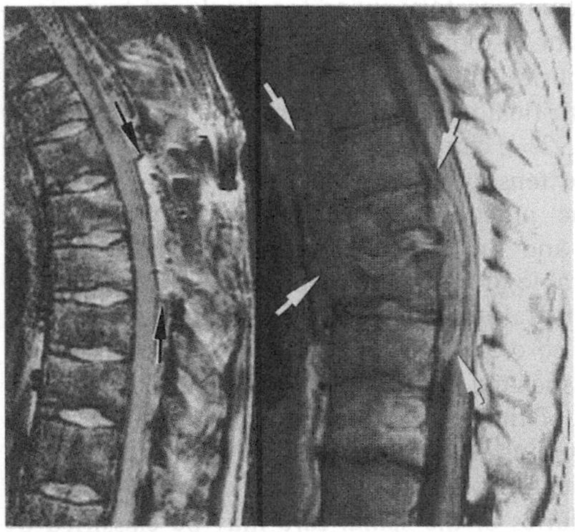

a b

Fig. 17.64. a Postoperative epidural hematoma in a 34-year-old man with recurrent transverse lesion of the cord 10 days after surgery. Hyperintense mass lesion of the dorsal epidural space at T5-7 *(arrows),* associated with slight cord compression. Metal artifacts (signal void) in dorsal soft tissue. Sagittal scan, SE 1.8 s/80 ms (1.5 T). **b** Subacute paravertebral and epidural hematoma *(arrows)* in a 28-year-old man after fracture of T7/8 with delayed development of paraparesis. Only small hyperintense rim surrounding the epidural portion of the otherwise still isointense hematoma 5 days after the injury. Sagittal scan, SE 0.45 s/15 ms (1.5 T)

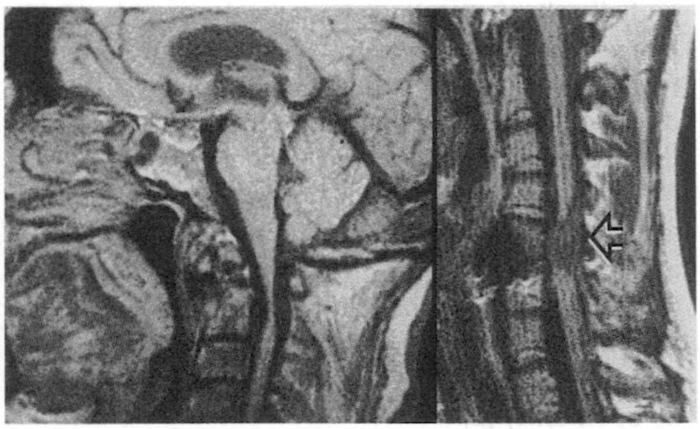

a b

Fig. 17.65. a Pseudarthrosis of the dens with atrophy of spinal cord at C2 in a 75-year-old man with marked spastic tetraparesis. Hourglass-shaped circumscribed atrophy of the cord at C2. Sagittal scan, SE 0.9 s/50 ms. **b** Post-traumatic myelomalacia in a 16-year-old girl with complete transverse lesion. Hypointense thickening of the cord at C5/6 without signs of cyst formation *(open arrow).* Metal artifacts (signal void) originating from surgical instruments used for ventral fusion of the vertebrae of this segment. Sagittal scan, SE 0.3 s/30 ms (1.5 T)

CT and MR Findings

The goals of diagnostic imaging in spinal injuries are:

- To demonstrate fractures of the vertebrae and the displacement of fragments
- To ascertain the effects of fractures on the vertebral canal and cord and reveal coexisting injuries of the ligaments and muscles
- To visualize injuries to the spinal cord itself in the acute and subacute stages and disclose their longer-term effects

Conventional roentgenography continues to be the mainstay for acute spinal injuries, especially if there is no clinical evidence of neurologic deficits.

CT is helpful in the evaluation of more obscure vertebral fractures, the identification and localization of small displaced bone fragments, and the detection of acute intraspinal hemorrhages. In this role it is superior to conventional roentgenography and MR imaging [46].

In the acute stage of spinal trauma, MR has as yet a very limited role in confirming or excluding intraspinal involvement because of the prohibitive length of the examination and the necessity of using ferromagnetic objects during primary care.

MR appears to have a larger role in the subacute stage, as it enables the spine to be examined on multiple planes without repositioning the patient. Sagittal images, like myelograms, can portray large segments of the vertebral canal and provide good visualization of regions that are not readily accessible to other modalities (e.g., the craniocervical and cervicothoracic junctions).

The technique for spinal examinations with MR is described in Sect. 17.1. Surface coils are recommended for improved spatial resolution. Figure 17.62 details the external anatomic features helpful in positioning the spinal segments that are to be examined [46, 61].

To keep the examination as brief as possible, it is best to start with sagittal T1-weighted images that afford good anatomic definition (e.g., TR 0.5 s/TE $\leq$30 ms). If necessary, these may be followed by sagittal images with T2 weighting (TR 1.5-2.0 s/TE 50/100 ms).

T1-weighted images demonstrate changes in the shape of the vertebral bodies, the displacement of fragments (see Figs. 17.57, 17.59, 17.60, 17.63), traumatic intervertebral disc herniation, and any associated compression of the subarachnoid space or damage to the cord (Fig. 17.65a, b). Small bone fragments are displayed better on CT scans.

Accompanying contusional edema, myelomalacia, and necrosis appear on T2-weighted images as areas of increased signal intensity, often spanning multiple segments. A subacute epidural or intramedullary hemorrhage is recognized by its high signal intensity on both T1-weighted and T2-weighted images [26] (Fig. 17.64).

Cervical nerve root avulsions secondary to trauma have been described by Enzmann et al. [20]. Coronal MR images show paravertebral signals isointense with CSF caused by dural injury with leakage of spinal fluid from the subarachnoid space into the often dilated root sleeves. Because the fluid pulsates less in these closed pockets, it produces a higher signal on T2-weighted images than the more mobile CSF in the vertebral canal (see also Sect. 5.3). Hemorrhages in these cases can shorten the relaxation times. Similar findings are seen on sagittal sections of pseudomeningocele (see Fig. 17.54).

Finally, MR is excellent in evaluating for late effects of spinal cord trauma such as atrophy, myelomalacia, and secondary syringomyelia (Fig. 17.65a, b).

MR is not considered advantageous for studies of laminar fractures, fractures of transverse and spinous processes, or minimally displaced fracture dislocations, which are displayed well by conventional X-ray tomograms or CT.

CT and MR imaging have made X-ray myelography virtually obsolete in evaluations of spinal trauma.

References

1. Aguila LA, Piraino DW, Modic MT, Dudley AW, Duchesnau PM, Weinstein MA (1985) The intranuclear cleft of the intervertebral disc: magnetic resonance imaging. Radiology 155: 155-158
2. Aschoff A, Löhlein A, Kunze ST (1986) Die posttraumatische Syringomyelie: Behandlungsergebnisse von sieben Drainageoperationen mit besonderer Berücksichtigung von prae- und postoperativen MR-Befunden.
3. Axel L (1984) Surface coil magnetic resonance imaging. J Comput Assist Tomogr 8: 381-384
4. Baleriaux O, Oeroover N, Hermanus N, Segebarth C (1986) MRI of the spine. Diagn Imag Clin Med 55: 66-71
5. Banna M (1985) Clinical radiology of the spine and the spinal cord. Aspen Systems, Rockville
6. Bedbrook G (1981) The care and management of spinal cord injuries. Springer, Berlin Heidelberg New York
7. Beltran J, Simon OC, Levy M, Herman L, Weis L, Mueller CF (1986) Aneurysmal bone cysts: MR imaging at 1.5 T. Radiology 158: 689-690
8. Beyer HK, Uhlenbrock D, Steiner G (1986) Die Diskushernie im LWS-Bereich. Radiologische Untersuchungsverfahren mit besonderer Berücksichtigung der Technik und Wertigkeit der Kernspintomographie. Röntgenblätter 39: 47-51

9. Brandt M, Schertel L, Roedig M, Fischer G (1986) Hodgkin-Manifestation des Zentralnervensystems. Klinikarzt 15: 838-848
10. Brocher JEW (1970) Die Wirbelsäulenleiden und ihre Differentialdiagnose, 5th edn. Thieme, Stuttgart
11. Bydder GM, Brown J, Niendorf HP, Young IR (1985) Enhancement of cervical intraspinal tumors in MR imaging with intravenous gadolinium DTPA. J Comput Assist Tomogr 9: 847-851
12. Chafetz NI, Genant HK, Moon KL, Helms CA (1984) Recognition of lumbar disc herniation with NMR. AJNR 5: 23-26
13. Cohen MD, Klatte EC, Baehner R, Smith JA, Martin-Simmermann P, Carr B, Provisor AJ, Weetman RM, Coates T, Siddiqui A, Weisman S, Berkow R, McKenna S, McGuire WA (1984) Magnetic resonance imaging of bone marrow disease in children. Radiology 151: 715-718
14. Costigan A, Winkelman MD (1985) Intramedullary spinal cord metastasis. A clinicopathological study of 13 cases. J Neurosurg 62: 227-233
15. DiChiro G, Doppman JL, Dwyer AJ, Patronas NJ, Knop RH, Bairamian D, Vermess M, Oldfield EH (1985) Tumors and arteriovenous malformations of the spinal cord: assessment using MR. Radiology 156: 689-697
16. Djindjian R, Merland JJ (1981) Angiography of the spinal cord and spinal tumors. Springer, Berlin Heidelberg New York
17. Easton EJ, Powers JA (1985) Musculoskeletal magnetic resonance imaging. Slack, Thorofare
18. Edelmann RR, Shoukimas GM, Stark DD, Davis KR, New PFJ, Saini S, Rosenthal DI, Wismer GL, Brady TJ (1985) High resolution surface-coil imaging of lumbar disc disease. AJR 144: 1123-1129
19. Von Einsiedel H, Stephan R (1985) Magnetic resonance imaging of spinal cord syndromes. Eur J Radiol 5: 127-132
20. Enzmann DR, Rubin JB, DelaPaz R, Wright A (1986) Cerebrospinal fluid pulsation: benefits and pitfalls in MR imaging. Radiology 161: 773-778
21. Freyschmidt J (1981) Knochenerkrankungen im Erwachsenenalter. Springer, Berlin Heidelberg New York
22. Friedburg H, Schumacher M, Hennig J (1986) Pathologie des kraniozervikalen Überganges in der magnetischen Resonanztomographie. RÖFO 145: 315-320
23. Friedmann G (1986) Sinnvoller Einsatz und Wandel bildgebender Verfahren bei Erkrankungen des Zentralnervensystems. Röntgenblätter 39: 303-307
24. Gonzales CF, Grossmann CB, Masdeu JC (1985) Head and spine imaging. Wiley, New York
25. Goy AMC, Pinto RS, Raghavendra DN, Epstein FJ, Kricheff II (1986) Intramedullary spinal cord tumors: MR imaging, with emphasis on associated cysts. Radiology 161: 381-386
26. Hackney DD, Asato R, Joseph PM, Carvlin MJ, McGrath JT, Grossman RI, Kassab EA, DeSimone D (1986) Hemorrhage and edema in acute spinal cord compression: demonstration by MR imaging. Radiology 161: 387-390
27. Han JS, Benson JE, Yoon YS (1984) Magnetic resonance imaging in the spinal column and craniovertebral junction. Radiol Clin North Am 22: 805-827
28. Heller H, Petsch R, Auberger T, Decker K (1985) Kernspintomographie der Wirbelsäule. RÖFO 142: 419-426
29. Heindel W, Friedmann G, Bunke J, Thomas B, Firsching R, Ernestus RI (1986) Artifacts in MR imaging after surgical intervention. J Comput Assist Tomogr 10: 596-599
30. Hennig J, Friedburg H, Ströbel B (1986) Rapid nontomographic approach to MR myelography without contrast agents. J Comput Assist Tomogr 10: 375-378
31. Holtas SI, Kido DK, Simon JH (1986) MR imaging of spinal lymphoma. J Comput Assist Tomogr 10: 111-115
32. Huckmann MS, Clark JW, McNeill TW, Whisler WW, Hejna WF, Russell EJ, Ramsey RG, David T (1987) Chemonucleolysis and changes observed on lumbar MR scan: preliminary report. AJNR 8: 1-4
33. Huk WJ, Heindel W, Deimling M, Stetter E (1983) Nuclear magnetic resonance (NMR) tomography of the central nervous system: comparison of two imaging sequences. J Comput Assist Tomogr 7: 468-475
34. Jeanmart I (1986) Radiology of the spine: tumors. Springer, Berlin Heidelberg New York
35. Kett H, Obletter N, Breit A (1987) Weiterentwicklung der diagnostischen Möglichkeiten in der MR-Tomographie: Kombination von 3D-Sequenzen mit schnellen Bildverarbeitungssystemen. RÖFO 147: 557-562
36. Kozlowski K, Beluffi G, Masel J, Diard F, Ferrariciboldi F, LeDosseur P, Labatut J (1986) Primary vertebral tumors. Pediatr Radiol 14: 129
37. Lanir A, Aghai E, Simon JS, Lee RGL, Clouse ME (1986) MR imaging in myelofibrosis. J Comput Assist Tomogr 10: 634-636
38. Lanz T, Wachsmuth W (1982) Praktische Anatomie, vol 2, part 7. Springer, Berlin Heidelberg New York
39. Laredo JD, Reizine D, Bard M, Merland JJ (1986) Vertebral hemangiomas: radiologic evaluation. Radiology 161: 183-189
40. Lee BCP, Deck MDF, Kneeland JB, Cahill PT (1985) MR iamging of the craniovertebral junction. AJNR 6: 209-213
41. Lochner B, Halbsguth A, Pia HW, Fischer PA (1985) Die spinale Kernspintomographie. Nervenarzt 56: 174-185
42. Mapstone TB, Kaufman B, Ratcheson RA (1983) Intradural chordoma without bone involvement: nuclear magnetic resonance appearance. J Neurosurg 59: 535-537
43. Maravilla KR, Weinreb JC, Suss R, Nunnally RL (1984) Magnetic resonance demonstration of multiple sclerosis plaques in the cervical cord. AJNR 5: 685-689
44. Masaryk TJ, Modic MT, Geisinger MA, Standefer J, Hardy RW, Boumphrey F, Duchesneau PM (1986) Cervical myelopathy: a comparison of magnetic resonance and myelography. J Comput Assist Tomogr 10: 184-194
45. Masaryk TJ, Boumphrey F, Modic MR, Tamborella C, Ross JS, Brown MD (1986) Effects of chemonucleolysis demonstrated by MR imaging. J Comput Assist Tomogr 10: 917-923
46. McArdle CB, Crofford MJ, Mirfakhree M, Amparo EG, Cahoun JS (1986) Surface coil MR of spinal trauma: preliminary experience. AJNR 7: 885-893
47. Mikhael MA, Ciric IS, Tarkington JA (1985) MR imaging in spinal echinococcosis. J Comput Assist Tomogr 9: 398-400
48. Modic MT, Feiglin OH, Piraino OW, Boumphrey F, Weinstein MA, Duchesneau PM, Rehm S (1985) Vertebral osteomyelitis: assessment using MR. Radiology 157: 157-166
49. Modic MT, Hardy RW, Weinstein MA, Duchesneau PM, Paushter DM, Boumphrey F (1984) Nuclear magnetic resonance of the spine: clinical potential and limitations. Neurosurgery 15: 583-592
50. Modic MT, Masaryk T, Boumphrey F, Goormastic M, Bell G (1986) Lumbar herniated disc disease and canal

stenosis: prospective evaluation by surface coil MR, CT, and myelography. AJNR 7: 709-717
51. Modic MT, Masaryk TJ, Mulopulos GP, Bundschuh C, Han JS, Bohlman H (1986) Cervical radiculopathy: prospective evaluation with surface coil MR imaging, CT with metrizamide, and metrizamide myelography. Radiology 161: 753-759
52. Modic MT, Masaryk T, Paushter D (1986) Magnetic resonance imaging of the spine. Radiol Clin North Am 24: 229-245
53. Modic MT, Pavlicek W, Weinstein MA, Boumphrey F, Ngo F, Hardy R, Duchesneau PM (1984) Magnetic resonance imaging of intervertebral disc disease: clinical and pulse sequence considerations. Radiology 152: 103-111
54. Monajati A, Spitzer RM, LaRue Wiley J, Heggeness L (1986) MR imaging of a spinal teratoma. J Comput Assist Tomogr 10: 307-310
55. Mulder DW, Dale AJD (1983) Tumors and discs. In: Barker LH (ed) Clinical neurology. Harper and Row, Philadelphia
56. Muller JA, Poppe H, von Bonnen JR (1981) Primäre Knochengeschwülste. In: Lehrbuch der Röntgendiagnostik, 6th edn, vol 2, part 12. Thieme, Stuttgart
57. Newton TH, Potts GD (1983) Computed tomography of the spine and spinal cord. Clavadel, San Anselmo
58. Nittner K (1972) Raumbeengende Prozesse im Spinalkanal. In: Handbuch der Neurochirurgie, vol 7, part 2. Springer, Berlin Heidelberg New York
59. Nittner K (1976) Spinal meningiomas, neurinomas and neurofibromas and hourglass tumors. In: Vinken PJ, Bruyn GW (eds) Handbook of clinical neurology. North Holand, Amsterdam
60. Norman D, Mills CM, Brant-Zawadzki M, Yeates A, Crooks IE, Kaufman I (1984) Magnetic resonance imaging of the spinal cord and canal: potentials and limitations. AJNR 5: 9-14
61. Panzky B, House EL (1975) Review of gross anatomy, 3rd ed, ed. Macmillan, New York
62. Paushter DM, Modic Mt, Masaryk TJ (1985) Magnetic resonance imaging of the spine: applications and limitations. Radiol Clin North Am 23: 551-562
63. Pech P, Daniels DI, Williams AL, Haughton VM (1985) The cervical neural foramina: correlation of microtomy and CT anatomy. Radiology 155: 143-146
64. Pech P, Haughton VM (1985) Lumbar intervertebral disc: correlative MR and anatomic study. Radiology 156: 699-701
65. Pernkopf E (1980) Brust, Bauch und Extremitäten. Urban und Schwarzenberg, München (Atlas der topographischen und angewandten Anatomie des Menschen 1, vol 2.)
66. Ramsey RG, Zacharias CF (1985) MRI of the spine after radation therapy - easily recognizable effects. AJR 144: 1131-1135
67. Reicher MA, Gold RH, Halbach VV, Rauschning W, Wilson GH, Lufkin RB (1986) MR imaging of the lumbar spine: anatomic correlations and the effects of technical variations. AJR 147: 891-898
68. Reiser M, Rupp N, Stetter F (1984) Erfahrungen bei der MR-Topographie des Skelettsystems. RÖFO 139: 365-373
69. Reiser M, Kahn Th, Weigert F, Lukas P, Büttner F (1986) Diagnostik der Spondylitis durch die MR-Tomographie. RÖFO 145: 320-325
70. Resnick D, Niwayama G (1981) Diagnosis of bone and joint disorders. Saunders, Philadelphia
71. Rosenthal DJ, Scott JA, Mankin HJ, Wismer GL, Brady TJ (1985) Sacrococcygeal chordoma: magnetic resonance imaging and computed tomography. AJR 145: 143-147
72. Rossier AB, Foo D, Shillito J, Dyro FM (1985) Posttraumatic cervical syringomyelia: incidence, clinical presentation, electrophysiological studies, syrinx protein and results of conservative and operative treatment. Brain 108 (2): 439-461
73. Rubin JM, Aisen AM, DiPietra MA (1986) Ambiquities in MR imaging of tumoral cysts in the spinal cord. J Comput Assist Tomogr 10: 395-398
74. Rubinstein LJ (1972) Tumors of the central nervous system. United States Armed Forces Institute of Pathology, Washington
75. Schaub T, Dittrich HM, Antoniadis A, Wolff P, Gutjahr P (1986) Diagnostik eines Ewing-Sarkoms im Bereich der Brustwirbelsäule - differentialdiagnostische Schwierigkeiten. Röntgenblätter 39: 287-290
76. Scheid W (1980) Lehrbuch der Neurologie. Thieme, Stuttgart
77. Schmorl G, Junghanns H (1968) Die gesunde und die kranke Wirbelsäule in Röntgenbild und Klinik. Thieme, Stuttgart
78. Scott JA, Rosenthal DI, Brady TJ (1984) The evaluation of musculoskeletal disease with magnetic resonance imaging. Radiol Clin North Am 22: 917-941
79. Scotti G, Scialfa G, Colombo N, Landoni L (1985) MR imaging of intradural extramedullary tumors of the cervical spine. J Comput Assist Tomogr 9: 1037-1041
80. Shapiro R (1975) Myelography, 3rd edn. Year Dook, Chicago
81. Siegel MJ, Jamroz GA, Glazer HS, Abramson CL (1986) MR imaging of intraspinal extension of neuroblastoma. J Comput Assist Tomogr 10: 593-595
82. Smith FW, Runge V, Permezel M, Smith CC (1984) Nuclear magnetic resonance (NMR) imaging in the diagnosis of spinal osteomyelitis. Magn Reson Imaging 2: 53-56
83. Sze G, Brant-Zawadzki M, Wilson CR, Norman D, Newton TH (1986) Pseudotumor of craniovertebral junction associated with chronic subluxation: MR imaging studies. Radiology 161: 391-394
84. Terwey B, Koschorek F, Jensen HP (1985) Kernspintomographie des Zervikalkanals. Röntgenpraxis 38: 422-432
85. Thurn P, Friedmann G (1986) Computertomographie der Wirbelsäule und des Spinalkanals, 2nd edn. Enke, Stuttgart
86. Treisch J, Schörner W (1986) Topographische Diagnostik von Chordomen mit der magnetischen Resonanztomographie (MRT). RÖFO 144: 232-234
87. Wackenheim A, Babin E (1980) The narrow lumbar canal. Springer, Berlin Heidelberg New York
88. Weinstein JB, Siegel MJ, Griffith RC (1984) Spinal Ewing sarcoma: misleading appearances. Skeletal Radiol 11: 262
89. Wimmer B, Friedburg H, Hennig J, Kauffmann GW (1986) Möglichkeiten der diagnostischen Bildgebung durch Kernspintomographie: Veränderungen an Wirbeln, Bändern und Bandscheiben im Vergleich mit der Computertomographie. Radiologe 26: 137-143
90. Yenerich DO, Haughton VM (1986) Oblique plane MR imaging of the cervical spine. J Comput Assist Tomogr 10: 823-826
91. Zanella FE, Steinbrich W, Friedmann G, Koulousakis A (1986) Magnetische Resonanztomographie (MR) bei spinalen Raumforderungen. RÖFO 145: 326-330

Glossary of Magnetic Resonance Terms

Acquisition time - see Image acquisition time.

ADC - see Analog to digital converter.

Adiabatic fast passage (AFP) - technique of producing rotation of the macroscopic magnetization vector by sweeping the frequency of an irradiating RF wave (for the strength of the magnetic field) through resonance (the Larmor frequency) in a time short compared to the relaxation times. Particularly used for inversion of the spins. A continuous wave MR technique.

Adiabatic rapid passage - see Adiabatic fast passage.

AFP - see Adiabatic fast passage.

Analog to digital converter (ADC) - part of the interface that converts ordinary (analog) voltages, such as the detected MR signal, into digital number form, that can be read by the computer.

Angular frequency (*ω*) - frequency of oscillation or rotation (measured, e.g., in radians/second) commonly designated by Greek letter ω: $\omega = 2\pi f$, where f is frequency (e.g., in hertz (Hz)).

Angular momentum - a vector quantity given by the vector product of the momentum of a particle and its position vector. In the absence of external forces, the angular momentum remains constant, with the result that any rotating body tends to maintain the same axis of rotation. When a torque is applied to a rotating body, the resulting change in angular momentum results in precession. Atomic nuclei possess an intrinsic angular momentum referred to as spin, measured in multiples of Planck's constant.

Antenna - device to send or receive electromagnetic radiation. Electromagnetic radiation per se is not relevant to MR, as it is the magnetic vector alone that couples the spins and the coils, and the term coil should be used instead.

Array processor - optional component of computer system specially designed to speed up numerical calculations like those needed in MR imaging.

Artifacts - false features in the image produced by the imaging process.

B_0 - a conventional symbol for the constant magnetic (induction) field in a MR system. (Although historically used, H_0 (units of magnetic field strength, ampere/meter) should be distinguished from the more appropriate B_0 (units of magnetic induction, tesla).)

B_1 - a conventional symbol for the radiofrequency magnetic induction field used in a MR system (another symbol historically used in H_1). It is useful to consider it as composed of two oppositely rotating vectors, usually in a plane transverse to B_0. At the Larmor frequency, the vector rotating in the same direction as the precessing spins will interact strongly with the spins.

Bloch equations - phenomenological "classical" equations of motion for the macroscopic magnetization vector. They include the effects of precession about the magnetic field (static and RF) and the T1 and T2 relaxation times.

Boltzmann distribution - if a system of particles which are able to exchange energy in collisions is in thermal equilibrium, then the relative number of particles, N_1 and N_2, in two particular energy states with corresponding energies, E_1 and E_2, is given by

$$\frac{N_1}{N_2} = \exp\left[-(E_1 - E_2)/kT\right]$$

where k is Boltzmann's constant and T is absolute temperature. For example, in MR of protons at room temperature in a magnetic field of 0.25 tesla, the difference in numbers of spins aligned with the magnetic field and against the field is about one part in a million; the small excess of nuclei in the lower energy state is the basis of the net magnetization and the resonance phenomenon.

Carr-Purcell (CP) sequence - sequence of a 90° RF pulse followed by repeated 180° RF pulses to produce a train of spin echoes; useful for measuring T2.

Carr-Purcell-Meiboom-Gill (CPMG) sequence - modification of Carr-Purcell RF pulse sequence with 90° phase shift in the rotating frame of reference between the 90° pulse and the subsequent 180° pulses to reduce accumulating effects of imperfections in the 180° pulses. Suppression of effects of pulse error accumulation can alternatively be achieved by alternating phases of the 180° pulses by 180°.

Chemical shift (σ) - the change in the Larmor frequency of a given nucleus when bound in different sites in a molecule, due to the magnetic shielding effects of the electron orbitals. Chemical shifts make possible the differentiation of different molecular compounds and different sites within the molecules in high-resolution MR spectra. The amount of the shift is proportional to magnetic field strength and is usually specified in parts per million (ppm) of the resonance frequency relative to a standard.

Coherence - maintenance of a constant phase relationship between rotating or oscillating waves or objects. Loss of phase coherence of the spins results in a decrease in the transverse magnetization and hence a decrease in the MR signal.

Coil - single or multiple loops of wire (or other electrical conductor, such as tubing, etc.) designed either to produce a magnetic field from current flowing through the wire, or to detect a changing magnetic field by voltage induced in the wire.

Computer - as used for MR, can be divided into central processing unit (CPU), consisting of instruction interpretation and arithmetic unit plus fast access memory, and peripheral devices such as bulk data storage and input and output devices (including, via the interface, the spectrometer). Under software control, the computer controls the RF pulses and gradients necessary to acquire data, and processes the data to produce spectra or images. (Note that devices such as the spectrometer may themselves incorporate small computers.)

Continuous wave MR (CW) - a technique for studying MR by continuously applying RF radiation to the sample and slowly sweeping either the RF frequency or the magnetic field through the resonance values; now largely superceded by pulse MR techniques.

Contrast - contrast can be defined as the relative difference of the signal intensities in two adjacent regions. In a general sense, we can consider image contrast, where the strength of the image intensity in adjacent regions of the image is compared, or object contrast, where the relative values of a parameter affecting the image (such as spin density or relaxation time) in corresponding adjacent regions of the object are compared. If the two intensities are J_1 and J_2, a useful quantitative definition of contrast is $(J_1-J_2)/(J_1+J_2)$. Relating image contrast to object contrast is more difficult in MR imaging than in conventional radiography, as there are more object parameters affecting the image and their relative contributions are very dependent on the particular imaging technique used. As in other kinds of imaging, image contrast in MR will also depend on region size, as reflected through the modulation transfer function (MTF) characteristics.

CP - see Carr-Purcell.

CPMG - see Carr-Purcell-Meiboom-Gill.

CPU - see Computer.

Crossed-coil - coil pair arranged with their magnetic fields at right angles to each other in such a way as to minimize their mutual electromagnetic interaction.

Cryomagnetic - see Superconducting magnet.

Cryostat - an apparatus for maintaining a constant low temperature (as by means of liquid helium). Requires vacuum chambers to help with thermal insulation.

CW - see Continuous wave.

DAC - see Digital to analog converter.

Data system - see Computer.

dB/dt - the rate of change of the magnetic field (induction) with time. Because changing magnetic fields can induce electrical fields, this is one area of potential concern for safety limits.

Demodulator - another term for detector, by analogy to broadcast radio receivers.

Detector - portion of the receiver that demodulates the RF MR signal and converts it to a lower frequency signal. Most detectors now used are phase sensitive (e.g., quadrature demodulator/detector), and will also give phase information about the RF signal.

Diamagnetic - a substance that will slightly decrease a magnetic field when placed within it (its magnetization is oppositely directed to the magnetic field, i.e., with a small negative magnetic susceptibility).

Diffusion - the process by which molecules or other particles intermingle and migrate due to their random thermal motion. MR provides a sensitive technique for measuring diffusion of some substances.

Digital to analog converter (DAC) - part of the interface that converts digital numbers from the computer into analog (ordinary) voltages or currents.

Echo - see Spin echo.

Echo planar imaging - a technique of planar imaging in which a complete planar image is obtained from one selective excitation pulse. The FID is observed while periodically switching the y-gradient field in the presence of a static x-gradient field. The Fourier transform of the resulting spin echo train can be used to produce an image of the excited plane.

Eddy currents - electric currents induced in a conductor by a changing magnetic field or by motion of the conductor through a magnetic field. One of the sources of concern about potential hazard to subjects in very high magnetic fields or rapidly varying gradient or main magnetic fields. Can be a practical problem in the cryostat of superconducting magnets.

Excitation - putting energy into the spin system; if a net transverse magnetization is produced, an MR signal can be observed.

f - see Frequency.

Faraday shield - electrical conductor interposed between transmitter and/or receiver coil and patient to block out electric fields.

Fast Fourier transform (FFT) - an efficient computational method of performing a Fourier transform.

Fast imaging - imaging with very short acquisition times in the range of seconds, using special pulse sequences.

Ferromagnetic - a substance, such as iron, that has a large positive magnetic susceptibility.

FFT - see Fast Fourier transform.

FID - see Free induction decay.

Field echo - see Gradient echo.

Field gradient - see Gradient magnetic field.

Field lock - a feedback control used to maintain the static magnetic field at a constant strength, usually by monitoring the resonance frequency of a reference sample or line in the spectrum.

Filling factor - a measure of the geometrical relationship of the RF coil and the body. It affects the efficiency of irradiating the body and detecting MR signals, thereby affecting the signal-to-noise ratio and, ultimately, image quality. Achieving a high filling factor requires fitting the coil closely to the body, thus potentially decreasing patient comfort.

Filtered back projection - mathematical technique used in reconstruction from projections to create images from a set of multiple projection profiles. It essentially involves "correcting" the projection profiles by convolving them with a suitable mathematical filter and then back projecting the filtered projections into image space. Widely used in conventional computed tomography (CT).

Flip angle (α) - amount of rotation of the macroscopic magnetization vector produced by an RF pulse, with respect to the direction of the static magnetic field.

Fourier transform (FT) - a mathematical procedure to separate out the frequency components of a signal from its amplitudes as a function of time, or vice versa. The Fourier transform is used to generate the spectrum from the FID in pulse MR techniques and is essential to most imaging techniques.

Fourier transform imaging - MR imaging techniques in which at least one dimension is phase encoded by applying variable gradient pulses along that dimension before "reading out" the MR signal with a gradient magnetic field perpendicular to the variable gradient. The Fourier transform is then used to reconstruct an image from the set of encoded MR signals. An imaging technique of this type is spin warp imaging.

Free induction decay (FID) - if transverse magnetization of the spins is produced, e.g., by a 90° pulse, a transient MR signal will result that will decay toward zero with a characteristic time constant T2 (or T2*); this decaying signal is the FID. In practice, the first part of the FID is not observable due to residual effects of the powerful exciting RF pulse on the electronics of the receiver.

Free induction signal (FIS) - see Free induction decay.

Frequency (f) - the number of repetitions of a periodic process per unit time. For electromagnetic radiation, such as radio waves, the old unit, cycles per second (cps), has been replaced, by the SI unit, hertz, abbreviated Hz. It is related to angular frequency, ω, by $f = \omega/2\pi$

FT - see Fourier transform.

G - see Gauss.

G_x, G_y, G_z - conventional symbols for gradient magnetic field. Used with subscripts to denote spatial direction component of gradient, i.e., direction along which the field changes.

Gauss (G) - a unit of magnetic flux density in the older (CGS) system. The Earth's magnetic field is approximately one half gauss to one gauss, depending on location. The currently preferred (SI) unit is the tesla (T), (1 T = 10000 G).

Golay coil - term commonly used for a particular kind of gradient coil, commonly used to create gradient magnetic fields, perpendicular to the main magnetic field.

Gradient - the amount and direction of the rate of change in space of some quantity, such as magnetic field strength.

Gradient coils - current carrying coils designed to produce a desired gradient magnetic field (so that the magnetic field will be stronger in some locations than others). Proper design of the size and configuration of the coils is necessary to produce a controlled and uniform gradient.

Gradient echo - spin echo produced by reversal of a gradient magnetic field without using an additional RF pulse. Especially used in fast imaging sequences.

Gradient magnetic field - a magnetic field which changes in strength in a certain given direction. Such fields are used in MR imaging with selective excitation to select a region for imaging and also to encode the location of MR signals received from the object being imaged. Measured (e.g.) in teslas per meter.

Gradient pulse - briefly applied gradient magnetic field.

Gyromagnetic ratio (γ) - the ratio of the magnetic moment to the angular momentum of a particle. This is a constant for a given nucleus.

H_0 - conventional symbol historically used for the constant magnetic field in a MR system; it is physically more correct to use B_0. A magnet provides a field strength, H; however, at a point in an object, the spins experience the magnetic induction, B.

H_1 - conventional symbol historically used for the radiofrequency magnetic field in a MR system; it is physically more correct to use B_1. It is useful to consider it as composed of two oppositely rotating vectors. At the Larmor frequency, the vector rotating in the same direction as the precessing spins will interact strongly with the spins.

Hardware - electrical and mechanical components of computer.

Helmholtz coil - pair of current carrying coils used to create uniform magnetic field in the space between them.

Hertz (Hz) - the standard (SI) unit of frequency; equal to the old unit cycles per second.

Homogeneity - uniformity. In MR, the homogeneity of the static magnetic field is an important criterion of the quality of the magnet. Homogeneity requirements for MR imaging are generally lower than the homogeneity requirements for MR spectroscopy, but for most imaging techniques must be maintained over a larger region.

Hz - see Hertz.

I - see Nuclear spin number.

Image acquisition time - time required to carry out a MR imaging procedure comprising only the data acquisition time. The additional image reconstruction time will also be important to determine how quickly the image can be viewed. In comparing sequential plane imaging and volume imaging techniques, the equivalent image acquisition time per slice must be considered, as well as the actual image acquisition time.

Inductance - measure of the magnetic coupling between two current carrying loops (mutual) (reflecting their spatial relationship) or of a loop (such as a coil) with itself (self). One of the principal determinants of the resonance frequency of an RF circuit.

Inhomogeneity - degree of lack of homogeneity, for example the fractional deviation of the local magnetic field from the average value of the field.

Interface - set of devices that enables the interaction of the computer and the spectrometer. Particularly, this includes an analog to digital converter (ADC), which turns the analog voltages, such as the output of the RF receiver, into numbers that can be read by the computer. It also includes a digital to analog converter (DAC), which does the reverse, enabling the computer to produce control voltages.

Interpulse time - times between successive RF pulses used in pulse sequences. Particularly important are the inversion time (TI) in inversion recovery, and the time between a 90° pulse and the subsequent 180° pulse to produce a spin echo, which will be approximately one half the spin echo time (TE). The time between repetitions of pulse sequences is the repetition time (TR).

Inversion - a nonequilibrium state in which the macroscopic magnetization vector is oriented opposite to the magnetic field; usually produced by adiabatic fast passage or 180° RF pulses.

Inversion-recovery (IR) - pulse MR technique which can be incorporated into MR imaging, wherein the nuclear magnetization is inverted at a time on the order of T1 before the regular imaging pulse-gradient sequences. The resulting partial relaxation of the spins in the different structures being imaged can be used to produce an image that depends strongly on T1. This may bring out differences in the appearance of structures with different T1 relaxation times. Note that this does not directly produce an image of T1. T1 in a given region can be calculated from the change in the MR signal from the region due to the inversion pulse compared to the signal with no inversion pulse or an inversion pulse with a different inversion time (TI).

Inversion time (TI) - time between inversion and subsequent 90° pulse to elicit MR signal in inversion-recovery.

Inversion transfer - see Saturation transfer.

IR - see Inversion recovery

k - Boltzmann's constant: appears in Boltzmann distribution.

kHz - see Kilohertz.

Kilohertz (kHz) - unit of frequency; equal to one thousand hertz.

Larmor equation - states that the frequency of precession of the nuclear magnetic moment is proportional to the magnetic field.
$\omega_0 = -\gamma B_0$ (radians per second)
or $f_0 = -\gamma B_0/2\pi$ (hertz)
where ω_0 or f_0 is the frequency, γ is the gyromagnetic ratio, and B_0 is the magnetic induction field. The negative sign indicates the direction of the rotation.

Larmor frequency (ω_0 or f_0) - the frequency at which magnetic resonance can be excited; given by the Larmor equation. By varying the magnetic field across the body with a gradient magnetic field, the corresponding variation of the Larmor frequency can be used to encode position. For protons (hydrogen nuclei), the Larmor frequency is 42.58 MHz/tesla.

Lattice - by analogy to MR in solids, the magnetic and thermal environment with which nuclei exchange energy in longitudinal relaxation.

Line imaging - see Sequential line imaging.

Line scanning - see Sequential line imaging.

Line width - width of line in spectrum; related to the reciprocal of the transverse relaxation time (T2* in practical systems). Measured in units of frequency, generally at the half-maximum points.

LMR - see Localized magnetic resonance.

Localized magnetic resonance (LMR) - a particular technique for obtaining MR spectra, for example, of phosphorus, from a limited region by creating a sensitive volume with inhomogeneous applied gradient magnetic fields, which may be enhanced with the use of surface coils.

Longitudinal magnetization (M_z) - component of the macroscopic magnetization vector along the static magnetic field. Following excitation by RF pulse, M_z will approach its equilibrium value M_0, with a characteristic time constant T1.

Longitudinal relaxation - return of longitudinal magnetization to its equilibrium value after excitation; requires exchange of energy between the nuclear spins and the lattice.

Longitudinal relaxation time - see T1.

Lorentzian line - usual shape of the lines in an MR spectrum, characterized by a central peak with long tails; proportional to $1/[(1/T2)^2 + (f-f_0)^2]$, where f is frequency and f_0 is the frequency of the peak (i.e., central resonance frequency).

M - conventional symbol for macroscopic magnetization vector.

$\mathbf{M_{xy}}$ - see Transverse magnetization

$\mathbf{M_z}$ - see Longitudinal magnetization.

$\mathbf{M_0}$ - equilibrium value of the magnetization; directed along the direction of the static magnetic field. Proportional to spin density, N (H).

Macroscopic magnetic moment - see Macroscopic magnetization vector.

Macroscopic magnetization vector - net magnetic moment per unit volume (a vector quantity) of a sample in a given region, considered as the integrated effect of all the individual microscopic nuclear magnetic moments. Most MR experiments actually deal with this.

Magnetic dipole - north and south magnetic poles separated by a finite distance. An electric current loop, including the effective current of a spinning nucleon or nucleus, can create an equivalent magnetic dipole.

Magnetic field (H) - the region surrounding a magnet (or current carrying conductor) is endowed with certain properties. One is that a small magnet in such a region experiences a torque that tends to align it in a given direction. Magnetic field is a vector quantity; the direction of the field is defined as the direction that the north pole of the small magnet points when in equilibrium. A magnetic field produces a magnetizing force on a body within it. Although the dangers of large magnetic fields are largely hypothetical, this is an area of potential concern for safety limits.
Formally, the forces experienced by moving charged particles, current carrying wires, and small magnets in the vicinity of a magnet are due to magnetic induction (B), which includes the effect of magnetization, while the magnetic field (H) is defined so as not to include magnetization. However, both B and H are often loosely used to denote magnetic fields.

Magnetic field gradient - see Gradient magnetic field.

Magnetic induction (B) - also called magnetic flux density. The net magnetic effect from an externally applied magnetic field and the resulting magnetization. B is proportional to H ($B=\mu H$), with the SI unit being the tesla.

Magnetic moment - a measure of the net magnetic properties of an object or particle. A nucleus with an intrinsic spin will have an associated magnetic dipole moment, so that it will interact with a magnetic field (as if it were a tiny bar magnet).

Magnetic resonance (MR) - the absorption or emission of electromagnetic energy by nuclei in a static magnetic field, after excitation by a suitable RF magnetic field. The peak resonance frequency is proportional to the magnetic field, and is given by the Larmor equation. Only nuclei with a non-zero spin exhibit MR. Another magnetic resonance phenomenon is electron spin resonance (ESR).

Magnetic susceptibility (χ) - measure of the ability of a substance to become magnetized.

Magnetization (see also Macroscopic magnetization vector) - the magnetic polarization of a material produced by a magnetic field (magnetic moment per unit volume).

Magnetogyric ratio - see Gyromagnetic ratio.

Maxwell coil - a particular kind of gradient coil, commonly used to create gradient magnetic fields along the direction of the main magnetic field.

Megahertz (MHz) - unit of frequency, equal to one million hertz.

Meiboom-Gill sequence - see Carr-Purcell-Meiboom-Gill sequence.

MHz - see Megahertz

MR imaging (see also Zeugmatography) - creation of images of objects such as the body by use of the magnetic resonance phenomenon. The immediate practical application involves imaging the distribution of hydrogen nuclei (protons) in the body. The image brightness in a given region is usually dependent jointly on the spin density and the relaxation times, with their relative importance determined by the particular imaging technique employed. Image brightness is also affected by motion such as blood flow.

MR signal - electromagnetic signal in the radiofrequency range produced by the precession of the transverse magnetization of the spins. The rotation of the transverse magnetization induces a voltage in a coil, which is amplified and demodulated by the receiver; the signal may refer only to this induced voltage.

Multiple line-scan imaging (MLSI) - variation of sequential line imaging techniques that can be used if selective excitation methods that do not affect adjacent lines are employed. Adjacent lines are imaged while waiting for relaxation of the first line toward equilibrium, which may result in decreased imaging time. A different type of MLSI uses simultaneous excitation of two or more lines with different phase encoding followed by suitable decoding.

Multiple plane imaging - variation of sequential plane imaging techniques that can be used with selective excitation techniques that do not affect adjacent planes. Adjacent planes are imaged while waiting for relaxation of the first plane toward equilibrium, resulting in decreased imaging time.

Multiple sensitive point - sequential line imaging technique utilizing two orthogonal oscillating magnetic field gradients, an SFP pulse sequence, and signal averaging to isolate the MR spectrometer sensitivity to a desired line in the body.

N (H) - see Spin density.

NMR - see Magnetic resonance (MR).

Nuclear magnetic resonance (NMR) - see Magnetic resonance (MR).

Nuclear signal - see MR signal.

Nuclear spin (see also Spin) - an intrinsic property of certain nuclei that gives them an associated characteristic angular momentum and magnetic moment.

Nuclear spin quantum number (I) - property of all nuclei related to the largest measurable component of the nuclear angular momentum. Non zero values of nuclear angular momentum are quantized (fixed) as integral or half-integral multiples of $(h/2\pi)$, where h is Planck's constant. The number of possible energy states for a given nucleus in a fixed magnetic field is equal to $2I+1$.

Nucleon - generic term for a neutron or proton.

Nutation - a displacement of the axis of a spinning body away from the simple coneshaped figure which would be traced by the axis during precession. In the rotating frame of reference, the nutation caused by an RF pulse appears as a simple precession, although the motion is more complex in the stationary frame of reference.

Orientation - a suggested standard orientation for the presentation of MR images is: 1) transverse: patient's right on the left side of the image, anterior or ventral on top, 2) coronal: patient's right to left side of image, superior or head to the top, 3) sagittal: patient's head to the top, anterior to the left side of image, R, L, S and A should be shown on the screen, as appropriate. In displaying sagittal images, it is helpful to indicate whether a slice is to the left or right of the midline.

Paramagnetic - a substance with a small but positive magnetic susceptibility (magnetizability). The addition of a small amount of paramagnetic substance may greatly reduce the relaxation times of water. Typical paramagnetic substances usually possess an unpaired electron and include atoms or ions of transition elements, rare earth elements, some metals, and some molecules including molecular oxygen and free radicals. Paramagnetic substances are considered promising for use as contrast agents in MR imaging.

Partial saturation (PS) - excitation technique applying repeated RF pulses in times on the order of or shorter than T1. In MR imaging systems, although it results in decreased signal amplitude, there is the possibility of generating images with increased contrast between regions with different relaxation times. It does not directly produce images of T1. The change in MR signal from a region resulting from a change in the interpulse time, TR, can be used to calculate T1 for the region. Although partial saturation is also commonly referred to as saturation recovery, that term should properly be reserved for the particular case of partial saturation in which recovery after each excitation effectively takes place from true saturation.

Permanent magnet - a magnet whose magnetic field originates from permanently magnetized material.

Permeability (μ) - tendency of a substance to concentrate magnetic field, $\mu = B/H$.

Phantom - an artificial object of known dimensions and properties used to test aspects of an imaging machine.

Phase - in a periodic function (such as rotational or sinusoidal motion), the position relative to a particular part of the cycle.

Phase sensitive detector - see Demodulator.

Pixel - acronym for a picture element; the smallest discrete part of a digital image display.

Planar spin imaging - one particular technique of planar imaging that creates an MR image of a plane from one excitation sequence by selectively exciting a grid of points within the plane and then applying a gradient magnetic field so that each point has a different Larmor frequency. Fourier transformation of the FID can then be used to separate the signals from each selected point and create the image.

Planar imaging - imaging technique in which image of a plane is built up from signals received from the whole plane. See also Sequential plane imaging.

Point imaging - see Sequential point imaging.

Point scanning - see Sequential point imaging.

Precession - comparatively slow gyration of the axis of a spinning body so as to trace out a cone; caused by the application of a torque tending to change the direction of the rotation axis, and continuously directed at right angles to the plane fo the torque. The magnetic moment of a nucleus with spin will experience such a torque when inclined at an angle to the magnetic field, resulting in precession at the Larmor frequency. A familiar example is the effect of gravity on the motion of a spinning top or gyroscope.

Precessional frequency - see Larmor frequency.

Probe - the portion of an MR spectrometer comprising the sample container and the RF coils, with some associated electronics. The RF coils may consist of separate receiver and transmitter coils in a crossed-coil configuration, or alternatively, a single coil to perform both functions.

Program - see Software.

Progressive saturation - see Saturation recovery.

Projection profile - spectrum of MR signal whose frequency components are broadened by a gradient magnetic field. In the simplest case (negligible line width, no relaxation effects, and no effects of prior gradients), it corresponds to a one-dimensional projection of the spin density along the direction of the gradient; in this form it is used in reconstruction from projections imaging.

PS - see Partial saturation.

Pulse, 90° ($\pi/2$ pulse) - RF pulse designed to rotate the macroscopic magnetization vector 90° in space as referred to the rotating frame of reference, usually about an axis at right angles to the main magnetic field. If the spins are initially aligned with the magnetic field, this pulse will produce transverse magnetization and an FID.

Pulse, 180° (π pulse) - RF pulse designed to rotate the macroscopic magnetization vector 180° in space as referred to the rotating frame of reference, usually about an axis at right angles to the main magnetic field. If the spins are initially aligned with the magnetic field, this pulse will produce inversion.

Pulse, RF - see RF pulse.

Pulse length (width) - time duration of a pulse. For an RF pulse near the Larmor frequency, the longer the pulse length, the greater the angle of rotation of the macroscopic magnetization vector will be (greater than 180° can bring it back toward its original orientation).

Pulse MR - MR techniques that use RF pulses and Fourier transformation of the MR signal; have largely replaced the older continuous wave techniques.

Pulse programmer - part of the spectrometer or interface that controls the timing, duration, and amplitude of the pulses (RF or gradient).

Pulse sequences - set of RF (and/or gradient) magnetic field pulses and time spacings between these pulses; used in conjunction with gradient magnetic fields and MR signal reception to produce MR images. See also Interpulse times.

Pulsed gradients - see Gradient pulse.

Q - see Quality factor.

Quadrature detector - a phase sensitive detector or demodulator that detects the components of the signal in phase with a reference oscillator and 90° out of phase with the reference oscillator.

Quality factor (Q) - applies to any electrical circuit component; most often the coil Q is limiting. Inversely related to the fraction of the energy in an oscillating system lost in one oscillation cycle. Q is inversely related to the range of frequency over which the system will exhibit resonance. It affects the signal-to-noise ratio, because the detected signal increases proportionally to Q while the noise is proportional to the square root of Q. The Q of a coil will depend on whether it is unloaded (no patient) or loaded (patient).

Quenching - loss of superconductivity of the current carrying coil that may occur unexpectedly in a superconducting magnet. As the magnet becomes resistive, heat will be released that can result in rapid evaporation of liquid helium in the cryostat. This may present a hazard if not properly planned for.

Radian - dimensionless unit of angular measure; $360° = 2\pi$, radians.

Radiofrequency (RF) - wave frequency intermediate between auditory and infra red. The RF used in MR studies is commonly in the megahertz (MHz) range. The principal effect of RF magnetic fields on the body is power deposition in the form of heating, mainly at the surface; this is a principal area of concern for safety limits.

Readout delay - see TE.

Receiver - portion of the MR apparatus that detects and amplifies RF signals picked up by the receiving coil. Includes a preamplifier, amplifier, and demodulator.

Receiver coil - coil of the RF receiver; "picks up" the MR signal.

Reconstruction from projections imaging - MR imaging technique in which a set of projection profiles of the body is obtained by observing MR signals in the presence of a suitable corresponding set of gradient magnetic fields. Images can then be reconstructed using techniques analogous to those used in conventional computed tomography (CT), such as filtered back projection. It can be used for volume imaging or, with plane selection techniques, for sequential plane imaging.

Refocusing - see Spin echo.

Relaxation rates - reciprocals of the relaxation times.

Relaxation times - after excitation, the spins will tend to return to their equilibrium distribution, in which there is no transverse magnetization and the longitudinal magnetization is at its maximum value and oriented in the direction of the static magnetic field. It is observed that in the absence of applied RF, the transverse magnetization decays toward zero with a characteristic time constant T2, and the longitudinal magnetization returns toward the equilibrium value M_0 with a characteristic time constant T1.

Repeated FID - a form of MR imaging in which repeated 90° pulses are applied. Results in partial saturation if interpulse times are of the order of or less than T1. Strictly speaking, applies only if MR signal is detected as an FID.

Repetition time - see TR.

Rephasing gradient - gradient magnetic field applied for a brief period after a selective excitation pulse, in the opposite direction to the gradient used for the selective excitation. The result of the gradient reversal is a rephasing of the spins (which will have got out of phase with each other along the direction of the selection gradient), forming an echo by "time reversal", and improving the sensitivity of imaging after the selective excitation process.

Resistive magnet - a magnet whose magnetic field originates from current flowing through an ordinary (nonsuperconducting) conductor.

Resolution, spatial - although generally referring to the ability of the imaging process to distinguish adjacent structures in the object (an important measure of image quality), the specific criterion of resolution to be used depends on the type of test used (e.g. bar pattern or contrast-detail phantom.). As the ability to separate or detect objects depends on their contrast, and the different MR parameters of objects will affect image contrast differently for different imaging techniques, care must be taken in comparing the results of resolution phantom tests of different machines and no single measure of resolution can be specified.

Resonance - a large amplitude vibration in a mechanical or electrical system caused by a relatively small periodic stimulus with a frequency at or close to a natural frequency of the system; in MR apparatus, resonance can refer to the MR itself or to the tuning of the RF circuitry.

Resonant frequency - frequency at which resonance phenomenon occurs; given by the Larmor equation for MR; determined by inductance and capacitance for RF circuits.

RF - see Radiofrequency.

RF coil - used for transmitting RF pulses and/or receiving MR signals. Most commonly used in saddle coil or solenoid configurations for MR imaging.

RF pulse - brief burst of RF magnetic field delivered to object by RF transmitter. For RF frequency near the Larmor frequency, it will result in rotation of the macroscopic magnetization vector in the rotating frame of reference (or a more complicated nutational motion in the stationary frame of reference.) The amount of rotation will depend on the strength and duration of the RF pulse; commonly used examples are 90° ($\pi/2$) and 180° (π) pulses.

Rotating frame of reference - a frame of reference (with corresponding coordinate systems) that is rotating about the axis of the static magnetic field B_0 (with respect to a stationary ("laboratory") frame of reference) at a frequency equal to that of the applied RF magnetic field, B_1. Although B_1 is a rotating vector, it appears stationary in the rotating frame, leading to simpler mathematical formulations.

Rotating frame zeugmatography - technique of MR imaging that uses a gradient of the RF excitation field (to give a corresponding variation of the flip angle along the gradient as a means of encoding the spatial location of spins in the direction of the RF field gradient) in conjunction with a static gradient magnetic field (to give spatial encoding in an orthogonal direction). It can be considered to be a form of Fourier transform imaging.

Saddle coil - RF coil configuration design commonly used when the static magnetic field is coaxial with the axis of the coil along the long axis of the body (e.g. superconducting magnets and most resistive magnets) as opposed to solenoid or surface coil.

Saturation - a nonequilibrium state in MR, in which equal numbers of spins are aligned against and with the magnetic field, so that there is no net magnetization. Can be produced by repeatedly supplying RF pulses at the Larmor frequency with interpulse times short compared to T1.

Saturation recovery (SR) - particular type of partial saturation pulse sequence in which the preceding pulses leave the spins in a state of saturation, so that recovery at the time of the next pulse has taken place from an initial condition of no magnetization.

Saturation transfer (or Inversion transfer) - nuclei can retain their magnetic orientation through a chemical reaction. Thus, if RF radiation is supplied to the spins at a frequency corresponding to the chemical shift of the nuclei in one chemical state so as to produce saturation or inversion, and chemical reactions transform the nuclei into another chemical state with a different chemical shift in a time short compared to the relaxation time, the MR spectrum may show the effects of the saturation or inversion on the corresponding, unirradiated, line in the spectrum. This technique can be used to study reaction kinetics of suitable molecules.

SE - see Spin echo.

Selective excitation - controlling the frequency spectrum of an irradiating RF pulse (via tailoring) while imposing a gradient magnetic field on spins, such that only a desired region will have a suitable resonant frequency to be excited. Originally used to excite all but a desired region; now more commonly used to select only a desired region, such as a plane, for excitation.

Selective irradiation - see Selective excitation.

Sensitive plane - technique of selecting a plane for sequential plane imaging by using an oscillating gradient magnetic field and filtering out the corresponding time dependent part of the MR signal. The gradient used is at right angles to the desired plane and the magnitude of the oscillating gradient magnetic field is equal to zero only in the desired plane.

Sensitive point - technique of selecting out a point for sequential point imaging by applying three orthogonal oscillating gradient magnetic fields such that the local magnetic field is time dependent everywhere except at the desired point, and then filtering out the corresponding time dependent portion of the MR signal.

Sensitive volume - region of the object from which MR signal will preferentially be acquired because of strong magnetic field inhomogeneity elsewhere. Effect can be enhanced by use of a shaped RF field that is strongest in the sensitive region.

Sequence time - see TR.

Sequential line imaging (Line scanning, Line imaging) - MR imaging techniques in which the image is built up from successive lines through the object. In various schemes, the lines are isolated by oscillating gradient magnetic fields or selective excitation, and then the MR signals from the selected line are encoded for position by detecting the FID or spin echo in the presence of a gradient magnetic field along the line; the Fourier transform of the detected signal then yields the distribution of emitted MR signal along the line.

Sequential plane imaging (Plane imaging) - MR imaging technique in which the image of an object is built up from successive planes in the object. In various schemes, the planes are selected by oscillating gradient magnetic fields or selective excitation.

Sequential point imaging (Point scanning) - MR imaging techniques in which the image is built from successive point positions in the object. In various schemes, the points are isolated by oscillating gradient magnetic fields (sensitive point) or shaped magnetic fields.

SFP - see Steady state free precession.

Shim coils - coils carrying a relatively small current that are used to provide auxiliary magnetic fields in order to compensate for inhomogeneities in the main magnetic field of an MR system.

Shimming - correction of inhomogeneity of the magnetic field produced by the main magnet of a MR system due to imperfections in the magnet or to the presence of external ferromagnetic objects. May involve changing the configuration of the magnet or the addition of shim coils or small pieces of steel.

SI (International System of Units) - the preferred international standard system of physical units and measures.

Signal-to-noise ratio (SNR or S/N) - used to describe the relative contributions to a detected signal of the true signal and random superimposed signals ("noise"). One common method to improve (increase) the SNR is to average several measurements of the signal on the expectation that random contributions will tend to cancel out. The SNR can also be improved by sampling larger volumes (with a corresponding loss of spatial resolution) or, within limits, by increasing the strength of the magnetic field used. S/N will depend on the electrical properties of the sample or patient being studied.

Simultaneous volume imaging - see Volume imaging.

Skin depth - time dependent electromagnetic fields are significantly attenuated by conducting media (including the human body); the skin depth gives a measure of the average depth of penetration of the RF field. It may be a limiting factor in MR imaging at very high frequencies (high magnetic fields). The skin depth also affects the Q of the coils.

S/N - see Signal-to-noise ratio.

SNR - see Signal-to-noise ratio.

Software - the set of instructions, or programs, that controls the activities of the computer. Programs may be written in machine language (sequences of numbers directly interpretable by the computer), assembly language, or higher level languages such as Fortran or Basic. The software includes overall supervising "executive" programs, data acquisition programs, data processing programs (including image reconstruction), and display programs.

Solenoid coil - a coil of wire wound in the form of a long cylinder. When a current is passed through the coil, the magnetic field within the coil is relatively uniform. Solenoid RF coils are commonly used when the static magnetic field is perpendicular to the long axis of the body.

Spectrometer - the portions of the MR apparatus that actually produce the MR phenomenon and acquire the signals, including the magnet, the probe, the RF circuitry, etc. The spectrometer is controlled by the computer via the interface under the direction of the software.

Spectrum - an array of the frequency components of the MR signal according to frequency. Nuclei with different resonant frequencies will show up as peaks at different corresponding frequencies in the spectrum, or "lines."

Spin - the intrinsic angular momentum of an elementary particle, or system of particles such as a nucleus, that is also responsible for the magnetic moment; or, a particle or nucleus possessing such a spin. The spins of nuclei have characteristic fixed values. Pairs of neutrons and protons align to cancel out their spins, so that nuclei with an odd number of neutrons and/or protons will have a net nonzero rotational component characterized by an integer or half integer quantum "nuclear spin number" (I).

Spin density (N/(H)) - the density of resonating spins in a given region; one of the principal determinants of the strength of the MR signal from the region. The SI units would be moles/m^3. For water, there are about 1.1×10^5 moles of hydrogen per m^3, or 0.11 moles of hydrogen/cm^3. True spin density is not imaged directly, but must be calculated from signals received with different interpulse times.

Spin echo - reappearance of an MR signal after the FID has died away, as a result of the effective reversal of the dephasing of the spins ("refocusing") by such techniques as reversal of a gradient magnetic field (often referred to as a form of "time reversal"), or by specific RF pulse sequences such as the Carr-Purcell sequence (applied in a time shorter than or on the order of T2). Multiple spin echoes or a series of spin echoes at different times can be used to determine T2 without contamination by effects of the inhomogeneity of the magnetic field.

Spin-echo imaging - any of many MR imaging techniques in which the spin echo MR signal rather than the FID is used. Can be used to create images that depend strongly on T2. Note that spin echoes do not directly produce an image of T2.

Spin-lattice relaxation time - see T1.

Spin number, nuclear - see Nuclear spin number.

Spin - Spin relaxation time - see T2.

Spin tagging - nuclei will retain their magnetic orientation for a time on the order of T1 even in the presence of motion. Thus, if the nuclei in a given region have their spin orientation changed, the altered spins will serve as a "tag" to trace the motion of any fluid that may have been in the tagged region for a time on the order of T1.

Spin warp imaging - a form of Fourier transform imaging in which phase encoding gradient pulses are applied for a constant duration but with varying amplitude. This is distinct from the original FT imaging methods in which phase encoding is performed by applying gradient pulses of constant amplitude but varying duration. The spin warp method, as other Fourier imaging techniques, is relatively tolerant of nonuniformities (inhomogeneities) in the static or gradient magnetic fields.

SR - see Saturation recovery.

SSFP - see Steady state free precession.

Steady state free precession (SFP or SSFP) - method of MR excitation in which strings of RF pulses are applied rapidly and repeatedly with interpulse intervals short compared to both T1 and T2. Alternating the phases of the RF pulses by 180° can be useful in obtaining maximal signal strength.

Superconducting magnet - a magnet whose magnetic field originates from current flowing through a superconductor. Such a magnet must be enclosed in a cryostat.

Superconductor - a substance whose electrical resistance essentially disappears at temperatures near absolute zero. A commonly used superconductor in MR imaging system magnets is niobium-titanium, embedded in a copper matrix to help protect the superconductor from quenching.

Surface coil MR - a simple flat RF receiver coil placed over a region of interest will have an effective selectivity for a volume approximately subtended by the coil circumference and one radius deep from the coil center. Such a coil can be used for simple localization of sites for measurement of chemical shift spectra, especially of phosphorus, and blood flow studies. Some additional spatial selectivity can be achieved with gradient magnetic fields.

Susceptibility - see Magnetic susceptibility.

T - see Tesla.

T1 ("T-one") - spin-lattice or longitudinal relaxation time; the characteristic time constant for spins to tend to align themselves with the external magnetic field. Starting from zero magnetization in the z direction, the z magnetization will grow to 63% of its final maximum value in a time T1.

T2 ("T-two") - spin-spin or transverse relaxation time; the characteristic time constant for loss of phase coherence among spins oriented at an angle to the static magnetic field, due to interactions between the spins, with resulting loss of transverse magnetization and MR signal. Starting from a non zero value of the magnetization in the xy plane, the xy magnetization will decay so that it loses 63% of its initial value in a time T2.

T2* ("T-two-star") - the characteristic time constant for loss of phase coherence among spins oriented at an angle to the static magnetic field due to a combination of magnetic field inhomogeneities, ΔB, and spin-spin transverse relaxation with resultant more rapid loss in transverse magnetization and MR signal. MR signal can still be recovered as a spin echo in times less than or on the order of T2.
$1/T2^* = 1/T2 + \Delta\omega/2$; $\Delta\omega = \gamma \Delta B$.

Tailored excitation - see Selective excitation.

Tailored pulse - shaped pulse whose magnitude is varied with time in a predetermined manner. Affects the frequency components of a RF pulse in a manner determined by the Fourier transform of the pulse.

TE - echo time. Time between middle of 90° pulse and middle of spin echo production. For multiple echoes, use TE1, TE2 ...

Tesla (T) - the preferred (SI) unit of magnetic flux density. One tesla is equal to 10000 gauss, the older (CGS) unit.

Thermal equilibrium - a state in which all parts of a system are at the same effective temperature, in particular where the relative alignment of the spins with the magnetic field is determined solely by the thermal energy of the system (in which case the relative numbers of spins with different alignments will be given by the Boltzmann distribution).

TI - inversion time. Time after middle of inverting RF pulse to middle of 90° pulse to detect amount of longitudinal magnetization.

Time reversal - technique of producing a spin echo by subjecting excited spins to a gradient magnetic field, and then reversing the direction of the gradient field. All methods of spin echo production can be viewed as effective time reversal.

Torque - the effectiveness of a force in setting a body into rotation. It is a vector quantity given by the vector product of the force and the position vector where the force is applied; for a rotating body, the torque is the product of the moment of inertia and the resulting angular acceleration.

TR - repetition time. The period of time between the beginning of a pulse sequence and the beginning of the succeeding (essentially identical) pulse sequence.

Transmitter - portion of the MR apparatus that produces RF current and delivers it to the transmitting coil.

Transmitter coil - coil of the RF transmitter.

Transverse magnetization (M_{xy}) - component of the macroscopic magnetization vector at right angles to the static magnetic field (B_0). Precession of the transverse magnetization at the Larmor frequency is responsible for the detectable MR signal. In the absence of externally applied RF energy, the transverse magnetization will decay to zero with a characteristic time constant of T2 or T2*.

Transverse relaxation time - see T2.

Two-dimensional Fourier transform imaging (2DFT) - a form of sequential plane imaging using Fourier transform imaging.

Tuning - process of adjusting the resonant frequency, e.g., of the RF circuit, to a desired value, e.g., the Larmor frequency. More generally, the process of adjusting the components of the spectrometer for optimal MR signal strength.

Tunnel - opening into MR imaging machine to place patient into imaging region.

Vector - a quantity having both magnitude and direction, frequently represented by an arrow whose length is proportional to the magnitude and with an arrowhead at one end to indicate the direction.

Volume imaging - imaging techniques in which MR signals are gathered from the whole object volume to be imaged at once, with appropriate encoding pulse/gradient sequences to encode positions of the spins. Many sequential plane imaging techniques can be generalized to volume imaging, at least in principle. Advantages include potential improvement in signal-to-noise ratio by including signal from the whole volume at once; disadvantages include a bigger computational task for image reconstruction and longer image acquisition times (although the entire volume can be imaged from the one set of data). Also called simultaneous volume imaging.

Voxel - volume element; the element of 3-D space corresponding to a pixel, for a given slice thickness.

x - dimension in the stationary (laboratory) frame of reference in the plane orthogonal (at right angles) to the direction of the static magnetic field (B_0 and H_0), z, and orthogonal to y, the other dimension in this plane.

x^1 - dimension in the rotating frame of reference in the plane orthogonal (at right angles) to the direction of the static magnetic field (B_0 and H_0), z, and orthogonal to y^1, the other dimension in this plane.

y - dimension in the stationary (laboratory) frame of reference in the plane orthogonal to the direction of the static magnetic field (B_0 and H_0), z, and orthogonal to x, the other dimension in this plane.

y^1 - dimension in the rotating frame of reference in the plane orthogonal (at right angles) to the direction of the static magnetic field (B_0 and H_0), z, and orthogonal to the other dimension in this plane, x^1.

z - dimension in the direction of the static magnetic field (B_0 and H_0), in both the stationary and rotating frames of reference.

Zeugmatography - term for MR imaging coined from Greek roots suggesting the role of the gradient magnetic field in joining the RF magnetic field to a desired local spatial region through magnetic resonance.

2DFT - see Two-dimensional Fourier transform.

γ - see Gyromagnetic ratio.

σ - see Chemical shift.

μ - see Permeability.

ζ - often used to denote different time delays between RF pulses. See Interpulse times.

χ - see Magnetic susceptibility.

ω - see Angular frequency.

ω_0 - see Larmor frequency.

Subject Index

Page numbers in *italics* refer to the principle discussion of subject

MIX
Papier aus verantwortungsvollen Quellen
Paper from responsible sources
FSC® C105338

If you have any concerns about our products,
you can contact us on
ProductSafety@springernature.com

In case Publisher is established outside the EU,
the EU authorized representative is:
Springer Nature Customer Service Center GmbH
Europaplatz 3, 69115 Heidelberg, Germany

Printed by Libri Plureos GmbH
in Hamburg, Germany